Nursing research

Denise F. Polit, Ph.D.

Humanalysis, Inc., Jefferson City, Missouri
Formerly of the Boston College School of Nursing
Chestnut Hill, Massachusetts

Bernadette P. Hungler, B.S.N., Ph.D.

Boston College School of Nursing
Chestnut Hill, Massachusetts

J. B. Lippincott Company
Philadelphia

London   Mexico City   New York   St. Louis   São Paulo   Sydney

Nursing research

principles and methods
Third edition

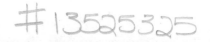

Sponsoring Editor: Paul Hill
Manuscript Editor: Helen Ewan
Indexer: Ellen Murray
Art Director: Tracy Baldwin
Designer: Anne O'Donnell
Production Manager: Kathleen P. Dunn
Compositor: Progressive Typographers
Printer/Binder: R. R. Donnelley and Sons

6   5   4   3   2   1

**Library of Congress Cataloging-in-Publication
Data**

Polit-O'Hara, Denise
   Nursing research.
   Includes bibliographies and index.
   1. Nursing — Research — Methodology.
I. Hungler, Bernadette P. II. Title. [DNLM:
1. Nursing. 2. Research. WY 20.5 P769n]
RT81.5.P64 1987   610.73'072   86-10251
ISBN 0-397-54631-9

To
Nana,
Paul-Paul,
and
Ellen Ferguson

Preface

The third edition of *Nursing Research: Principles and Methods,* like the earlier two editions, was shaped by a number of basic convictions. First, we are convinced that, more than ever before, the development of research skills is critical to the nursing profession. Nurses are increasingly expected to actively engage in inquiries that enhance nurses' ability to serve their clients effectively. Furthermore, nurses are expected to keep abreast of relevant research in nursing, medicine, and other disciplines related to their areas of specialization. Second, we are convinced that research is an intellectually rewarding enterprise. For anyone who is curious about the world and its inhabitants, research can be challenging and stimulating. We try to reflect our enthusiasm for the research process throughout this text. And third, we believe that learning about research methods need not be a drudgery.

As in earlier editions, we have tried to present the fundamentals of research methods in a way that both facilitates understanding and stimulates interest. We know of no better way to accomplish both aims than to incorporate — liberally — actual and hypothetical research studies that illustrate concepts under discussion. We have also maintained other aspects of our basic teaching style: concepts are introduced carefully and systematically; difficult ideas are presented with some redundancy, but from several vantage points; and no assumptions are made about the reader's prior exposure to technical terms.

We have tried to keep in mind the needs of both consumers and producers of nursing research. The uses to which the first two editions have been put suggest that we continue to reach both audiences. In the text, we have paid attention to the problems frequently encountered by students in reading, understanding, and evaluating research reports. However, the organization of the book is intended as a guide to those nursing students who are learning to conduct their own research projects.

Despite these similarities with earlier editions, this third edition improves on earlier editions in several important respects. The first and most pervasive change is the substantial expansion of discussions relating to qualitative research. Major portions of the chapters on data collection are now devoted to the collection of unstructured or semistructured data, and an entire chapter on the analysis of qualitative data is now included. This edition also includes an expanded discussion of theories, with particular emphasis on conceptual frameworks in nursing. Another important change is the inclusion of material on powerful new techniques, such as meta-analysis, path analysis, and power analysis. The presentation on power analysis in Chapter 22 is expected to be an especially valuable tool for nurse researchers, whose sample sizes are frequently too small to test adequately their research hypotheses. Lastly, the final chapter on proposal development has been completely revamped and offers step-by-step information on the submission of grant applications through the Public Health Service.

The third edition is organized into six main sections that lead the reader sequentially through the steps in the research process. Part I introduces the reader to the rationale underlying the scientific approach in general and to the basic aims of nursing research in particular. The principal goal of the first two chapters is to help students understand and appreciate the manner in which the scientific approach can be applied to the solution of problems and to develop an enthusiasm for the kinds of discoveries and knowledge that research can produce. Chapter 3 describes the basic steps in

conducting research and serves as an overview of many of the remaining chapters.

In Part II, the preliminary steps of a research project are discussed. Chapter 4 explores some of the contexts within which research topics arise and gives some practical suggestions for the selection and evaluation of a research problem. Chapter 5 presents a guide for performing a literature review, including suggestions for locating sources, organizing materials, and writing up the review. Chapter 6 contains materials that, we have found, create difficulties for students: the identification of a theoretical framework for a research problem. In this chapter we discuss the advantage of a strong conceptual scheme and present a number of examples of theories, with particular emphasis on contextual frameworks developed by nurses. Chapter 7 concentrates on the formulation of hypotheses and stresses the link between this step in the research process and both previous and subsequent steps.

Various kinds of nursing research are examined in Part III, and some basic research design considerations are introduced. Chapter 8 focuses on experiments and quasi-experiments. Quasi-experimental techniques are seldom treated in nursing research textbooks and yet probably are better suited to the realities of the nursing research situation than are classical experimental designs. Chapter 9 discusses various kinds of nonexperimental research, including ex post facto/correlational and descriptive studies. Chapter 10 introduces some specific forms of research, including survey research, evaluation, needs assessments, case studies, field studies, historical research, meta-analyses, and methodological research. Chapter 11 presents an overview of some important design principles, including control of extraneous variables, the notion of maximizing experimental variance, and the issue of cross-sectional versus longitudinal designs. The final chapter of Part III discusses sampling designs and strategies, sample size considerations, and practical problems of sampling.

Part IV covers the major techniques in the collection of data for nursing research studies, as well as principles of measurement. Chapter 13 discusses the collection of data through self-report techniques, and includes both unstructured and structured approaches. Basic considerations in the design and use of questionnaires and interview schedules are reviewed. Various types of psychosocial self-report instruments are covered in Chapter 14, with particular emphasis on scales for the measurement of attitudes. The techniques of observational research are presented in Chapter 15. Chapter 16 reviews other types of data collection approaches. Biophysiological measures are given lengthy coverage in this chapter; also included are descriptions of the use of records, projective techniques, Q methodology, Delphi surveys, and vignettes. Chapter 17 deals with various criteria for evaluating measuring tools. The concepts of reliability and validity are extensively treated. The final chapter of Part IV deals with the fundamentals of measurement, including the different levels of measurement.

Part V is devoted to the analysis of research data. The first chapter in this section is new to this edition, and deals with the analysis of qualitative materials. Chapters 20 to 22 present some fundamental principles of statistical analysis. In these chapters, the emphasis is less on the computation of statistics than on an understanding of how statistics can be useful, what they mean, and which statistics are appropriate in a given situation. Chapter 20 presents basic information on descriptive statistics. Chapter 21 deals with the commonly used tests of statistical significance. Chapter 22 introduces some advanced statistical procedures such as multiple regression, analysis of covariance, factor analysis and power analysis. Multivariate statistics are playing an increasingly prominent role in nursing research reports, so that a treatment of them, on an elementary level at least, was considered important. The final two chapters in this section focus on the use of computers in the data analysis task. Chapter 23 presents a discussion of how computers work and how a user interacts with a computer, particularly through the use of existing software packages. In Chapter 24, the steps in preparing data for computer analysis are outlined.

The final section of the book is devoted to communication in research. Chapter 25 explores the problems of interpreting research results and offers some suggestions for preparing a research report. Chapter 26 was designed as a comprehensive guide for the preparation of a research critique. The concluding chapter provides guidelines for the development of a research proposal.

We hope that the content and organization of this book will continue to meet the needs of a broad spectrum of nursing students and nurse researchers.

Denise F. Polit, PH.D.
Bernadette P. Hungler, B.S.N., PH.D.

Acknowledgments

This third edition, like the first two, depended on the contribution of many individuals. We are deeply appreciative of those who made all three editions possible. In addition to all those who assisted us with the earlier editions, the following individuals deserve special mention.

Many faculty and students who used the text during the past decade have made invaluable suggestions for its improvement, and to all of you we are very grateful. In particular, we would like to acknowledge the continuing feedback from the nursing students at Boston College, and from nursing faculty in Massachusettes and Missouri. Beth Geden provided constructive suggestions regarding the inclusion of qualitative materials. Mary Pekarski, Anne Lippman, and Marilyn Grant made important contributions to Chapter 5. Several of the examples used in the text and in the accompanying study guide were developed from ideas provided by Sarah Cimino, Susan Kelly, and Jean Weyman. Thomas Knapp made several excellent comments that improved the chapters on statistical analysis. Cheryl Stetler and her colleagues had a strong influence on the test questions in the instructor's manual. We again wish to note our deep appreciation for the mentorship of Peter W. Airasian, without whose fine teaching and clear writing this book would not be possible.

We also extend our warmest thanks to those who helped to turn the manuscript into a finished product. Susan Hoefener diligently and single-handedly typed all of the new materials. The staff at J. B. Lippincott has given us ongoing support. We would like to express our gratitude to Paul Hill, Helen Ewan, Kathy Dunn, and all the others behind the scenes for their contributions.

Finally, we thank our friends and family, who provided support and encouragement throughout this enterprise.

Contents

Part I

The scientific research process

Chapter 1 □ Nursing and the role of research

Nursing research has experienced remarkable growth in the past two decades. During this time, the focus of nursing research has been directed toward problems relating to nursing practice. Nurses today are being schooled in the scientific method to a greater degree than ever before. Today, there appears to be a more orderly progression of research functions demanded of graduates from associate, baccalaureate, master's and doctoral programs in nursing.

To produce scientific research it is necessary to develop skills in the scientific method. But it is not only nursing researchers who need to understand the scientific approach and methods of research. Nurses engaged in the practice of nursing, nursing administrators, and nursing educators all have a responsibility to identify problems that warrant scientific investigation. Professional accountability demands that nurses utilize the findings of research to perform their roles. In addition, as consumers of research nurses are called upon to evaluate the methods used to carry out research projects in order to estimate the confidence that can be placed in the results. The purpose of this text is to acquaint potential consumers and producers of nursing research with the fundamentals of scientific research methods.

In this introductory chapter, we discuss the important role that research plays in establishing a scientific base for the practice of nursing, the historical development of nursing research, the current status of nursing research, and possible future directions of nursing research as suggested by nursing leaders.

☐
Importance of research in nursing

The ultimate goal of any profession is to improve the practice of its members so that the services provided to its clientele will have the greatest impact. Any profession seeking to enhance its professional image undertakes the continual development of a scientific body of knowledge fundamental to its practice. The emergence of such a body of scientific knowledge can be instrumental in fostering a commitment and accountability to the profession's clientele.

Many nurses use the Standards of Nursing Practice established by the American Nurses' Association (1973) not only to evaluate the quality of their nursing care but also as their method of clinical practice. The process requires nurses to engage in many decision-making activities. What will be assessed? What nursing diagnoses result from the assessment? What plan of care is most likely to produce the desired outcomes? What nursing interventions are necessary? How will the results be evaluated in terms of their effectiveness? Research has an important role to play at each phase of the nursing process. The findings from research aid nurses in making more informed decisions in the delivery of nursing care and help document the unique role that nursing has in the health-care system.

Assessment phase

The assessment phase of the nursing process dictates the systematic collection of information. The information may come from a variety of sources, such as clients, families, records, or nurses' observations. At present, many different forms and methods exist for collecting assessment information. For example, Gordon (1982) has suggested using a functional pattern assessment. Bates (1983) focuses on a body systems approach. Nursing research can help nurses select alternative methods or forms for particular types of clients, settings and situations. Research can help to determine the extent to which the forms produce comparable information.

Diagnosis phase

Based upon an analysis of the information collected at the assessment phase of the nursing process, nurses are expected to develop nursing diagnoses. Research can play an important role in helping nurses make more accurate nursing diagnoses by validating the etiology of each diagnosis against the recorded assessment information. In addition, nursing research can help determine the frequency of occurrence for each defining characteristic or cue associated with each diagnosis. The documentation will be helpful to the profession of nursing, which has only recently begun the task of building up its taxonomy of diagnoses.

Planning phase

The planning phase of the nursing process involves decisions concerning *what* nursing actions or interventions are needed and *when* the nursing actions are most appropriately instituted for each nursing diagnosis. The last step of this phase generally involves the delineation of behavioral outcomes for the client. Nursing research can help nurses evaluate the holism of the plan of care and make more informed decisions as to whether the goals set are realistic for the type of facility and the characteristics of the client involved.

Intervention phase

Professionally accountable nurses base as many of their nursing interventions as possible on research findings. Consider, for example, the many decisions made by night nurses working in a nursing home. At what point do they decide that the nursing interventions are no longer producing the desired results for a resident in the process of dying? When is it time to notify the family or physician? What alterations in nursing interventions are available that facilitate, with as much ease as is possible, the transition from a state of life to a state of death? What approach might be used with families? What response might be expected from other residents of the home and how might their stresses be appropriately helped? The systematic documentation of nursing interventions that have been found to be helpful may benefit other nurses facing the same kind of situation.

Evaluation phase

The last stage of the nursing process evaluates the degree to which the behavioral outcomes or goals developed at the planning stage have been met. Research can help document success or failure in meeting the various outcomes. When success occurs with relative frequency, it offers other nurses the opportunity to implement the plan in other comparable situations with a fair degree of confidence. When the plan has not been successful, then nurses are redirected to examine the accuracy of the assessment, the nursing diagnoses, the goals, the plan, and the nursing interventions. Such information, collected systematically, may aid other nurses in avoiding the same dilemmas and should lead to improvements in nursing care.

In summary, research conducted by nurses can play a critical role in improving both the quality of care delivered and the process of delivering that care. Although most nursing studies of the 1980s involve inquiries into the nursing process, this focus is relatively recent. The next section provides an overview of the history of nursing research.

Historical evolution of nursing research

Most people would agree that research in nursing began with Florence Nightingale, who maintained detailed, recorded observations about the effects of nursing actions during the Crimean War and, on the basis of her observations, was able to effect some changes in nursing care. For a number of years following her work, however, little is found in the nursing literature concerning nursing research.

The pattern that nursing research followed, subsequent to Nightingale, was closely aligned to the problems confronting nursing. For example, as more nurses received university-based education and advanced academic preparation, studies concerning students — their differential characteristics, problems, satisfactions — became more numerous. Most of the early nursing leaders received their advanced nursing preparation in the field of education and, thus, it is not surprising that the studies conducted by them focused on the nurse or nursing student rather than on the practice of nursing. Also, tests and other tools from education were already available for these early nursing researchers to use. It has been only recently that research on the practice of nursing has become a high priority.

Early years

Most of the studies conducted between 1900 and 1940 concerned nursing education. During these years much of the nursing students' preparation was service-oriented rather than education-oriented and nurse educators did not hold advanced educational preparation. One group (Committee for the Study of Nursing Education, 1923), at the request of the National Organization for Public Health Nursing and financed by the Rockefeller Foundation, studied on the national level the educational preparation of nurse teachers, administrators, and public health nurses and the clinical experiences of nursing students. They identified many inadequacies in the educational backgrounds of the groups studied and concluded that advanced educational preparation was essential for teachers, administrators, and public health nurses. The report of this group is referred to as the Goldmark Report. Simmons and Henderson (1964) pointed out that the school of nursing at Yale University came into being as a result of this investigation. Partly as a result of this study, hospitals began employing registered nurses to give nursing care that freed student nurses from heavy service demands.

The 1940s

During the 1940s, studies concerning nursing education continued. However, the Second World War and the increase in the number of hospital admissions created an unprecedented demand for nursing personnel, and researchers began to investigate the supply and demand of nurses, the hospital environment and the status of staff nurses in various regions of the country.

For example, Brown (1948), a social anthropologist, reassessed nursing education in her study initiated at the request of the National Nursing Council for War Service and funded by the Carnegie Foundation. The findings from this study, like those of Winslow-Goldmark, revealed that inadequacies existed in nursing education. She recommended that the education of nurses occur in collegiate settings. Many subsequent research investigations concerning the functions performed by nurses, nurses' roles and attitudes, hospital environments, and nurse-patient interactions stemmed from the Brown report (Abdellah and Levine, 1978).

Simmons and Henderson (1964) reported that almost every state nurses' association conducted its own fact-finding study concerning nursing needs and resources during this period. Comparisons of the findings from these studies revealed that wide variations in the quantity and quality of nursing care existed; that personnel policies varied greatly for staff nurses; and the functions of nurses were often ill defined. These studies initiated further research by bringing together nurses and other groups to promote more uniform and systematic research on the national level, by pointing out areas and issues in nursing that were in need of further research, and by establishing a beginning point for periodic state checks on the changing needs and resources in nursing.

The 1950s

A number of forces combined during the 1950s to put nursing research on a rapidly accelerating upswing that is still being experienced today. An increase in the number of nurses with advanced educational degrees, the establishment of a nursing research center by the government, an increase in the availability of funds from the government and private foundations, the inception of the American Nurses' Foundation, and the appearance of the journal *Nursing Research* occurred during this period and provided impetus to the research movement in nursing.

Not only were more nurses enrolling in undergraduate nursing programs during the 1950s, but, also, more master's programs in nursing were being developed with courses in research methods being included in the curriculum. Funding from the federal government during the late 1950s enabled more nurses to pursue master's level preparation, and most of the programs required a thesis or research project as part of the program. A growing awareness of the need for nursing research was being introduced to an ever-increasing number of nurses.

The first nursing unit to focus its efforts on research in nursing practice, established at the Walter Reed Army Institute of Research, hoped to parallel the research conducted by other professionals, such as physicians and dentists, at the institution. Werley (1972) noted that, despite the unique opportunity, nursing research did not flourish to the same extent as research in other professions. She attributed the lack of growth of nursing research, in part, to lack of experienced nurse researchers able to cope with the issues and problems and able to develop research projects. Nonetheless, research in nursing practice was becoming established as an important area.

The American Nurses' Association (ANA) undertook a five-year research project in which it studied the activities and functions performed by nurses. The report of this lengthy study served as the basis for the functions, standards, and qualifications statements for nurses prepared by the ANA (Hughes, 1958). Individual nurses provided the financial support for this particular study, demonstrating the belief that nursing had something to gain from systematic study of its activities.

The ANA created the American Nurses' Foundation, which is devoted exclusively to the promotion of nursing research. The increasing number of research studies being conducted during the 1950s created the need for a vehicle in which the findings from these studies could be published; thus, *Nursing Research* came into being in 1952.

In education, Montag (1954) developed and evaluated the effectiveness of establishing two-year programs leading to an associate degree in nursing. Funding from the federal government provided universities the opportunity to develop curricula (Sands and Belcher, 1958) and to increase the research competencies in faculty.

Nursing research took a twist in the 1950s not experienced by research in other professions, at least not to the same extent as in nursing. Nurses studied themselves: Who is the nurse? What does the nurse do? Why do individuals choose to enter nursing? What are the characteristics of the ideal nurse? How do other groups perceive the nurse?

The 1960s

The 1960s was the period during which terms such as conceptual framework, conceptual model, nursing process, and theoretical base of nursing practice began to appear in nursing literature. Nurse researchers collaborated more than in the past with members of other professions on nursing research projects. Funding continued to be available both for the educational preparation of nurses and for nursing research projects. Nursing leaders expressed concern about the lack of research in nursing practice, and the professional nursing organizations established priorities for research investigations.

A collaborative research project involving a nurse and social scientists studied dying patients and hospital personnel. The findings from this study revealed that interaction between a dying patient and hospital personnel changes according to the awareness level the dying person has of his or her condition (Glaser and Strauss, 1966). The findings from this study served as the basis for further investigations into the area of death and dying.

The five-year study undertaken by Hall (1963) focused on an alternative to acute care hospitalization for a carefully selected group of chronically ill elderly persons. Only professional nurses gave nursing care, and the nurses and patients decided when the services of a physician were needed. At a time when staff nurse shortages were acute, the Loeb Center, where this study was conducted, had no difficulty in recruiting nurses.

The findings from scientific investigations such as these have been used to improve the quality of care to patients. The results from other basic research studies, such as investigations on sensory deprivation and pain, have been incorporated into the curricula of nursing schools. The trend seems to be that the findings from research are being used by nurse educators as well as nurse practitioners in improving the quality of nursing practice.

During the 1960s, nurse educators continued to study nursing students' characteristics. Councils of nurse educators received funds to conduct workshops for faculties and to examine the characteristics of graduate nursing education. Nurse investigators compared students enrolled in the various types of nursing programs and compared nursing students with other students, such as education students, in terms of personality and attitudinal characteristics. The Western Interstate Council for Higher Education in Nursing (WICHEN) developed content for graduate education in the clinical areas of community health, maternal–child, medical-surgical, and psychiatric nursing, and WICHEN conducted workshops for faculty on the application of scientific knowledge.

The Mugar Library at Boston University established a nursing archive in the late 1960s; one purpose of the archive is to foster nursing research. This is the first archive for nursing history and was initially supported through a grant from the federal government.

The 1970s

The decade of the 1970s witnessed a series of accomplishments in a number of areas germane to nursing research. The ANA and the National League for Nursing (NLN) had established a National Commission for the study of nursing and nursing education in the late 1960s. The Commission's report, completed in 1970, recommended that increased research should be undertaken in both the areas of nursing practice and nursing education. The Commission urged that funding be sought for nursing research (Lysaught, 1970).

Various groups discussed what direction nursing research should take. Lindeman (1975), for example, conducted a study to ascertain the views of nursing leaders concerning the focus of scientific nursing studies. Clinical problems were identified as the highest priorities for nursing research. Similar themes emerged in the resolution passed by the delegates to the 1974 ANA convention. Actual research appeared to be consistent with these views: Carnegie (1978) reported a steady increase in the number of clinical investigations published in *Nursing Research.*

The research preparation of nurses received attention from a number of sources. Both the ANA and the NLN addressed the importance of research in the education of nurses. The Commission on Nursing Research of the ANA (1976) recommended preparation for research in undergraduate, graduate, and continuing education programs. The NLN began reviewing the research component of curricula as part of the accreditation process. The cadre of nurses with earned doctorates steadily increased, especially during the later part of the decade. The availability of both predoctoral and postdoctoral research fellowships facilitated advanced preparation in research skills.

The rapidly accelerating pace of nursing research was also evident in the number and types of activities undertaken by regional groups of nurses. Regional meetings and workshops provided nurses who shared mutual interests with both support and an opportunity to exchange ideas. For example, the Western Interstate Council for Higher Education in Nursing began a seven-year project that focused on increasing the quality and quantity of clinical nursing research. Other activities of the western regional group included the compilation of a two-volume work that contained data collection tools for measuring various aspects of health care and a similar compendium of data collection instruments for measuring nursing education-related concepts (Elliott, Krueger and Kearns, 1980).

The growing number of nurses conducting research studies and the discussions of theoretical and contextual issues surrounding nursing research created the need for additional sources of communication. Examples of nursing journals that focus on nursing research established during the 1970s are *Advances in Nursing Science, Research in Nursing and Health,* and the *Western Journal of Nursing Research.*

In the 1970s, the change in emphasis from such areas as teaching, administration, curriculum, recruitment, and nurses themselves to the improvement of client or patient care may be attributed to the growing awareness by nurses of the need for a scientific base from which to practice. Many questions might be raised as to the role that research currently plays in nursing: If the knowledge of a discipline is best investigated by members of the discipline, are nurses studying nursing? Have nurse researchers produced any knowledge that is applicable to the practice of nursing? We can say with increasing confidence that the answers to these questions are "yes."

The 1980s

In the first year of this decade, the ANA Commission on Nursing Research (1980) identified priorities for the 1980s that have helped research to focus more precisely on aspects of nursing practice. The group recommended that the generation of knowledge for the practice of nursing should be in the areas of health promotion, prevention of illness, development of cost-effective health-care delivery systems, and the development of strategies that provide effective nursing care to high-risk

groups. Many nurse researchers have responded to these recommendations.

Nurses at all levels are increasingly being called upon to develop research skills. The ANA Commission on Nursing Research (1981) issued several guidelines relating to the ability of nurses to integrate research into clinical practice. For example, they suggested that baccalaureate nurses, as consumers of research, be able to evaluate research in terms of its applicability to nursing practice, to identify problems for future investigation, to incorporate research findings in their practice, and to share research findings with their colleagues. The group also suggested that nurses with master's degrees conduct scientific investigations, assist others in their research endeavors, help others apply research findings in their practice, and work toward developing a climate that is conducive to the conduct of research.

Several other trends are discernible among nursing studies of this decade. The conceptual models of nursing that were developed in the 1960s and 1970s began to receive increasing attention by researchers. In particular, the conceptual models of such nursing theorists as Dorothea Orem, Dorothy Johnson, Martha Rogers, Sister Callesta Roy, and Betty Neuman have been subjected to validation efforts by nurse researchers (see Chap. 6).

There has also emerged in the 1980s a growing interest in intensive, process-oriented studies that try to gain an in-depth understanding of a given problem or situation through naturalistic observation of people in their environments. This research approach often has its roots in such disciplines as anthropology or ethnography. This emerging interest has given rise to a debate about whether the "appropriate" research approach for nurse researchers lies in these descriptive, qualitative methods or in more controlled, quantitative procedures. Nursing leaders are suggesting that both major types of research approaches are needed in developing a scientific base for nursing practice.

Future directions of nursing research

Several recent events should provide impetus in directing future nursing research. First, legislation is currently pending for the establishment of a nursing research center at the National Institutes of Health (Solomon, 1985). The creation of such a center would put nursing research more into the mainstream of research activities currently enjoyed by other health disciplines. Second, the National Institutes of Health have announced a new funding program that supports feasibility, pilot, and other small-scale research studies. The purpose of the grants is to stimulate research activities in colleges or universities that have not been the traditional recipients of funding (Federal Register, September 26, 1985). Such support from sources external to nursing is essential to the development of knowledge that is fundamental to the practice of nursing.

The trend toward clinical research is destined to continue in the future. The ANA Standards of Practice will be evaluated in terms of their application to nursing. Studies will compare various assessment tools in terms of their ability to collect comparable information and their suitability for different types of clients and clinical situations. Jones, Lepley, and Baker (1984) have suggested that nursing diagnoses could be used as a framework for clinical research. The validation of the diagnoses could help identify nursing actions that are within the realm of nursing practice and help delineate nursing's unique role in health care.

Studies concerning the effect of nursing interventions on client or patient outcomes will undoubtedly continue. There is also a growing interest in building a firmer knowledge base by repeating studies, using the identical procedures of previous research but with different clients, in various types of clinical settings and at different times. When findings from several studies are similar, nurses will be able to develop greater confidence that their nursing actions have an effect on client outcomes.

It is likely that research will be increasingly directed toward the continuing development of nursing theories that are grounded in practice. Efforts to develop theories capable of guiding nursing practice will be encouraged. An increasing number of studies will focus on testing the applicability of current frameworks for practice proposed by nursing leaders to various types of clinical situations.

The development of tools that adequately and accurately measure client or patient outcomes is also likely to be a high priority of the future. Tool construction will be directed toward the measurement of both short- and long-term outcomes. Valid and effective instruments are sorely needed to collect information about the effectiveness of nursing interventions.

In essence, the future of nursing research looks bright and challenging. In the future nursing research is more likely to be directed toward the practice of nursing than it was in the past. Perhaps such direction will not only improve the quality of nursing practice but also alter existing curricula of nursing schools. Future nursing students may learn the art and science of nursing practice from perspectives that are completely different from those of today.

Summary

Research has an important role to play in helping nursing establish a scientific base for its practice. The ANA Standards of Practice provide nurses with a method of clinical practice, a means to evaluate the quality of nursing care, and a rich variety of clinical research problems.

Nursing research began slowly. Most people trace its roots to the work of Florence Nightingale during the Crimean War. The early focus of nursing research closely paralleled the problems faced by the nursing profession. The majority of early research studies were conducted in the areas of nursing education and nursing administration. Only in recent years has the major focus of nursing research shifted toward nursing practice.

The last two decades have continued the rapidly accelerating acceptance of nursing research begun during the 1950s. The educational preparation of nurses as consumers and producers of research has been better delineated; the number of nursing journals devoted to the dissemination of research findings has increased; nursing leaders have identified priorities for nursing research; and increasing numbers of nurses are investigating problems of a clinical nature.

The future direction of nursing research seems sure to continue in the area of nursing practice. The establishment of a scientific base of nursing knowledge will permit nurses to make more informed decisions in their practice and will have implications for the education of future nursing students.

☐
Study suggestions

1. What are some of the current changes occurring in the health-care delivery system and how could these changes influence nursing research?
2. Read the article by the American Nurses' Association concerning priorities in nursing research listed in the references. How many of the articles published in *Nursing Research* between 1980 and 1985 concern each of these priorities?
3. Of what benefit to nursing would collabora-

tive research efforts among health professionals be?

☐
Suggested readings

Abdellah, F.G. & Levine, E. (1978). *Better patient care through nursing research* (2nd Ed.). New York: Macmillan. (Chapter 1).

American Nurses' Association Commission on Nursing Research (1980). Generating a scientific basis for nursing practice: Research priorities for the 1980s. *Nursing Research, 29,* 219.

American Nurses' Association Commission on Nursing Research (1981). *Guidelines for the investigative function of nurses.* Kansas City: American Nurses' Association.

American Nurses' Association Commission on Nursing Research (1976). *Preparation of nurses for participation in research.* Kansas City: American Nurses' Association.

American Nurses' Association Congress for Practice (1973). *Standards for practice.* Kansas City: American Nurses' Association.

American Nurses' Association (1974). Resolutions of priorities in nursing research. *American Nurse, 6,* 5.

Bates, B. (1983). *A guide to physical examination.* (3rd Ed.). Philadelphia: J.B. Lippincott.

Brown, E.L. (1948). *Nursing for the future.* New York: Russell Sage.

Carnegie, M.E. (1978). Quo vadis? *Nursing Research, 27,* 277–278.

Elliott, J.E., Krueger, J.C., & Kearns, J.M. (1980). Update on nursing research in the West. *Nursing Research, 29,* 184–188.

Federal Register (1985, September 26). *Grants programs for Baccalaureate degree-granting institutions; Academic Research Enhancement Award* (p. 39046)

Glaser, B.C. & Strauss, A.L. (1966). *Awareness of dying.* Chicago: Aldine.

Gordon, M. (1982). *Nursing diagnosis: Process and applications.* New York: McGraw-Hill Book Company.

Hall, L.E. (1963). A center for nursing. *Nursing Outlook, 11,* 805–806.

Hughes, E.C. (1958). *Twenty thousand nurses tell their story.* Philadelphia: J.B. Lippincott.

Jones, D., Lepley, M., & Baker, B. (1983). *Health assessment across the life span.* New York: McGraw-Hill Book Company.

Lindeman, C.A. (1975). Delphi survey of priorities in clinical nursing research. *Nursing Research, 24,* 434–441.

Lysaught, J. (1970). *An abstract for action.* New York: McGraw-Hill Book Company.

Montag, M. (1954). Experimental programs in nursing education. *Nursing Outlook, 2,* 620–621.

Sands, O. & Belcher, H. (1958). *An experience in basic nursing education.* New York: G.P. Putnam's Sons.

Simmons, L.W. & Henderson, V. (1964). *Nursing research: Survey and assessment.* New York: Appleton-Century-Crofts. (Chapters 2 & 8).

Solomon, S. (1985, October 21). *Important dated news.* New York: National League for Nursing.

Werley, H. (1972). Nursing and research. Paper presented at the National Commission for the Study of Nursing and Nursing Education, Georgia.

Chapter 2
☐
The scientific approach

The human experience in this world of physical, chemical, biological, social, and psychological forces is a complex affair, defying total comprehension. In our daily private lives and in our work, we strive to make sense of our experience, to understand regularities, and to predict future circumstances. The scientific researcher, similarly, endeavors to understand, explain, predict, or control phenomena. The scientist, however, goes about this task in a more orderly and systematic fashion than is typical of most of our everyday efforts to solve problems. The scientific method involves the formal application of systematic, logical procedures that guide the investigation of phenomena of interest. All sciences, though they differ in content or in specialized techniques, employ the same general approach in arriving at knowledge and understanding. The purpose of this text is to acquaint potential consumers and producers of nursing research with the fundamentals of scientific research methodology. In this chapter we discuss the rationale, characteristics, goals, assumptions, and limitations of the scientific method of inquiry.

☐
Sources of human knowledge

Human knowledge has many roots. Think for a moment about some facts relating to the practice of nursing. What is the source of this information? Some of it is derived from scientific research, but some of it is not. A brief discussion of some alternative sources of understanding shows how scientific information is different.

Tradition

Many questions are answered and problems solved on the basis of inherited customs or tradition. Within our culture, certain "truths" are accepted as givens. For example, as citizens of the United States, most of us accept, without demanding "proof," that democracy is the highest form of government. This type of knowledge often is so much a part of our heritage that few of us seek verification. The discipline of nursing, like other disciplines, also has its store of information passed on to us by tradition or custom. For example, one of the tasks traditionally performed by nurses is the "change of shift" report for each and every patient, whether the patient's condition has changed or not. The question of whether it might be more productive or effective under certain circumstances to make a report for only those patients whose conditions have changed has not been seriously addressed.

Tradition offers some advantages as a source of knowledge. It is efficient in the sense that each individual is not required to begin anew in an attempt to understand the world or certain aspects of it. Tradition or custom also facilitates communication by providing a common foundation of accepted "truth." Nevertheless, tradition poses some problems for human inquiry. Many traditions have never been evaluated for their validity. Indeed, by their very nature, traditions may interfere with the ability to perceive the possibility of challenging customs. Walker's (1967) research on ritualistic practices in nursing suggests that some traditional nursing practices, such as the routine taking of a patient's temperature, pulse, and respirations, may be dysfunctional. The Walker study illustrates the potential value of critical appraisal of custom and tradition before accepting them as truth.

Authority

In our complex society, there are "authorities," or people with specialized expertise, in every field. We are constantly faced with making decisions about matters with which we have had no direct experience and, therefore, it seems natural to place our trust in the judgment of persons who are authoritative on an issue by virtue of specialized training or experience. As a source of understanding, however, authority has shortcomings. Authorities are not infallible, particularly if their expertise is based primarily on personal experience; yet, like tradition, their knowledge often goes unchallenged. While nursing practice would flounder if every piece of advice from nursing educators were challenged by students, nursing education would be incomplete if students never had occasion to pose the questions: How does the authority (the instructor) know? What evidence is there that what I am learning is true?

Experience and trial and error

Our own experiences represent a familiar and functional source of knowledge. The ability to generalize, to recognize regularities, and to make predictions based upon observations is an important characteristic of human behavior. Despite the obvious utility of experience, it has limitations as a basis of understanding. First, each individual's experience may be too restricted to develop generalizations. A nurse may notice, for example, that two or three cardiac patients follow very similar postoperative sleep patterns. This observation may lead to some interesting discoveries with implications for nursing interventions, but does the one nurse's observation and experience justify widespread changes in nursing care? A second limitation of experience as a source of knowledge lies in the fact that the same objective event generally is experienced or perceived differently by two individuals. Whose experience constitutes truth?

Closely related to experience is the method of trial and error. In this approach alternatives are tried successively until we find one that answers our questions or solves our problems. Probably we have all used the trial and error method at some time in our lives, including in our professional work. For example, many patients dislike the taste of potassium chloride solution. Nurses try to disguise the taste of the medication in various ways until one method meets with the approval of the patient. Trial and error may offer a practical means of securing knowledge, but it is fallible and inefficient. This method is haphazard and unsystematic, and the knowledge obtained is often unrecorded and, hence, inaccessible to subsequent problem-solvers.

Logical reasoning

The solutions to many of our perplexing problems are developed by means of logical thought processes. Logical reasoning as a method of knowing combines experience, our intellectual faculties, and formal systems of thought. *Inductive reasoning* is the process of developing generalizations from specific observations. For example, a nurse may observe the behavior of (specific) hospitalized children and conclude that children's separation from their parents is (in general) very stressful. *Deductive reasoning* is the process of developing specific predictions from general principles. For example, if we assume that separation anxiety does occur in hospitalized children (in general), then we might predict

that the children in Hospital X whose parents do not room-in (a specific) would manifest symptoms of stress.

Both systems of reasoning are useful as a means of understanding and organizing phenomena, and both play a role in the scientific approach. Neither system of thought, however, is without limitations when used alone as a basis of knowledge. The quality of knowledge arrived at through inductive reasoning is highly dependent upon the representativeness of the specific examples used as the basis for generalization. The reasoning process itself offers no mechanism for evaluating this criterion and has no built-in checks for self-correction. Deductive reasoning is not itself a source of new information; it is, rather, an approach to illuminating relationships as one proceeds from the general (an assumed truth) to the specific. Deductive logic depends, furthermore, on the truth of the generalizations (called premises) in order to arrive at valid conclusions.

Scientific method

The scientific approach is the most sophisticated method of acquiring knowledge that humans have developed. The scientific method combines important features of induction and deduction, together with several other characteristics, to create a system of obtaining knowledge that, though fallible, is generally more reliable than tradition, authority, experience, or inductive or deductive reasoning alone. One important aspect that distinguishes the scientific approach from other methods of understanding is its capacity for self-evaluation. That is, scientific research uses checks and balances that minimize the possibility that the researcher's emotions or biases will affect the conclusions.

☐
Characteristics of the scientific approach

The scientific approach to inquiry refers to a general set of orderly, disciplined procedures used to acquire dependable and useful information. The term research designates the application of this scientific approach to the study of a question of interest. Kerlinger, a leader in the field of research methodology, has defined scientific research as "systematic, controlled, empirical, and critical investigation of hypothetical propositions about the presumed relations among natural phenomena" (1973, p. 11). This definition is complex (as is the concept it refers to), so let us briefly examine some characteristics to provide a firmer basis for understanding.

Order and control

The scientific method is a *systematic* approach to problem-solving and to the expansion of knowledge. In a scientific study, the researcher moves in an orderly and systematic fashion from the definition of a problem, through the design of the study and collection of information, to the solution of the problem. By systematic, we mean that the investigator progresses logically through a series of steps, according to a prespecified plan of action. An overview of the steps taken in a scientific study is provided in Chapter 3.

Control is another critical characteristic of the scientific approach. Control involves imposing conditions on the research situation so that biases and confounding factors are minimized. The problems that are of interest to scientists, for example, lung cancer, obesity, mental retardation, or perceptions of pain, are highly complicated phenomena, often representing the effects of various factors. In trying to isolate relationships between phenomena, the scientist must attempt to control factors that are not under direct investigation. For example, if a scientist is interested in exploring the relationship between diet and heart disease, steps must be taken to control other potential contributors to coronary disorders, such as stress and cigarette smoking, as well as additional factors that might be relevant, such as a person's age and sex. The mechanisms of scientific control are the subject of a large part of this text.

Empiricism

The term empiricism refers to the process whereby evidence rooted in objective reality and gathered directly or indirectly through the human senses is used as the basis for generating knowledge. This requirement causes findings of a scientific investigation to be grounded in reality rather than in the personal beliefs of the researcher. Empirical inquiry imposes a certain degree of objectivity on the research situation because ideas or hunches are exposed to testing in the real world.

Empirical evidence, then, consists of observations made known to us by way of our sense organs. The observations are verified through sight, hearing, taste, touch, or smell. Observations of the presence or absence of skin inflammation, the color of a person's eyes, or the number of victims of an automobile accident are all examples of empirical observations.

Generalization

An important goal of science is to understand phenomena. This pursuit of knowledge, however, is focused not on isolated events or situations but rather on a more generalized understanding of relationships. For example, the scientific researcher is typically not as interested in understanding why Ann X has cervical cancer as in understanding what general factors led to this form of carcinoma. Of course, a health practitioner would want to take advantage of the general knowledge obtained in the course of scientific research in an effort to assist a particular individual. The ability to go beyond the specifics of the situation at hand is an important characteristic of the scientific approach. Generalizability of research findings is an important criterion for assessing the quality of an investigation.

☐
Assumptions of the scientific approach

Assumptions refer to basic principles that are accepted on faith, or assumed to be true, without proof or verification. In this section our discussion of the characteristics of the scientific approach is extended by paying specific attention to the assumptions upon which science is founded.

The nature of reality

The scientist assumes that there is an objective reality that exists independent of human discovery or observation. That is, the world is assumed to be real and not a creation of the human mind; the processes of the universe would continue to exist even if humans were not capable of observing or recording them.

A related assumption is the belief that nature is basically orderly and regular. Events in nature are assumed to be, at least to a certain extent, consistent. If this principle were not assumed, it would make little sense to conduct scientific research.

Determinism

The assumption of determinism refers to the belief that all phenomena have antecedent (preceding) causes. Natural events or conditions are assumed to not be haphazard, random, or accidental. Given the presumed orderliness of nature, events must have causes. If a pregnant woman has a premature delivery, there must be a reason that can potentially be identified and understood. If an individual has a cerebral vascular accident, there must be a cause or perhaps several causes.

Much of the activity in which a scientific researcher engages is directed toward an understanding of cause-and-effect relationships. Scientists believe that antecedent factors relating to all phenomena exist and can be discovered. Science does, however, accept the concept of multiple causation. A particular phenomenon may have several different causes. For example, heart disease may be caused by smoking habits, diet, stress, and additional factors or combinations of factors. The identification of these causes, that is, the search for an explanation of *why* things are the way they are, is one of the chief goals of science.

☐
Purposes of scientific research

The scientific approach has been discussed in a general way as a method of solving problems or a system for acquiring knowledge. In this section we examine some of the more specific reasons for conducting research in the context of the nursing profession.

Description

Many nursing research studies have as their main objective the description of phenomena relating to the nursing process. The researcher who conducts a descriptive investigation observes, describes, and, perhaps, classifies. Descriptive studies can be of considerable value to the nursing profession. The phenomena that nursing researchers have been interested in describing are varied: stress in patients, grieving behavior, sleep patterns, nutritional habits, health beliefs, time patterns of temperature readings, to mention only a few.

Exploration

Exploratory research is an extension of descriptive research that focuses more directly on the discovery of relationships. In descriptive studies the researcher selects a specific event, condition, or behavior and makes observations and records of the phenomenon. The final result of such an investigation is a list, a catalogue, a classification, or some other type of description. Exploratory research also focuses on a phenomenon of interest, but pursues the question: What factor or factors influence, affect, cause, or relate to this phenomenon? For example, a descriptive study might examine patients' satisfaction with the nursing care they received. Such a study might reveal that 75 percent of the hospitalized patients who were questioned indicated that they were satisfied with the quality of nursing care. The purpose of such a descriptive study would probably be to document the need (or the absence of a need) to improve the quality of care currently available in hospitals. An exploratory study, on the other hand, would try to identify important relationships. What kinds of factors are related to a patient's degree of satisfaction? Is the patient's diagnosis an important factor? Do the patient's age, sex, or prior hospitalization record play a role? Or is patient satisfaction related to characteristics of the hospital, such as size, geographic location, or staff traits?

Researchers may engage in exploratory research for two basic reasons. First, the investigator may simply be curious and desire a richer understanding of the phenomenon of interest than a straightforward descriptive study could provide. This reason is particularly salient when a new area or topic is being investigated. Second, exploratory studies are sometimes conducted to estimate the feasibility and cost of undertaking a more rigorous or extensive research project on the same topic. When large-scale studies are anticipated, it is usually wise to explore potential difficulties with a smaller version of the study.

Explanation

The third basic purpose for conducting research is to explain things. Explanations of natural phenomena are referred to as *theories*. Theories represent a method of organizing, integrating, and deriving abstract conceptualizations about the manner in which phenomena are interrelated. In its aim to understand and explain phenomena, the scientific approach unites empirical observations, logical reasoning, order, and control to formulate systematic, abstract, and generalized interpretations concerning natural phenomena. Theories, then, offer an opportunity for bringing together observed events and relationships, for explaining how and why phenomena are associated with one another, and for predicting the occurrence of future events and relationships.

Many writers on the scientific process argue that theory formation is the ultimate aim of science. It might be said that, whereas descriptive and exploratory research provide new information, theoretical or explanatory research offers us understanding. Reinforcement theory, for example, asserts that when a behavior is positively reinforced, that is, rewarded in some way, then that behavior will tend to be repeated. This generalized explanation of human behavior offers the possibility of understanding a broader scope of activity than would the more specific proposition that children who are praised (reinforced) for taking their medications will tend to be more compliant in following a medications regimen. A theory gets us much closer to the "why" of phenomena.

Prediction and control

Although the goal of explanation epitomizes the spirit and nature of scientific inquiry, there are unfortunately numerous problems that, with our current level of knowledge and technology, defy absolute comprehension. Yet it is frequently possible to use the scientific approach to make reliable predictions, and to develop control mechanisms, in the absence of total understanding. For example, various scientific studies have demonstrated an association between the age of mothers and the incidence of Down's syndrome in their infants. Such an association makes it possible to predict that women beyond the age of 35 are at a greater risk of bearing infants with Down's syndrome than are younger women. The ability to predict, in turn, offers the possibility of control. That is, through appropriate education, women can learn to have an amniocentesis performed after they turn 35. Note that the ability to predict and control in this example does not depend upon the scientist's complete explanation of *why* older women are at a higher risk of having an abnormal child than younger women. There are many examples of medical and nursing research investigations in which prediction and control are key objectives.

Basic versus applied research

We have seen that scientific research strives to describe, explore, explain, predict, or control phenomena. A second approach to classifying the functions of research is based upon the degree to which the findings have direct practical utility or application. *Basic research* is concerned with making empirical observations that can be used to accumulate information or to formulate or refine a theory. Basic

research is not designed to solve immediate problems but, rather, to extend the base of knowledge in a discipline for the sake of knowledge and understanding itself. Of course, many of the findings from basic research endeavors are ultimately applied to practical problems. For example, advances in the practice of nursing have resulted from basic research in biochemistry, psychology, and nursing itself. But basic research is not directly concerned with the social utility of its findings, and many years may pass before a relevant application is developed. Whipple, who studied the bleeding tendency in liver disease, and Dam, who studied cholesterol metabolism, probably could not have envisioned that their independent and seemingly unrelated basic research endeavors would combine for the practical application of treating bleeding tendencies with vitamin K.

The researchers who engage in *applied research* concentrate on finding a solution to an immediate practical problem. Applied research has as its final goal the scientific planning of induced change in a troublesome situation. We need basic research for the discovery of general laws about human behavior and bodily functioning, but applied research tells us how these laws operate in, say, a hospital environment. Just as the possibility of practical application is not ruled out in basic research, applied research may also contribute to general knowledge in a field. In fact, it is perhaps more meaningful to think of applied and basic research as two endpoints on a continuum, because in a given study there may be multiple goals and multiple lessons.

Much of the research conducted in nursing tends to be more applied in nature. For example, the question of how long a rectal, oral, or axillary thermometer must be in place to record accurately is a problem for which the solution has immediate application in practice. Yet nursing researchers are demonstrating increasing interest in the conduct of theory-based research designed to enhance a general understanding of the nursing process and the role of nurses. In nursing, as in medicine, the feedback process between basic and applied research seems to operate more freely than in the case of other disciplines. The findings from applied research almost immediately pose questions for basic research, and the results of basic research many times suggest clinical application to a practical problem.

☐
Limitations of the scientific method

The scientific approach to inquiry is regarded by many as the highest form of attaining knowledge that human beings have devised. This is not to say, however, that scientific research can solve all human problems or that scientists are immune from making mistakes. There are a number of limitations of applying the scientific approach to nursing problems that should be mentioned lest the impression be given that scientific research is infallible. Some of the limitations discussed here are common to all scientific endeavors, whereas others are more prevalent in the social scientific disciplines (psychology, sociology, education), with which nursing research sometimes overlaps.

General limitations

Perfectly designed and executed studies are unattainable. Virtually every research study contains some flaw. Every research question can be addressed in an almost infinite number of ways. The researcher must make decisions about how best to proceed. Invariably, there are trade-offs. The best methods are often very expensive and time-consuming. Even when tremendous resources are expended, there are bound to be some flaws. This does not mean that small, simple studies are worthless. It

means that *no single study can ever definitively prove or disprove our hunches*. Each completed study adds to a body of accumulated knowledge. If the same question is posed by several researchers, each of whom obtains the same or similar results, increased confidence can be placed in the answer to the question. This is especially true if the researchers' studies have different types of shortcomings.

Moral or ethical issues

Moral or ethical issues create limitations for scientific research in two respects. The first concerns constraints on what is considered acceptable in the name of science with regard to the rights of living organisms. The researcher must be careful to avoid violating the rights of those who participate in a scientific investigation. Research ethics are discussed in greater detail in the next section of this chapter.

The second issue concerns the kind of problems that can be solved using the scientific method. Questions that focus on ethical or value-laden matters cannot be empirically tested. Many of our most persistent and intriguing questions about the human condition fall into the category of moral/ethical problems. Consider, for example, the issue of euthanasia. Descriptive research concerning how nurses feel about euthanasia is certainly possible. Studies concerning the characteristics of nurses with different points of view are also feasible. Similarly, a researcher could explore the extent to which nurses' attitudes concerning euthanasia affect their behavior toward terminally ill patients. All of these hypothetical studies lend themselves to a scientific approach. But no specific investigation could be expected to answer the question "Should euthanasia be practiced?" The nursing process may increasingly incorporate scientific knowledge into its problem-solving strategies. However, it is probable that the nursing process will never rely completely upon scientific information because some decisions involve moral, ethical, or value issues that are not addressed by scientific research.

Human complexity

One of the major obstacles to conducting nursing studies using the scientific paradigm is the complexity of the central topic of investigation—human beings. This problem is much less troublesome in clinical research dealing with bodily processes than in research concerning human behavior or attitudes. Biological and physical functioning is considerably more regular and consistent and less susceptible to external influences than is psychological functioning. Each human being is essentially unique with respect to his or her personality, social environment, mental capacities, values, and lifestyle. This fact makes it relatively more difficult to detect regularities in, say, human eating behavior than to make generalizations concerning the functioning of, say, the pancreas. In other words, there appear to be fewer individual biological/chemical differences than there are individual social/psychological differences. Thus, it has been impossible to achieve the same level of order and discipline over the research situation in studies focusing on human behavior and thought than is the case in studies dealing with biological or physical phenomena.

The inability of the scientific approach to meaningfully capture the human experience holistically has led some nurse researchers to adopt an alternative approach of investigation. This emerging school of thought, which has as its intellectual roots the tradition known as *phenomenology,* offers an alternative to the scientific method, whose philosophical underpinnings are *logical positivism.* The phenomenological approach rests on different assumptions about the nature of humans and how that nature is to be understood. Phenomenologists emphasize the complexity of humans, the ability of humans to shape and create their own experiences, and the idea that "truth" is a composite of realities. Investigations in the phenomenological tradition place a heavy emphasis on understanding the human experience as it is actually experienced, generally through the careful collection and analysis of narrative, subjective materials. According to phenomenologists, a major limitation of the scientific approach is that it is *reductionist,* that is, it reduces human experience to only the few concepts under investigation, and those concepts are defined in advance by the researcher rather than emerging from the experience of those under study.

In this text, we take the view that both the phenomenological and scientific approaches represent valid and important paradigms for the study of nursing problems. We have devoted more attention to methods normally associated with the scientific approach because the vast majority of nursing research studies have adopted this approach. However, there is some overlap in the activities undertaken in phenomenological and scientific research, and so much of the discussion is applicable to both approaches.

Measurement problems

Another limitation of the scientific approach that is related to the issue of human complexity concerns problems of measurement. In order to study, for example, patient morale, we must be able to observe or measure it; that is, we must be able to assess whether a patient's morale is high or low, or higher under certain conditions than under others. While there are reasonably accurate measures of such physiological phenomena as blood pressure, temperature, and cardiac activity, comparably accurate measures of such psychological phenomena as anxiety, pain, self-confidence, or aggression have not been developed. The problems associated with measurement are often the most perplexing in the research process.

Control problems

In discussing the characteristics of the scientific approach, it was pointed out that the scientist attempts to control the research situation in order to have confidence in the outcomes. Because scientists accept the principle of multiple causation, they generally attempt to control factors that are not under direct investigation.

Adequate control, however, is often difficult to achieve. Confounding factors may be difficult to even identify, let alone control, if the phenomenon of interest is complex. Control over confounding factors is especially problematic in research with human beings in naturalistic settings.

Despite the various obstacles mentioned above, nurse researchers have made outstanding progress in contributing knowledge and understanding about the practice and theory of nursing. Even further progress can be anticipated in the years to come as information accumulates and forms a foundation for more sophisticated theories, as data collection methods and research design become more refined, and as nurses integrate findings from phenomenological and scientific studies.

□
Ethical considerations in scientific research

When human beings are used as subjects of research investigations, as is generally the case in nursing research, great care must be exercised in ensuring that the rights of those human beings are protected. The requirement for ethical conduct may strike the reader as so self-evident as to require no further comment, but the fact is that conflicts often arise in structuring research that is both ethical and scientifically rigorous. This discussion is designed to alert researchers to such potential conflicts so that neither the rights of individuals nor the worth of the research will be compromised. Appendix A of this book presents some supplementary information relating to the rights of human research subjects. It is beyond the scope of this text on research methods, however, to do complete justice to this complex and important issue. A number of books, including guidelines issued by professional organizations and federal funding agencies, have been devoted to a consideration of research ethics and should be consulted by those readers who intend to design and conduct their own studies.

Informed consent

One of the key principles of ethical conduct in research is that participation in studies must be voluntary. The medical experiments carried out by Nazi physicians in Germany during World War II were criticized not only for their cruelty but also for the fact that participants could not refuse to participate. The ethically correct procedure, then, is to inform prospective participants about the study and to secure their voluntary consent.

While the requirement of informed consent appears as easy to implement as it is justifiable, this, unfortunately, is not always the case. This seemingly straightforward principle often conflicts directly with practical arrangements or scientific concerns. Sometimes, for example, the researcher is faced with the possibility that the information would result in atypical behavior on the part of the participants and would distort the processes being studied. For example, if we were conducting a descriptive, observational study of nurses' behavior in intensive care units, the nurses' knowledge of being observed could alter their behavior and render the resulting description invalid. Furthermore, we have said that scientific research strives to develop generalized principles concerning phenomena or the relationships between phenomena. Yet if we use in our studies only individuals who volunteer, how can we be sure that our results can be generalized to nonvolunteers?

Clearly, these are thorny issues. The scientific researcher is ethically obligated to obtain informed consent from prospective participants, but the scientist is also obligated to contribute scientific knowledge, which ultimately improves human welfare. When the requirement of voluntary participation threatens the value of a research study, the investigator is forced to evaluate the consequences of such involuntary participation to the subjects and weigh these consequences against the potential contribution of the study. If the scientist believes that the study's findings would be beneficial without making undue impositions on unknowing participants, he or she may feel justified in violating the principle of informed consent. In such a case, however, it is especially important to adhere to other ethical restrictions.

Freedom from harm

Researchers should take every precaution to protect the people being studied from physical or mental harm or discomfort. It should be perfectly obvious that exposing participants to experiences that result in serious or permanent harm is unacceptable. For example, almost all scientists would question the right of a researcher to administer drugs with unknown properties and consequences to human beings before extensive tests with laboratory animals.

However, some of the psychological consequences of participating in a study are typically more subtle and, thus, require critical attention and sensitivity. Sometimes, for example, individuals are asked questions about their personal views, their weaknesses, their fears. Such queries might require people to admit to aspects of themselves that they dislike and would perhaps rather forget. The point is not that the researcher should refrain from asking *any* questions but, rather, that it will often be necessary to think very carefully about the nature of the intrusion upon people's psyches. As a rough guideline, sometimes it is suggested that researchers design their studies in such a way that they would feel comfortable if a family member participated.

Privacy, anonymity, and confidentiality

Virtually all research with human beings constitutes some type of an intrusion, however small. Nursing researchers are fortunate in that the acquisition of information from patients is often required and serves the personal interests of the participants, thereby posing no ethical problems. At other times, however, requests for information in the course of a research study serve the function of helping the researcher rather than the participants. The procedures used to obtain the information, and the information itself, should not be used to the disadvantage of the person providing it. Individuals who divulge their personal views and affairs should be protected from public disclosure.

Two mechanisms that act as safeguards of participants' identities are known as *anonymity* and *confidentiality*. A participant in a study is regarded as anonymous if even the researcher cannot link the participant with the information provided. When research is conducted in a hospital setting with patients, anonymity may well be impossible to achieve. However, if questionnaires were distributed to a group of hospital nurses and respondents were not requested to indicate their names, we could say that the anonymity of participants had been assured.

In face-to-face situations in which anonymity is difficult, the researcher should offer participants a guarantee of confidentiality. This means that the researcher promises that any information that the participant divulges will not be publicly reported. It is the researcher's responsibility to ensure that any such pledges of confidentiality be strictly honored; this often may require the adoption of some very elaborate procedures, particularly if the information the participant provides involves illegal or deviant behavior (for example, drug addiction or child abuse).

This brief discussion has demonstrated that ethical issues in the context of scientific research are not clear-cut. The considerations raised here point out some of the major moral dilemmas that a researcher must face, and above all be sensitive to, in carrying out an investigation of human beings. In many cases, ethical considerations are subject to the scrutiny of not only individual researchers but also of one or more review panels, such as an *Institutional Review Board* (IRB).

Each issue of the *Western Journal of Nursing Research* contains excellent essays on the ethics of nursing research. These essays and other references listed at the end of this chapter should be consulted if you need assistance in resolving an ethical dilemma. Some examples of research materials relating to the protection of human subjects are included in Appendix A.

□

Summary

Nurse researchers are increasingly utilizing the scientific approach to extend their knowledge about nursing theory and practice. The scientific approach may be contrasted with other sources of truth and understanding. Certain "truths" are passed on to us by tradition or custom—that is, they are accepted as cultural givens without demands for verification. Authority figures or specialists are another common source of information or knowledge. Our own experiences, together with trial and error procedures, are familiar to all of us as a method of acquiring understanding. Some of our problems can be dealt with by logical reasoning. *Inductive reasoning* is the process of establishing generalizations from specific observations, while *deductive reasoning* is the pro-

cess of developing specific predictions from general principles. These approaches suffer various limitations as techniques for solving problems. The scientific method offers several advantages as a method of inquiry.

The scientific approach may be described in terms of a number of characteristics. It is, first of all, a systematic, disciplined, and controlled process. Scientists base their findings on *empirical* observations, which means that evidence is rooted in objective reality and collected by means of the human senses. Unlike many other problem-solving techniques, the scientific approach strives for generalizability and for the development of conceptual explanations or theories concerning the relationships among phenomena.

The scientist assumes that there is an objective reality that is not dependent upon human observation for its existence. A related belief is that natural phenomena are basically regular and orderly. The assumption of *determinism* refers to the belief that events are not haphazard but, rather, are the consequence of prior causes. The search for an understanding of cause-and-effect relationships is an activity basic to many scientific endeavors.

Scientific research can be categorized in terms of its functions or objectives. Description, exploration, explanation, prediction, and control of natural phenomena represent the most common goals of a research investigation. It is also possible to describe research in terms of the direct practical utility that it aspires to achieve. *Basic research* is designed to extend the base of knowledge in a discipline for the sake of knowledge itself. *Applied research* focuses on discovering solutions to immediate practical problems.

Although the scientific approach offers a number of distinct advantages as a system of inquiry, it is not without its share of difficulties and shortcomings. In general, researchers must make compromises in the face of limited time and resources, so that no single study can ever definitively answer a given question. The design of studies with human beings is constrained not only by resources but also by standards of professional ethics. In addition, there are numerous questions of interest to nurse researchers that are difficult to study because they deal with complex social or psychological functioning, such as pain, fear, guilt, anxiety, motivation, and the like. Such phenomena are difficult to measure (in comparison with aspects of biological functioning such as blood pressure or body temperature) and difficult to control in a natural setting. In fact, phenomenologists have argued that the scientific approach is overly reductionist and cannot adequately capture the human experience in all of its complexity. Although this text emphasizes methods that have emerged in connection with the scientific approach, methods consistent with phenomenological inquiry are also described.

In dealing with human beings in research situations, a number of ethical issues must be raised. Three common ethical requirements are voluntary participation, freedom from physical or psychological harm and distress, and anonymity or confidentiality of information. Ethics in research is a continually perplexing concern because ethical demands often conflict with scientific requirements. The researcher needs to develop great sensitivity to ethical considerations.

□
Study suggestions

1. Consider one or two nursing "facts" that you possess and then trace the fact back to some source. Is the basis for your knowledge tradition, authority, experience, or scientific research?
2. Explain the ways in which scientific knowledge differs from knowledge based on tradition, authority, trial and error, and logical reasoning.
3. How does the assumption of scientific determinism conflict with or coincide with superstitious thinking? Take, as an example, the superstition associated with four-leaf clovers or a rabbit's foot.
4. How does the ability to predict phenomena offer the possibility of their control?
5. Below are a few research problems. For each problem, specify whether you think it is essentially a basic or applied research question. Justify your response.
   a. Is the stress level of patients related to the level of information they possess about their medical status?
   b. Do students who get better grades in nursing school become more effective nurses than students with lower grades?
   c. Does the early discharge of maternity patients lead to later problems with breastfeeding?
   d. Can the incidence of decubitus ulcers be affected by a certain massaging technique?
   e. Is individual contraceptive counseling more effective than group-based instruction in minimizing unwanted pregnancies?
6. Point out the ethical considerations that might emerge in the following studies:
   a. A study of the relationship between sleeping patterns and acting-out behaviors in hospitalized psychiatric patients.
   b. A study of the effects of a new drug on human subjects.
   c. An investigation of an individual's psychological state following an abortion.

□
Suggested readings

References concerning science and the scientific approach

Braithwaite, R. (1955). *Scientific explanation.* Cambridge, England: Cambridge University Press.
Hacking, I. (1981). *Scientific revolutions.* Oxford, England: Oxford University Press.

Hesse, M.B. (1974). *The structure of scientific inference*. Berkeley: University of California Press.

Kerlinger, F. (1973). *Foundations of behavioral research* (2nd Ed.). New York: Holt, Rinehart and Winston. (Chapter 1).

Kuhn, T.S. (1970). *The structure of scientific revolutions* (2nd ed.). Chicago: University of Chicago Press.

Madden, E. H. (Ed.) (1974). *The structure of scientific thought*. Boston: Houghton Mifflin.

Meyers, S.T. (1982). The search for assumptions. *Western Journal of Nursing Research, 4,* 91–98.

Newton, D.E. (1974). *Science and society*. Boston: Holbrook Press.

Oiler, C. (1982). The phenomenological approach in nursing research. *Nursing Research, 31,* 178–181.

Popper, K. R. (1959). *The logic of scientific discovery*. (Rev. Ed.). New York: Harper & Row.

Simon, H.M. (1968). Panel discussion: The position of the pure and applied scientist. Conference on the nature of science and nursing. *Nursing Research, 17,* 507–509.

Wysocki, A.B. (1983). Basic versus applied research: Intrinsic and extrinsic considerations. *Western Journal of Nursing Research, 5,* 217–224.

References concerning ethical considerations

American Nurses' Association (1975). *Human Rights Guidelines for Nurses in Clinical and Other Research*. Kansas City, MO: ANA.

American Psychological Association (1982). *Ethical principles in the conduct of research with human participants*. Washington: APA.

Arminger, B., Sr. (1977). Ethics of nursing research: Profile, principles, perspective. *Nursing Research, 26,* 330–336.

Berthold, J.S. (1969). Advancement of science and technology while maintaining human rights and values. *Nursing Research, 18,* 514–522.

Bower, R.T. & De Gasparis, P. (1978). *Ethics in social research: Protecting the interests of human subjects*. New York: Praeger Press.

Code of Federal Regulations (1983). *Protection of human subjects: 45CFR46,* revised as of March 8, 1983. Washington: Department of Health and Human Services.

Davis, A.J. (1979). Informed consent. *Western Journal of Nursing Research, 1,* 145–147.

Diener, E. & Crandall, R. (1978). *Ethics in social and behavioral research*. Chicago: University of Chicago Press.

Freund, P.A. (1970). *Experimentation with human subjects* (Ed.). New York: George Braziller.

Jacobson, S.F. (1973). Ethical issues in experimentation with human subjects. *Nursing Forum, 12,* 58–71.

May, K.A. (1979). The nurse as researcher: Impediment to informed consent? *Nursing Outlook, 27,* 36–40.

Packard, J.S. (1981). Human subjects protection in hospital field studies. *Western Journal of Nursing Research, 3,* 216–230.

Regan, C.E. (1971). *Ethics for scientific researchers* (2nd ed.). Springfield, IL: Charles C. Thomas.

Robb, S.S. (1983). Beware of the informed consent. *Nursing Research, 32,* 132–135.

Wilson, H.S. (1985). *Research in nursing*. Menlo Park, CA: Addison-Wesley. (Chapter 3).

Other reference cited in chapter

Walker, V.H. (1967). *Nursing and ritualistic practice*. New York: Macmillan.

Chapter 3
☐
Overview
of the research
process

Basic research terminology

Scientific research, though complex, is based upon logical principles and proceeds in an orderly fashion through a number of steps. In this chapter an overview of the major steps in research is presented so that the reader can gain some understanding of how a research study is planned and executed. In a sense, this chapter represents an outline of the issues that will be addressed in the remainder of the book.

Like any other discipline, scientific research has its own language and terminology. Therefore, before turning to the description of the steps involved in research, some important ideas and terms that will be discussed throughout the text are introduced here. Although a more thorough familiarization with research terminology will be acquired as the reader progresses through this book, it is recommended that this section be read with particular care before proceeding to more advanced chapters.

Scientific concepts and constructs

Conceptualization refers to the process of refining general or abstract ideas. Scientific research almost always is concerned with abstract rather than tangible phenomena. For example, the terms good health, pain, emotional disturbance, patient care, and grieving are all abstractions that are formulated by generalizing from particular manifestations of certain behaviors or characteristics. These abstractions are referred to as *concepts*.

The term *construct* is also encountered frequently in the scientific literature. Like the term concept, a construct refers to an abstraction or a mental representation inferred from situations, events, or behaviors. Kerlinger (1973) distinguishes concepts from constructs by noting that constructs are terms that are deliberately and systematically invented (or constructed) by researchers for a specific scientific purpose. In practice, however, the two terms are often used interchangeably.

Variables

When concepts are put into operation in a research study, they are usually referred to as *variables* rather than concepts. A variable is, as the name implies, something that varies. Weight, height, body temperature, educational attainment, and medical diagnosis all are variables. That is, each of these properties varies or differs from one individual to another. When one considers the variety and complexity of human and situational characteristics, it becomes clear that nearly all aspects of individuals and our environment can be considered variables. If everyone had black hair and weighed 125 pounds, hair color and weight would not be variables. If it rained continuously and the outdoor temperature was a constant 70°F., weather would not be a variable. But it is precisely because individuals and conditions *do* vary that most research is conducted. The bulk of all research activity is aimed at trying to understand how or why things vary, to gain insights into how differences in one variable are related to differences in another. For example, lung cancer research is concerned with the variable of lung cancer. It is a variable because not everybody has lung cancer. Researchers in this area are concerned with learning what other variables can be linked to lung cancer. They have discovered that cigarette smoking appears to be related to lung cancer. Again, this is a variable because not everyone smokes.

A variable, then, is an abstract quality that takes on different values. Age, for instance, can take on values from zero to over one hundred when we are referring to the age in years of human beings. For some variables, a system of assigning values may have to be devised by the researcher. For example, gender is a variable that has no "natural" numerical values assigned to it. Variables of this type, which take on only two values are referred to as *dichotomous variables.* Other examples of dichotomous variables include smoker/nonsmoker, presence of allergic reaction/absence of allergic reaction, alive/dead, and pregnant/nonpregnant.

Active versus attribute variables

Variables are not restricted to preexisting attributes of individuals, organisms, events, or environments. In many research situations the investigator creates or designs a variable. For example, if a researcher is interested in testing the effectiveness of ice chips as opposed to effervescent ginger ale to refresh the mouth after vomiting, some individuals might be given ice chips and others would receive ginger ale. For the purposes of this study, the type of mouth care may be considered a variable because different individuals will receive ice chips or ginger ale. Kerlinger (1973) refers to these variables that the researcher creates or manipulates as *active variables. Attribute variables,* on the other hand, are preexisting characteristics that the researcher simply observes and measures.

Dependent versus independent variables

One further distinction between two types of variables needs to be made, and the distinction is important enough to merit rather extensive coverage here. Many research studies are aimed at unraveling and understanding the causes underlying phenomena. Does a drug *cause* improvement of a medical problem? Does a nursing intervention *cause* more rapid recovery? Does smoking *cause* lung cancer? The presumed cause is referred to as the *independent variable,* while the presumed effect is referred to as the *dependent variable.* Variability in the dependent variable is presumed to *depend* upon variability in the independent variable. For example, the researcher investigates the extent to which lung cancer (the dependent variable) depends upon smoking behavior (the independent variable). In another study, a researcher might examine the effects of two special formulas (the independent variable) on weight gain in premature infants (the dependent variable). Or, an investigator may be concerned with the extent to which patients' perception of pain (the dependent variable) is dependent upon different types of nursing approaches (the independent variable).

The terms independent and dependent variable are frequently used to indicate directionality of influence rather than a causal connection. For example, let us say that a researcher is studying nurses' attitudes toward abortion and finds that older nurses hold less favorable opinions about abortion than younger nurses. The researcher might be unwilling to take the position that the nurses' attitudes were *caused* by their age. Yet, the direction of influence clearly runs from age to attitudes. That is, it would make little sense to suggest that the attitudes caused or influenced age. Even though in this example the researcher does not infer a causal relationship between age and attitudes, it is appropriate to conceptualize attitudes toward abortion as the dependent variable and age as the independent variable.

The dependent variable usually is the variable the researcher is interested in understanding, explaining, or predicting. In lung cancer research, it is the carcinoma that is of real interest to the research scientist, not smoking behavior per se. In studies of therapeutic treatments for alcoholics, it is the drinking behavior of the subjects that is under investigation (the dependent variable). Although a great deal of time, effort, and resources may be devoted to designing new therapies (the independent variable), they are of no interest in and of themselves but, rather, as they relate to improvements in drinking behavior and overall functioning of alcoholics.

Many of the dependent variables that are studied by researchers have a multiplicity of causes or antecedents. If we are interested in studying the factors that influence the weight of a person, for example, we might consider the sex, age, height, and eating habits of the individual as the independent variables. Note that some of these independent variables are attribute variables (sex, age, and height), while eating patterns can be manipulated by the investigator, in which case it would be an active variable. Just as a study may examine more than one independent variable, two or more dependent variables may be of interest to the researcher. For example, an investigator may be concerned with comparing the effectiveness of two methods of nursing care delivery (primary versus functional) for children with cystic fibrosis. Several dependent variables could be designated as measures of treatment effectiveness, such as length of stay in the hospital, number of recurrent respiratory infections, presence of cough, dyspnea on exertion, and so forth. In short, it is quite common to design studies with multiple independent and dependent variables.

The reader should not get the impression that variables are *inherently* dependent or independent. A variable that is classified as dependent in one study may be considered an independent variable in another study. For example, a researcher may find that the religious background of a nurse (the independent variable) has an effect on his or her attitude toward death and dying (the dependent variable). Another study, however, may analyze the extent to which attitudes of nurses toward death and dying (the independent variables) have an impact on their job performance (the dependent variable). To illustrate this point with another example, consider a study that examines the relationship between contraceptive counseling (the independent variable) and unwanted pregnancies (the dependent variable). Yet another research project could study the effect of unwanted pregnancies (the independent variable) on the incidence of child abuse (the dependent variable). In short, the designation of a variable as independent or dependent is a function of the role that the variable plays in a particular investigation.

It should be pointed out that some researchers use the term *criterion variable* (or criterion measure) rather than dependent variable. In studies that analyze the consequences of a treatment, therapy, or some other type of intervention, it is usually necessary to establish criteria against which the success of the intervention can be assessed and, hence, the origin of the expression criterion variable. The term dependent variable, however, is broader and more general in its implications and applicability. For example, in the previously mentioned hypothetical study of age of nurses and abortion attitudes, the use of the term criterion variable in relation to the attitudes does not seem particularly applicable, although dependent variable is perfectly appropriate. We therefore use the term dependent variable more frequently than criterion variable, although in many situations the two are equivalent and interchangeable.

A term that is frequently used in connection with variability is *heterogeneity.* When an attribute is extremely varied in the group under investigation, the group is said to be *heterogeneous* with respect to that variable. If, on the other hand, the amount of variability is limited, the group is described as *homogeneous.* For example, with respect to the variable height, two-year-old children are generally more homogeneous than 18-year-old adolescents. The degree of variability of a group has implications for the design of a study.

Operational definitions

Before a study progresses, the researcher usually clarifies and defines the variables under investigation. In order to be precise, the definition should specify how the variable will be observed and measured in the actual research situation. Such a definition of a concept, termed an *operational definition,* is a specification of the operations that the researcher must perform in order to collect the required information.

Variables differ considerably in the facility with which they can be operationalized. The variable weight, for example, is easy to define and measure. We may use as our definition of weight "the heaviness or lightness of an object in terms of pounds." Note that this definition designates that weight will be determined according to one measuring system (pounds) rather than another (grams). The operational definition might specify that the weight of participants in a research study would be measured to the nearest pound using a spring scale with subjects fully undressed after ten hours of fasting. This operational definition spells out what the investigator must do to measure weight in such a way that an individual not associated with the study would know precisely what the term "weight" meant.

Unfortunately, many of the variables of interest in nursing research are not operationalized as easily and straightforwardly as weight. Often there are multiple methods of measuring a variable, and the researcher must choose the method that best captures the variable as he or she conceptualizes it. For example, "patient well-being" may be defined in terms of both physiological and psychological functioning. If the researcher chooses to emphasize the physiological aspects of patient well-being, the operational definition will involve a measure such as heart rate, white blood cell count, blood pressure, vital capacity, and so forth. (Furthermore, it will specify what is meant by "patient.") If, on the other hand, well-being is conceptualized for the purposes of research as primarily a psychological phenomenon, the operational definition will need to identify the method by which emotional well-being will be assessed, as for example the responses of the patient to certain questions or the behavior of the patient as observed by the researcher.

Not all readers of a research report may agree with the way that the investigator has conceptualized and operationalized the concepts. Nevertheless, precision in defining the terms conceptually and operationally has the advantage of communicating *exactly* what the terms mean. If the researcher is reluctant to be explicit, it will be impossible for others to gauge the full meaning and implications of the research findings.

Researchers operating in a phenomenological framework generally do not define the concepts in which they are interested in operational terms prior to the gathering of information. This is because of their desire to have the meaning of concepts defined by the subjects themselves. Nevertheless, in summarizing the results of a study, all researchers should be careful in describing the conceptual and methodological basis of key research concepts.

Relationships

Researchers are rarely interested in single, isolated variables, except perhaps in some descriptive studies. For example, a study might focus on the percentage of women who elect to breast-feed their babies. In this example,

there is only one variable: breast-feeding versus bottle-feeding. Usually, however, researchers study two or more variables simultaneously. What scientists are most often interested in is the *relationship* between the independent and dependent variables of a study.

But what exactly is meant by the term "relationship" in scientific terms? Generally speaking, a relationship refers to a bond or connection between two entities. Let us consider as a possible dependent variable a person's body weight. What variables are related to (associated with) a person's weight? Some possibilities include height, bone structure, metabolism, caloric intake, and exercise. For each of these five independent variables we can make a tentative relational statement:

Height: Tall people, in general, weigh more than short people.
Bone Structure: The finer the bone structure, the lower the person's weight.
Metabolism: The lower a person's metabolic rate, the more he or she will weigh.
Caloric Intake: People with high caloric intake are heavier than those with lower caloric intake.
Exercise: The greater the amount of exercise, the lower the person's weight.

Each of these statements expresses a presumed relationship between weight and an independent variable. The terms "more than" and "lower than" imply that as we observe a change in one variable, we are likely to observe a corresponding change in the other. If Jane were taller than Jean, we would expect (in the absence of any other information) that Jane would be also heavier than Jean.

Research is essentially devoted to establishing that relationships do or do not exist among variables. Is there a relation between nursing shift assignments and absentee rates? Or between the frequency of turning patients and the incidence and severity of decubiti? One might predict that such relationships exist, but one would need to verify these hunches empirically.

The concept of relations among variables is so fundamental to the research process that it is worth pursuing a bit further. Variables can be related to one another in different ways. Scientists are often interested in what is referred to as *cause-and-effect relationships.* As noted in the introductory chapter, the scientist assumes that natural phenomena are not random or haphazard, but rather that all phenomena have antecedent factors or causes that are discoverable. If variable X causes the occurrence or manifestation of variable Y, then it can be said that those variables are causally related; there exists a causal relationship between variables X and Y. For instance, in the example presented above we might say that there is a causal relationship between caloric intake and weight: eating more calories causes weight gain.

Causality, however, is a tricky business. Unfortunately, we are rarely in a position to make definitive assertions concerning cause-and-effect relationships. However, two variables can be related to one another in a noncausal way if there is a systematic connection between their values. There is a relationship, for example, between a person's sex and weight; men tend to be heavier than women, on the average. The relationship is not perfect; some women are heavier than some men. Nevertheless, if we had to guess whether Keith Jones or Debbie Jones were heavier, we would be likely to say Keith, because men generally weigh more than women. We cannot really say, however, that a person's sex causes his or her weight, despite the relationship that exists between the two variables. This type of relationship is sometimes referred to as a *functional* rather than a causal relationship.

Control

The concept of *research control* is central to scientific inquiry. It is a topic to which much of this text is devoted. Chapter 11, in particular, discusses methods of achieving control in scientific research. The concept is so important, however, that some basic ideas about control are presented here.

Essentially, research control is concerned with holding constant the possible influences on the dependent variable under investigation so that the true relationship between the independent and dependent variables can be understood. In other words, research control attempts to eliminate any contaminating factors that might otherwise obscure the relationship between the variables that are really of interest. A detailed example should clarify this point.

Let us suppose that a researcher is interested in studying whether teenage women are at higher risk of having low-birthweight infants than are older mothers because of their age. In other words, the researcher wants to test whether there is something about the physiological development of women that causes differences in the birthweights of their babies. Existing studies have shown that, in fact, teenagers have a higher rate of low-birthweight babies than women in their 20s. The question, however, is whether age itself causes this difference or whether there are other mechanisms that mediate the relationship between maternal age and infant birthweight.

The researcher in this example must design the study in such a way that these other factors are controlled. But what are the other variables that must be controlled? To answer this, one must ask the following critical question:

What variables could affect the dependent variable under study while at the same time be related to the independent variable?

In the present study the dependent variable is infant birthweight and the independent variable is maternal age. Two variables are prime candidates for concern (although there are several other possibilities): the nutritional habits of the mother and the amount of prenatal care received. Teenagers are not always as

Table 3-1
Fictitious example of controlling two variables in a research study

Age of Mother	Rating of Nutritional Practices	Number of Prenatal Visits	Infant Birthweight
15–19	33% Good 33% Fair 33% Poor	33% 1–3 visits 33% 4–6 visits 33% > 6 visits	20% ≤ 2500 grams 80% > 2500 grams
25–29	33% Good 33% Fair 33% Poor	33% 1–3 visits 33% 4–6 visits 33% > 6 visits	9% ≤ 2500 grams 91% > 2500 grams

careful as older women about their eating patterns during pregnancy and are also less likely to obtain adequate medical care. Both nutrition and the amount of care could, in turn, affect the baby's birthweight. Thus, if these two factors are not controlled, then any observed relationship between the mother's age and her baby's weight at birth could be caused by the mother's age itself, her diet, or her prenatal care.

These three possible explanations are shown schematically below:

1. Mother's age → infant birthweight
2. Mother's age → prenatal care → infant birthweight
3. Mother's age → nutrition → infant birthweight

The arrows here symbolize a causal mechanism or an influence. The researcher's task is to design a study in such a way that the true explanation is made clear. Both nutrition and prenatal care must be controlled in order to see if explanation 1 is valid.

How can the researcher impose such control? There are a number of ways, as discussed in Chapter 11, but the general principle underlying each alternative is the same: the competing influences—often referred to as *extraneous variables*—must be held constant. The extraneous variables to be controlled must somehow be handled in such a way that they are not related to the independent or dependent variable. Again, an example should help make this point more clear. Let us say we want to compare the birthweights of infants born to two groups of women: those aged 15 to 19 and those aged 25 to 29. We must then design a study in such a way that the nutritional and health-care practices of the two groups are comparable, even though, in general, the two groups are not comparable in these respects. Table 3-1 illustrates how groups could be selected in such a way that both older and younger mothers have similar eating habits and amounts of prenatal attention. By building this comparability into the two groups, we are holding nutrition and prenatal care constant. If the babies' birthweights in the two groups continue to differ (as they in fact did in Table 3-1), we will be in a position to conclude that age (and not diet or prenatal care) influenced the birthweight of the infants. If the two groups do not differ, however, we will be left to tentatively conclude that it is not their age per se that causes young women to have a higher percentage of low-birthweight babies, but either nutrition, prenatal care, or both variables.

By exercising research control in this example, we have taken a step toward one of the most fundamental aims of science, which is to explain the relationship between variables. Control is essential because the world is extremely complex and many variables are interrelated in complicated ways. When studying a

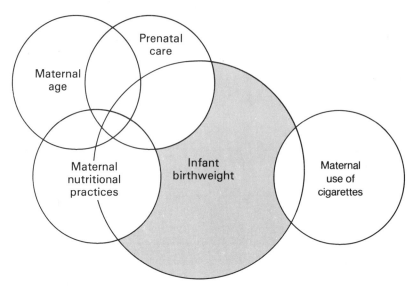

Figure 3-1. Hypothetical representation of factors affecting infant birthweight.

particular problem, it is almost never possible to examine this complexity directly: we must be content to analyze a couple of relationships at a time and put the pieces together like a jigsaw puzzle. That is why even modest research studies can make important contributions to science. The extent of the contribution, however, is strongly related to how well a researcher is able to control contaminating influences. A controlled study allows a researcher to understand the nature of the relationship between the dependent and independent variables.

In the present example, we identified three variables that could affect a baby's birthweight, but dozens of others could have been suggested, such as maternal stress, mothers' use of drugs or alcohol during the pregnancy, and so on. Researchers need to isolate the independent and dependent variables in which they are interested and then pinpoint from the dozens of possible candidates those that need to be controlled. It is not often possible to control all the variables that affect the dependent variable, nor is it necessary to do so. It is essential to control a variable only if it is simul-taneously related to both the dependent and independent variables.

Figure 3-1 illustrates this notion. In this figure, each circle represents the variability associated with a particular variable. The large circle in the center represents the dependent variable, infant birthweight. Overlapping variables indicate the degree to which the variables are related to each other. In this hypothetical example, four variables are shown as possibly being related to infant birthweight: the mother's age, the amount of prenatal care she receives, her nutritional practices, and her smoking practices during pregnancy. The first three variables are also related to each other: this is shown by the fact that these three circles overlap not only with infant birthweight but also with each other. That is, younger mothers tend to have different patterns of prenatal care and nutrition than older mothers. The mother's prenatal use of cigarettes, however, is unrelated to these three variables. In other words, women who smoke during their pregnancies (according to this hypothetical representation) are as likely to be young as old, to eat properly as not, and to get a lot of prenatal care as not. If this representation is accurate, then it would not be essential to control smoking in a study of the effect of maternal age on infant birthweight. If this scheme is incorrect — if teenage mothers smoke more or less than older mothers — then the mother's smoking practices should be controlled.

Figure 3-1 does not represent infant birthweight as being totally determined by the four other variables. The darkened area of the birthweight circle designates unexplained variability in infant birthweight. That is, other "circles" or determinants of birthweight are needed in order for us to fully understand what causes babies to be born weighing different amounts. Genetic characteristics, events occurring during the pregnancy, and medical treatments administered to the pregnant woman are all examples of other factors contributing to an infant's weight at birth. Dozens, and perhaps hundreds, of circles would need to be sketched onto Figure 3-1 in order for us to fully understand the complex interrelationships between infant birthweight and other variables. In designing a study we might be interested in the effect of only one variable (such as maternal age) on the dependent variable. This is perfectly respectable — indeed, often necessary. However, researchers need to control those variables that overlap with both the independent and dependent variables. In Figure 3-1, if there are other variables that belong in the darkened area that are also related to maternal age, then those extraneous variables should be controlled. Because uncontrolled extraneous variables can lead to erroneous or misleading conclusions, the researcher designing a study must plan how best to control these extraneous variables to maximize the usefulness of the research. Also, the careful consumer of research studies needs to question whether the investigator has properly designed the study so that the true relationship between the independent and dependent variables is not obscured by the influence of contaminating factors.

Research rooted in the phenomenological paradigm is usually less concerned with the issue of control. With its emphasis on a holistic perspective and the individuality of human experience, the phenomenological approach holds that to impose controls on a research setting is to irrevocably remove some of the meaning of reality. However, critics of the phenomenological approach argue that lack of control often makes it impossible to rule out numerous alternative explanations to the findings, in which case firm conclusions about the relationships among variables cannot be reached.

Data

The *data* (singular, datum) of a research study are the pieces of information obtained in the course of the investigation. The researcher identifies the variables of interest, develops operational definitions of those variables, and then collects the necessary data. The variables, because they vary, take on different values. The *actual* values of the study variables constitute the data for a research project.

For example, suppose we were interested in studying the relationship between sodium consumption and blood pressure. That is, we want to learn if people who consume more sodium are particularly susceptible to high blood pressure, or whether these variables are unrelated. The data for this study would consist of three pieces of information for all participants: their average daily intake of sodium (in milligrams), their diastolic blood pressure, and their systolic blood pressure. Some hypothetical data for ten subjects are shown in Table 3-2. These numerical values associated with the variables of interest represent the data for a research project. The collection and analysis of data are typically the most time-consuming parts of a study.

In phenomenological studies, the pieces of data are usually narrative descriptions rather than numerical values. Narrative descriptions

Table 3-2
Hypothetical data for blood pressure study

Subject Number	Daily Sodium Intake (Milligrams)	Systolic Blood Pressure	Diastolic Blood Pressure
1	8125	130	90
2	7530	126	80
3	1000	140	90
4	4580	118	78
5	2810	114	76
6	4150	112	78
7	6000	120	80
8	2250	110	70
9	5240	114	76
10	3330	116	74

can be obtained by having conversations with subjects, by making detailed notes of how subjects behave in naturalistic settings, or by obtaining narrative records from subjects, such as diaries. Because of the nature of data obtained, phenomenological studies are generally described as qualitative, as opposed to quantitative, investigations.

☐
Major steps in the research process

A researcher typically moves from the beginning point of a study (the posing of a question) to the end point (the obtaining of an answer) in a logical sequence of steps. True, in some cases the steps overlap; in other cases some steps are interchangeable; in yet other cases some are unnecessary. Still, there is a general flow of activities that is typical of a scientific investigation. That flow is briefly described below. The remainder of the text provides more detail about these research activities in roughly the same sequential order.

1. Formulating and delimiting the problem

Good research depends to a great degree on good questions. Sometimes the importance of

securing an interesting and meaningful topic gets lost in the concern for utilizing appropriate and sophisticated research procedures. Yet without a good, workable, significant topic, the most carefully and skillfully designed research project will be of no value.

Once a general topic is selected, the specific problem to be investigated should be defined. One of the most common difficulties for beginning researchers is the development of a manageable, researchable problem statement. Initial statements of the problem are typically too broad and too vague, mirroring perhaps the enthusiasm and reluctance of the researcher to limit the area of research on the one hand and her or his own fuzziness concerning what is to be accomplished on the other. Problem statements that are hazy and broad, however, may ultimately lead to confusion if they cannot provide direction to the pursuit of the project.

2. Reviewing the related literature

Good research does not exist in a vacuum. In order for research findings to be useful, they should be an extension of previous knowledge and theory as well as a guide for future research activity. In order for a researcher to build on existing work, it is essential to understand what is already known about a topic. A thorough review of the literature provides a foundation upon which to base new knowledge.

Nursing research, which is a rapidly expanding field, is, nevertheless, a relatively wide-open area for research activity. There are very few nursing research topics about which *the* definitive study can be said to have been done. In any event, previous work on a problem should not discourage the researcher from pursuing a topic of interest, because no two studies are ever identical. However, a thorough familiarization with previous studies can be useful in suggesting aspects of a problem about which less is known and where, therefore, greater contributions can be made.

3. Developing a theoretical framework

A *theory* is a generalized, abstract explanation of the interrelationships among phenomena, with the primary purpose of explaining and predicting those phenomena. Theory is the ultimate aim of science in that it transcends the specifics of a particular time, place, and set of individuals and aims to identify regularities in the relationships among variables. When research is performed in the context of a theoretical framework, it is more likely that its findings will be useful in improving our ability to understand or control events, situations, and individuals.

4. Formulating hypotheses

A *hypothesis* is a statement of the researcher's expectations concerning relationships between the variables under investigation. In other words, a hypothesis is a prediction of expected outcomes; it states the relationships that the researcher anticipates finding as a result of the study. The problem statement identifies the phenomena under investigation; a hypothesis predicts how those phenomena will be related. For example, a problem state-

ment might be phrased "Is preeclamptic toxemia in pregnant women associated with stress factors present during pregnancy?" This might be translated into the following hypothesis or prediction: "Pregnant women with preeclamptic toxemia will report a higher incidence of emotionally disturbing or stressful events during pregnancy than asymptomatic pregnant women." Thus, problem statements represent the initial effort to give a research project direction; hypotheses represent a more formalized focus for the collection and interpretation of data.

5. Selecting a research design

Once a researcher has developed testable hypotheses, a number of decisions have to be made concerning how the study will be conducted. Sometimes the nature of the study will dictate the approach to be used. More often, however, the investigator will have a number of options from which to choose.

The research design is the overall plan for how to obtain answers to the questions being studied and how to handle some of the difficulties encountered during the research process. The design should specify which of the various types of research approach will be adopted and how the researcher plans to implement a number of scientific controls to enhance the interpretability of the results.

A wide variety of research approaches are available to nurse researchers. A basic distinction is the difference between *experimental* designs (in which the researcher actively introduces some form of intervention) and *nonexperimental* designs (in which the researcher passively collects data without trying to make any changes or introduce any treatments). For example, if a researcher gave bran flakes to one group of people and prune juice to another each morning, the study would involve an intervention and would be considered experimental. If the researcher compared elimination patterns for a group who normally took foods that stimulated bowel elimination with another group that did not, the study would not involve an intervention and would be considered nonexperimental. Experimental designs generally offer the possibility of greater control over extraneous variables than nonexperimental designs. However, if the researcher's primary interest is understanding some human behavior in naturalistic contexts (as in the case of phenomenological research), the design will inevitably be nonexperimental.

6. Specifying the population

The term *population* refers to the aggregate or totality of all the objects, subjects, or members that conform to a designated set of specifications. For example, we may specify "nurses" (RNs) and "living in the United States" as the attributes of interest: our population would then consist of all licensed RNs who reside in the United States. We could in a similar fashion define a population consisting of *all* children under 10 years of age with muscular dystrophy in the state of California; or *all* the patient records in a particular hospital; or *all* the individuals who had a fatal coronary during a particular year.

The requirement of defining a population for a research project arises from the need to specify the group to which the results of a study can be applied. It is seldom possible to study an entire population, unless it is quite small. Research studies typically involve only a small fraction of the population referred to as a *sample*. Before one selects actual study participants, (often referred to as *subjects*), it is essential to know what characteristics the sample should possess in order to be able to generalize the findings to the broader population.

7. Developing a data collection plan

In order to meaningfully address a research problem, some method must be developed to observe or measure the research variables as accurately as possible. In most situations the researcher begins by carefully defining the research variables to clarify exactly what each one means. Then the researcher needs to select or design an appropriate method of measuring the variables — that is, of collecting the data. A variety of measurement approaches exist. *Physiological measurements* often play an important role in nursing research. Another popular form is *self-reports,* wherein subjects are directly asked about their feelings, behaviors, attitudes, and personal traits. Another method of measuring variables is through *observational techniques.* Here the researcher collects data by observing people's behavior and recording relevant aspects of it. Data collection methods vary in the structure imposed on the research subjects. Qualitative methods tend to be loosely structured, permitting subjects full opportunity to express themselves and behave in naturalistic ways. Quantitative approaches are more structured and controlled. Thus, developing a data collection plan is a complex and challenging process that permits a great deal of creativity and choice.

8. Conducting the pilot study and making revisions

Unforeseen problems often arise in the course of a project. The effects of such problems may be negligible but in other cases may be so severe that the study has to be stopped so that modifications can be introduced. In order to minimize the possibility of major difficulties, several procedures can be adopted. One useful approach is to have individuals external to the project check your preliminary work, particularly the data collection instruments. An experienced researcher with a fresh perspective on a research problem can often be invaluable in identifying pitfalls and shortcomings that might otherwise have not been recognized.

Whenever possible, it is advisable to carry out a *pilot study,* which is a small-scale version, or trial run, of the major study. The function of the pilot study is to obtain information for improving the project or for assessing its feasibility. The pilot study may reveal that revisions are needed in one or more aspects of the project. For example, the pilot study may provide information suggesting that the target population was defined too broadly. Or it may reveal that the initial conceptualization was somehow inadequate or that the hypotheses as stated are untestable. From a more practical point of view, a trial run may reveal that it will not be possible to secure the cooperation of people by the intended procedures or that the study is more costly than anticipated. Very often, the principle focus of a pilot study is the assessment of the adequacy of the data collection plan. The researcher may need to know, for example, if technical equipment is functioning properly. In the case of interview schedules and questionnaires, it is important to know whether respondents understand the questions and directions, or if they find certain questions objectionable in some way.

It should be pointed out that a pilot test should be carried out with as much care as the major study so that any weaknesses that are detected will be truly representative of inadequacies inherent in the major study. Subjects for a pilot study should possess the same characteristics as individuals who will compose the main sample. That is, pilot subjects should be chosen from the same population as subjects for the major study. It is often useful to question the individuals who participate in a pilot study concerning their reactions to and overall impressions of the project.

When the data from the test run have been collected and scrutinized, the researcher should make the revisions and refinements that in her or his judgment would eliminate or reduce problems encountered during the pilot study. If extensive revisions are required, it may prove advisable to have a second trial run that incorporates those revisions.

9. Selecting the sample

Data are generally collected from a sample rather than from an entire population. The advantage of using a sample is that it is more practical and less costly than collecting data from the population. The risk is that the sample selected might not adequately reflect the behaviors, traits, symptoms, or beliefs of the population.

Various methods of obtaining a sample are available to the researcher. These methods vary in cost, effort, and level of skills required, but their adequacy is assessed by the same criterion: the representativeness of the selected sample. That is, the quality of the sample is a function of how typical, or representative, the sample is of the population with respect to the variables of concern in the study. Sophisticated sampling procedures can produce samples that have a high likelihood of being representative. The most sophisticated sampling methods are referred to as *probability sampling,* which employs random procedures for the selection of the sample. In a probability sample, every member of the population has the possibility of being included in the sample. With *nonprobability sampling* techniques, by contrast, there is no way of ensuring that each member of the population could be selected; consequently, the risk of a biased (unrepresentative) sample is greater.

10. Collecting the data

The actual collection of data normally proceeds according to a preestablished plan in order to minimize confusion, delays, and mistakes. That is, the procedures to be used in describing the study to the participants, in administering the measuring instruments, in answering the questions of participants, and so forth, should generally be specified in advance. This step may sometimes involve the training of research personnel in the case of complicated experiments or detailed interview studies.

A considerable amount of both clerical and administrative work is required in the data collection task. The investigators must be sure, for example, that enough materials are available to complete the study, that participants are informed of the time and place that their presence may be required, that research personnel (such as interviewers) are conscientious in keeping their appointments, that schedules do not conflict, or that a suitable system of assigning an identification numbr to maintain subject anonymity has been implemented.

The collecting of data is typically the most time-consuming phase of a study, although the actual amount of time spent varies considerably from project to project. If data are collected by administering the measuring instrument to an intact group, this task may be accomplished in a day or so. More often, however, the data collection requires several weeks, or even months, of work.

11. Preparing the data for analysis

After the data are collected, a few preliminary activities must be performed before the actual analysis of the data can begin. For instance, it is normally necessary to look through questionnaires and interview schedules to determine if they are usable. Sometimes such forms are left almost entirely blank or contain other indications of misinterpretation or noncompliance. Another step that should be taken at this point is to assign identification numbers to the responses or observations of different subjects, if this has not been done previously.

Generally, the data collected in a study are not directly amenable to analysis. Some preliminary steps are usually necessary before the

analysis can proceed. One such step that is typically needed is known as *coding,* which refers to the process of "translating" verbal data into categories or numerical form. For example, patients' responses to a question about the quality of nursing care they received during hospitalization might be coded into positive reactions, negative reactions, neutral reactions, and mixed reactions.

Another preliminary step that is increasingly common is the preparation of data for computer analysis. The procedures involved in the use of computers are briefly discussed in Chapter 23.

12. Analyzing the data

The data themselves do not provide us with answers to our research questions. Ordinarily the amount of data collected in a study is rather extensive and, therefore, needs to be processed and analyzed in some orderly, coherent fashion so that patterns and relationships can be discerned. There are two basic types of data analysis. *Qualitative analysis* involves the integration and synthesis of narrative, non-numerical data, such as the analysis of historical materials. *Quantitative* information is generally analyzed through statistical procedures.

Statistical analyses cover a broad range of techniques, from some very simple procedures to complex and sophisticated methods. The underlying logic of statistical tests, however, is relatively simple and should, therefore, be no cause for concern to the beginning researcher. Computers and pocket calculators have virtually eliminated the need to get bogged down with detailed arithmetic operations.

13. Interpreting the results

Before the results of a study can be communicated effectively, they must be organized and interpreted in some systematic fashion. By interpretation, we refer to the process of making sense of the results and of examining the implications of the findings within a broader context. The process of interpretation begins with an attempt to explain the findings.

If the research hypotheses have been supported, an explanation of the results is usually straightforward, because the findings fit into a previously conceived argument. If the hypotheses are not supported, the investigator must develop some possible explanations. Is the underlying conceptualization wrong, or perhaps inappropriate for the research problem? Or do the findings reflect problems with the research methods rather than the theory (*e.g.,* was the sample biased)? In order to provide sound explanations for obtained findings, then, the researchers must not only be familiar with the literature on a topic and with the conceptual underpinnings of the problem, but must also be able to understand the methodological weaknesses of the study design. In other words, a researcher should be in a position to critically evaluate the decisions he or she made in designing the study and to recommend alternatives to others interested in the same research problem.

14. Communicating the findings

The results of a research investigation are of little utility if they are not communicated to others. Even the most compelling hypothesis, the most careful and thorough study, the most dramatic results are of no value to the scientific community if they are unknown. The final task of a research project, therefore, is the preparation of a research report. There are various forms of research reports: term papers, dissertations, journal articles, books, and so on. Journal articles — that is, short reports appearing in such professional journals as *Nursing Research*— are generally the most useful because such reports are available to a broad audience.

□
Organization of a research project

The model of research steps presented in the preceding section is an idealized conception of what researchers do. The research process rarely follows a neatly prescribed pattern of sequential procedures. Developments in one step, for example, may require some backtracking to make accommodations in earlier activities. This fact does not obviate the need for careful planning in advance; indeed, it makes the need for organization even more salient. Although we cannot hope to alert beginning researchers to even a majority of the obstacles they are likely to encounter (even the most experienced researcher normally runs into some difficulties), we can perhaps offer a few suggestions for minimizing potential problems.

Almost all research projects are conducted under some time pressure. Students in research courses may have end-of-term deadlines; government-sponsored research involves funds granted for a specified time period; and researchers performing an applied research study ordinarily must supply decision-makers with information relatively quickly. Those who may not have such formal time constraints — such as graduate students working on dissertations — normally have their own goals for project completion. Setting up a timetable in advance may be an important step toward meeting such goals. This means that the investigator should make projections about which tasks should be completed by what point in time. Of course, initial projections often have to be modified, but estimates made at the outset of a project often help in setting subgoals.

Unfortunately it is not possible for us to give even approximate figures for the relative percentage of time that should be spent on each task. Some projects require many months to develop and pilot test the measuring instru-

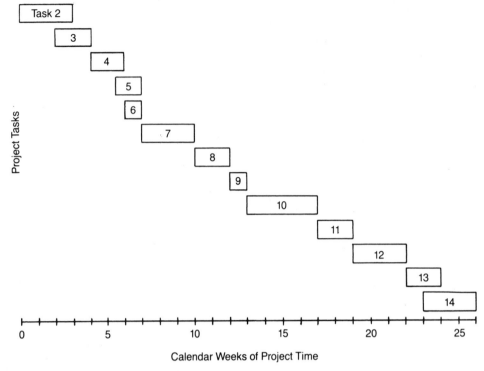

Figure 3-2. *Breakdown of project tasks by time allotted.*

ments whereas other studies use previously existing instruments. The write-up of the study may take many months or only a few days. Clearly, however, not all 14 of these steps will be equally time-consuming. If the researcher knew that there was a specified deadline, it would make little sense to simply divide the time available by 14. But having a deadline, or at least a tentative one, does have the function of imposing some structure and limits on tasks that might otherwise continue indefinitely, such as the selection of a problem and review of the literature.

Let us suppose that during a six-month period we were studying the problem "Does the presence of fathers in the delivery room affect the mothers' perception of pain?" Figure 3-2 presents a hypothetical time schedule for the research tasks to be completed. The selection

of the problem (Task 1) is not included because the research topic has already been identified. Note that many activities overlap and that some tasks are projected to involve very little time in terms of time elapsed on the calendar.

In developing a time schedule of this sort, a number of considerations should be kept in mind. The level of knowledge and competence of the researcher are certainly contributing factors, but inexperienced investigators should in any event avoid complex projects requiring extensive technical skills. Resources available to the researcher, in the form of research funds and personnel, will greatly influence the time estimates. It is also important to consider the practical aspects of performing the study, which were not all enumerated in the preceding section. Obtaining supplies, securing the necessary permissions, having forms or instruments approved by granting agencies or supervisors, holding meetings, and the like are all time-consuming, but often necessary, activities.

Individuals differ in the kinds of tasks that are appealing to them. Some people greatly enjoy the preliminary phases that have a strong intellectual component, while others are more eager to collect the data, a task that is often more interpersonal in nature. The researcher should attempt, however, to allocate a reasonable amount of time to do justice to each activity. Inadequately conceived and hastily designed studies are doomed to failure, or at best mediocrity, no matter how much care and time are given to the collection and analysis of data. On the other hand, the person who lingers too long in the library may never reach the final goal.

□
Summary

Scientific research focuses on abstract *concepts* or *constructs*. In research studies, the concepts under investigation are referred to as *variables*. A variable is a characteristic or quality that takes on different values; that is, a variable is something that varies from one person or object to another. The blood type, blood pressure, grip strength, and hair color of a person are variables. These variables, which are inherent characteristics of a person that the researcher only measures or observes, are referred to as *attribute variables*. In some situations, a researcher actively creates or manipulates a variable, as when bran flakes are given to some research subjects and prune juice is given to others (an *active variable*).

An important distinction for researchers is differentiation between the dependent and independent variables of a study. The *dependent variable* is the behavior, characteristic, or outcome that the researcher is interested in understanding, explaining, predicting, or affecting. The dependent variable (or *criterion variable*) is the presumed consequence or effect of the *independent variable*. The independent variable is the presumed cause of, antecedent to, or influence on the dependent variable. Groups that are highly varied with respect to some attribute are described as *heterogeneous;* groups with limited variability are described as *homogeneous*.

In an actual investigation, the variables are generally clarified and defined in such a way that they are amenable to observation or measurement. The *operational definition* of a concept is the specification of the procedures and tools required to make the needed measurements.

Except in rare cases, researchers are not interested in studying variables in isolation, but rather in learning about the *relationship* between two or more variables simultaneously. A relationship refers to a bond or connection between two variables. Researchers focus on the relationship between the independent and dependent variables. When the independent variable causes the occurrence, manifestation, or alteration of the dependent variable, a *cause-and-effect relationship* is said to exist. Variables that are not causally related can be linked by a *functional relationship*.

In attempting to understand how variables are related, researchers generally attempt to design a study that controls contaminating factors. Research *control* involves holding constant contaminating influences, known as *extraneous variables,* that might otherwise mask the true relationship between the independent and dependent variables.

The term *data* is used to designate the information that is collected during the course of a study. Because variables take on different values, the record of those values for the subjects in the study constitutes the data.

The steps involved in the conduct of a scientific investigation are fairly standard. The following steps are often performed in a roughly sequential fashion:

1. *Formulating and Delimiting the Problem*—the identification of a research topic, statement of the problem, and assessment of its feasibility.
2. *Reviewing the Literature*—the reading and organization of previously written materials relevant to (1) the specific problem to be investigated, (2) the theoretical framework, and (3) methods appropriate to perform the study.
3. *Developing a Theoretical Framework* — the integration of the specific problem into a broader scientific context that seeks to explain regularities in the relationship among variables.
4. *Formulating Hypotheses*—the development of predictions concerning the outcomes of the study; the specification of testable expected relationships among variables.
5. *Selecting a Research Design*—the formulation of a strategy for answering the research questions and for implementing controls over the research situation.
6. *Specifying the Population*—the identification of the target group to whom the researcher hopes to generalize the results of the study; the term *population* refers to the totality of some class of objects or individuals that have one or more characteristic in common.
7. *Developing a Data Collection Plan*—the development or selection of suitable instruments and methods to measure the variables of interest, via some data collection approach such as self-reports, observational techniques, or physiological measurements.
8. *Conducting the Pilot Study and Making Revisions*—the carrying out of a small-scale trial run to detect any unforeseen problems in the research methods.
9. *Selecting the Sample*—the development and implementation of a sampling procedure (using either *probability* or *nonprobability* sampling procedures) to obtain a sample or subset to represent the whole population and from whom data will be collected.
10. *Collecting the Data*—the gathering together of the information needed to answer the research questions and test the hypotheses.
11. *Preparing the Data for Analysis*—the performance of preliminary steps, such as coding, to prepare the data for analysis.
12. *Analyzing the Data*—the organization and summary of the information obtained in the study through qualitative or statistical procedures designed to enhance the interpretability of the findings.
13. *Interpeting the Results*—the task of making sense of the findings, of explaining how the results relate to the conceptual framework and to other findings, and of suggesting further research in the area.
14. *Communicating the Findings*—the written description of what was done, why it was done, to whom or with whom it was done, what was found, and what the implications could be.

These steps represent an idealized model of the research process. There is often a considerable amount of shifting back and forth, rethinking, and reorganizing. Certain steps may be unnecessary in certain types of projects whereas in others there may be a need for supplementary steps.

There are, in addition to these theoretical and methodological concerns, a number of practical matters to be dealt with in the course of a project. Furthermore, unanticipated difficulties are inevitable. The researcher cannot avoid all problems but can minimize their impact through careful planning and organization. The preparation of a timetable with expected deadlines for task completion can be extremely useful in establishing subgoals and in helping the researcher to be more realistic in the allocation of time to different tasks.

□
Study suggestions

1. Suggest ways of operationally defining the following concepts: nursing competency; patients' time to first voiding after surgery; aggressive behavior; patients' level of pain; home health hazards; psychogenic sterility; social class; and body image.
2. Name five dichotomous variables.
3. Identify which of the following variables are active variables and which are attribute variables (some might be both): height; degree of fatigue; cooperativeness; noise level on hospital units; length of stay in hospital; educational attainment; self-esteem; nurses' job satisfaction.
4. In the following research problems, identify the independent and dependent variables:
   a. How do nurses and physicians differ in the way they view the extended role concept for nurses?
   b. Does problem-oriented recording lead to more effective patient care than other recording methods?
   c. Do elderly patients have lower pain thresholds than younger patients?
   d. How are the sleeping patterns of infants affected by different forms of stimulation?
   e. Can home visits by nurses to released psychiatric patients reduce readmission rates?
5. Suppose that you were planning to study the following question: "Does a patient's body position affect the measurement of vital bodily signs?" You would like to collect data for at least five physiological measurements and four body positions from 100 subjects. The project must be completed in 9 months. Prepare a time schedule such as the one shown in Figure 3-2 for the completion of the required research steps.

□
Study readings

Methodological references

Abdellah, F. & Levine, E. (1978). *Better patient care through nursing research* (2nd ed.). New York: Macmillan. (Chapter 5).

Fox, D.J. (1982). *Fundamentals of research in nursing* (4th ed.). New York: Appleton-Century-Crofts. (Chapter 3).

Kerlinger, F. (1973). *Foundations of behavioral research* (2nd ed.). New York: Holt, Rinehart and Winston. (Chapter 3).

Sweeney, M.A. & Olivieri, P. (1981). *An introduction to nursing research.* Philadelphia: J.B. Lippincott. (Chapters 2 & 3).

Wilson, H.S. (1985). *Research in nursing.* Menlo Park, CA: Addison-Wesley. (Chapters 1 & 4).

Substantive references *

Atkinson, L.D. (1979). Prenatal nipple conditioning for breastfeeding. *Nursing Research, 28,* 267–271.

Broom, B.L. (1984). Consensus about the marital relationship during transition to parenthood. *Nursing Research, 33,* 223–228.

---

* In this chapter and in subsequent chapters, studies that illustrate the concepts discussed in the text are listed in the section designated as "Substantive References." The inclusion of a study is not intended to imply that it is technically excellent in all respects but rather that it contains a concept or methodological element that has relevance for the issues discussed in the chapter. These are examples of studies with explicit operational definitions of variables and/or identification of independent and dependent variables.

Derdiarian, A.K. & Forsyth, A.B. (1983). An instrument for theory and research development using the Behavioral Systems Model for nursing. *Nursing Research, 32,* 260–266.

Fehring, R.J. (1983). Effects of biofeedback-aided relaxation on the psychological stress symptoms of college students. *Nursing Research, 32,* 362–366.

Geden, E. *et al.* (1985). Self-report and psychophysiological effects of Lamaze preparation. *Research in Nursing and Health, 8,* 155–165.

Hoskins, C.N. (1979). Level of activation, body temperature, and interpersonal conflict in family relationships. *Nursing Research, 28,* 154–160.

Kurzuk-Howard, G., Simpson, L., & Palmieri, A. (1985). Decubitus ulcer care: A comparative study. *Western Journal of Nursing Research, 7,* 58–79.

Munro, B.H. (1983). Job satisfaction among recent graduates of schools of nursing. *Nursing Research, 32,* 350–355.

Papa, L.L. (1980). Responses to life events as predictors of suicidal behavior. *Nursing Research, 29,* 326–369.

Part II

Preliminary research steps

Chapter 4
□
Selecting and defining a nursing research problem

For many beginning researchers, the selection of a problem for study is the most difficult task of the research endeavor. The difficulty of selecting a problem for study does not stem from a dearth of things to be studied. Nothing has been researched in its entirety. Sometimes researchers find it difficult to select a particular topic for study because there are so many things to be known and it is perplexing to choose only one. Other researchers may experience difficulty in selecting a topic because they are unfamiliar with previous research. Beginning researchers experience an additional dilemma. They must choose a problem for study at a time when they are unsure of what the research process entails and what constitutes a researchable problem.

Ideally, this first step in the research process should not be hurried. Many hours will be devoted to investigating the problem that is selected and the time will be more profitably spent if the researcher is devoting his or her efforts to a problem that is of real interest. The identification of a researchable problem is not an easy matter, but it is a crucial one. It is simply not possible to proceed in an orderly, intelligent fashion on a research project unless a clear notion of the problem has been developed. Much as health professionals do not administer medications or perform surgery without some understanding of a person's ailment, so a researcher should not attempt to solve a research problem until it has been stated in a concise and unambiguous form. Researchers must know what they are trying to do before they can succeed at doing it.

☐
Sources of problems

Beginning researchers often are puzzled and perhaps even threatened by a requirement to develop a research problem. Where do ideas for research problems come from? How can a topic be selected? In this section we will suggest some sources for locating a problem or topic. The three most common sources are experience, the nursing literature, and theories.

Experience

The nurse's everyday experience provides a rich supply of problems for investigation. Whether you are a student nurse, practicing nurse, nurse educator, or nursing administrator, there are sure to be occurrences or situations that you have found puzzling or problematic. If you have ever asked yourself such questions as "Why are things done this way?" "I wonder what would happen if . . . ?" "What approach would work better?" or "Who is most likely to benefit from this?" you may be well along the way to developing a research idea. For the beginning researcher in particular, experience is often the most compelling source for topics. Immediate problems that are in need of solution or that excite the curiosity are relevant and interesting and, thus, may generate more enthusiasm than abstract and distant problems inferred from a theory.

An important ingredient for a successful research project is the investigator's curiosity. If you look around you as you are performing your nursing functions, you are bound to find a wealth of research ideas if you are curious about why things are the way they are, or how things could be improved if something were to change. Here are a few hints:

- Watch for recurring problems and see of you can discern a pattern in situations that lead to the problem.
  Example: Why do many patients complain of being tired after being transferred from a coronary care unit to a progressive care unit?
- Think about aspects of your work that are irksome, frustrating, or do not result in the intended outcome—then try to identify factors that may contribute to the problem that could be changed.
  Example: Why is supper-time so frustrating in a nursing home?
- Critically examine some of the decisions you make in the performance of your functions. Are these decisions based on tradition or are they based on scientific evidence that supports their efficacy? Many practices in nursing that have become custom might be challenged.
  Example: What would happen if visiting hours in ICU were changed from ten minutes every hour to the regularly scheduled hours existing in the rest of the hospital?

Nursing literature

Ideas for research projects often come from reading the nursing literature. The beginning nurse researcher would profit from regularly reading nursing journals, especially ones that report the results of nursing studies, such as *Nursing Research, Advances in Nursing Science, Research in Nursing and Health,* and the *Western Journal of Nursing Research.* Such reading may not only help the neophyte researcher find a problem amenable to scientific investigation but may also help to familiarize the beginning researcher with the wording of research problems and the actual conduct of research studies.

Published research reports may suggest

problem areas indirectly by stimulating the reader's imagination and directly by specifying further areas in need of investigation. For example, Brandt (1984) found that stress and social support influenced maternal discipline of young children with a developmental delay. Her findings led her to suggest further study of the type and amount of social support that enables parents to cope with acute and chronic stresses and to provide optimal caretaking. She also suggested observation of caretaking and limit-setting interactions between the parent and child.

Inconsistencies in the findings reported in nursing literature often generate new ideas for research studies. A researcher may also wonder whether a study similar to one reported in a journal article would yield comparable results if applied in a different setting or with different subjects. Sometimes problems can be identified not by what is in the literature but rather by what is not. That is, gaps in the research literature may provide a rich area for research. For example, many articles have appeared in relation to the nursing process as a method of clinical practice. The Standards of Nursing Practice published by the American Nurses' Association (1973) for evaluating the quality of nursing care are formulated according to the steps of the nursing process. A large number of nursing educators teach students according to these steps. Yet, few studies have actually investigated the effectiveness of the nursing process as a method of clinical practice, as a way of evaluating nursing care, or as a method of teaching nursing.

In sum, a familiarity with existing research, or with problematic and controversial nursing issues that have yet to be understood and investigated scientifically, is an important route to developing a research topic. The student who is actively seeking a problem to study, such as the student required to do an empirical thesis, will find it most useful to read widely in areas of interest. In the next chapter we deal more extensively with the procedures of actually doing a thorough literature review.

Theory

The third major source of problems lies in the theoretical systems and conceptual schemes that have been developed in nursing and other related disciplines. As we pointed out in the previous chapter, a theory is an abstract, generalized explanation of phenomena. Theories are not in themselves rooted to practical problems or concrete situations, but a theory that is not translated to real-world conditions and scientifically tested is of little value. In order to be useful in nursing practice, research must be conducted to test the applicability of the theory to the hospital unit, the emergency room, the classroom, and other nursing environments.

If a researcher decides to base a research project on an existing theory, deductions from the theory must be developed. This deductive process is explained in greater detail in Chapters 6 and 7. Essentially, the researcher must ask the questions "If this theory is correct, what kind of behavior would I expect to find in certain situations or under certain conditions?" and "What kind of evidence would support this theory?" This process would eventually result in a specific problem that could be subjected to scientific investigation.

Let us look at an example of how a problem can be derived from a conceptual system. Levine (1973) has postulated a conceptual framework for nursing that concerns conservation. She explains nursing as conserving the patient's energy, structural integrity, personal integrity, and social integrity. From this theory, the researcher could formulate specific predictions about expected findings. For example, it might be hypothesized that primary nursing is more effective in conserving the patient's energy and social integrity than team nursing. By developing measures of energy expenditure and social integration, this hypothesis could be tested scientifically.

The 1970s and 1980s have witnessed a proliferation of conceptual frameworks and theories of nursing. Few studies have been conducted to substantiate whether or not the theories or conceptual frameworks hold up in actual nursing practice. It seems likely that these theoretical systems will play a growing role in the formulation of future nursing research problems.

☐
Developing and refining a research topic

The actual procedures for developing a research topic are difficult to identify, inasmuch as the process is not a smooth and orderly one. There probably will be many false starts, several inspirations, and several disappointments in the first efforts to devise a problem statement. The few suggestions offered here are not intended to imply that there are techniques for making this first step easy but, rather, to encourage the beginning researcher to persevere in the absence of instant success.

Selecting a topic

The development of a research problem is essentially a creative process, dependent upon imagination, insight, and ingenuity. Research on creativity has revealed that the creative process can be impeded or stifled by tension and by an early evaluation of ideas. In the early stages, when research ideas are being generated, it is wise not to be critical of them immediately. It is much better to begin by just relaxing and jotting down general areas of interest

as they come to mind. At this point it matters very little if the terms used to remind you of your ideas are abstract or concrete, broad or specific, technical or colloquial—the important point is to put some ideas on paper. Examples of some broad topics that may come to mind include "communications with patients," "reducing stress in hospitalized children," "needs of a grieving spouse," "postnatal care," "styles of leadership of nurse administrators," and "postoperative loss of orientation."

After this first step, the ideas can be sorted in terms of interest, the researcher's knowledge of the area, and the perceived promise that they hold as a research topic. When the most fruitful idea has been selected, the rest of the list should not be discarded; it may be necessary to return to it.

Narrowing the topic

Once you have identified one or more general topics of interest, you will need to begin asking questions that will lead to a researchable problem statement. Some examples of question stems that may help you focus your inquiry include the following:

- What causes . . . ?
- What is the extent of . . . ?
- Why do . . . ?
- When do . . . ?
- What factors lead to . . . ?
- What influences . . . ?
- How intense are . . . ?
- What conditions prevail before . . . ?
- What characteristics are associated with . . . ?
- What are the consequences of . . . ?
- What is the relationship between . . . ?
- How effective is . . . ?
- How do you know when . . . ?
- What differences exist . . . ?

Here again, early criticism of ideas is often inappropriate and counter-productive in this basically creative endeavor. Try not to jump to the conclusion that an idea sounds "silly" or "trivial" without giving it more careful consideration. Discussing one's thoughts with fellow students, colleagues, or advisors can be helpful. Not too much energy should be wasted in concern over whether some other researcher has already done a similar study. Totally original and unique problems are rare, despite the almost infinite range of possible topics. At the same time, no two studies are ever identical, so that every study has the potential of making some contribution to knowledge.

Beginning researchers typically develop problems that are too broad in scope or too complex and unwieldy for their level of methodological expertise. The transformation of the general topic into a workable problem is typically accomplished in a number of uneven steps, involving a series of successive approximations. Each step should result in progress toward the goals of narrowing the scope of the problem and sharpening and defining the concepts.

As the researcher moves from a general topic of interest to more specific researchable problems, it is likely that more than one potential problem area will emerge. Let us consider an example. Suppose you were working on a medical unit and observed that some patients always complained about having to wait for pain medication when certain nurses were assigned to them and yet, these same patients offered no complaints when other nurses were assigned to them. You wonder why this phenomenon occurs. The general problem area is discrepancy in complaints from patients regarding pain medications administered by different nurses. You might ask "What accounts for this discrepancy?" or "How can I improve the situation?" Such questions are not actual research questions because they are too broad and vague. They may, however, lead you to ask other questions such as "How do the two groups of nurses differ?" or "What characteristics are unique to each group of nurses?" or "What characteristics do the group of complaining patients share?" At this point you may observe that the cultural background of the patients and nurses appears to be a relevant factor. This may direct you to a review of the literature for studies concerning ethnic subcultures in relation to nursing interventions or it may provoke you to discuss the observations with peers. The result of these efforts may be several researchable problems, such as the following:

Is there a relationship between the ethnic background of nurses and the frequency with which they dispense pain medication?

Is there a relationship between the ethnic background of patients and their complaints of having to wait for pain medication?

Does the number of patient complaints increase when the patients are of dissimilar ethnic backgrounds as opposed to when they are of the same ethnic backgrounds as the nurse?

Do nurses' dispensing behaviors change as a function of the similarity between their own ethnic background and that of the patients?

All of these problems have a similar theme, yet each would be studied in a different manner. How does one choose the final problem to be studied? Tentative problems usually vary considerably in their feasibility and worth. It is at this point that a critical evaluation of ideas is appropriate. The factors that should be considered in the final selection of a problem are discussed in the next section.

□
Criteria for evaluating research problems

There are no fixed rules for making a final selection of a research problem. There are, however, some criteria that should be kept in mind in the decision process. The four most important considerations are the significance, researchability, and feasibility of the problem and its interest to the researcher.

Significance of the problem

A crucial factor in selecting a problem to be studied is its significance to nursing. The research question should have the potential of contributing to the body of knowledge in nursing in a meaningful way. The researcher should pose the following kinds of questions: Is the problem an important one? Will patients, nurses, or the broader health care community or society benefit by the knowledge that will be produced? Will the results lead to practical applications? Will the results have theoretical relevance? Will the findings challenge (or lend support to) untested assumptions? Will the study help to formulate or alter nursing practices or policies? Will anyone *care* what the findings are? If the answer to all of these questions is "no," the problem should probably be abandoned.

The problem does not need to be of Nobel Prize caliber in order to be useful, but trivial questions should be avoided. It would be technically possible to study, for example, the relationship between surgical patients' hair color and their length of stay in a hospital, but who would be interested in learning the results of such a study? If blondes as a group were found to have a longer hospital stay, on the average, than brunettes, would this finding have any implications for nursing care? The problem is trivial because it has little signifi-

cance for nursing practice, nor does it have any theoretical relevance.

Researchability of the problem

Not all questions are amenable to study through scientific investigation. Problems or issues of a moral or ethical nature, although provocative, are not capable of being researched. An example of a philosophically oriented question is: "Should nurses join unions?" The answer to such a question is ultimately based on a person's values. There are no "right" or "wrong" answers, only points of view. The question as stated is more suitable to a debate than to scientific research. To be sure, it is possible to modify the question so that aspects of the issue could be researched. For instance, each of the following questions could be investigated in a research project:

What are nurses' attitudes toward unionization?

Do younger nurses hold more favorable opinions of unions than older nurses?

Does a person's role (nurse vs. nursing administrator vs. hospital administrator) affect her or his perceptions of the consequences of unions on the delivery of health care?

Is opposition to unionization for nurses based primarily on perceived outcomes to patients and clients or on outcomes to the nursing profession?

The findings from these hypothetical projects would have no bearing, of course, on the answer to the original question of whether or not nurses *should* join unions, but the information could be useful in developing a comprehensive understanding of the issues and in facilitating decision-making.

Generally, researchable problems are ones that involve variables capable of being precisely defined and measured. For example, suppose the researcher was trying to determine what effect early discharge had on the general well-being of a patient. General well-being is too broad and fuzzy a concept to measure as it is stated. The researcher would have to find a means of sharpening the concept so that it could be observed and measured before proceeding to subsequent steps in the research process. One would have to establish criteria against which the patients' progress toward well-being would be assessed. In other words, the researcher would need to answer the question "How will I be able to distinguish those who have attained 'general well-being' from those who have not?" On the other hand, if the researcher has identified a problem that involves complex concepts that are difficult to measure but important to the advancement of nursing, it may be appropriate to address the problem using in-depth qualitative research. In such cases, the problem is often stated in broad terms to permit full exploration of the concept of interest. However, it is generally wise to delimit the problem in some way in order to make it manageable. For example, if the investigator were interested in studying through qualitative procedures empathic behavior in nurses, it might be judicious to set some limits on the type of situations to be studied (such as empathy with parents of hospitalized children or empathy with severely disfigured burn patients). The generalizability of the conclusions regarding the dimensions of nurses' empathy could then be studied by others in different contexts.

Feasibility of the problem

Problems that are both significant and researchable may still be inappropriate if they are not feasible. The issue of feasibility is a complex one and encompasses a variety of considerations. Not all of these factors are relevant for every problem, but most of them should be kept in mind in making a final decision.

1. Time and timing

As pointed out in the previous chapter, most studies have deadlines or at least informal goals for their completion. The problem must, therefore, be one that can be adequately studied within the time allotted. This means that the scope of the problem should be sufficiently restricted that enough time will be available for the various steps reviewed in Chapter 3. It is usually wise to allocate more time to the performance of the tasks than originally anticipated. Research activities almost always require more time to accomplish than one thinks.

A related consideration is the timing of the project. Some of the research steps are more readily performed at certain times of the day, week, or year than at other times. This consideration is particularly relevant for the data collection task. For example, if the problem focused on patients with peptic ulcers, the research might be more easily conducted in the fall and spring because of the increase in the number of patients with peptic ulcers during these seasons than in the summer or winter months. When the timing requirements of the tasks do not match or overlap with the time periods available for their performance, the feasibility of the project may be seriously jeopardized.

2. Availability of subjects

In any study involving human beings, the researcher needs to consider whether individuals with the desired characteristics will be available *and* willing to cooperate. Securing people's cooperation may be relatively easy, as in the case of studies conducted in classrooms. Other situations may pose more difficulties for the researcher: some people may not have the time or interest to participate in a study that has little personal relevance or benefit, and others may be suspicious of the researcher's motives or even hostile to research in general.

Fortunately people are usually willing to co-operate with a researcher if the demands upon their time and comfort are minimal. However, if the research is time-consuming, additional effort may be necessary to obtain a sufficiently large and representative sample of subjects. In research funded by a sponsor, subjects are often offered a stipend (usually $10 to $25) in compensation for the time they commit to the study, and this stipend may serve as a needed incentive.

An additional problem may be that of identifying and locating subjects with the needed characteristics. For example, suppose we were interested in studying the health care needs of individuals who had lost an intimate friend or relative through suicide. Such individuals may not present themselves for treatment — indeed, that is precisely the reason that such an investigation might be necessary. There are procedures for locating individuals with specialized attributes, but these methods are often time-consuming and expensive.

3. Cooperation of others

Often it is not sufficient to obtain the cooperation of prospective subjects alone. If the sample includes children, the mentally retarded or mentally incompetent, or senile individuals, it is almost always necessary to secure the permission of parents or guardians. In institutional settings, such as hospitals, clinics, public schools, or industrial firms, access to clients, members, personnel, or records usually requires administrative approval. Many health care facilities require that any project be presented to a panel of reviewers for approval before permitting the study to be conducted.

4. Facilities and equipment

All research projects have some resource requirements, although in some cases the needs will be quite modest. It is prudent to consider what facilities and equipment will be needed,

and whether or not they will be available, before embarking on a project in order to prevent disappointments and frustration. Here is a partial list of considerations that fall in this category:

Will space be required and can it be obtained?

Will telephones, typewriters, or other office supplies be required?

If technical equipment and apparatus are needed, can they be secured and are they functioning properly?

Are reproducing or printing services available and are they reliable?

Will transportation needs pose any difficulties?

Will a computer be required for the analysis of the data and are computing facilities easily obtainable?

The researcher who has given some thought to the feasibility of the study in terms of these requirements usually will be rewarded for his or her efforts.

5. Money

Monetary requirements for research projects vary widely, ranging from $10 to $20 for small student projects to hundreds of thousands of dollars for large-scale, federally sponsored research. The investigator on a limited budget should think very carefully about projected expenses before the final selection of a problem is made. Some major categories of research-related expenditures include:

a. literature costs — index cards, books and journals, reproduction of articles, computerized literature search service charges.

b. personnel costs — payments to individuals hired to help with the interviewing, coding, keypunching, typing, and so forth.

c. Subject costs — payment to subjects for their cooperation.

d. supplies — paper, envelopes, typewriter ribbons, pens, and so forth.

e. equipment — laboratory apparatus, typewriters, calculators, and the like.

f. computer service charges.

g. other service charges, such as the costs of printing and duplicating materials.

h. transportation costs.

In assessing the feasibility of a study in terms of monetary considerations, researchers should ask themselves not only "Will I have enough money to complete this project?" but also "Does the anticipated cost outweigh the value of the expected findings?"

6. Experience of the researcher

The problem should be chosen from a field about which the investigator has some prior knowledge or experience. The researcher will have a difficult time in adequately preparing and designing a study on a topic that is totally new and unfamiliar. In addition to substantive knowledge of existing concepts, findings or theories, the issue of technical expertise should not be overlooked. A beginning researcher usually has limited methodological skills and should, therefore, avoid research problems that require the development of sophisticated measuring instruments or that involve complex statistical analyses.

7. Ethical considerations

A research problem may not be feasible because the investigation of the problem would pose unfair or unethical demands upon the participants. The ethical responsibilities of researchers should not be taken lightly. Persons engaged in research activities should acquaint themselves with ethical guidelines that are issued by various professional organizations and by federal agencies. An overview of major ethical considerations was presented in an earlier chapter and should be reviewed in considering the feasibility of a prospective topic. Research protocols may also need to be reviewed by the Institutional Review Board (IRB) of the institution in which the research will be conducted. The primary function of the IRB is to review procedures for protecting the rights of human subjects.

Interest to the researcher

If the tentative problem passes the tests of researchability, significance, and feasibility, there is still one more criterion for its selection, and that is the researcher's own interest in the problem. Genuine interest in and curiosity about the chosen research problem are important prerequisites to a successful study. A great deal of time and energy are expended in any scientific investigation and interest as well as enthusiasm ebb and flow throughout the time required for completion of the project. The problem selected should be of sufficient importance that the findings will extend the researcher's personal knowledge as well as the base of knowledge for others.

Beginning research students often hope that their instructors or advisors will suggest a problem for them to investigate. There is no doubt that such advice might be quite useful to those who are unfamiliar with what research involves. Nevertheless, it is often a mistake to be talked into a research topic toward which you are not personally inclined. If you do not find a problem attractive or stimulating during the beginning phases of a study — when the opportunity for creativity and intellectual reasoning is at its highest — then you are bound to regret your choice later in the project.

☐
Statement of the research problem

It is clear that a study cannot progress without the choice of a problem; it is less clear, but

Table 4-1
Examples of problem statements for nursing research

General topic	Formal problem statement
1. Early discharge	Is early discharge for hemorrhoidectomy patients related to postoperative problems?
2. Chloasma gravidarum	Are women with chloasma gravidarum more likely to have premature infants than those who do not?
3. Bladder catheterization	Is there a relationship between bladder catheterization and urinary infection in patients?
4. Decubitus ulcers	Is there a relationship between the incidence of decubitus ulcers in comatose patients and the frequency of turning?
5. Blood pressure variations	Are month-to-month blood pressure variations predictive of cerebral vascular accidents in the elderly?
6. Effects of visitors	Do hospitalized patients who have daily visitors express fewer somatic complaints than patients without daily visitors?
7. Attitudes toward the mentally ill	Are nurses' attitudes toward the mentally ill related to the nurses' length of experience in working with them?
8. Nursing diagnoses	Do nursing diagnoses for surgical patients differ from those for medical patients?
9. Malpractice risks	How aware are nurses of their liabilities with respect to malpractice?
10. Children's hospital adjustment	Do children who are instructed about pain manifest better adjustment to hospitalization than those who are not?

nonetheless true, that the problem should be carefully and concisely stated in written form before proceeding with the design of the study. Putting one's ideas in writing is often sufficient to illuminate ambiguities and uncertainties.

A good statement of the problem should serve as a guide to the researcher in the course of designing the study. The statement should normally identify the key variables in the study, specify the nature of the population being studied, and suggest the possibility of empirical testing.

Form of the statement

Researchers differ in their opinions concerning the form the problem statement should take. The two basic alternatives are declarative and interrogative. The following example illustrates these two options:

Declarative: The purpose of this research is to investigate the relationship between the dependency level of renal transplant patients and their rate of recovery.

Interrogative: What is the relationship between the dependency level of renal transplant patients and their rate of recovery?

The question form has the advantage of simplicity and directness. Questions invite an answer, and help psychologically to focus the researcher's attention on the kinds of data that would have to be collected in order to provide that answer. We, therefore, recommend the interrogative form for the statement of the problem.

In order to familiarize the reader with researchable problem areas and appropriate forms for the problem statement, a number of examples are presented in Table 4-1. The left column of this table gives examples of the original topics, while the right-hand column presents the more formal statements of the problem. In real-life situations, the transition from the broad topic to the final statement usually requires many intermediary attempts.

Defining terms in a problem statement

The problem statements in Table 4-1 would be incomplete without an accompanying set of definitions of the variables involved. Sometimes the definition and clarification of concepts can be inserted in the statement of the problem itself, but it is likely that this practice would make the statement inordinately complex and clumsy.

Without further clarification, many of the concepts in Table 4-1 are inadequate for precise and unambiguous communication. For instance, what exactly does the researcher mean by "early discharge" in the first example? Dictionary definitions of terms and concepts are almost always inadequate for research purposes. The definition provided by the researcher must imply or specify a method of operationalizing (observing and measuring) the variables. To pursue the same example, "early discharge" might be defined as "discharged on the first postoperative day"; "postdischarge problem" might be defined, in part, as "the patient's inability to have a bowel movement within three postoperative days." If adequate definitions are appended to a well-formulated problem statement, there should be little confusion as to what is being studied.

□
Research example

Research reports, unfortunately, do not always identify the problem under investigation in a concise, articulate fashion. When the study problem is formally stated in a manner such as suggested above, the reader is in a good posi-tion to judge the adequacy of the research methods.

Chang and her colleagues (1984) tested preferences for types of nursing care among elderly ambulatory women by showing simulated patient/nurse encounters on videotape to a sample of women at senior citizen nutrition sites. Three aspects of nursing care (medical-technical care; psychosocial aspects of care; and patient involvement through self-care) were systematically varied in the videotaped presentations. The research report carefully delineated the problem statements and the definition of terms used in this investigation. One of the three research questions was as follows: "What are the effects of different levels (high and low) of three components of care (technical quality, psychosocial, patient participation) on patients' global satisfaction?" The investigators increased the precision of their problem by presenting clear definitions of terms. For example, patients' global satisfaction "was measured by adaptations of Section III of the Patient Satisfaction Questionnaire (PSQ)." (p. 371). Seven items designed to capture the subject's satisfaction with the nursing care depicted on the videotape were used to measure the dependent variable.

The care that a researcher takes in carefully and methodically stating a problem and defining the concepts is often a good index of the thoroughness of the overall design and conceptualization. It is extremely difficult to evaluate the methods used to collect research data if one does not have a clear picture of what the study was attempting to accomplish in the first place.

□
Summary

The selection of a problem in a scientific investigation frequently is an arduous task, particularly for novice researchers. The most common sources of ideas for research questions are experience, relevant literature, and theory. Nurses, nursing students, nurse educators, and nurse administrators are likely to have an abundance of experiences in their daily activities that are puzzling, problematic, or provoke curiosity. Any situation that is poorly understood or any condition that gives you cause to wonder if a better method could be devised represents a potential research topic. Readings in areas of interest constitute a second method of generating ideas for a scientific study. Finally, theories and conceptual frameworks often serve as a springboard for empirical studies: the utility and viability of any theory ultimately depend upon its ability to withstand tests in real-life situations.

The process of developing a research problem is not a smooth and direct one. The researcher usually starts with the identification of several topics of broad interest. The researcher should be open-minded about the possibilities that are developed at this early phase because a hasty evaluation may result in the rejection of several potentially valuable ideas. After a topic has been tentatively selected, the researcher must begin the task of successively narrowing the scope of the problem. This task begins by posing a series of questions linked to the topic of interest.

A number of criteria should be considered in making the final selection of the problem. First, the problem should be a significant one. That is, the research question should contribute to nursing practice or nursing theory in a meaningful way. Second, the problem should be researchable. Questions of a moral or ethical nature are inappropriate, and concepts that defy precise definition and measurement should usually be avoided. Third, a problem may have to be abandoned if the investigation is not feasible. Feasibility involves the issues of timing, availability of subjects, cooperation of other individuals, availability of facilities and equipment, monetary requirements, experience and competencies of the researcher,

and ethical considerations. Finally, the research question should be one that is of interest to the researcher.

The selected problem should be stated formally (in writing) before proceeding to the design of the study. A good statement of the problem will serve as a guide throughout the study. The problem may be stated in either declarative or interrogative form; the latter is preferred because it is more simple and concise and because it leads more directly to a solution. The statement of the problem should identify the major variables under consideration, specify the characteristics of the population being studied, and suggest the possibility of empirical testing. The problem statement should be accompanied by a set of clear definitions of the concepts involved in order to facilitate communication of the research ideas and to help bridge the gap between abstract phenomena and measurable variables.

☐
Study suggestions

1. Think of a frustrating experience you have had as a student nurse or as a practicing nurse. Identify the problem area. Ask yourself a series of questions until you have one that you feel is researchable. Evaluate the problem in terms of the criteria of a researchable problem discussed in this chapter.

2. Examine the following five problem statements. Are they researchable problems as stated? Why or why not? If a problem statement is not researchable, modify it in such a way that the problem could be studied scientifically.
   a. What are the factors affecting the attrition rate of nursing students?
   b. What is the relationship between humidity and heart rate in humans?
   c. Should nurses be responsible for inserting nasogastric tubes?
   d. How effective are walk-in clinics?

e. What is the best approach for conducting patient interviews?

3. Identify a researchable problem from one of the conceptual frameworks or theories of nursing. Of what relevance is the problem to scientific nursing knowledge?

4. Examine one issue of the journal *Nursing Research*. Find an article that does not present a formal, well-articulated problem statement. Write a problem statement for that study in both declarative and interrogative form.

5. Below are three general topics that could be investigated. Develop at least one problem statement for each. Assess the adequacy of the problems in terms of their researchability and feasibility.
   a. nurse-patient interaction
   b. sleep disturbances
   c. preoperative anxiety

□
Suggested readings

Methodological references

Abdellah, F.G. & Levine, E. (1978). *Better patient care through nursing research* (2nd ed.). New York: Macmillan. (Chapter 5).

Adebo, E.O. (1974). Identifying problems for nursing research. *International Nursing Review, 21,* 53–54, 59.

American Nurses' Association Congress for Practice (1973). *Standards for Practice.* Kansas City: American Nurses' Association.

Beckingham, A.C. (1974). Identifying problems for nursing research. *International Nursing Review, 21,* 49–52.

Fox, D.J. (1982). *Fundamentals of research in nursing* (4th ed.). New York: Appleton-Century-Crofts (Chapter 3).

Kerlinger, F.N. (1973). *Foundations of behavioral research* (2nd ed.). New York: Holt, Rinehart and Winston. (Chapter 2).

Levine, M.E. (1973). *Introduction to clinical nursing* (2nd ed). Philadelphia: F.A. Davis Co.

Selltiz, C., Wrightsman, L.S., & Cook, S.W. (1976).

Research methods in social relations (3rd ed.). New York: Holt, Rinehart and Winston.

Sweeney, M.A. & Olivieri, P. (1981). *An introduction to nursing research.* Philadelphia: J.B. Lippincott. (Chapter 1).

Treece, E.W. & Treece, J.W., Jr. (1982). *Elements of research in nursing* (2nd ed.). St. Louis: C.V. Mosby. (Chapter 7).

Wilson, H.S. (1985). *Research in Nursing.* Menlo Park, CA: Addison-Wesley. (Chapter 5).

Substantive References*

Anderson C.J. (1981). Enhancing reciprocity between mother and neonate. *Nursing Research, 30,* 89–93.

Baun, M.M. *et al.* (1984). Physiological effects of human/companion animal bonding. *Nursing Research, 33,* 126–129.

Brandt, P.A. (1984). Stress-buffering effects of social support on maternal discipline. *Nursing Research, 33,* 229–234.

Chang, B.L. *et al.* (1984). The effect of systematically varying components of nursing care on satisfaction in elderly ambulatory women. *Western Journal of Nursing Research, 6,* 367–379.

Killeen, M.L. (1985). Taking risks with health. *Western Journal of Nursing Research, 7,* 116–124.

McKeever, P. & Galloway, S.C. (1984). Effects of nongynecological surgery on the menstrual cycle. *Nursing Research, 33,* 42–46.

Mitchell, J.R. (1980). Male adolescents' concern about a physical examination conducted by a female. *Nursing Research, 29,* 165–169.

O'Rourke, M.W. (1983). Subjective appraisal of psychological well-being and self-reports of menstrual and nonmenstrual symptomatology in employed women. *Nursing Research, 32,* 288–292.

Uphold, C.R. & Susman, E.J. (1985). Childrearing, marital, recreational, work role integration and climacteric symptoms in midlife women. *Research in Nursing and Health, 8,* 73–81.

Walker, L.O., Crain, H., and Thompson, E. (1986). Maternal role attainment and identity in the postpartum period. *Nursing Research, 35,* 68–71.

Wineman, N.M. (1980). Obesity: Locus of control, body image, weight loss, and age-at-onset. *Nursing Research, 29,* 231–237.

* The references cited were chosen because they include a clearly labeled problem statement.

Chapter 5
☐
*Locating
and summarizing
existing
information
on a problem*

A review of related research and theory on a topic has become a standard and virtually essential activity of scientific research projects. A literature review involves the systematic identification, location, scrutiny, and summary of written materials that contain information on a research problem. The beginning researcher is undoubtedly familiar with locating library documents and organizing them. However, inasmuch as a review of research literature differs in a number of respects from other kinds of term papers or summaries that students are often called upon to prepare, a separate chapter is devoted to this topic.

This chapter covers several related areas: first, the functions that a literature review can play in a research project; second, the kinds of materials covered in a literature review; third, suggestions concerning where to find appropriate references and how to record the information once it is located; and finally, the organization and summary of a written literature review.

☐
Purposes of a literature review

Usually beginning researchers are required by their instructors to read materials related to their research topic before actually conducting a study. The fact that a literature review is a standard requirement may obscure the purposes and importance of this task. By examining some specific functions of a literature review, we hope to shed some light on its potential value.

Source for research ideas

Familiarizing oneself with practical or theoretical issues relating to a problem area often helps the researcher to generate ideas or focus on a research topic. A review of the literature may, in some cases, precede the identification of a topic. Readings in areas of general interest to the researcher can be extremely useful in alerting him or her to unresolved research problems or to new applications suitable for a project. When a general topic has already been selected, readings on that topic help to bring the problem into sharper focus and aid in the formulation of appropriate research questions.

Orientation to what is already known

One of the major functions of the literature review is to ascertain what is already known in relation to the problem of interest. Acquaintance with the current state of knowledge should enable the researcher to avoid unintentional duplication of effort and may, thus, lead to aspects of the problem about which there is relatively little knowledge. Of course, there are situations in which a deliberate decision to *replicate* a study is made but, here too, the researcher needs to be thoroughly familiar with existing research in order to make that type of decision.

A search of related research is also useful in identifying truths or assumptions about certain aspects of the phenomena being studied. An *assumption* is a proposition or statement whose truth is either considered self-evident or has been satisfactorily (at least tentatively) established by earlier research. Research studies necessarily build upon a series of assumptions. Without a foundation of accepted knowledge and theory, little scientific progress would be possible. However, the beginning researcher needs to be extremely careful not to assume that a fact is proven or established simply because one researcher or author reported it.

Provision of a conceptual context

Reviewing the literature is important in broadening the understandings and insights necessary for the development of a broad conceptual context into which a problem fits. It is only within such a context that the findings of a project can make a contribution to a body of knowledge. The more one's study is linked with other research, the more of a contribution it is likely to make. The accumulation of scientific knowledge is very much analogous to the fitting together of a jigsaw puzzle. Your piece of the puzzle, small though it may be, may help to join together other parts of the puzzle.

The review also serves the essential function of providing the individual researcher with a perspective on the problem in terms of interpreting the results of his or her study. The comparison of the results of a study with earlier findings is often a good point of departure for suggesting new research to either resolve conflicts or extend the base of knowledge. Finally, a written review included in a research report is useful to the nursing community in that it makes explicit to readers the context within which the study was conducted.

Information on research approach

A very important role of the literature review, particularly for students engaged in their first research project, is to suggest ways of going about the business of conducting a study on a topic of interest. In other words, the review can be useful in pointing out the research strategies and specific procedures, measuring instruments, and statistical analyses that might be productive in pursuing one's problem. Research reports differ considerably in the amount of detail they include concerning specific procedures, but it is not unusual for a report to provide complete documentation for the investigator's methods, including the measuring instruments used. When the actual instrument is not published with the report, it is almost always possible to obtain a copy by writing to the author.

□
Scope of a literature review

The previous section demonstrated that a literature review is a multifaceted task that serves a variety of purposes. In this section the type of information that should be sought in conducting the review of the literature is examined, and other issues relating to the breadth and depth of the review are considered.

Types of information to seek

Written materials vary considerably in their quality, their intended audience, and the kind of information they contain. The researcher performing a review of the literature ordinarily comes in contact with a wide range of materials and, thus, has to be selective in deciding what to examine or include. How are such decisions to be made? There is, unfortunately, no easy answer to this question, but we can offer a number of suggestions that might prove useful.

The first step in selecting appropriate materials is to make sure that you have been thorough in tracking down all (or most) of the relevant references. It is irksome (and embarrassing) to learn of good references *after* the completion of a study. The next main section of this chapter addresses the issues of locating good source materials.

The type of information included in academic or other nonfictional documents can be classified roughly into five categories: (1) facts, statistics, or findings; (2) theory or interpretation; (3) methods and procedures; (4) opinions, beliefs, or points of view; and (5) anecdotes, clinical impressions, or narrations of incidents and situations. Table 5-1 summarizes the functions that each type of information normally serves in a literature review. A brief description of the utility of the various kinds of information follows.

1. *Research Findings.* This category of information represents the results of other research efforts and documents the progress on a specific topic or problem. This first category of materials clearly constitutes one of the most important types of information for a research review. As Table 5-1 indicates, published studies can suggest topics to be investigated, and can help in the development of the conceptualization and design of new research. Normally, research findings are available in a variety of sources including textbooks, encyclopedias, reports, conference proceedings, publications, and, especially, scholarly journals such as *Nursing Research.* Depending on the topic, it is usually useful to review research findings in the nursing literature, as well as in the literature of related disciplines, such as sociology, psychology, medicine, or physiology.

2. *Theory.* The second type of information deals with broader, more conceptual issues of relevance to the topic of interest. Descriptions of theory are useful in providing a conceptual context for a research problem, but may also be useful for suggesting a research topic. Sometimes discussions of a body of theory are briefly presented in research reports and

Table 5-1
Summary of the uses of various types of information

Type of information	Review function			
	Source of Research Ideas	*Information on What Is Known*	*Conceptual Context*	*Research Approach*
Research findings	✓	✓	✓	✓
Theoretical explications	✓		✓	
Methodology				✓
Opinions	✓			
Clinical anecdotes	✓			

journal articles, but they are more likely to be found in developed form in books.

3. *Methodological Information.* The third type of information that should be sought in a literature review concerns the methods of conducting a study on the topic of interest. That is, in reviewing the literature the researcher should pay attention not only to what has been found, but also *how* it was found. What approaches have other researchers used? How have they operationalized or measured their variables? How have they controlled the research situation to enhance interpretation? What statistical procedures have they used to analyze their data? Although we may have to greatly modify existing approaches and instruments, it usually is possible to find techniques that can serve as a foundation for our research activities. Articles and reports concerning similar research problems should be useful in this regard. Articles and texts on methods and statistics may be helpful. There are also several references dealing exclusively with various tests, measures, and instruments that may be useful. Several of these sources are cited in the bibliographies of the chapters in Part IV.

4. *Opinions and Viewpoints.* The general and specialty nursing literature contains numerous papers and articles that focus on an author's opinions or attitudes concerning the topic of interest. Such articles are inherently subjective, presenting the suggestions and points of view of one or more individual. Opinion articles are often an important source of ideas for studies that focus on controversial or emerging issues in nursing.

5. *Anecdotes and Clinical Descriptions.* There are numerous reports of an anecdotal nature that appear frequently in nursing, medical, and health-related literature. These articles relate the experiences and clinical impressions of the authors. For instance, Julia Malcomb (1985) described, in an article that appeared in *Nursing 85,* her experience in dealing with a difficult nursing home patient and gave advice on how to help elderly patients handle their dependency. Anecdotes or other types of nonresearch literature (such as opinion articles) may serve to broaden the researcher's understanding of the problem, particularly if the researcher is relatively unfamiliar with the underlying issues. Such sources may also illustrate a point or demonstrate

a need for rigorous research. However, these two categories have limited utility in literature reviews for research studies because of their highly subjective nature. Beginning researchers should avoid the temptation of relying very heavily on such sources in their review of the literature, particularly if they are preparing a written review. This is not to say that such materials are uninteresting or unimportant, but generally they are inappropriate in summarizing scientific knowledge and theories concerning a research question.

Depth and breadth of literature coverage

Beginning students often are troubled by the question of how limited or broad their literature review should be. Once again, there is no convenient formula giving a precise number of references to be tracked down. The extensiveness of the literature review depends on a number of factors. For written reviews, one determinant is the nature of the document being prepared. Doctoral dissertations often include a very thorough and extensive review that covers materials directly and indirectly related to the problem area. Reports in research journals, on the other hand, tend to have a much more selective bibliography covering only highly pertinent findings from other studies. Another factor to consider is the researcher's own level of knowledge and expertise. Inexperienced researchers who are relatively unfamiliar with a topic may have to cover more materials than more experienced researchers, in order to feel more comfortable and secure about their level of understanding.

Finally, the breadth of a literature review will depend quite heavily on how well-researched the topic is. If there have been 50 studies on a specific problem, it would be difficult for the researcher to come to conclusions about the current state of knowledge on a topic without reading all 50 reports. However, it is not necessarily true that the literature task is more easily accomplished if the topic has not been heavily researched. Literature reviews on new topics or little-researched problems may need to review a broad spectrum of peripherally related studies in order to develop a meaningful context.

The beginning student should strive for relevancy and quality rather than quantity in selecting references for a written review of the literature. A very common misconception is that the quality of the review is dependent upon the amount of references included. A small review covering pertinent studies and organized in a coherent fashion is of more value than a rambling presentation of questionably relevant information.

With respect to the depth of coverage in a written review, the most important criterion is, once again, that of relevancy. Research that is highly related to your problem or theory usually merits rather detailed coverage, including a description of the purpose, research approach, instruments, sample, target population, findings, and conclusions. Studies that are only indirectly related can often be summarized in a sentence or two.

☐
Sources for the literature review

The ability to identify and locate documents on a topic of interest is an important skill that is not as easily acquired as one might suspect. It is, nevertheless, a skill worth cultivating because it is clearly indispensable for a researcher or scholar to know how to access previous work on a topic. In this section some general issues concerning the mechanics of locating references are discussed, and some specific major sources commonly used by nursing researchers are presented.

Primary and secondary sources

References can be categorized as being either primary or secondary sources. While this distinction probably is familiar to most readers, it is sufficiently important to merit a comment here. A *primary source,* from the point of view of the research literature, is the description of an investigation written by the person who conducted it. For example, most of the articles appearing in the journals *Nursing Research, Advances in Nursing Science, Research in Nursing and Health,* and *Western Journal of Nursing Research* are original research reports and, therefore, are primary sources. A *secondary source* is a description of a study or studies prepared by someone other than the original researcher. Review articles, which summarize the literature on a topic, are secondary sources. When you have completed and written up a review of the literature on a topic, your presentation will be considered a secondary reference. If you go on to collect new data on the same topic, however, your description of the hypotheses, methods, and results of the study will be a primary reference.

Both primary and secondary sources play important roles in the literature review task, but they play different roles. Secondary sources are useful in providing bibliographical information on relevant primary sources. However, secondary descriptions of studies should not be considered substitutes for the primary sources. Secondary sources typically fail to provide sufficient detail about research studies. An even more serious limitation of secondary sources is the fact that it is rarely possible to achieve complete objectivity in summarizing and reviewing written materials. We must accept our own values and biases as one filter through which information passes (although we should certainly make every effort to control such biases). However, we should not have to accept as a second filter the

biases of the person who prepared a secondary summary of research studies. The literature review task should utilize primary sources whenever possible.

Bibliographical aids for nursing research problems

The number of individual books, journals, and reports that could be consulted in compiling information on a nursing research topic is overwhelming. Fortunately, there are various indexes, abstracting services, and other retrieval mechanisms that facilitate the process of locating pertinent references. Several major sources that can be consulted in performing the review of the literature are identified here. However, these materials by no means exhaust the possibilities. Librarians are a particularly valuable resource inasmuch as they are knowledgeable about the literature, literature retrieval tools, and services in their own and other libraries.

Table 5-2 is presented to aid in the selection of an appropriate literature retrieval index for locating references from books, periodicals, government documents, and abstracts. This table also indicates whether the source can be searched by computer. The chart is not meant to imply that these are the only sources but, rather, its intent is to aid the beginning researcher who is initiating a literature search. Two additional aids that serve as detailed guides to the nursing literature are *Lippincott's Guide to Nursing Literature: A Handbook for Students, Writers and Researchers* (Binger and Jensen, 1980) and *Guide to Library Resources for Nursing* (Strauch and Brundage, 1980).

Indexes
Health science indexes are the key to the vast health science literature. It is a wise practice in using any index to begin the search for rele-

(Text continues on p. 70)

Table 5-2
A quick guide to selected abstracts and indexes for nursing and related subjects

TITLE	Type of Index		Frequency	Date coverage	Subject Coverage				Type of Materials Covered										Can be Searched by Computer	
	Abstract	Index			Medicine	Nursing	Hospital	Other	Books	Studies	Technical report	Periodical	ANA NLN Publ	Gov't Publ	Pamphlet	Dissertation	Book review	AV	Data Base Name	Date
Books																				
Card catalog of the library		●			●	●	●		●				X	X	X	X		X		
National Library of Medicine Current Catalog @ Catalog—		●	Qa	1880	●	●	●	H	●	●	●	●							CATLINE	1801+
Sophia F. Palmer Memorial Library, AJN Co		●	2 vol	1922–1973	●	●	●		●				●							
Medical Books in Print		●	A	1986	●	●	●		●										Books in Print	Current
Periodicals																				
Annual or cumulative indexes to individual periodical titles (e.g., AJN, Public Health Nursing)		●				●						●								
INI (International Nursing Index)		●	Qa	1966	●	●						●	X	X	X				MEDLINE	1966+
CINAHL (Cumulative Index to Nursing and Allied Health Literature) @		●	B–Ma	1956		●			○			●	○	○	○	○	X		CINAHL	1983+
Nursing Studies Index (V. Henderson)		●	4 vol	1900–1959	●	●			●	●		●								
Index Medicus/Cumulated Index Medicus @		●	Ma	1927+	●	⊕	⊕		○		○	●	⊕	○	○	⊕			MEDLINE	1966+
Hospital Literature Index/ Cumulative Index of Hospital Literature		●	Qa	1945		⊕	●	H	○			●	⊕	⊕					HEALTH	1975+
History of Nursing. Index to Adelaide Nutting, Teachers' College, Columbia U. Collection.		●	1 vol			●			○			●								
Bibliography of Bioethics		●	A	1973/75+		●	⊕	M e	●●	⊕⊕	⊕	⊕ ●	⊕ X	⊕	⊕⊕				BIOETHICS	1973+

Table of nursing and health-related indexes and abstracts

Title	Frequency	Coverage	Online database	Online dates
Bibliography of the History of Medicine	Aa	1965+	HISTLINE	1970+
Gov't.				
NTIS—SRIM INDEX to HEALTH PLANNING	Qa	1978+	NTIS	1964+
MEDOC	Qa	1968+	MEDOC	1976–9
Monthly Catalog—U.S. Government Publications	Msa	1895+	Monthly Catalog	1976+
Abstracts				
Annual Review of Nursing Research	A	1983+		
Nursing Abstracts	B-Ma	1979+		
Abstracts of Reports of Studies in Nursing (in each issue of Nursing Research)				
Abstracts of Studies in Public Health Nursing (in Nursing Research 8 45115, Spring, 1957)	B-M	1960–1978 / 1924–1957		
Nursing Research Abstracts (England)	Qa	1979+		
Abstracts of Health Care Management Studies @	Qa	1965+	PARADEX (offline)	
ERIC (Educational Resources Information Center)	Qa	1966+	ERIC	1966+
Psychological Abstracts	Msaa	1927+	Psyc INFO	1967+
Dissertation Abstracts International @	Ma	1938+	DISS ABS	1861+
Excerpta Medica	Msa	1947+	EXCERPTA MEDICA	1974+

Key
@ — title varies
● — primary focus
⊕ — some coverage included
O — included in special appendices, etc.
X — may be included

Frequency
A — annual
M — monthly
B-M — bi-monthly
Q — quarterly
a — with annual or multiyear cumulation
sa — with semiannual cumulation

Subject Coverage
e — ethics
E — education
H — health
M — multidiscipline
P — psychology/psychological aspects
SC — science
SO — social science
SP — special subject

Some titles listed in this chart under periodical indexes also include books and other materials. This table is printed with the permission of its author, ML Pekarski, Coordinator, Special Projects, O'Neill Library (which contains Nursing collection) Boston College, Chestnut Hill, MA 02167.

vant references with the most recent issue of the index and proceed backward. Several indexes particularly useful to nurse researchers are the *International Nursing Index, Index Medicus, Nursing Research Index, Nursing Studies Index,* and *Current Index to Journals in Education.* Additional sources of information may be found in "References Sources for Nursing," prepared by a committee of the Interagency Council on Library Resources for Nursing and published in *Nursing Outlook* every two years.

1. The *International Nursing Index* is one of the major sources for locating references from both nursing and non-nursing journals. Articles from over 200 nursing journals as well as nursing articles appearing in more than 2600 non-nursing journals are listed alphabetically by subject heading and author. Foreign journal articles appear at the end of each subject heading and are enclosed in brackets.

Although the *International Nursing Index* is primarily a periodical index, it also lists in special appendices publications of professional organizations and agencies, nursing books published during the year, and doctoral dissertations by nurses. It is published quarterly with an annual cumulative index and covers articles beginning with 1966 to the present.

The procedure for locating references through an index is described in the preliminary pages of each volume. Because the procedures tend to be similar, only those for accessing information in the *International Nursing Index* will be described here. The *International Nursing Index* begins with a thesaurus, which lists commonly used terms, not all of which are actual subject headings. The thesaurus directs the reader to the actual subject heading, by means of a "see" reference, if the term is not one used. An example may help to clarify this characteristic of the thesaurus. Suppose you are looking for references on "nursing care plans." This phrase, although

common in nursing, is not one of the subject headings. "Nursing care plans" would be listed and followed by a "see" reference directing you to look under the subject heading of "Patient Care Planning."

In addition to "see" references, the thesaurus also suggests, at times, other subject headings that are pertinent to your particular topic. It does this by means of a "see also" reference. Sometimes both "see" and "see also" references appear for a particular term.

The researcher proceeds to the subject section of the index following use of the thesaurus. The subject heading lists the actual references. Each reference contains the following information: title of article, author, journal, volume number, issue number, page numbers, and date of issue. A recent reference found under "Patient Care Planning" is:

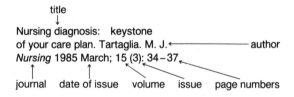

If the researcher is seeking articles published by a particular author, the procedure would be to go directly to the author section of the index. Each researcher must decide whether the references cited might be pertinent to the topic under study. Once references are identified, the particular journal is obtained and the article read.

2. CINAHL, the Cumulative Index to Nursing and Allied Health Literature is published bimonthly with an annual cumulation. It indexes over 300 nursing, allied health and health-related journals published in English and also the publications of the American Nurses' Association and the National League for Nursing. It includes pertinent articles from the 2600 biomedical journals indexed in *Index Medicus* and relevant material from popular journals. CINAHL started publication

in 1956, before the International Nursing Index, and is the only index to the nursing journals from 1960 to 1965. Articles not available through local sources or the Regional Medical Library and its area libraries may be obtained for a fee from the CINAHL or American Journal of Nursing Libraries.

3. The *Nursing Studies Index* is a four-volume index prepared by Virginia Henderson and others. It is an annotated guide to reported studies, research methods, and historical and biographical materials in periodicals, books, and pamphlets published in English. The *Nursing Studies Index* constitutes the only means of access to nursing literature for the 1900 to 1959 period. Originally published by J.B. Lippincott, this index is now available in reprint format from Garland Publishing.

4. The *Index Medicus* is one of the most well-known biomedical indexes. Over 2000 worldwide biomedical journals are indexed. A small number of nursing journals are also indexed. It is published monthly and cumulated annually. Foreign language articles appear at the end of a subject and are enclosed in brackets. An additional feature included as a separate entity in both the monthly and annual cumulated volumes is the *Bibliography of Medical Reviews,* an index to the latest review articles that have appeared in biomedical journals.

5. The *Nursing Research Index* appears annually in the last issue of *Nursing Research.* It contains alphabetical listings of research studies by subject heading and author. The index is more selective than the *International Nursing Index* because only research investigations having pertinence to nursing are listed. Because its focus is solely on research, it has been singled out from other journals such as the *American Journal of Nursing* and *Nursing Outlook,* which also have annual cumulated indexes.

6. Educational Resources Information Center (ERIC) was established in 1964 by the U.S. Office of Education and is of invaluable assistance to the researcher concerned with educational issues. Access to ERIC is by *The Thesaurus of ERIC Descriptors* found in most libraries. The *Current Index to Journals in Education* is a monthly publication produced by ERIC. The index references articles, by subject and author, from more than 500 educational journals. Another publication of ERIC is the monthly *Research in Education,* which abstracts reports of research projects funded by the U.S. Office of Education. These abstracts are indexed by subject and author.

Abstracts

Abstract journals summarize articles that have appeared in other journals. Abstracting services are generaly more useful than indexes in that they provide a summary (abstract) of a study rather than just a title. The title of an article often is not fully indicative of its contents. Having an abstract helps in deciding whether a particular reference is worth pursuing.

1. Each issue of *Nursing Research* for the 1960 to 1978 period contained abstracts of research studies having relevance to nursing. The articles are classified alphabetically by author under alphabetical subject headings. The subject headings are listed at the beginning of the abstract section. The journals from which articles are abstracted are listed in the September–October issue each year. Sometimes only the title of a particular article is given, and the reader is referred to the journal in which the original article appears. There is an author–subject guide to these abstracts in the annual index.

2. Abstracts of books and journal articles in the field of psychology and other behavioral and social sciences appear in *Psychological Abstracts.* Articles from selected nursing journals, such as *Nursing Research,* which are psychologically oriented are abstracted. To use this tool, the researcher first employs the cu-

mulative index and looks up the appropriate subject heading. Under each subject heading are listed, in alphabetical order, the titles of research reports pertaining to the subject area of interest and an abstract number. The abstract number can then be located in the abstract section of this work.

Computer searches

As an alternative to searching indexes or abstracts manually, computerized literature searches have become increasingly popular. A computer search provides the researcher with a list of references with complete bibliographic information and, in many cases, abstracts as well. References to new literature may be available by way of the computer up to 1 month before their appearance in the printed index or abstract. In addition, computer searches may save some of the researcher's time and energy, thereby providing more time for reading the original publications.

No knowledge of computers is necessary for requesting a computer literature search. The researcher typically fills out a request form indicating the topic of interest and any limitations on the search, such as dates of publication. If the researcher has done some manual searching of the literature, subject headings found to be useful can be indicated. The librarian confers with the researcher, devises the best search strategy, and then performs the actual search.

Most computer searches are able to produce an immediate search, generating references at the same time the request is received. This is called an *on-line search*. Generally, if more than a small number of citations is obtained, the bulk of them will be printed *off-line* because this process is less expensive. The off-line print is sent by mail and usually arrives three to five days after the computer search is conducted. The cost of a computer search varies depending upon the type of search (the

extensiveness of the bibliography requested) and the data base used in the search.

Table 5-2 includes a selected listing of data bases available for computer literature searches relevant for nursing. MEDLINE is the data base most commonly used by nurse researchers. MEDLINE centers are located at the libraries of major research centers, medical schools, nursing schools, and hospitals. It covers all areas of biomedical literature and corresponds to *Index Medicus* with added coverage of nursing, hospital, and dental literature. All journals currently indexed in the *International Nursing Index* are included in MEDLINE. Several subfiles relating to specific subject areas or types of materials are also included. For example, CANCERLINE contains literature on all aspects of cancer.

The Combined Health Information Database (CHID) is a combination of files of books, periodicals, and other materials from various clearinghouses on arthritis, diabetes, health, digestive diseases, and high blood pressure.

The *PSYCHOLOGICAL ABSTRACTS* data base provides worldwide coverage of the literature of psychology and other behavioral sciences, including journals monographs, dissertations, and some technical reports and treatises. The *SOCABS* data base, corresponding to *Sociological Abstracts,* provides international coverage of sociological references.

ERIC is another data base that may be of great help to the nurse researcher. It contains the complete file of educational materials from the U.S. Office of Education and corresponds to the publications, *Current Index to Journals in Education* and *Research in Education.* Additional related data bases of potential interest are *AIM/ARM* for vocational and technical educational material and *Exceptional Child Abstracts* for information on the education of handicapped and gifted children.

SOCIAL SCISEARCH and SCISEARCH are data bases that correspond to the printed *So-*

cial Science Citation Index and the *Science Citation Index*, respectively. These data bases may be useful to nurse researchers in obtaining references in scientific and social scientific disciplines.

Finally, the NTIS data base covers all publications contained in the weekly *Government Reports Announcements*. This service covers technical reports released by over 240 government and other agencies and encompasses completed research in a wide range of disciplines, including nursing and health planning.

Although the traditional data base search systems generally require the services of a librarian, a new and intensifying trend is *end user* searching. End-user systems are designed to allow researchers without computer expertise to conduct their own computer search in the library or in other locations with a personal computer or terminal without the assistance of a search specialist. Selected examples of end-user systems include BRS AFTER DARK, BRS COLLEAGUE, BRS BRKTHRU, and DIALOG KNOWLEDGE.

Books

Books should not be overlooked by the researcher conducting a literature search. Although periodicals contain more up-to-date information than books, books do provide more extensive coverage of a particular topic by treating more than one facet or aspect of the isue in depth. Books are a particularly valuable resource for locating discussions of theoretical issues. Books are also useful in that they usually contain numerous references to other sources of information.

Bibliographies

Bibliographies are compilations of references found in books, periodicals, and reports on some particular topic. Annotated bibliographies provide comments concerning the purposes or findings of the references and, sometimes, concerning their quality. Examples of bibliographies include *Bibliography on Bioethics, Bibliography on Suicide and Suicide Prevention, International Bibliography of Studies on Alcoholism, Selected Bibliography on Death and Dying,* and *A Classified Bibliography of Gerontology and Geriatrics.*

□
Preparing and writing the literature review

The task of identifying and locating relevant references is just the first step in performing a literature review. The next step is to peruse, summarize, and classify the references in such a way that the information required will be preserved in accessible form. This section provides some advice on taking notes and preparing a written review.

Abstracting and recording notes

Not all of the references obtained through the various abstracts, indexes, or computerized literature searches will prove to be valuable. Titles of papers and reports are very often misleading, and their content may be disappointing. Thus, it usually is useful to first examine the abstract or summary of a report in order to determine its potential value. An *abstract* of a paper is a brief (usually 100 to 200 words) synopsis appearing at the beginning of a report; a *summary* presents the highlights of the findings of a study and is placed at the end.

Once the document is considered relevant, the entire report should be read critically, identifying material that is sufficiently important to warrant note-taking as well as observing flaws or gaps in the report. (Chapter 26 presents some tips on evaluating research papers.) Notes should be made on index cards and should synthesize the contents of the reference. If the reference is a research report, the following kinds of information should usually be recorded: the problem statement or hypotheses, the theoretical framework, the procedures and methodology, and the results and conclusions. It is a good idea to note any of the researcher's own criticisms or comments while the article is being read. If the article is not a research report but is a discussion of theory or opinion, the main points of the author's arguments should be abstracted and recorded together with collaborating or supporting evidence.

Organizing the review

If the end product of your literature search is to be a written review, a critical task is the organization of the gathered information. Most writers find it helpful to work from an outline. If the review is lengthy, it will be useful to write out the outline on paper. For shorter reviews, a mental outline might be sufficient. The important point is to sit back for a minute before starting to write and work out a structure so that the presentation has a meaningful and understandable organization. Lack of organization is perhaps the most common weakness of students' first attempts at reviewing the literature. Once the main topics and their order of presentation have been identified, a review of the notes is in order. This will not only help recall materials read earlier, but will also lay the groundwork for decisions about where a particular reference fits in terms of the outline. If certain references do not seem to fit anywhere, the outline may need to be revised or the references discarded. It is best not to try to "force" a reference into the review if it does not make a contribution. The number of references used in the review is much less important than the relevance of the reference, the quality of the summary, and the overall organization.

Content of the review

A review of the literature should be neither a series of quotes nor a series of abstracts. The central task is to organize and summarize the references so as to lay a systematic foundation for new research. The review should point out both consistencies and contradictions in the literature as well as offer possible explanations for the inconsistencies in terms of, say, different conceptualizations or methods.

Studies that are particularly relevant should be described in detail. However, reports that result in comparable findings can usually be grouped together and briefly summarized, as in the following fictitious example: "A number of studies have found that the incidence of phlebitis is directly related to the method of administering intravenous infusions and to certain parameters of materials used in the infusions (Moody and Tate, 1986; Kendrick, 1985)."

It is important to paraphrase, or summarize, a report in one's own words. The review should demonstrate that thoughtful consideration has been given to the materials. Stringing together quotes from various documents fails to show that previous research and thought on the topic have been assimilated and understood.

Another point to bear in mind is that the review should be as objective as possible. Studies that conflict with personal values should not be omitted. It is not unusual to find studies with contradictory results. The review should not deliberately ignore a study simply because its findings contradict other studies. Analyze inconsistent results and evaluate the supporting evidence as objectively as possible.

The literature review should conclude with a summary or overview of the "state of the art" of the problem under consideration. The summary should point out not only what has been studied and how adequate the investigations have been, but should also make note of any gaps or areas of research inactivity. In other words, the summary requires some critical judgment concerning the extensiveness and dependability of information on a topic. If the

Table 5-3
Examples of stylistic difficulties for research reviews

Inappropriate Style or Wording	Recommended Change
1. It is known that unmet expectations engender anxiety.	1. A number of commentators have asserted that unmet expectations engender anxiety (Thompson, 1984; Bradford, 1986)*
2. The woman who does not undertake preparation for childbirth classes tends to manifest a high degree of stress during labor.	2. Previous studies have demonstrated that women who participate in preparation for childbirth classes manifest less stress during labor than those who do not (Andrew, 1981; Chase, 1978).
3. Studies have proven that doctors and nurses do not fully understand the psychobiological dynamics of beastfeeding.	3. The studies by O'Hara (1982) and Jenkins (1985) suggest that doctors and nurses do not fully comprehend the psychobiological dynamics of breastfeeding.
4. Attitudes cannot be changed overnight.	4. Attitudes presumably are enduring attributes that cannot be changed overnight.
5. Responsibility is an intrinsic stressor.	5. Responsibility is an intrinsic stressor, according to Doctor A. Cassard, an authority on stress (Cassard, 1982).

* All references are fictitious

literature review is conducted as part of a research project, this critical summary should demonstrate the need for the new study and should clarify the context within which the hypotheses will be developed.

Style of a literature review

One of the most frequent problems for the student researcher preparing a written review for the first time is adjusting to the style of writing that is appropriate for research reviews. There is a tendency, for example, for students to accept the results of previous research as a fact or as proof that a theory is correct. This tendency is understandable; it is the style of presentation commonly used in many texts, opinion articles, and other nonresearch papers. This style may derive from a desire for clarity and unambiguity for pedantic purposes, but it is also, in part, the result of a common misunderstanding about the degree of conclusiveness that results from empirical research. *No hypothesis or theory can be definitively proved or disproved by empirical testing.* This statement may come as a surprise to most indi-

viduals who, throughout their education, have been taught to accept as givens many research findings. The fact that theories and hypotheses cannot be ultimately proved or disproved does not, of course, mean that we must disregard evidence or challenge every idea we encounter. The problem is partly a semantic one: hypotheses are not proved, they are supported by research findings; theories are not verified, but they may be tentatively accepted if there is a substantial body of evidence demonstrating their legitimacy. The researcher must learn to adopt this language of tentativeness in presenting the review of the literature.

A related stylistic problem is the inclination of beginning researchers to liberally intersperse opinions (their own or someone else's) with the findings of research investigations. The review should use statements of opinions very sparingly, if at all, and should be explicit about the source of the opinion. A description of the point of view of a knowledgeable or influential individual may be useful in establishing the need to investigate the problem or in providing a perspective on the topic, but it should occupy a relatively small section of the review. The researcher's own opinions do not belong in a review section, with the exception of an assessment of the quality of existing studies.

The left-hand column of Table 5-3 presents several examples of the kinds of stylistic difficulties we have been discussing in this section. The right-hand column offers some recommendations for rewording the sentences to conform to a more generally acceptable form for a research literature review. Many alternative phrasings are possible.

□
Example of a literature review

The following excerpt was taken from a literature review in connection with a study by Joan Austin and colleagues (1984).* In this study, reported in *Nursing Research,* the aim was to assess parental attitudes and adjustments to childhood epilepsy. Austin and her co-authors provided a context for the study with the following review:

> Research regarding parenting the school-age child with epilepsy is almost nonexistent in the nursing literature. . . . The majority of nursing articles on epilepsy focus on the different types of seizures, their treatment, and physical nursing care (Muehl, 1979; Norman & Browne, 1981; Willis & Oppenheimer, 1977). The remainder describes the psychosocial problems associated with epilepsy, including parental reactions believed to lead to emotional problems in children with epilepsy (Ozuna, 1979; Slimmer, 1979).
>
> The few research studies found in related professional literature suggest that parent-

ing may be adversely affected by childhood epilepsy. In a study of 12 families, Mulder and Suurmeijer (1977) found evidence of disruption in every family and that the parents experienced stress due to the epilepsy. In a study of 19 families, Long and Moore (1979) found that parents expected their child with epilepsy to have more emotional problems, to be more unpredictable, and to be more highly strung ($p < .05$) than a sibling without epilepsy. Ferrari, Matthews, and Barabas (1983) reported families of children with epilepsy to have less cohesion and poorer communication patterns than those families of healthy children or children with diabetes.

Only three empirical studies purported to investigate parental attitudes to epilepsy in a child. In two of the studies (Hartlage & Green, 1972; Hartlage, Green, & Offutt, 1972), the Parental Attitude Research Instrument (PARI), developed by Schaeffer and Bell (1958), was used to measure parental attitudes. Unfortunately, the PARI lacks validity because of response-set problems (Becker & Krug, 1965). Hartlage and Green (1972) did, however, find support for a positive relationship between parental attitudes and social maturity in children with epilepsy. Parental attitudes were not found to be significantly correlated with dependency in the Hartlage, Green, and Offutt study (1972), but children with epilepsy were found to be more dependent ($p < .001$) than children who had had recent tonsillectomies or cystic fibrosis.

In the third study, Bagley (1971) conducted interviews with parents of 118 children with epilepsy in order to measure parental attitudes and behavior. Bagley, however, did not use a theoretical model to measure parental attitude and subsequently conflated parental attitude and adjustment. Psychiatric social workers conducted extensive interviews with one or both parents. In-

---

* From Austin, J.K., McBride, A.B., and Davis, H.S.: Parental atitude and adjustment to childhood epilepsy. *Nursing Research,* 1984, *33,* 92–96. Copyright © 1984 by American Journal of Nursing Company. Used by permission. The reader is referred to this source for the full article and references cited in the literature review.

formation on parental attitude and behavior, including manifestation of anxiety, coping ability, evidence of depression and guilt, support of the child, family dynamics, understanding and response to the implications of epilepsy, discipline, and overprotection, were extracted from the interviews to operationalize attitude and behavior. No attempt was made to separate parental attitude from behavior. Results did show negative parental attitude and behavior to be strongly correlated with behavior disorders in children with epilepsy. . . .

In the literature there is a confluence of opinion that negative parental attitudes lead to negative parental adjustment to epilepsy. The increased incidence of emotional problems in children with epilepsy is assumed to be caused by negative parental attitude and adjustment. Available research in this area is both sparse and of limited value due to small samples, invalid measures of parental attitudes, or the failure to differentiate between attitude and adjustment. Descriptive research on parental attitude and adjustment to childhood epilepsy is needed as a first step toward better understanding parental influence on the increased incidence of emotional problems in children with epilepsy.

□

Summary

The task of reviewing literature involves the identification, selection, critical analysis, and reporting of existing information on the topic of interest. It is almost always necessary to examine previous literature on a subject before actually undertaking a research project. Such a review can play a number of important roles. First, in the start-up phase of a project, a review of work conducted in an area of general interest can help in the formulation or clarification of a research problem. Second, a study of pre-

vious work acquaints the researcher with what has been done in a field, thereby minimizing the possibility of unintentional duplication. Third, the review provides a conceptual context or framework for the reseacher and for the research community, thereby facilitating the cumulation of scientific knowledge. Fourth, the researcher may be in a better position to assess the feasibility of a proposed study by becoming familiar with related work. Finally, the review can be highly useful in providing methodological suggestions for the actual conduct of the investigation.

The kinds of information available in written documents can be categorized into five broad classes: facts, findings, or results; theory; research procedures or methods; opinions, points of view, or personal commentaries; and anecdotes or impressions of a particular event or situation. Another way of categorizing literature is in terms of its being either a primary or secondary source. A *primary source* with respect to the research literature is the original description of a study prepared by the researcher who conducted it, while a *secondary source* is a description of the study by a person not connected with the investigation. Primary sources should be consulted whenever possible in performing the literature review task.

The search for existing writings on a topic is greatly facilitated by the use of various abstracting and indexing services. Since more than a million scientific and technical articles are published in hundreds of journals, reports, and periodicals annually, it is obvious that the location of all the papers on a given topic would be impossible without such services. An important bibliographic development to emerge in recent years is the increasing availability of various computerized information retrieval systems. It is useful to search for related literature in reverse chronological order. That is, it is best to begin with the most recent studies, which incorporate the findings of earlier works and which provide references to those works.

Skillful note-taking and organization of the notes can greatly simplify the task of analyzing, summarizing, and evaluating literature on a given topic. In preparing a written review, it is important to organize materials in a logical, coherent fashion. An outline is usually useful in this regard. The review should be developed in such a way that the rationale for conducting a new study clearly emerges. The review should not be a succession of quotes or abstracts. The role of the reviewer is to point out what has been studied to date, how adequate and dependable those studies are, what gaps there are in the existing body of research, and what contribution the new study will make. The reviewer should present "facts" and "findings" in the tentative language that befits scientific inquiry and should remember to identify the source of opinions, points of view, and generalizations.

Study suggestions

1. Read Mary M. Zeimer's (1983) study entitled "Effects of information on postsurgical coping," which appeared in the September–October issue, volume 32, of *Nursing Research*. Write a summary of the problem, methods, findings, and conclusions of this study. Your summary should be capable of serving as notes for a review of the literature.

2. Suppose that you are planning to study counseling practices and programs for rape trauma victims. Make a list of several key words relating to this topic that could be used with indexes or information retrieval systems for identifying previous work.

3. Below are five sentences from literature reviews that require stylistic improvements. Rewrite these sentences to conform to considerations mentioned in the text. (Feel free to give fictitious references if desired.)

   a. Parents who abuse their children have psychopathological disturbances.
   b. Young adolescents are not prepared to cope with complex issues of sexual morality.
   c. More structured programs to use part-time nurses are needed.
   d. Intensive care nurses need so much emotional support themselves that they can provide insufficient support to patients.
   e. Most nurses have not been adequately educated to understand and cope with the reality of the dying patient.

4. Suppose you are studying factors relating to the discharge of chronic psychiatric patients. Obtain five bibliographical references for this topic. Compare your references and sources with those of other students.

Suggested readings

Methodological references

Abdellah, F.G. & Levine, E. (1978). *Better patient care through nursing research* (2nd Ed.). New York: Macmillan. (Chapter 5).

American Psychological Association (1983). *Publication manual* (3rd ed.). Washington: American Psychological Association.

Binger, J.L. & Jensen, L.M. (1980). *Lippincott's guide to nursing literature: A handbook for students, writers and researchers*. Philadelphia: J.B. Lippincott.

Cooper, H.M. (1984). The integrative research review. Beverly Hills, CA: Sage.

Fox, R.N. & Ventura, M.R. (1984). Efficiency of automated literature search mechanisms. *Nursing Research, 33,* 174–177.

Light, R.J. & Pillemer, D.B. (1984). *Summing up: The science of reviewing research.* Cambridge, MA: Harvard University Press.

Pavlovich, N. (1978). *Nursing research: A learning guide.* St. Louis: C.V. Mosby. (Chapter 2).

Selltiz, C., Wrightsman, L.S., & Cook, S.W. (1976). *Research methods in social relations.* (2nd ed.).

New York: Holt, Rinehart and Winston. (Chapter 3).

Strauch, K.P. & Brundage, D.J. (1980). *Guide to library resources for nursing.* New York: Appleton-Century-Crofts.

Taylor, S.D. (1975). Bibliography on nursing research, 1950–1974. *Nursing Research, 24,* 207–225.

Turabian, K.L. (1973). *A manual for writers of term papers, theses, and dissertations* (4th ed.). Chicago: University of Chicago Press.

Substantive references*

Austin, J.K., McBride, A.B., & Davis, H.W. (1984). Parental attitude and adjustment to childhood epilepsy. *Nursing Research, 33,* 92–96.

Choi-Lao, A.T.H. (1981). Trace anesthetic vapors in hospital operating-room environments. *Nursing Research, 30,* 156–161.

Flaskerud, J.H. (1984). A comparison of perceptions of problematic behavior by six minority groups and mental health professionals. *Nursing Research, 33,* 190–197.

Harris, R.B. (1984). Clean vs. sterile tracheotomy care and level of pulmonary infection. *Nursing Research, 33,* 80–85.

Hilbert, G.A. (1985). Spouse support and myocardial infarction patient compliance. *Nursing Research, 34,* 217–220.

Keane, A., Ducette, J., and Adler, D.C. (1985). Stress in ICU and non-ICU nurses. *Nursing Research, 34,* 231–236.

La Montagne, L.L. (1984). Children's locus of control beliefs as predictors of preoperative coping behavior. *Nursing Research, 33,* 76–79.

Newport, M.A. (1984). Conserving thermal energy and social integrity in the newborn. *Western Journal of Nursing Research, 6,* 175–188.

Schraeder, B.D. & Cooper, B.M. (1983). Development and temperament in very low birth weight infants—the second year. *Nursing Research, 32,* 331–335.

Van Bree, N., Hollerbach, A.D., & Brooks, G.P. (1984). Clinical evaluation of three techniques for administering low-dose heparin. *Nursing Research, 33,* 15–19.

Weisman, C.S., Dear, M.R., Alexander, C.S., & Chase, G.A. (1981). Employment patterns among newly hired hospital staff nurses: Comparison of nursing graduates and experienced nurses. *Nursing Research, 30,* 188–199.

Ventura, J.N. (1986). Parental coping, a replication. *Nursing Research, 35,* 77–80.

* These studies are cited because they include an explicitly labeled "Literature Review" section.

Chapter 6
□
Placing
the problem
in a theoretical
context

Scientists are fact-finders, but they cannot be content with the accumulation of isolated facts. Scientific researchers strive to integrate the findings into an orderly, coherent system. Theories constitute the mechanism by which researchers organize empirical findings into a meaningful pattern.

A theory is an abstract generalization that presents a systematic explanation about the relationships among phenomena. Theories embody principles for explaining, predicting, and controlling phenomena. Thus, theory construction and testing are intimately related to the advancement of scientific knowledge, and it may even be claimed that theory is the ultimate goal of science. Regardless of the nature of the discipline, theory serves essentially the same functions in scientific endeavors. Theoretical and conceptual systems represent the highest and most advanced efforts to understand the complexities of the world in which we live.

□
Purposes of theories

The development of theories is not an end in and of itself; theories must ultimately be of some utility. Theory plays several interrelated roles in the progress of a science. The overall purpose of theory is to make scientific findings meaningful and generalizable. Several subgoals are subsumed under this broader objective — summarization, explanation, and stimulation.

Summarization of existing knowledge

Theories allow scientists to knit together observations and facts into an orderly system.

They are efficient mechanisms for drawing together and summarizing accumulated facts from separate and isolated investigations. The linkage of findings into a coherent structure makes the body of accumulated knowledge more accessible and, thus, more useful both to practitioners who seek to implement findings and to researchers who seek to extend the knowledge base. The summarizing aspects of a theory are critical to the organization and advancement of scientific knowledge. For example, consider the theory of hypertension in renal disease. This theory states that (1) the degree of renal hypertension varies directly with the degree of sodium retention, (2) the degree of sodium retention varies with the amount of dietary sodium intake, and (3) therefore, the degree of renal hypertension varies with the amount of sodium intake. This sequence of propositions represents a summary of previous observations concerning patients with renal hypertension.

Explanation of observations and prediction and control of outcomes

Theory guides the scientist's understanding of not only the "what" of natural phenomena but also the "why" of their occurrence. The power of theories to explain lies in their specification of which variables are related to one another and the nature of that relationship.

The explanatory principles embodied in a theory provide a framework for predicting the occurrence of phenomena. Although the summarization and explanation functions are concerned with what has occurred and has been established, a theory is also expected to forecast facts and relationships that would be observed under specified circumstances. Prediction, in turn, has implications for the control of those phenomena. A theory should ideally provide the capability of bringing about desirable changes in our environment. To pursue

the example of a theory of renal hypertension, relationships are specified between the variables in the theory (degree of renal hypertension, degree of sodium retention, and amount of dietary sodium intake). The theory predicts conditions under which renal hypertension would be high. The theory also has implications for controlling renal hypertension and the degree of sodium retention.

Stimulation of new discoveries

Theories help to stimulate research and the extension of knowledge by providing both direction and impetus. On the basis of a theory, scientists draw inferences (formulate hypotheses) about what will occur in specific situations. These hypotheses are then subjected to empirical testing in research studies. The outcome of the study may lend support to the theory or may suggest the need for modification. Theories, thus, serve as a springboard for scientific advances.

To illustrate this point, consider the theory of social facilitation proposed in the 1960s by the social psychologist Robert Zajonc. The theory of social facilitation postulates that the presence of others in a performance situation facilitates well-learned responses or behavior but impairs the acquisition of new, yet-to-be learned responses. His theory integrated seemingly contradictory results from earlier research in which the presence of others was sometimes found to be debilitating to and other times enhancing of task performance. Zajonc's proposition has stimulated hundreds of investigations that have sought to refine, clarify, and extend social facilitation theory. For example, social facilitation effects have been extended to nonperformance situations. Davidson and Kelley (1973) used social facilitation theory as a basis for testing the effect of the presence of a nurse on anxiety levels in hospitalized psychiatric patients who watched a stressful film.

☐
The nature and characteristics of theory

Nursing instructors and students frequently use the term "theory" to refer to the content covered in classrooms, as opposed to the actual practice of performing nursing activities. This usage is not incorrect in that it connotes the involvement of abstraction and generalization. However, in its broader scientific meaning, the term *theory* refers to a series of propositions regarding the interrelationships among concepts, from which a large number of empirical observations can be deduced. In this section we will attempt to make this distinction clearer by describing various aspects of a scientific theory. Although we will not discuss the formal calculus and deductive logic that have been developed in connection with theoretical systems, several references at the end of this chapter are recommended for the student who wishes to pursue theory development.

Origin of theories

Theories are not discovered by scientists; they are created and invented by them. The building of a theory depends not only upon the observable facts in our environment but also on the scientist's ingenuity in pulling those facts together and making sense of them. Theory construction, in short, is a creative and intellectual enterprise that can be engaged in by anyone with sufficient imagination. But imagination alone is not an adequate qualification; theories must be congruent with the realities of the world around us and with existing knowledge.

Components of a theory

In the writings on scientific theory, one encounters a variety of terms such as "proposi-

tion," "postulate," "premise," "axiom," "law," "concept," "principle," and so forth, some of which are used interchangeably, and others of which introduce subtleties that are too complex for the beginning researcher. We, therefore, present a simplified analysis of the components of a theory, for the sake of clarity.

Theories consist, first of all, of a set of concepts. As we noted in Chapter 3, concepts are abstract characteristics of the objects that are being studied. Examples of nursing concepts are adaptation, health, self-care, nurse – client interaction, and social support. Concepts are the basic ingredients in the formulation of a theory.

Secondly, theories consist of a set of statements or propositions, each of which indicates a relationship. Relationships are denoted by such terms as "is associated with," "varies directly with," or "is contingent upon." Thirdly, the propositions must form a logically interrelated deductive system. This means that the theory must provide a mechanism for logically arriving at new statements from the original propositions.

Let us consider an example to illustrate these three points. Selye (1978) developed a theory of adaptation to stress. This theory postulates that a person's body responds to the nonspecific demands of stress by means of the General Adaptation Syndrome, which continues until adaptation occurs or death ensues. Stress may be internal or external to the individual and is manifested by the syndrome, which consists of nonspecifically induced changes occurring within the person's body. The General Adaptation Syndrome consists of three phases — the alarm phase, the phase of adaptation or resistance, and the phase of exhaustion — all of which are reversible if adjustment to stress occurs. A greatly simplified construction of Selye's theory might consist of the following propositions, which correspond to the various phases:

1. Humans seek to attain a desired state (e.g., the reduction of stress) by mobilizing the body's general defense mechanisms to overact in order to maintain life.
2. When the specific defense mechanism is identified by the body for dealing with the sources of stress (such as increased muscular activity), the overactivity of the general mechanisms subsides and the specific mechanisms overact (such as increasing the oxygen supply in muscular activity).
3. If the specific defense mechanisms are unable to cope with the stress, then the general defense mechanisms reactivate to help the body adjust, or death ensues.
4. During the alarm and exhaustion phases, there is an increase in the production of adrenocortical hormones, which subsides during the resistance phase when specific defense mechanisms come into play.

The concepts that form the basis of Selye's theory include stress, General Adaptation Syndrome, the body's general defense mechanisms and specific defense mechanisms. His theory postulates that relationships occur between stress and the body's defense mechanisms, which are activated to cope with the stress. For example, the theory claims that the level of adrenocortical hormones varies with the stage of the General Adaptation Syndrome. Selye's propositions readily lend themselves to empirical verification by providing a mechanism for deductive hypothesis generation. We might hypothesize on the basis of Selye's theory that the level of ACTH will be greater before a meal than it is after a meal or that ACTH production is less during an intravenous infusion than it is immediately prior to its inception. On the basis of his theory, we should be able to identify how well the person is coping with the stress by measuring changes in ACTH production. Several nursing studies have been based on Selye's theory of stress and adaptation. For example, Erickson and Swain (1982) studied hospitalized medical-surgical patients to determine the relationship between their adaptive potential and length of hospital stay.

Types of theories

Theories differ extensively in their level of generality. So-called grand theories or "macrotheories" purport to describe and explain large segments of the environment or of human experience. Some learning theorists, such as Clark Hull, or sociologists, such as Talcott Parsons, have developed highly general theoretical systems that claim to account for broad classes of behavior and social functioning. On the whole, macrotheories have not been shown to be particularly useful in the behavioral and applied sciences.

Within nursing and fields like psychology, sociology, and education, theories are usually somewhat restricted in scope, focusing only upon a narrow range of phenomena. Theories that focus on only a piece of reality and that incorporate a selected number of concepts are sometimes referred to as *middle-range theories*. For example, there are middle-range theories that focus on decision-making behavior, leadership behavior, attitude change, and so forth. This limited scope is consistent with the state of scientific developments in these fields and is, therefore, appropriate and realistic. In the physical sciences macrotheories such as the theory of mechanics are feasible and provide a goal toward which the younger social and applied sciences may aspire.

Theories also vary in their complexity. Here we refer to the number and intricacy of the concepts involved and the complexity of relationships presumed. Concepts can, like the theories they form, be hierarchically arranged in terms of their generality and abstractness. "Suicide" is a concept that is less abstract than "alienation." Theories in the sciences dealing with human beings often tend to be complex, not only because the subject matter is inherently complex but also because conditional relationships and multiple variables are required at the current level of understanding and conceptualization.

Tentative nature of theories

It cannot be stressed too strongly that a theory can never be "proved" or "confirmed." A theory represents a scientist's best efforts to describe and explain phenomena; today's successful theory may be relegated to tomorrow's intellectual garbage dump. It is not only that new evidence or observations "disprove" a previously useful theory; it is also possible that a new theoretical system can integrate new observations with the observations that the old theory "explained." There are also other reasons beside utility and parsimony for the rejection of a theory. Theories that are not congruent with a culture's values and philosophical orientation may be discredited. It is not unusual for a theory to lose supporters because its implications are not in vogue. For example, the emergence of feminism and the changing status of women in our society have resulted in attacks on psychoanalytical and structural social theories. This link between theory and values may surprise those who think of science as being completely objective. It should be remembered, however, that theories are deliberately invented by humans; they can, thus, never be freed totally from the human perspective, which is amenable to change over time. In sum, no theory, no matter what its subject matter, can ever be considered final and verified. There always remains the possibility that a theory will be modified or discarded. Many theories in the physical sciences have received considerable empiri-

cal support, and their well-accepted propositions are often referred to as *laws,* such as Boyle's law of gases. Nevertheless, we have no way of knowing the ultimate accuracy and utility of any theory and should, therefore, treat all theories as tentative. This caveat is nowhere more relevant than in the emerging sciences such as nursing.

Relationship between theory and research

The relationship between theory and research is a reciprocal and mutually beneficial one. A theory must be built inductively from observations, and there is no better source for those observations than scientific research. Concepts and relations that are validated in the empirical arena become the foundation for theory development. The theory, in turn, must be tested by subjecting deductions from it (hypotheses) to further scientific inquiry. Thus research plays a dual and continuing role in theory building and testing. Theory guides and generates ideas for research; research assesses the worth of the theory and provides a foundation for new ones.

It would be unreasonable to assert that research without any theoretical underpinnings is useless. In nursing research, there are still many "facts" that need to be accumulated, and descriptive inquiries may well form the basis for subsequent theoretical developments. Nontheoretical research can potentially be linked to theory at a later time. This is not to say, however, that nurse researchers need not strive to develop a theoretical framework for their research problems. The time is ripe for the discipline to enter a new phase in which theory development and testing are major goals. It is not always easy to place one's research problems into a theoretical context, particularly because nursing theory per se is in its embryonic stages. There are, however, useful *conceptual frameworks* from nursing and other disciplines that can be utilized in the conduct of nursing investigations.

☐
Conceptual frameworks and models

The terms "theory," "theoretical framework," "conceptual framework," "conceptual scheme," "conceptual model," and "model" are sometimes used synonymously in the research literature. We have been very careful in the preceding discussion to restrict our terminology to "theory" and "theoretical framework" and to use these terms to refer to a well-formulated deductive system of abstract formal statements. In this section we distinguish theories from conceptual frameworks and models.

Conceptual frameworks

Conceptual frameworks, models, or schemes (we will use the terms interchangeably) represent a less formal and less well-developed attempt at organizing phenomena than theories. As the name implies, conceptual frameworks deal with abstractions (concepts) that are assembled by virtue of their relevance to a common theme. Both conceptual schemes and theories use concepts as building blocks. What is absent from conceptual schemes is the deductive system of propositions that assert a relationship between the concepts. As Fawcett (1984) has observed, conceptual models also tend to be more global than theories. Homans (1964), in noting the virtual absence of formal theory in the field of sociology, pointed out the following with regard to conceptual schemes: "Concepts and their definitions are certainly part of a theory, but they are not sufficient by themselves to constitute a theory. Concepts are names for properties of nature, and a theory does not even begin to exist until propositions are stated about contingent rela-

tionships of the general form *x* varies as *y* between properties" (1964, p. 957).

Most of the conceptual work that has been done in connection with nursing practice is more rightfully designated as conceptual models or frameworks than as theories. This label in no way diminishes the importance and value of these endeavors. Indeed, many existing conceptual frameworks will undoubtedly serve as the preliminary steps in the construction of more formal theories. In the meantime, conceptual frameworks can serve to guide research that will further support theory development. Conceptual frameworks, like theories, can serve as a springboard for the generation of research hypotheses. The next section of this chapter describes a few of the major conceptual models in nursing and illustrates how these models have been used in nursing research.

Schematic and statistical models

The term *model* is often used to denote a symbolic representation of phenomena. Within a research context, the models that one is most likely to encounter are mathematical or statistical models and schematic models. These two basic types share one important attribute in common: these models attempt to represent reality with *minimal use of words.*

Language is, and probably always will be, a problem for scientists. A word or phrase that designates a concept can convey different meanings to different individuals, or to the same individual when used in different contexts. The creation of a dictionary of conceptual terms to accompany theoretical propositions does help some, but the definitions are still made up of words whose imprecision can interfere with effective communication. A visual or symbolic representation of a theory or conceptual framework often helps to express abstract ideas in a more readily understand-

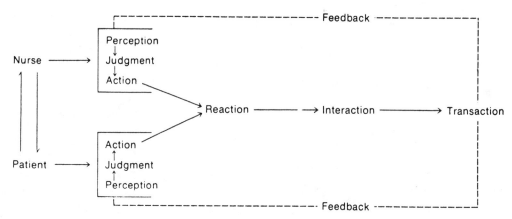

Figure 6-1. Human interaction process. (After King, I.M. [1981]. A Theory for Nursing. *New York: John Wiley & Sons, p. 145. Used with permission.)*

able or precise form than the original conceptualization.

Schematic models are quite common and undoubtedly are familiar to all readers. A schematic model or diagram represents the phenomena of interest figuratively. Concepts and the linkages between them are represented diagrammatically through the use of boxes, arrows, or other symbols. An example of a schematic model is presented in Figure 6-1. This model is described by its designer as "a human interaction diagram showing nurse and client interactions" (King, 1981, p. 145). The author noted that the perception, judgment, and reaction activities are not directly observable. However, the interactions are directly observable behaviors that can be recorded and analyzed to determine what transactions have occurred. Schematic models of this type can be quite useful in the research process in clarifying concepts and their associations, in enabling researchers to place a specific problem into an appropriate context, and in revealing areas of inquiry.

Statistical models are playing a growing role in research endeavors in nursing and related sciences. These models use symbols to express quantitatively the nature of relationships among variables. There are few relationships in the behavioral sciences that can be summarized as elegantly as in the mathematical model $F = ma$ (Force = mass × acceleration). Because human behavior is so complex and subject to so many influences as yet poorly understood, it is typically possible to model it only in a probabilistic manner. This means that we are not yet able (and perhaps never will be able) to develop equations, such as the example of force from mechanics, in which a human behavior can be simply described as the product of two other phenomena. What we can do, however, is describe the probability that a certain behavior will be performed, given the occurrence of specified phenomena. This is the function of statistical models. An example of a statistical model is shown below:

$$Y = \beta_1 X_1 + \beta_2 X_2 + \beta_3 X_3 + \beta_4 X_4 + e$$

where Y = nursing effectiveness, as measured by a supervisor's evaluation

X_1 = nursing knowledge, as measured by the licensure examination

X_2 = past achievement, as measured by grades in nursing school

X_3 = decision-making skills, as measured by number of nursing diagnoses made

X_4 = empathy, as measured by timing between patient's request for pain medication and actual administration of pain medication

e = a residual, unexplained factor

$\beta_1, \beta_2, \beta_3$, and β_4 = weights indicating the importance of X_1, X_2, X_3, and X_4, respectively, in determining nursing effectiveness

Note that each term in this model is quantified or quantifiable; that is, every symbol can be replaced by a numerical value, such as an individual's score on the nursing licensure exam (X_1).

What does this equation mean and how does it work? This model constitutes a mechanism for understanding and predicting nursing effectiveness. The model proposes that on-the-job effectiveness is affected primarily by four factors: the nursing knowledge, past achievement, decision-making skill, and empathy of the nurse. These influences are not presumed to be equally important. The weights (βs) associated with each factor represent a sort of recipe for designating the relative importance of each. If empathy were much more important than past achievement, for example, the weights might be 2 to 1 respectively (that is, two parts empathy to one part past achievement). The "e" at the end of the model represents all those unknown or unmeasurable other attributes that affect one's performance as a nurse. In the quantitative equation, "e" would be set equal to some constant value; it would not vary from one nurse to another, because it really constitutes an unknown element in the equation. Once the values of the weights and "e" have been established

(through statistical procedures), the model can be used to predict the nursing effectiveness of any nurse for whom we have gathered information on the four Xs (licensure exam scores, etc.). Our prediction will not always be perfectly accurate, in part because of the influence of those unknown factors summarized by "e." Perfect forecasting is seldom attainable with probabilistic statistical models, but such a model makes prediction less haphazard than mere guesswork.

In summary, it may not always prove possible to identify a formal theory that is relevant to a nursing research problem, but conceptual schemes and models of the type discussed here can also be used to clarify concepts and to provide a context for findings that might otherwise be isolated and meaningless. Conceptual schemes in nursing are very much in need of testing if theories for nursing are to be formulated.

☐
Conceptual models in nursing

In the past few decades, nurses have formulated a number of conceptual models of nursing and for nursing practice. These models constitute formal explanations of what the nursing discipline is according to the model developer's point of view. As Fawcett (1984) has noted, there is general agreement that there are four central concepts of the nursing discipline: person, environment, health, and nursing. However, the various conceptual models define these concepts differently, link them in diverse ways, and give different emphasis to the relationships among them.

The conceptual models were not developed solely as a base from which nursing research could be launched. Indeed, these models have thus far had more impact on nursing education, administration, and clinical practice than on nursing research. Nevertheless, nurse researchers are turning increasingly toward these conceptual models for their inspiration and theoretical foundations in formulating research questions and hypotheses. In this section we briefly examine some of the major conceptual models in nursing and give examples of research that claimed its intellectual roots in these models.

Johnson's Behavioral Systems Model

Like other systems models, Johnson's (1980) model focuses on a system, its subsystems, and its environment. The system of central interest in Johnson's model is the patient as a behavioral system. According to this model, each individual behavioral system is a collection of seven interrelated subsystems the response patterns of which form an organized and integrated whole. The seven subsystems are: (1) attachment or affiliation; (2) dependency; (3) ingestion; (4) elimination; (5) sexuality; (6) aggression; and (7) achievement. Each subsystem carries out specialized tasks for the integrated system, and each is structured by four motivational elements: goal, set, choice, and action/behavior.

The model is concerned with behavioral functioning that results in the equilibrium of the integrated system. Behavioral system balance reflects adjustments and adaptations that are successful in the achievement of a steady state. Johnson indicates that the seven subsystems must be stimulated to grow and adapt, but must also be protected from malfunctions and noxious influences. The function of nursing is to help restore the balance of each subsystem in the event of disequilibrium and to help prevent future system disturbances.

Several researchers have designated Johnson's Behavioral Systems Model as their conceptual basis. For example, Derdiarian and Forsythe (1983) described the development of an instrument (the Derdiarian Behavioral System Model Instrument) to measure the perceived behavioral changes of cancer pa-

tients. Holaday (1981) focused on Johnson's concept of "behavioral set" in her study of the crying bouts of chronically ill infants and their mothers' responses. Johnson's model also guided Small's (1980) investigation of the body image and spatial awareness of visually impaired children.

King's Open System Model

King's conceptual model (1981) includes three types of interacting systems. The first type of system, personal systems, is represented by individuals. The key concepts included in personal systems are perception, self, body image, growth and development, time, and space. Interpersonal systems are the second type in the network of interacting systems (see Fig. 6-1). When individuals interact (e.g., client and nurse), they form interpersonal systems. Concepts relevant to interpersonal interactions include role, interaction, communication, transaction, and stress. The third major category in the framework is social systems. Any social systems in which the nurse interacts with health care consumers, such as a family or a hospital, belongs to this category of systems. Concepts relevant for functioning in social systems include organizations, role, power, authority, and decision-making.

Within King's model, the domain of nursing includes promoting, maintaining, and restoring health. Nursing is viewed as "a process of action, reaction, and interaction whereby nurse and client share information about their perceptions of the nursing situation. Through purposeful communication they identify specific goals, problems, or concerns. They explore means to achieve a goal and agree to means to the goal" (King, 1981, p. 2).

King's model has not been used as the basis for many studies. However, King herself (1981) conducted a descriptive observational study of nurse-client encounters that yielded a classification of elements in nurse-client interactions. The study provided preliminary support for the proposition that goal attainment was facilitated by accurate nurse-client perceptions, satisfactory communication, and mutual goal setting.

Levine's Conservation Model

Levine's (1973) model focuses on individuals as holistic beings, and the major area of concern is maintenance of the person's wholeness. The model identifies adaptation as the process by which the integrity or wholeness of individuals is maintained.

Levine suggested four principles of conservation that aim to facilitate patients' adaptation processes:

1. Conservation of patient energy, that is, the conservation of the individual's physiologic and psychological energy resources
2. Conservation of structural integrity, that is, the conservation of patients' body form and function
3. Conservation of personal integrity, that is, the conservation of patients' self-esteem and psychological identity
4. Conservation of social integrity, that is, the conservation of patients' familial, community, and subcultural affiliations

Through these four conservation principles the model emphasizes the nurse's responsibility to maintain the client's integrity in the threat of assault through illness or environmental influences.

Levine noted that her model is appropriate for investigating the interface between the internal and external environments of the person. In one of the few published studies based on Levine's model, Newport (1984) investigated two alternative methods of conserving newborn thermal energy and social integrity.

Neuman's Health Care Systems Model

Neuman's (1982) model focuses on the person as a complete system, the subparts of which are interrelated physiologic, psychological, sociocultural, and developmental factors. These interacting variables determine the amount of resistance an individual can mount against stressors. The stressors may be intrapersonal, interpersonal, or extrapersonal.

The central core of protection the person has for his or her first-line defense against stressors is a flexible line of resistance — internal factors that help defend against the stressor. The next protective barrier is the normal line of defense, which includes such factors as the person's coping style, developmental stage, and so on. The final buffer against stressors is the flexible line of defense, composed of dynamic factors that can fluctuate in response to circumstances.

In Neuman's model, the person maintains balance and harmony between internal and external environments by adjusting to stress and by defending against tension-producing stimuli. Wellness is equated with equilibrium, which is maintained when the person's flexible line of defense has prevented stressors from penetrating the normal line of defense. The primary goal of nursing is to assist in the attainment and maintenance of client system stability. Nursing interventions include activities to strengthen flexible lines of defense, to strengthen resistance to stressors, and to maintain adaptation.

The Neuman Health Care Systems Model has led to some applications in nursing research. For example, Craddock and Stanhope (1980) applied Neuman's scheme in a study of clients' and health-care providers' perceptions of stressors. Ziemer (1983) operationalized many of Neuman's concepts in a study of the effects of preoperative information on the postoperative outcomes of clients who have had abdominal surgery.

Orem's Model of Self-Care

Orem's (1985) model focuses on each individual's ability to perform self-care, defined as "the practice of activities that individuals initiate and perform on their own behalf in maintaining life, health, and well-being" (p. 35). One's ability to care for oneself is referred to as self-care agency, and the ability to care for others is referred to as dependent-care agency.

According to the model, there are three categories of self-care requisites, purposes to be attained through self-care actions: universal requisites (associated with life processes and the maintenance of integrity of human structure and functioning); developmental requisites (associated with developmental processes at various stages of the life cycle); and health-deviation requisites (arising from structural/functional deviations or constitutional/genetic defects). Therapeutic self-care demand refers to the self-care actions needed to address these requisites. Self-care deficits are said to occur when a person does not have the capacity for continuous self-care.

In Orem's model, the goal of nursing agency is to help people meet their own therapeutic self-care demands. Orem identified three types of nursing systems: (1) wholly compensatory—wherein the nurse compensates for the patient's total inability to perform self-care activities; (2) partially compensatory —wherein the nurse compensates for the patient's partial inability to perform self-care activities; and (3) supportive-educative —wherein the nurse assists the patient in making decisions and acquiring skills and knowledge.

Orem's Self-Care Model has generated considerable interest among nurse researchers. For example, Chang and colleagues (1985) examined components of nurse practitioners' care in the context of Orem's model to determine what aspects of the care contributed most to the elderly patients' intentions to adhere to the care plan. Kearney and Fleischer (1979) described a study the purpose of which was to develop an instrument measuring a person's exercise of self-care agency. Patterson and Hale (1985) based their study of menstrual care practices on Orem's Self-Care Model. A fuller description of other research based on this model is provided in a subsequent section of this chapter.

Rogers' Model of the Unitary Person

Rogers' model (1970) focuses on individuals as a unified whole in constant interaction with the environment. The unitary person is viewed as an energy field that is more than, and different from, the sum of the biologic, physical, social, and psychological parts. The environment constitutes another energy field. The human and environmental energy fields have pattern and organization, but are continuously and creatively changing.

Three principles of homeodynamics define the nature and direction of human change and development: (1) helicy—characterized by the diversity of the human and environmental field emerging from their interactions and manifesting nonrecurring rhymicities; (2) resonancy—characterized by ongoing change from lower to higher frequency wave patterns in the human and environmental fields; and (3) complementarity/integrality—the continuous, mutual, and simultaneous interaction between human and environmental fields.

In Rogers' model, nursing is concerned with the unitary person as a synergistic phenomenon. Nursing science is devoted to the study of the nature and direction of unitary human development. Nursing practice helps individuals achieve maximum well-being within their potential.

Several nursing studies have been based on

Rogers' Model of the Unitary Person. For example, Fitzpatrick (1980), focusing on the principle of resonancy, described a series of studies relating to patients' temporal experiences. Gill and Atwood (1981) linked Rogers' principles of helicy and reciprocy to the relationship between epidermal growth factor and wound healing, using a sample of domestic pigs. Floyd (1983) tested a theorem of sleep-wake patterns based on Rogers' model with samples of rotating shift workers and hospitalized psychiatric patients.

Roy's Adaptation Model

In Roy's (1980) Adaptation Model, human beings are biopsychosocial adaptive systems who cope with environmental change through the process of adaptation. Within the human system there are four subsystems: physiologic needs; self-concept; role function; and interdependence. These subsystems constitute adaptive modes that provide mechanisms for coping with environmental stimuli and change. The adaptive mode relating to physiologic needs is concerned with the need for physiologic integrity. The adaptive mode of self-concept addresses the need for psychic integrity. The adaptive modes of role function and interdependence focus on the need for social integrity.

The goal of nursing, according to this model, is to promote patient adaptation in all four modes during health and illness. Nursing also regulates stimuli affecting adaptation. Nursing interventions generally take the form of increasing, decreasing, modifying, removing, or maintaining internal and external stimuli that affect adaptation.

Roy's Adaptation Model has been used as the conceptual framework in several nursing studies. For example, Norris, Campbell, and Brenkert (1982) used Roy's concepts of focal, contextual, and residual stimuli in their study of the effect of nursing procedures on transcutaneous oxygen tension in premature infants. Fawcett and Burritt (1985) analyzed responses to questions dealing with reactions to a cesarean birth experience according to Roy's adaptive modes. Shannahan and Cottrell (1985) invoked Roy's concept of manipulation of contextual stimuli in their assessment of the effects of delivering in a birth chair versus a traditional delivery table.

□
Testing, using and developing theory

In a previous section, we described the strong interrelationship between theory and research. The manner in which theory and conceptual frameworks are used by researchers is elaborated upon in the following section. In the discussion, the term "theory" will not be restricted to its narrow, formal connotation but will refer to its broader meaning as something conceptual, abstract, and general. In other words, the procedures discussed will almost always be equally applicable to conceptual frameworks and models and formal theories.

Testing a theory

As noted earlier, theories often stimulate new research investigations. For example, a nurse may have read several papers relating to Orem's Self-Care Model. As the nurse's reading progresses, the following types of conjectures might arise: "If Orem's self-care model is valid, one might expect that nursing effectiveness might be enhanced in environments more conducive to self-care (for example, a birthing room versus a delivery room)" or "Given this conceptual framework, it might be expected that the dependency level of patients (in terms of either their age of physical or psychological characteristics) would affect the nature and intensity of effective interventions." These conjectures, derived from the theory or conceptual framework, can serve as a point of departure for testing the adequacy of the theory.

In testing a theory, the researcher deduces implications (as in the above example) and develops research hypotheses. These hypotheses are predictions about the manner in which variables would be related, if the theory were correct and useful. The hypotheses are then subjected to empirical testing through systematic research. A theory is never tested directly. It is the hypotheses deduced from a theory that are subjected to scientific investigations. Comparisons between the observed outcomes of research and the relationships predicted by the hypotheses are the major focus of the testing process. Through this process, the theory is continually subjected to potential disconfirmation. Repeated failures of research endeavors to disconfirm a theory result in increasing support for and acceptance of a theoretical position. The testing process continues until some piece of evidence cannot be interpreted within the context of the theory but *can* be explained by a new theory that also accounts for all previous findings. From the point of view of theory testing, the goal of a serviceable research project is to develop a research design that reduces the credibility of alternative explanations for observed relationships, to devise logically adequate deductions from theory, and to select methods that assess the theory's validity under maximally heterogeneous situations so that potentially competing theories can be ruled out. The theory-testing aspect of research is described in more detail in the next chapter, which deals with hypotheses.

It should be noted that before using a theory as a basis for a research study, the investigator should first evaluate the theory. Stevens (1984) presents a useful set of standards for assessing conceptual frameworks in nursing that uses the principles of internal and external criticism.

Fitting a problem to a theory

The preceding discussion was concerned with the situation in which a researcher begins with a specific theory or conceptual framework of interest and utilizes that theory as a basis for developing a research problem and design. Circumstances sometimes arise in which the problem is formulated before consideration is given to a theoretical framework. Even in such situations researchers may strive to (or may be required to) devise a theoretical context to enrich the value and meaningfulness of their inquiry. An after-the-fact linkage of theory to a research question is considerably more problematic than the testing of a particular theory of interest. This is particularly true for neophyte researchers who may lack a thorough grounding in the theoretical positions of their own or related disciplines.

The search for relevant existing theories can be greatly facilitated by first conceptualizing on a sufficiently abstract level what the nature of the problem is. For example, take the problem statement "Do daily telephone conversations between a psychiatric nurse and a patient for 2 weeks following discharge from the hospital result in lower rates of readmission by short-term psychiatric patients?" This is a relatively concrete example but might profitably be viewed as a subproblem for Orem's self-care model, or a theory of reinforcement, or a theory of social influence, or a theory of crisis resolution. Part of the difficulty in finding a theory is that a single phenomenon of interest can be conceptualized in a number of ways and, depending on the manner chosen, may refer the researcher to conceptual schemes from a wide range of disciplines. Furthermore, even with a single conceptualization a number of alternatives may exist, particularly in nursing and the social sciences. The multiplicity of conceptual frameworks to explain nursing behavior is just one example.

Once the researcher has conceptualized the research problem on an abstract level, the search for existing theories can proceed relatively efficiently because the difficult part of the task will have been completed. Textbooks, handbooks, and encyclopedias in the chosen discipline usually are a good starting point for the selection of a theory. These sources usually summarize the status of a theoretical position and document the efforts to confirm and disconfirm it. Journal articles contain more current information but are usually restricted to descriptions of specific studies rather than to broad expositions or evaluations of theories. When a theoretical position has been developed at length and/or has been supported by extensive empirical observations, whole books may be devoted to their description.

The task of fitting a problem to a theory should be done with caution. It is true that having a theoretical context enhances the meaningfulness of a research study, but artificially cramming a problem into a theory is not the route to scientific utility. There are many published studies that purport to have a conceptual framework, when in fact the *post hoc* nature of the conceptualization is all too evident. If a conceptual framework is really linked to a research problem, then the design of the study, the selection of appropriate data collection strategies, and the analysis and (especially) the interpretation of data *flow* from that conceptualization. We advocate a balanced and reasoned perspective on this issue: Researchers should not shirk their intellectual duties by failing to make an attempt to link their problem to broader theoretical concerns, but there is no point in fabricating such a link when it really does not exist.

Developing a theory

Many beginning researchers may think of themselves as unqualified to develop a theory or conceptual scheme of their own. But theory development depends much less on one's knowledge of research methods and experience in the conduct of investigations than on one's powers of observation, understanding of a problem, and readings about a substantive issue. There is, therefore, nothing to prevent an imaginative and sensitive person from formulating an original conceptual framework for a study. The conceptual scheme may or may not be a full-fledged formal theory with well-articulated postulates; the scheme should, however, place the issues of the study into some broader perspective. In the field of nursing research, where there has not yet been extensive theoretical work, the beginning researcher may have an easier task in devising an original framework than in finding one that is really appropriate for the problem of interest.

The basic intellectual process underlying theory development is induction, which refers to the process of reasoning from particular observations and facts to generalizations. The inductive process involves integrating what one has experienced or learned into some concise and general conclusion. If one has observed that Virginia C., Joseph P., Patricia M., and Edward R. (all of whom are tonsillectomy patients) have refused to eat any of their first postoperative meal, one might arrive at the conclusion that loss of appetite characterizes those who have just had a tonsillectomy operation. The "observations" used in the inductive process need not be personal observations; they may be (and often are in formal theories) the findings and conclusions from research investigations. When relationships among variables are arrived at this way, one has the makings of a theory that can be put to a more rigorous scientific test. The first step in theory

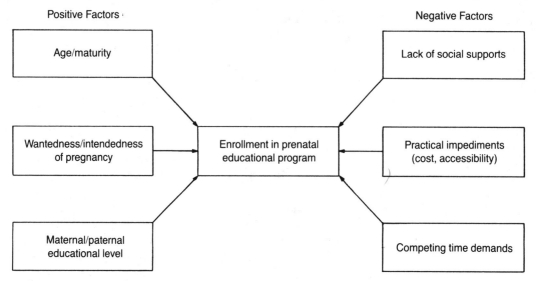

Figure 6-2.   *Conceptual model — factors that influence enrollment in a prenatal education program.*

development, then, is to formulate a generalized scheme of relevant concepts, that is, to perform a conceptual analysis. The product of this step should be a conceptual framework, whose worth can be assessed according to the criteria presented in the previous section.

Let us look at a simple example. Suppose that we were interested in understanding the factors influencing enrollment in a prenatal education program. We might begin by considering two basic sets of forces: those that promote enrollment and those that hinder it. After reviewing the literature, discussing the problem with colleagues, and developing ideas from our own experiences, we might arrive at a conceptual scheme such as the one presented in Figure 6-2. This framework is undoubtedly incomplete and imperfect, but it does allow us to study a number of research questions *and* to place those problems in perspective. For example, the conceptual scheme suggests that as the availability of social supports declines, the obstacles to participation in a prenatal education program increase. We might then make the following hypothesis:

"Single pregnant women are less likely to participate in a prenatal education program than married pregnant women," on the assumption that husbands are an important source of social support to women in their pregnancy.

The translation of conceptual schemes into formal theories is considerably more complex and intellectually formidable than the initial conceptual analysis. To date, few such theories have been devised in nursing and fewer yet have been subjected to rigorous confirmatory efforts. Theory development remains a critical challenge to this generation of nursing researchers.

☐
Theoretical contexts and nursing research

As noted earlier, theory and research have reciprocal, beneficial ties. Fawcett (1978) described the relationship between theory and research as a double helix, with theory as the impetus of scientific investigations and findings from research shaping the development of theory. However, this relationship has not always characterized the progress of nursing science. Many have criticized nursing researchers for producing numerous pieces of isolated research that are not placed in a theoretical context.

This criticism was more justified a decade ago than it is today. As we saw in an earlier section, many researchers are developing studies on the basis of conceptual models of nursing. However, nursing science is still struggling to integrate accumulated knowledge within theoretical systems. This struggle is reflected, in part, in the number of controversies surrounding the issue of theoretical frameworks in nursing.

One of these controversies concerns whether there should be one single, unified model of nursing, or multiple, competing models. Fawcett (1984) has argued against combining different models, noting that "before all nurses follow the same path, the competition of multiple models is needed to determine the superiority of one or more of them" (p. 9). Research can play a critical role in testing the utility and validity of alternative nursing models.

Another controversy involves the desirability and appropriateness of developing theories unique to nursing. Some commentators argue that theories relating to human beings developed within other disciplines (e.g., physiology, psychology, anthropology, sociology) can and should be applied to nursing problems. Others advocate the development of unique nursing theories, claiming that only through such development can knowledge to guide nursing practice be generated.

Until these controversies are resolved, nursing research is likely to continue on its current path of conducting studies within a multidisciplinary and multitheoretical perspective. We are inclined to see the use of multiple frameworks as a healthy and unavoidable part of the development of nursing science. We conclude this chapter by presenting several nursing research applications using both "borrowed" and nursing-specific theoretical schemes.

□
Research examples

Example 1: Social learning theory

The psychologist Julian Rotter developed a theoretical position known as social learning theory, which has generated extensive research interest in a number of disciplines, including nursing research. Briefly, social learning theory postulates that human behaviors in specific situations are contingent upon the individual's expectancy that a particular behavior will be reinforced (rewarded). A key concept in social learning is locus of control, which is conceptualized as the degree to which a person perceives that rewards are a function of his or her own actions, efforts, or characteristics as opposed to external forces. Internal controllers are those who perceive themselves and their behavior as the major determinants of the reinforcement, while external controllers are those who tend to see little if any relationship between their own actions and subsequent reinforcement.

Lowery and DuCette (1976) investigated the relationship between patients' response to diabetes and their locus of control orientation. A sample of 90 diabetics between the ages of 25 and 65 who differed in terms of duration of diabetes was selected. These subjects were administered an instrument to measure locus of control orientation and a "Diabetes and Health Information Test" developed for the study. The latter instrument included control items directly related to the management of a health or disease situation. Internally oriented diabetics were found to have more diabetic information than external diabetics, consistent with results from other studies in which internal individuals are more active seekers of information than externals. On the other hand, internals showed no decrease in the number of problems associated with their disease over time, unlike the externals. The investigators interpreted this unexpected finding as the possible result of the external's greater dependence on, and compliance with, medical authority and prescribed regimen.

LaMontagne (1984) conducted a study to examine the relationship between children's locus of control beliefs and their preoperative coping behaviors. Based on earlier research, it was argued that one's internal-external locus of control affects the way a stressful event is interpreted, and thus affects one's coping strategies. In other words, the belief that one has control can reduce the threat of a noxious stimuli, and increase information-seeking. The sample consisted of 51 children aged 8 to 12 who were scheduled for minor elective surgery. The subjects were administered the Nowicki-Strickland Locus of Control Scale and were interviewed to determine their mode of coping. Based on a series of 26 questions, the children's coping style was classified along a dimension labeled avoidant-active. The results indicated that children rated as active copers were more internally oriented than children rated as avoidant. The "internal" children in the sample knew more about their medical problems and the nature of the surgery than children who were "external," consistent with the theory and with previous research that had shown that internality and information-seeking (active coping) are related.

Example 2: The health belief model

The Health Belief Model (HBM) has become a popular conceptual framework in studies focusing on patient compliance. The model integrates psychological theories of goal setting, decision making, and social learning. The model postulates that health-seeking behavior is influenced by a person's perception of a threat posed by a health problem and the value associated with actions aimed at reducing the threat (Becker, 1978). The major components of the HBM include perceived susceptibility, perceived severity, perceived benefits and costs, motivation, and enabling or modifying factors. Perceived susceptibility refers to a person's perception that a health problem is personally relevant or that a diagnosis of illness is accurate. Even when one recognizes personal susceptibility, action will not occur unless the individual believes that becoming ill would have serious organic or social implications. Perceived benefits refers to the patients' beliefs that a given treatment will cure the illness or help prevent it, whereas perceived costs refers to the complexity, duration, and accessibility of the treatment. Motivation includes desire to comply with a treatment, belief that people should do what is prescribed by health-care personnel, concern about health matters in general, willingness to seek and accept health care, and engagement in positive health activities. Among the modifying factors that have been identified are personality variables, the patient-practitioner relationships, patient satisfaction, and sociodemographic factors.

Itano and her colleagues (1983) studied factors related to compliance with therapy among cancer patients. Among the factors considered were the patients' self-esteem, anxiety, locus of control, understanding of the illness, perception of the severity of the symptoms, and perception of the nurses' care and concern. The sample consisted of 66 patients from two hospital-based chemotherapy clinics. Compliance was determined by a retrospective 3-month audit of the patients' records. Subjects also completed a questionnaire that included measures of the other study variables. The findings indicated that noncompliers had higher scores on a measure of external locus of control. Compliers were found to be less anxious than noncompliers, but the two groups did not differ in terms of self-esteem. Differences were also observed with respect to perceived severity of symptoms, with noncompliers rating their symptoms more severely, contrary to expectations. Both groups perceived nurses as being very caring and concerned.

DeVon and Powers (1984) used the Health Belief Model in their study of compliance and psychosocial adjustment in two groups of hypertensive patients. Subjects were classified as being either "controlled" or "uncontrolled" with respect to their hypertension, based on the clinical judgment of their physicians. The study sample involved 30 subjects (15 in each group). The subjects completed a compliance questionnaire (based on the HBM) and the Psychosocial Adjustment to Illness Scale. Blood pressure and hypertension-related information were obtained from the patients' records. Contrary to expectations, the two groups did not differ in their health beliefs affecting compliance, but differences were found with respect to psychosocial adjustment to illness. Uncontrolled hypertensives showed less illness-related adjustment and reported more psychological distress. Lower adjustment to illness was found to be related to both lower compliance and to a more complex medication regimen. The investigators concluded that the findings supported the notion that psychosocial distress may be an important moderating variable to consider in further development of the Health Belief Model.

Example 3: Orem's Self-Care Model

Earlier in this chapter we reviewed the major features of Orem's Self-Care Model. In this section we examine several studies that used this model as their conceptual framework.

Rothlis (1984) investigated whether persons with reactive depression exposed to a self-help group experience greater decrease in their feelings of hopelessness and helplessness than persons not participating in a self-help group. Rothlis viewed reactive depression within Orem's framework as a health-deviation self-care deficit. Rothlis further identified the intervention (the introduction of the self-help groups) as a nursing activity within the educative-supportive-developmental domain. Self-help groups were conceptualized as a means of creating a milieu wherein therapeutic processes could occur. These processes were believed to increase the capacity for self-care agency and hasten the process of separating the patient from the health professional. The sample consisted of 28 patients with a primary diagnosis of reactive depression. Half the subjects were randomly assigned to participate in a self-help group while the other subjects did not participate. Subjects were administered a measure of hopelessness and helplessness prior to the implementation of the self-help groups and 4 days later. The findings indicated that although the two groups were comparable at the beginning of the study, patients who participated in the self-help groups had significantly lower scores of helplessness and hopelessness at the end of the study.

Dodd (1984) studied the self-care behaviors of cancer patients in chemotherapy. She argued that because there is little information on how patients manage an illness, studies of self-care in disease are needed. The subjects in the study (48 cancer patients in chemotherapy) were assigned at random to four types of treatment that were hypothesized to influence patients' capabilities for self-care. The first group received drug information only; the second group received information on side-effect management techniques; the third group received both types of information; and the fourth group received no special intervention. Information on chemotherapy knowledge, self-care behavior, and overall psychological well-being was obtained both prior to and after the completion of the interventions. Subjects who received the drug information scored higher than other subjects on the chemotherapy knowledge test. Subjects who received information on side-effect management techniques (either alone or with drug information) performed more self-care behaviors after the intervention than subjects who did not receive this information.

☐
Summary

A *theory* is an abstract generalization that systematically explains the relationships among phenomena. The overall objective of theory is to make scientific findings meaningful and generalizable. In addition, theories help to summarize existing knowledge into coherent systems, stimulate new research by providing both direction and impetus, and explain the nature of relationships between or among variables, which provides a framework for predicting and, in turn, controlling the occurrence of the phenomena.

Theories are created or developed by scientists. Their creation requires imagination on the part of the scientist and congruence with reality and existing knowledge. The basic components of a theory are concepts. Theories consist of a set of statements, each of which expresses a relationship. The statements are arranged in a logically interrelated system that permits new statements to be derived from them.

Theories vary in their level of generality and level of complexity. Some theories attempt to describe large segments of the environment and are called "grand" or "macro" theories whereas other theories are more restricted in scope. Theories that are more specific to certain phenomena are sometimes referred to as *middle-range theories.* The complexity of a theory refers to the number and abstractness of the concepts contained in the theory. All theories are considered tentative and are never "proved."

Conceptual schemes are less well-developed attempts at organizing phenomena than are theories. As in the case of theories, concepts are the basic elements of a conceptual scheme. However, the concepts are not linked to one another in a logically ordered deductive system. Much of the conceptual work in nursing is more rightfully described as conceptual schemes than as theories. Conceptual frameworks are highly valuable in that they often serve as the springboard for theory development.

Models are symbolic representations of phenomena. Models depict a theory or conceptual scheme through the use of symbols or diagrams. The two types of models most frequently used in research are mathematical or statistical models and schematic models. Models are useful to scientists because they use a minimal amount of words, which tend to be ambiguous, in representing reality.

A number of conceptual models of nursing have evolved and have been used in nursing research. Among the major conceptual models of nursing are Johnson's Behavioral Systems Model, King's Open System Model, Levine's Conservation Model, Neuman's Health Care Systems Model, Orem's Model of Self-Care, Rogers' Model of the Unitary Person, and Roy's Adaptation Model.

Conceptual schemes and theories can be integrated with empirical research in a number of ways. The investigator may design a scientific study specifically to test a theory of interest. In other situations, a problem may be developed first and a theory selected to "fit" the problem. An after-the-fact selection of a theory usually is more problematic and less meaningful than the systematic testing of a particular theory.

Nursing research is increasingly drawing upon conceptual frameworks and models in its efforts to integrate accumulated knowledge and advance nursing science. At present, many investigations are based on theories borrowed from other disciplines, but an increasing number of studies have conceptual models of nursing as their frameworks.

☐
Study suggestions

1. Read the article by S.I. Laffrey in the August 1985, issue of *Western Journal of Nursing Research,* pages 279–300. What theoretical basis does the author develop for health conception and health behavior choice? Would you classify the theoretical basis as a theory or as a conceptual framework? Draw a schematic model of the major concepts used in the study.
2. Select one of the nursing conceptual frameworks or models described in the chapter. Formulate a research question and two hypotheses that could be used to empirically test the utility of the conceptual framework or model in nursing practice.
3. Four researchable problems are:
   a. What is the relationship between angina pain and alcohol intake?
   b. What effect does rapid weight gain during the second trimester have on the outcome of pregnancy?
   c. Do multiple hospital readmissions affect the achievement level of children?
   d. To what extent do coping mechanisms of individuals differ in health and illness?

Abstract a generalized issue or issues for each of the above problems. Search for an existing theory that might be applicable and appropriate.

☐
Suggested readings

Theoretical references

Batey, M.V. (1977). Conceptualization: Knowledge and logic guiding empirical research. *Nursing Research, 26,* 324–329.

Becker, M. (1978). The Health Belief Model and sick role behavior. *Nursing Digest, Spring,* 35–40.

Braithwaite, R.B. (1962). Models in the empirical sciences. In E. Nagel, P. Suppes, & A. Tarski (eds.): *Logic methodology and philosophy of science* (pp. 224–231). Stanford, CA: Stanford University Press.

Craig, S.L. (1980). Theory development and its relevance for nursing. *Journal of Advanced Nursing, 5,* 349–355.

Fawcett, J. (1978). The relationship between theory and research: A double helix. *Advances in Nursing Science, 1,* 49–62.

Fawcett, J. (1984). *Analysis and evaluation of conceptual models of nursing.* Philadelphia: F.A. Davis Co.

Flaskerud, J.H. & Halloran, E.J. (1980). Areas of agreement in nursing theory development. *Advances in Nursing Science, 3,* 1–7.

Flaskerud, J.H. (1984). Nursing models as conceptual frameworks for research. *Western Journal of Nursing Research, 6,* 153–155.

Hardy, M.E. (1974). Theories: Components, development, evaluation. *Nursing Research, 23,* 100–107.

Homans, G.C. (1964). Contemporary theory in sociology. In R.E.L. Farris (ed.), *Handbook of modern sociology* (pp. 951–977). Chicago: Rand McNally.

Hurley, B.A. (1979). Why a theoretical framework in nursing research? *Western Journal of Nursing Research, 1,* 28–41.

Jacox, A. (1974). Theory construction in nursing. *Nursing Research, 23,* 4–13.

Johnson, D.E. (1980). The behavioral system

model for nursing. In J.P. Riehl & C. Roy (eds.), *Conceptual models for nursing practice* (2nd ed.). Appleton-Century-Crofts.

Kim, H.S. (1983). *The nature of theoretical thinking in nursing.* Norwalk, CT: Appleton-Century-Crofts.

King, I.M. (1981). *A theory for nursing: Systems, concepts, process.* New York: John Wiley and Sons.

Levine, M.E. (1973). *Introduction to clinical nursing* (2nd ed.). Philadelphia: F.A. Davis, Co.

McFarlane, E.A. (1980). Nursing theory: The comparison of four theoretical proposals (King, Rogers, Roy, Orem). *Journal of Advanced Nursing, 5,* 3–19.

Neuman, B. (1982). *The Neuman systems model: Application to nursing education and practice.* New York: Appleton-Century-Crofts.

Orem, D.E. (1985). *Concepts of practice* (3rd ed.). New York: McGraw-Hill.

Rogers, M.E. (1970). *An introduction to the theoretical basis of nursing.* Philadelphia: F.A. Davis Co.

Rotter, J.B. (1954). *Social learning and clinical psychology.* Englewood Cliffs, NJ: Prentice-Hall.

Roy, C. (1980). The Roy adaptation model. In J.P. Riehl and C. Roy (eds.): *Conceptual models for nursing practice* (2nd ed.). New York: Appleton-Century-Crofts.

Roy, C., Sr. & Roberts, S.L. (1981). *Theory construction in nursing: An adaptation model.* Englewood Cliffs: Prentice Hall.

Selye, H. (1978). *The stress of life* (2nd ed.). New York: McGraw-Hill.

Stevens, B.J. (1984). *Nursing theory: Analysis, application, evaluation.* (2nd ed.). Boston: Little, Brown.

Substantive References*

Chang, B.L. *et al.* (1984). The effect of systematically varying components of nursing care on satisfaction in elderly ambulatory women. *Western Journal of Nursing Research, 6,* 367–379. (Orem's Self-Care Model).

* These studies have a formally stated conceptual framework, which is specified in parentheses.

Chang, B.L. *et al.* (1985). Adherence to health care regimens among elderly women. *Nursing Research, 34,* 27–31 (Orem's Self-Care Model).

Craddock, R.B. & Stanhope, M.K. (1980). The Neuman health-care systems model: Recommended adaptation. In J.P. Riehl & C. Roy (eds.), *Conceptual models for nursing practice* (2nd ed.). New York: Appleton-Century-Crofts (Neuman's Health Care Systems Model).

Davidson, P.O. & Kelley, W.R. (1973). Social facilitation and coping with stress. *British Journal of Social Clinical Psychology, 12,* 130–136. (Social facilitation).

Derdiarian, A.K. & Forsythe, A.B. (1983). An instrument for theory and research development using the Behavioral Systems Model for Nursing: The cancer patient. *Nursing Research, 32,* 260–266 (Johnson's Behavioral Systems Model).

DeVon, H.A. & Powers, M.J. (1984). Health beliefs, adjustment to illness, and control of hypertension. *Research in Nursing and Health, 7,* 10–16 (Health Belief Model).

Dodd, M.J. (1984). Measuring informational intervention for chemotherapy knowledge and self-care behavior. *Research in Nursing and Health, 7,* 43–50 (Orem's Self-Care Model).

Erickson, H. & Swain, M.A. (1982). A model for assessing potential adaptation to stress. *Research in Nursing and Health, 5,* 93–101 (Selye's Stress and Adaptation Theory).

Fawcett, J. & Burritt, J. (1985). An exploratory study of antenatal preparation for cesarean birth. *Journal of Obstetric, Gynecologic, and Neonatal Nursing, 14,* 224–230 (Roy's Adaptation Model).

Fitzpatrick, J.J. (1980). Patients' perceptions of time. *International Nursing Review, 27,* 148–153. (Rogers' Model of the Unitary Person).

Floyd, J.A. (1983). Research using Rogers' conceptual system: Development of a testable theorem. *Advances in Nursing Science, 5,* 37–48 (Rogers' Model of the Unitary Person).

Gill, B.P. & Atwood, J.R. (1981). Reciprocity and helicy used to relate MEFG and wound healing. *Nursing Research, 30,* 68–72 (Rogers' Model of the Unitary Person).

Holaday, B.J. (1974). Achievement behavior in chronically ill children. *Nursing Research, 23,* 25–30 (Social Learning Theory).

Holaday, B. (1981). Maternal response to their

chronically ill infants' attachment behavior of crying. *Nursing Research, 30,* 343–348 (Johnson's Behavioral Systems Model).

Itano, J. *et al.* (1983). Compliance of cancer patients to therapy. *Western Journal of Nursing Research, 5,* 5–16 (Health Belief Model).

Kearney, B.Y. & Fleischer, B.J. (1979). Development of an instrument to measure exercise of self-care agency. *Research in Nursing and Health, 2,* 25–34 (Orem's Self-Care Model).

LaMontagne, L.L. (1984). Children's locus of control beliefs as predictors of preoperative coping behavior. *Nursing Research, 33,* 76–79 (Social Learning Theory).

Lowery, B.J. & DuCitte, J.P. (1976). Disease-related learning and disease control in diabetes as a function of locus by control. *Nursing Research, 25,* 358–362 (Social Learning Theory).

Newport, M.A. (1984). Conserving thermal energy and social integrity in the newborn. *Western Journal of Nursing Research, 6,* 175–188 (Levine's Conservation Model).

Norris, S., Campbell, L., & Brenkert, S. (1982). Nursing procedures and alterations in transcutaneous oxygen tension in premature infants. *Nursing Research, 31,* 330–336. (Roy's Adaptation Model).

Patterson, E.T., & Hale, E.S. (1985). Making sure: Integrating menstrual care practices into activities of daily living. *Advances in Nursing Science, 7,* 18–31 (Orem's Self-Care Model).

Rothlis, J. (1984). The effect of a self-help group on feelings of hopelessness and helplessness. *Western Journal of Nursing Research, 6,* 157–168. (Orem's Self-Care Model).

Shannahan, M.D. & Cottrell, B.H. (1985). Effect of the birth chair on duration of second-stage labor, fetal outcome, and maternal blood loss. *Nursing Research, 34,* 89–92 (Roy's Adaptation Model).

Small, B. (1980). Nursing visually impaired children with Johnson's model as a conceptual framework. In J.P. Riehl & C. Roy (eds.), *Conceptual models for nursing practice* (2nd ed.). New York: Appleton-Century-Crofts (Johnson's Behavioral Systems Model).

Toth, J.C. (1980). Effect of structured preparation for transfer on patient anxiety on leaving coronary care unit. *Nursing Research, 29,* 28–34 (Orem's Self-Care Model).

Watts, R.J. (1982). Sexual functioning, health beliefs, and compliance with high blood pressure medications. *Nursing Research, 31,* 278–283 (Health Belief Model).

Ziemer, M.M. (1983). Effects of information on postsurgical coping. *Nursing Research, 32,* 282–287 (Neuman's Health Care Systems Model).

Chapter 7
□
Formulating hypotheses

A hypothesis is a tentative prediction or explanation of the relationship between two or more variables. A hypothesis, in other words, translates the problem statement into a prediction of expected outcomes. It is the hypothesis, rather than the problem statement, that is subjected to empirical testing through the collection and analysis of data.

The researcher normally formulates one or more hypotheses following identification of the problem, a review of the literature, the final conceptualization of the research variables, and identification of a suitable theoretical framework. Research problems, as we have seen, are typically phrased in the form of questions concerning how phenomena are related and interact. Hypotheses, on the other hand, are tentative solutions or answers to such research queries. For instance, the problem statement might ask: Does room temperature affect the optimal placement time of rectal temperature measurements in adults? As a tentative solution to this problem, the researcher might predict the following: "Cooler room temperatures will require longer placement times for rectal temperature measurements in adults than warmer rooms." Hypotheses should generally be developed *before* the conduct of the study itself because it is the hypothesis that gives direction to the gathering and interpretation of data. In the following section we will briefly examine the role of the hypothesis in the research process.

□
Purposes of the research hypothesis

Generally speaking, the function of the hypothesis is to guide scientific inquiry. Various aspects of this function include unifying theory and reality, extending knowledge, and directing research.

Unification of theory and reality

Hypotheses often follow directly from a theoretical framework. The scientist reasons from theories to hypotheses, and tests those hypotheses in the real world. Hypotheses are the conclusions that follow from the premises or assumptions inherent in the theory. Thus, hypotheses are the vehicle through which theories are linked to real-world situations.

Let us take as an example the general theory of reinforcement. This theory maintains that behavior or activity that is positively reinforced (rewarded) will tend to be learned or repeated. Because nurses play an important teaching and guiding role in hospitals or clinical settings, there are many opportunities for this general theory to be incorporated into the context of nursing practice. However, the theory itself is untestable. It makes no explicit prediction, nor does it specify measurable or observable variables. In short, it is too abstract to be put to an empirical test. However, *if* the theory is valid, then it should be possible to make accurate predictions (hypotheses) about certain kinds of behavior in hospitals. For example, the following hypotheses have been deduced from reinforcement theory: (1) Elderly patients who are praised (reinforced) by nursing personnel for self-feeding will require less assistance in feeding than patients who are not praised; and (2) hyperactive children who are given a reward (e.g., cookies or permission to watch television) when they perform a 15-minute motor task without disruption will tend to display less acting-out behavior during task-performance than nonrewarded peers. Both of these propositions can be put to a test in the real world. If the hypotheses are confirmed, the theory will be supported, and we can place more confidence in it.

Extension of knowledge

Not all hypotheses are derived from theory. Even in the absence of a theoretical framework, however, the researcher who proceeds to collect data without having made predictions about the outcome may jeopardize the contribution that the findings can make to human knowledge. Well-conceived hypotheses offer direction and suggest explanations.

Even when hypotheses fail to be confirmed, their presence provides a greater possibility for the advancement of understanding than the absence of hypotheses. Perhaps an example will clarify this point. Suppose we were to hypothesize that nurses who have received a baccalaureate education are more likely to experience stress in their first nursing job than nurses with diploma school education. We could justify our speculation on the grounds of theory (role conflict, cognitive dissonance theory, reality shock theory), on the basis of earlier studies, on personal observations, on the basis of logic, or on the basis of some combination of these. *The need to develop justifications in and of itself forces the researcher to think logically, to exercise critical judgment, and to tie together earlier research findings.* Now let us suppose the above hypothesis is not confirmed by the evidence collected; that is, we find that baccalaureate and diploma nurses demonstrate an equal amount of stress in their first nursing assignment. *The failure of data to support a prediction forces the investigator to critically analyze theory or previous research, to carefully review the limitations of the study's methods, and to explore alternative explanations for the findings.* The use of hypotheses, in other words, induces critical thinking and, hence, promotes understanding.

To pursue the same example, suppose we conducted the investigation without formulating an explicit prediction and were guided only by a problem statement: "Is there a relationship between a nurse's basic preparation and the degree of stress experienced on the first job?" The investigator without a hypothesis is, apparently, prepared to accept any results. The problem is that it is almost always possible to explain something superficially after-the-fact, no matter what the findings are. Hypotheses guard against superficiality and minimize the possibility that spurious results will be misconstrued.

Research direction

Problem statements typically are more vague than research hypotheses. A critical function of hypotheses is to provide direction to the research design and to the collection, analysis, and interpretation of data. Without a hypothesis (or, as is often the case, a set of hypotheses), there is sometimes a tendency for investigators to gather isolated pieces of information that are as unwieldy to analyze as they are meaningless. Hypotheses interconnect variables of interest through statements of formal relationships; it is these relationships that are subjected to an empirical test.

□
Characteristics of workable hypotheses

An essential characteristic of a workable research hypothesis is that it states the predicted relationship between two or more variables. The variables that are related to one another through the hypothesis are the independent variable (the presumed cause or antecedent) and the dependent variable (the presumed effect or phenomenon of primary interest). One of the most common flaws of the predictions of beginning researchers is the failure to make a relational statement. The prediction "Pregnant women who receive prenatal training will have favorable reactions to the labor and delivery experience" is not a hypothesis that can be tested using the scientific approach. This statement expresses no anticipated relationship; in fact, there is only one variable (the woman's

reactions to the labor and delivery experience), and a relationship by definition requires at least two variables. This prediction can, however, be altered to make it a suitable hypothesis with an independent and dependent variable: "Pregnant women who receive prenatal training will have *more* favorable reactions (the dependent variable) to the labor and delivery experience *than* pregnant women with no prenatal training." Here the second variable (the independent variable) is the woman's status with respect to prenatal training: some will have received it and others will not have received it.

The relational aspect of the prediction is embodied in the phrase "more than." If a hypothesis lacks a phrase such as "more than," "less than," "greater than," "different from," "related to," or something similar, it is not amenable to scientific testing. As an example of why this is so, consider the original prediction: Pregnant women who receive prenatal training will have favorable reactions to the labor and delivery experience. How would we know whether the women's reactions are favorable? That is, what absolute standard could be used for deciding whether the women's reactions to their labor and delivery experiences were favorable or not? Perhaps this point will be clearer if we illustrate it more specifically. Suppose that we ask a group of women who have taken an 8-week prenatal training course to respond to the following question*:

On the whole, how would you describe your labor and delivery experience?

1. Very favorably
2. Rather favorably
3. Neither favorably nor unfavorably
4. Rather unfavorably
5. Very unfavorably

---

* This rather simple question is provided primarily for the sake of illustrating the need to have a relational statement in a hypothesis. Normally, a measure of a dependent variable would be somewhat more complex than this example suggests.

Based on this question, how could we compare the actual outcome with the predicted outcome that the women would have favorable responses? Would *all* of the women questioned have to respond "very favorably?" Would our prediction be supported if *half* the women say "very favorably" or "favorably"? There is simply no adequate way of testing the accuracy of the prediction. If we modify the prediction, as suggested above, to "Pregnant women who receive prenatal training will have more favorable reactions to the labor and delivery experience than pregnant women with no prenatal training," a test is quite simple. We could simply ask two groups of women with different prenatal training experiences to respond to the question and then compare the responses of the two groups. The absolute degree of favorability of either group would not be at issue.

Hypotheses, ideally, should be based on a sound, justifiable rationale. The most defensible hypotheses follow from previous research findings or are deduced from a theory. When a new area is being investigated, the researcher may have to turn to logical reasoning or personal experience in order to justify the predictions. There are, however, very few topics for which research evidence is totally lacking.

A good hypothesis should be consistent with an existing body of research findings. This requirement may in some cases be difficult to satisfy since it is not uncommon to find conflicting results on some topics in the research literature. For example, Clark and Clark (1984) critically reviewed the research literature relating to the effectiveness of therapeutic touch as a treatment modality, and found inconsistent findings. Some investigators have found that therapeutic touch results in an increase of hemoglobin levels, increased relaxation, and reduced anxiety, while other investigators have found no differences among those treated and those not treated with therapeutic touch. Obviously, when the findings from previous research are inconsistent, it is impossible for the hypothesis to be consistent with all the findings! The researcher must then make a decision, and a good solid basis for such a decision is the critical evaluation of the methods used in earlier studies. The investigator should attempt to understand *why* conflicting results occurred through an examination of the research approach.

□
The derivation of hypotheses

Many students ask the question "How do I go about the task of developing hypotheses?" There are no formal rules for deriving hypotheses, but we can perhaps offer some suggestions by discussing two broad types of approach. Like the development of problem statements, the sources most likely to be fruitful as a basis for the formulation of hypotheses are theoretical systems, experience and observation of practical problems, or readings in related literature. However, two basic processes — induction and deduction — constitute the intellectual machinery involved in deriving hypotheses.

An *inductive hypothesis* is a generalization based on observed relationships. The researcher observes certain patterns, trends, or associations among phenomena and then uses these observations as a basis for a tentative explanation or prediction. Related literature should be examined in order to learn what is already known on a topic, but an important source of ideas for inductive hypotheses is the researcher's own experiences, combined with intuition and critical analysis. For example, a nurse may notice that presurgical patients who ask a lot of questions relating to pain or express many pain-related apprehensions have a more difficult time in learning appropriate postoperative procedures. The nurse could then formulate a hypothesis that could be tested through more rigorous scientific procedures. The following hypothesis might be derived: "Patients who are stressed by fears of pain will have more difficulty in deep breathing and coughing after their surgery than patients who are not stressed."

The other mechanism for deriving hypotheses is through *deduction*. As pointed out earlier, theories of how phenomena behave and interrelate cannot be tested directly. Through deductive reasoning a researcher can develop scientific expectations or hypotheses based on general theoretical principles. Inductive hypotheses begin with specific observations and move toward generalizations; deductive hypotheses have as a starting point general "laws" or theories that are applied to particular situations.

While a full explication of deductive logic is beyond the scope of this text, the following syllogism illustrates the reasoning process involved:

All human beings have red and white blood cells.
John Doe is a human being.
Therefore, John Doe has red and white blood cells.

In this simple example, the "hypothesis" is that John Doe does, in fact, have red and white blood cells, a deduction that could be verified.

If a nurse researcher is familiar with a theory relating to phenomena of interest, the theory can serve as a valuable point of departure for the development of hypotheses. The researcher must ask the question, "If this theory is correct or valid, what would the logical consequences be in terms of a situation that interests me?" In other words, the researcher *deduces* that if the general law is true, specific outcomes or consequences can be expected. The specific predictions derived from general principles must then be subjected to further testing through the collection of empirical data. If these data are in fact congruent with hypothesized outcomes, then the theory is strengthened.

The advancement of scientific research depends on both inductive and deductive hypotheses. Ideally, a cyclical process is set in motion, wherein the researcher makes observations; formulates hypotheses inductively; makes systematic, controlled observations; develops theoretical systems; deduces hypotheses; seeks new systematic observations; rethinks the hypotheses or theories; modifies them inductively; and so forth. The scientific researcher needs to be an organizer of concepts (think inductively), a logician (think deductively) and, above all, a critic and a skeptic of resulting formulations.

☐
Wording the hypothesis

As previously noted, a workable hypothesis is one that is congruent with existing theory and research, states a relationship between two (or more) variables, and is testable. In this section we will look at how the hypothesis should be stated and provide examples of various kinds of hypotheses.

A good hypothesis is worded in simple, clear, and concise language and provides a definition of the variables in concrete, operational terms. These two requirements may in some cases be conflicting if the operational definition needs extensive explanation. If it is not too awkward to incorporate the operational definition of terms within the statement of the hypothesis itself, the researcher should attempt to do so. However, if the hypothesis is too unwieldy or unclear, the variables should be operationally defined separately, following the hypothesis statement. The hypothesis should, however, be specific enough so that the reader understands what the variables are and whom the researcher will be studying.

Simple versus complex hypotheses

For the purpose of this text, we will define *simple hypotheses* as hypotheses that express an expected relationship between *one* independent and *one* dependent variable. A *complex hypothesis* refers to a prediction of a rela-

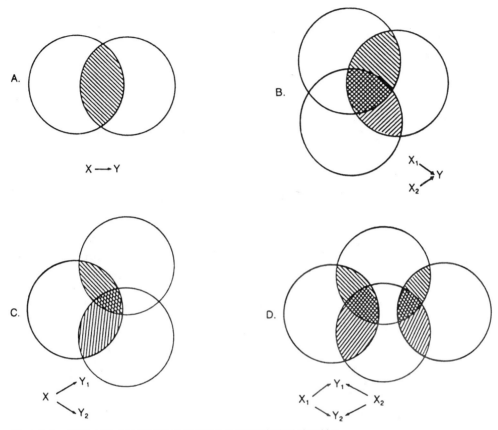

Figure 7-1. Schematic representation of various hypothetical relationships.

tionship between two (or more) independent variables and/or two (or more) dependent variables. Sometimes complex hypotheses are referred to as *multivariate hypotheses* (because they involve multiple variables).

We will give some concrete examples of both types of hypotheses, but let us first explain the differences in abstract terms. Simple hypotheses state a relationship between a single independent variable, which we will call "X," and a single dependent variable, which we will label "Y." Our Y variable is the predicted effect, outcome, or consequence of our X variable, which is the presumed cause, antecedent, or precondition. The nature of this relationship is presented graphically in Figure

7-1,A. In Figure 7-1,A, the hatched area of the circles, representing variables X and Y, can be taken to signify the strength of the relationship between these two variables. If there were a one-to-one correspondence between variables X and Y, the two circles would completely overlap and the entire area would be hatched. If the variables were totally unrelated, the circles would not converge or overlap at all.

In the real world, the majority of phenomena are the result, not of one variable, but of a complex network of many variables. A person's weight, for example, is affected simultaneously by such factors as the person's height, diet, bone structure, and metabolism. If the

Table 7-1
Examples of Hypotheses

Hypothesis

1. Infants born to heroin-addicted mothers have lower birth weights than infants of nonaddicted mothers.
2. There is a relationship between tactile and auditory stimulation and heart rate response in premature infants.
3. Older nurses are less likely to express approval of the expanding role of nurses than younger nurses.
4. Structured preoperative support is more effective in reducing surgical patients' perception of pain and requests for analgesics than structured postoperative support.
5. Teenage girls are better informed about the risks of venereal disease than teenage boys.
6. Nurses who are scheduled by the block rotation method will have a lower number of reported sick days and express a higher level of job satisfaction than nurses scheduled by a random rotation method.
7. Nursing students who have been with a patient who dies will be more likely to report a physical complaint within 72 hours than students who have not had this experience.
8. Patients who have a primary nurse assigned to them on admission report a more favorable impression of their nursing care than patients who do not have a primary nurse assigned on admission.
9. Patients who receive a copy of the "Patient's Bill of Rights" ask more questions about their treatment and diagnosis than those who do not receive this document.
10. Patients with a leg amputation who practice the prone lying position will develop fewer contractures than patients with a leg amputation who do not lie prone.

dependent variable (Y in Figure 7-1,A) is weight and the independent variable (X) is a person's caloric intake, we would not be able to completely explain or understand individual variation in weight. Knowing that Mr. A's daily caloric intake averaged 2500 calories would not allow us to predict with much precision what his weight is. Knowledge of other factors, such as Mr. A's height, would improve the accuracy with which his weight could be predicted.

Figure 7-1,B presents a schematic representation of a design that examines the simultaneous effect of two independent variables on a single dependent variable. The complex hypothesis would state the nature of the relationship between Y on the one hand and X_1 and X_2 on the other. To pursue the example above,

the hypothesis might be "Taller people (X_1) and people with higher caloric intake (X_2) will weight more (Y) than shorter people and individuals with lower caloric intake." As the figure shows, a larger proportion of the area of Y is hatched when there are two independent variables than when there is only one. This means that caloric intake *and* height do a better job in helping us understand weight (Y) than caloric intake alone. Complex hypotheses thus have the advantage of allowing researchers to capture some of the complexity of the real world. It is not always possible, of course, to design a study with complex hypotheses. A number of practical considerations, including the researcher's technical skills, resources, and time, may render the testing of complex hypotheses impossible or

Independent Variable	Dependent Variable	Simple or Complex
Addiction or nonaddiction of infant's mother	Birth weight	Simple
a. Tactile stimulation; b. auditory stimulation	Heart rate response	Complex
Age of nurses	Approval of nurses' expanding role	Simple
Timing of nursing intervention	a. Surgical patients' pain perception; b. requests for analgesics	Complex
Gender of teenager	Knowledge about venereal disease	Simple
Schedule method	a. Absenteeism; b. level of job satisfaction	Complex
Experiencing death of patient	Physical complaint	Simple
Assignment of primary nurse	Impression of nursing care	Simple
Receipt of "Patient's Bill of Rights"	Number of questions asked by patients	Simple
Type of position	Development of contractures	Simple

inadvisable. It should be understood, however, that an important goal of research is to explain the dependent variable as thoroughly as possible and that two or more independent variables are typically more successful than one alone.

Just as a phenomenon can be understood as resulting from more than one independent variable, so a single independent variable can have an effect on, or can be antecedent to, more than one phenomenon. Part C of Figure 7-1 illustrates this type of relationship. A number of studies have found, for example, that cigarette smoking (X) can lead to lung cancer (Y_1) and coronary disorders (Y_2). This type of an approach is very common in studies that try to assess the impact of a nursing intervention on a variety of criterion measures of patient

well-being. Finally, the most complex type of hypothesis,* which links two or more independent variables to two or more dependent variables, is shown in Figure 7-1,D.

Table 7-1 presents ten specific examples of simple and complex hypotheses. Most of these hypotheses would need further elaboration in terms of the specification of operational definitions, but each of these hypotheses is potentially testable and each delineates a predicted relationship. Beginning research students should carefully scrutinize this table in order to familiarize themselves with the language and style of scientific hypotheses. The first column specifies the hypotheses them-

* A special kind of complex hypothesis, known as an *interaction hypothesis,* is described in Chapter 8.

selves, while the last three columns indicate the independent and dependent variable for each hypothesis and designate whether it is simple or complex.

It should be pointed out that, although researchers typically adopt a certain style in the phrasing of hypotheses, there is some degree of flexibility allowed. The same hypothesis can generally be stated in a variety of ways, so long as the researcher specifies (or implies) the relationship that will be tested. As an example of how a hypothesis can be reworded while maintaining its integrity and usefulness, let us state hypothesis 3 from Table 7-1 in a variety of ways:

1. Older nurses are less likely to express approval of the expanding roles of nurses than younger nurses.
2. There is a relationship between the age of a nurse and approval of the nurse's expanding role.
3. The older the nurse, the less likely it is that she or he will approve of the nurse's expanding role.
4. Older nurses will differ from younger nurses with respect to approval of the nurse's expanding role.
5. Younger nurses will tend to be more approving of the nurse's expanding role than older nurses.
6. Approval of the nurse's expanding role decreases as the age of the nurse increases.

A number of other variations of the wording of this hypothesis are also possible. The important point to remember is that the statement should specify the independent and dependent variables and the anticipated relationship between them.

Directional versus nondirectional hypotheses

Sometimes hypotheses are described as being either directional or nondirectional. A *direc-*

tional hypothesis is one that specifies the expected direction of the relationship between variables. That is, the researcher predicts not only the existence of a relationship, but also the nature of the relationship. In the six versions of the same hypothesis above, versions 1, 3, 5, and 6 are all directional because there is an explicit expectation that older nurses will be less approving of the expanding role of nurses than younger nurses.

A *nondirectional hypothesis,* by contrast, does not stipulate the direction of the relationship. Such a hypothesis predicts that two or more variables are related but makes no projections concerning the exact nature of the association. The second and fourth variations in the example illustrate the wording of nondirectional hypotheses. These hypotheses state the prediction that a nurse's age and degree of approval of the nurse's changing role are related; they do not stipulate, however, whether the researcher thinks that older nurses or younger nurses will be more approving.

Deductive hypotheses derived from theory will almost always be directional, because theories attempt to explain phenomena and, hence, provide a rationale for expecting variables to behave in certain ways. Existing studies also supply, typically, a basis for directional hypotheses. When there is no theory or related research, when the findings of related studies are contradictory, or when the researcher's own experience results in ambivalent expectations, the investigator may use nondirectional hypotheses. Some people argue, in fact, that nondirectional hypotheses are generally preferable because they connote a degree of impartiality or objectivity. Directional hypotheses, it is said, carry the implication that the researcher is intellectually committed to a certain outcome, and such a commitment might lead to bias. This argument fails to recognize that researchers typically do have specific expectations or hunches concerning the outcomes, whether they state those expectations explicitly or not. Directional hypotheses have three distinct advantages: (1) they demonstrate that the researcher has thought critically and carefully about the phenomena under investigation; (2) they make clear to the readers of a research report the framework within which the study was conducted; and (3) they may permit a more sensitive statistical test of the hypothesis. This last point, which refers to whether the researcher chooses a one-tailed or two-tailed statistical test, is a rather fine point that is discussed in Chapter 21.

Research versus statistical hypotheses

Hypotheses are sometimes classified as being either research hypotheses or statistical hypotheses. *Research hypotheses* (also referred to as substantive, declarative, or scientific hypotheses) are statements of expected relationships between variables. All of the hypotheses in Table 7-1 are research hypotheses. Such hypotheses indicate what the researcher expects to find as a result of conducting the study.

The logic of statistical inference operates on principles that are somewhat confusing to many beginning students. This logic requires that hypotheses be expressed such that *no* relationship is expected. *Statistical hypotheses* (also known as *null hypotheses*) state that there is no relationship between the independent and dependent variables. The null form of Hypothesis 1 in Table 7-1 would be: "Infants born to heroin-addicted mothers have birth weights comparable to those of infants born to nonaddicted mothers." As another illustration, the null hypothesis for example 2 would read: "There is no relationship between tactile and auditory stimulation and heart rate response in premature infants." The null hypothesis might be compared to the assumption of innocence of an accused criminal in our system of justice: the variables are assumed to be "innocent" of any relationship until they can be shown "guilty" through appropriate statistical procedures. The null hypothesis represents the formal statement of this assumption of innocence.

In designing a study, the researcher is typically concerned only with the research hypotheses. While some research reports do express the hypotheses in null form, it is more common (and more desirable) to state the researcher's actual expectations. When statistical tests are performed, the underlying null hypothesis is usually assumed without being explicitly stated.

☐
Testing the hypothesis

The testing of hypotheses constitutes the heart of empirical investigations. It must again be emphasized, however, that neither theories nor hypotheses are ever proven in an ultimate sense through hypothesis testing. It is inappropriate to say that the data "proved" the validity of the hypothesis, or that the conclusions "proved" the worthiness of the theory. Such statements are inappropriate not only because they are not congruent with the limitations of the scientific approach but also because they are inconsistent with the fundamentally skeptical attitudes of scientists. Scientists are basically doubters and skeptics, who are constantly seeking objective, replicable evidence as a basis for understanding natural phenomena. Findings are always considered tentative. Certainly, if the same results are repeatedly produced in a large number of investigations, then greater confidence can be placed in the conclusions. Hypotheses, then, come to be increasingly accepted or believed with mounting evidence, but ultimate proof is rarely possible. Nor, for that matter, is ultimate falsification of a hypothesis possible.

Let us look more closely at why this is so. Suppose we hypothesize that there is a relationship between height and weight. We predict that, on the average, tall people weigh more than short people. We would then take a sample of people, obtain height and weight measurements, and analyze the results. Now suppose we happened by chance to choose a sample that consisted of short, fat people, and tall, thin people. Our results might then indicate that there is no relationship between an individual's height and weight. Would we then be justified in stating that "this study proved that height and weight in humans are not related?" A second example illustrates the converse principle. Suppose we hypothesize that taller persons are better nurses than shorter persons. This hypothesis is used here only to illustrate a point, since, in reality, one might suspect that there is no relationship between height and nurse's job performance. Now suppose that, by chance again, we hit upon a sample of nurses in which the taller nurses happen to receive better job evaluations by their supervisors than short nurses. Could we conclude definitively that height is related to a nurse's performance? These two examples illustrate the difficulty of using observations from a sample to generalize to the broader group (the population) from which the sample has been taken. Other problems, such as the accuracy of our measures, the validity of underlying assumptions, the reasonableness of our logical deductions, and rapid changes in technologies and in society, prohibit us from concluding with finality that our hypotheses are proven.

☐
Concluding note: are hypotheses required?

In the first section of this chapter we reviewed the various important functions that scientific hypotheses play in the research process. The reader may be wondering: Is a hypothesis always necessary? Most research that can be classified as descriptive proceeds without an explicit hypothesis. Descriptive research, that is, research that aims predominantly at describing phenomena rather than explaining them, is very common in the emerging field of nursing research. Examples of descriptive investigations include studies of the health needs of elderly citizens, studies of the coping patterns of mothers of handicapped children, and surveys of the nutritional status of low-income pre-school children. This type of study is often extremely important in laying a foundation for later research. When a field is new, it may be quite difficult to provide adequate justification for the development of explanatory hypotheses because of a dearth of facts or previous findings. Studies that have a phenomenological perspective generally proceed without hypotheses because their aim is to provide an opportunity for the human experience to be revealed without preconceived restrictions. Thus, there are some studies of a descriptive or exploratory nature for which hypotheses may not be required.

However, initial efforts to investigate phenomena using the scientific approach are often strengthened by the formulation of hypotheses. Even when related literature on a topic is lacking, a nurse's experience is an extremely valuable source of ideas for predicting outcomes. Descriptive studies whose goal is to depict the status quo of some situation typically have some broader purpose in mind. A study that aims to describe nursing students' attitudes toward the mentally ill, for example, could have implications for nursing education. It seems likely that the ability to understand how attitudes toward mental illness are related to various characteristics of the students would have much more meaningful educational implications than a pure attitudinal description. Do nursing students in different specialty areas have more favorable attitudes than others? Does personal contact with a mentally ill person affect attitudes? What role do the student's age, social class, academic record, or emotional stability play? The answers to these questions might not only be interesting but also could lead to more useful approaches to making the student's attitudes toward mental illness more positive. These questions go beyond pure description; they deal with relationships. Where there is a relationship, there is a potential hypothesis.

☐
Research example

Earlier in this chapter we mentioned a research review that found conflicting findings regarding the effectiveness of therapeutic touch. Randolph (1984) conducted a study designed to shed additional light on this topic. Her study examined the physiological responses to therapeutic touch as opposed to normal physical touch among subjects exposed to a stressful stimulus (viewing of a stress-invoking film). Sixty healthy female subjects watched the film; half were touched by therapeutic touch practitioners, and the remaining half were touched by nurses not trained in therapeutic touch. Randolph developed three hypotheses regarding expected differences in the physiological response of subjects in the two groups. For example, it was hypothesized that the "Muscle tension level of female college students treated with physical touch will exceed the muscle tension level of female college students treated with therapeutic touch." (p. 33). All three hypotheses were simple, directional hypotheses. None of the hypotheses was supported. Nevertheless, the care that Randolph took in developing the hypotheses provided overall direction for the study. The hypotheses guided her in performing the data collection, in identifying the kind of sample she had to obtain, and in selecting the types of comparisons and analyses she was to perform. Randolph's findings add to the challenge of those advocating therapeutic touch to demonstrate the effectiveness of this procedure as a treatment modality.

☐
Summary

A hypothesis is a statement concerning predicted relationships among variables. The successful progression from initial problem statement to the final collection and analysis of data is often intimately associated with the development of one or more clear, workable hypotheses. Hypotheses are important because (1) they serve as a link between theory and real-world situations, (2) they provide an effective mechanism for extending knowledge, and (3) they offer overall direction for the investigation.

A workable hypothesis must specify the anticipated *relationship* between two or more variables. That is, the researcher must state the hypothesized association between the independent and dependent variables. A hypothesis that projects a result for only one variable is essentially untestable because there is typically no criterion for assessing absolute, as opposed to relative, outcomes. A good hypothesis should also be justifiable. In other words, it should be consistent with existing theory or knowledge (or with the researcher's own experiences) and with logical reasoning.

Knowledge and experience in an area and familiarity with related research and theory are important sources for the development of hypotheses. Hypotheses are derived either through inductive, observational processes or through deductive, theory-based processes.

Hypotheses can be classified according to various characteristics. *Simple hypotheses* express a predicted relationship between one independent and one dependent variable, while *complex hypotheses* state an anticipated relationship between two or more independent and/or two or more dependent variables. Complex hypotheses are powerful because they offer the possibility of mirroring the complexity of the real world. A *directional hypothesis* specifies the expected direction or nature of a hypothesized relationship. *Nondirectional* hypotheses denote a relationship but do not stipulate the precise form that the relationship will take. Directional hypotheses are generally preferable. Sometimes a distinction between research and statistical hypotheses is made. *Research hypotheses* predict the existence of relationships; *statistical* or *null* hypotheses express the absence of any relationships. This latter type is related to the logic of statistical inference and is often assumed without being formally stated. These classifications illustrate the fact that there is some flexibility in the wording of hypotheses.

After hypotheses are developed and refined, they are subjected to an empirical test through the collection, analysis, and interpretation of data. It must be stressed, however, that hypotheses are never proved or disproved in an ultimate sense. Scientists say that hypotheses are "accepted" or "rejected," "supported" or "not supported." Through replication of studies, hypotheses and theories can gain increasing acceptance, but scientists, who are essentially skeptics, avoid the use of the word "proof."

It was noted in conclusion that not all investigations are designed to test hypotheses. Descriptive research, which focuses on a depiction of the status quo of some situation rather than on explanation, often proceeds without a hypothesis. Exploratory research and phenomenological research may also not require hypotheses. However, many exploratory studies that adopt the scientific approach can be strengthened by a statement of predicted outcomes.

☐
Study suggestions

1. Below are five hypotheses. For each hypothesis, give a possible problem statement from which the hypothesis might have been developed.
   a. Absenteeism is higher among nurses in intensive care units than among nurses on other wards.
   b. Patients who are not told their diagnosis report more subjective feelings of stress than do patients who are told their diagnosis.
   c. Patients receiving intravenous therapy will report greater nighttime sleep pattern disturbances than patients not receiving intravenous therapy.
   d. Patients with roommates will call for a nurse less often than patients without roommates.
   e. Women who have participated in Lamaze classes will request pain medication less often than will women who have not undergone these classes.
2. For each of the five hypotheses in Suggestion 1, indicate whether the hypothesis is simple or complex, and directional or nondirectional.
3. For each hypothesis in Suggestion 1, state the independent and dependent variables.
4. State the five hypotheses in Suggestion 1 in null form.
5. Below are five problem statements. Develop a hypothesis based on each one. Try to state each hypothesis in more than one way.
   a. Are verbalized feelings of helplessness by patients related to the amount of ambulation permitted by the patients' conditions?
   b. Is the clinical specialty of nurses related to their attitudes toward alcoholism?
   c. Are nutritional habits related to a person's age and sex?
   d. Is there a relationship between the prematurity of an infant and the mother's smoking behavior?
   e. Do nurse practitioners perform triage functions as well as physicians?
6. Read one or more articles of the readings suggested for the "Substantive References." Discuss the adequacy of the hypotheses cited in terms of the existence of a relational statement and the justifiability of the hypotheses.

□
Suggested readings

Methodological references

Abdellah, F. & Levine, E. (1978). *Better patient care through nursing research* (2nd ed.). New York: Macmillan. (pp. 122–137).

Kerlinger, F. (1973). *Foundations of behavioral research* (2nd ed.). New York: Holt, Rinehart and Winston. (Chapter 2).

Pavlovich, N. (1978). *Nursing Research: A learning guide.* St. Louis: C.V. Mosby. (Chapter 3).

Popper, K.R. (1959). *The logic of scientific discovery* (Rev. ed.). New York: Basic Books. (Chapter 10).

Smith, M. (1971). Hypothesis versus problem solving in scientific investigation. In B.J. Franklin & H.W. Osborne (eds.). *Research methods: Issues and insights.* Belmont, CA: Wadsworth Publishing. (pp. 111–117).

Treece, E.W. & Treece, J.W., Jr. (1982). *Elements of research in nursing* (3rd ed.). St. Louis: C.V. Mosby. (Chapter 8).

Wilson, H.S. (1985). *Research in Nursing.* Menlo Park, CA: Addison-Wesley. (Chapter 9).

Substantive references*

Beck, C.T. (1983). Parturients' temporal experiences during the phases of labor. *Western Journal of Nursing Research, 5,* 283–294.

Brouse, S.H. (1985). Effect of gender role identity on patterns of feminine and self-concept scores from late pregnancy to early postpartum. *Advances in Nursing Sciences, 7,* 32–48.

Byrne, T.J. & Edeani, D. (1984). Knowledge of medical terminology among hospital patients. *Nursing Research, 33,* 178–181.

Dawson, C. (1985). Hypertension, perceived clinical empathy, and patient self-disclosure. *Research in Nursing and Health, 8,* 191–198.

Dooher, M.E. (1980). Lamaze method of childbirth. *Nursing Research, 29,* 220–224.

Douglas, S. & Larson, E.L. (1985). The effect of a positive end expiratory pressure adapter on oxygenation during endotracheal suctioning. *Heart & Lung, 14,* 396–400.

Laffrey, S.C. (1985). Health behavior choice as related to self-actualization and health conception. *Western Journal of Nursing Research, 7,* 279–300.

Lewandowski, L.A. & Kramer, M. (1980). Role transformation of special care unit nurses. *Nursing Research, 29,* 170–179.

Randolph, G.L. (1984). Therapeutic and physical touch: Physiological response to stressful stimuli. *Nursing Research, 33,* 33–36.

Thompson, T. (1980). An ordinal evaluation of the consumer participation process in community health programs. *Nursing Research, 29,* 50–54.

Tompkins, E.S. (1980). Effect of restricted mobility and dominance on perceived duration. *Nursing Research, 29,* 333–338.

Other reference cited

Clark, P.E. & Clark, M.J. (1984). Therapeutic touch: Is there a scientific basis for the practice? *Nursing Research, 33,* 37–41.

* These studies are included here because they present clearly stated hypotheses.

Part III

Designs
for
nursing
research

Chapter 8
□
Experiments and quasi-experiments

The choice of an overall research approach constitutes one of the many major decisions that must be made in conducting a research study. In some cases the nature of the research problem will dictate the approach to be taken. More often, however, there is considerable flexibility in the decision-making process. While this flexibility can introduce complications — in the sense that the reseachers must be familiar with the options and must exercise judgment in the selection — it also provides the investigators with ample opportunity to exercise their creativity.

This section of the text examines some of the basic kinds of research strategies that have been used in nursing research. In this chapter we will examine two research approaches that are typically more scientifically rigorous than other types of research. Experiments and quasi-experiments differ from nonexperimental research activities in one very important respect: the researcher is an active agent in experimental work rather than a passive observer. Early physical scientists learned that while observation of natural phenomena is valuable and instructive, the complexity of the events occurring in the natural state often obscures understanding of important relationships. This problem was handled by isolating the phenomenon of interest in a laboratory setting and controlling the conditions under which it occurred. The procedures developed by physical scientists were profitably adopted by biologists during the nineteenth century, resulting in many achievements in physiology and medicine. The twentieth century has witnessed the utilization of experimental methods by scholars and researchers interested in human behavior and psychological states.

☐
Characteristics of true experiments

In methodological parlance an experiment has a very precise and unambiguous meaning. An experiment is a scientific investigation characterized by the following properties:

1. *Manipulation*—the experimenter *does* something to at least some of the subjects in the study.
2. *Control*—the experimenter introduces one or more controls over the experimental situation, including the use of a control group.
3. *Randomization*—the experimenter assigns subjects to a control or experimental group on a random basis.

Each of these properties is discussed here in detail. It might be well to mention, however, that the controlled experiment is considered the ideal of science. Except for purely descriptive research, the aim of scientific research is to understand the relationships between phenomena: Does a certain drug cause the cure of a certain disease? Do certain nursing techniques produce a decrease in patient anxiety? The strength of the true experiment over other methods lies in the fact that the experimenter can achieve greater confidence in the genuineness and interpretability of relationships because they are observed under carefully controlled conditions. As we have pointed out in earlier chapters, hypotheses are never ultimately proved or disproved by scientific methods, but true experiments offer the most convincing evidence concerning the effects one variable can have on another.

Manipulation

It was mentioned above that manipulation involves *doing* something to at least one group of subjects. The introduction of that "something" (often referred to as the *experimental treatment* or *experimental intervention*) constitutes the independent variable. The experimenter manipulates the independent variable by administering it to some subjects and withholding it from others (or by administering some other treatment such as a placebo). The experimenter, in other words, consciously *varies* the independent variable and observes the effect that the manipulation has on the dependent variable of interest.

A couple of examples should help to clarify this point. Let us say we have hypothesized that the color of a pediatric nurse's uniform affects the degree to which children display positive and negative affective behaviors (e.g., smiling, laughing, crying, whining) during hospitalization. The independent or presumed causative variable in this example is uniform color, which can be manipulated by assigning some nurses (for instance) white uniforms and other nurses brightly colored uniforms. Thus, in this study we could compare the affective behaviors (the dependent variables) of two groups of children: those cared for by white-uniformed nurses and those cared for by nurses in colored uniforms. This simple design is sometimes referred to as an *after-only* or *posttest-only* experimental design because data are only collected after the experimental treatment is completed.

A second example serves to illustrate a slightly more complex design. Let us suppose that we are interested in investigating the effect on heart rate of being physically restrained by posey belt. We might choose to begin our experimentation with some subhuman species such as the rat. We decide to use an experimental scheme such as the one shown in Figure 8-1. This design involves imposing restraint by posey belt on one group of rats (the experimental group) while imposing no restraint on another (the control group). In this design the dependent variable is measured at two points in time, before and after the experimental intervention (physical re-

Before   After

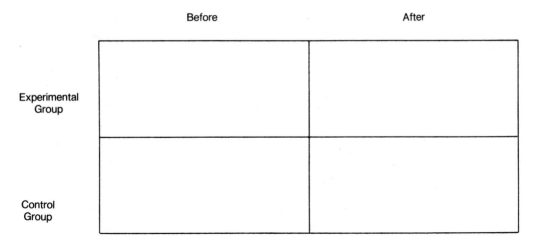

Experimental
Group

Control
Group

Figure 8-1. Before–after experimental design.

straint). This scheme permits us to examine what changes in heart rate were produced as a result of being physically restrained, our independent variable. This design, because of its two measurement points, is referred to as a *before-after* or *pretest-posttest* experimental design.

Control

The notion of control in an experimental context actually summarizes all of the major experimental activities: control is acquired by manipulating, by randomizing, by the careful preparation of the experimental protocols, and by the use of a comparison group or groups. This section will focus on the function of the control group.

As Campbell and Stanley (1963) have observed, obtaining scientific evidence requires making at least one comparison. If we were to supplement the diet of a group of premature neonates with a particular combination of vitamins and other nutrients every day for two weeks, the weight of these infants at the end of the two-week period would give us absolutely no information about the effectiveness of the

treatment. At a bare minimum we would need to compare their posttreatment weight with their pretreatment weight to determine if, at least, their weight had increased. But let us assume for the moment that we find an average weight gain of one pound. Does this finding support the conclusion that there is a causative relationship between the vitamin supplements (the independent variable) and weight gain (the dependent variable)? No, it does not. Babies will normally gain weight as they mature. Without a control group—a group that does *not* receive the nutritional supplements —it is impossible to separate the effects of maturation from those of the treatment. The introduction of a control group permits us to design our research study according to the scheme in Figure 8-1. The term control group, in other words, refers to a group of subjects whose performance on a dependent variable is used as a basis for evaluating the performance of the experimental group (the group that receives the treatment of interest to the researcher) on the same dependent variable.

One further aspect of control groups should be noted. In some biological, medical, and psychological research the experimenter administers the treatment of interest to the experimental group while the control group receives no treatment at all and is merely observed with respect to behavior on the dependent variable. This kind of situation probably is not feasible for many nursing research projects because it may not be possible to isolate a control group and do nothing to it. For example, if we wanted to evaluate the effectiveness of some nursing intervention on hospital patients, it would be unlikely that we would devise an experiment in which one group of patients received no nursing care at all. We would have to evaluate our new intervention not against the total absence of care but, rather, against a control group receiving conventional methods of care. This type of an arrangement is perfectly acceptable and in no way diminishes the status of the study as an experiment.

Randomization

Earlier in the chapter it was said that randomization involves the assignment of subjects to groups on a random basis. The term random essentially means that every subject has an equal chance of being assigned to any group. If subjects are placed in groups randomly, there is no *systematic bias* in the groups with respect to attributes that may affect the dependent variable under investigation.

Before going on to discuss the mechanics of random assignment, we should pause to consider the function of randomization. Suppose a researcher wishes to study the effectiveness of a hospital-based contraceptive counseling program for a group of multiparous women who have just given birth. Two groups of subjects are established, one of which will be counseled and the other of which will receive no counseling. The women as a whole may be expected to differ on a number of characteristics, such as age, marital status, financial situa-

tion, attitude toward the parent role, and the like. Any of these chacteristics could have an effect on the diligence with which a woman practices contraception, quite independent of whether or not she receives counseling. The researcher naturally wants to have the "counsel" and "no counsel" groups equal with respect to these extraneous characteristics in order to adequately assess the impact of the counseling. The random assignment of subjects to one group or the other is designed to perform this equalization function. One method might be to flip a coin for each woman (more elaborate procedures are discussed later). If the coin is "heads" the woman would be assigned to one group, and if the coin is "tails" she would be assigned to the other group.

The reader must be warned, however, that while randomization is the preferred scientific method for equalizing groups, there is no guarantee that they will, in fact, be equal. Let us take as an extreme example the case in which only ten women, all of whom have given birth to at least four children, have volunteered to participate in the study. Five of the ten women are aged 35 or older and the remaining five are under 35. One would anticipate that a random assignment of women to a control and experimental group would result in approximately two or three women from the two age ranges in each group. But let us suppose that by chance alone the older five women ended up in the experimental group. Because these women are nearing the end of their childbearing years, the likelihood of their conceiving is diminished. Thus, followups on their subsequent reproductive behavior (the dependent variable) might suggest that the counseling program was successful for the experimental group; however, a higher birth rate for the control group may only reflect the age and, hence, fecundability difference and not the lack of exposure to counseling.

Despite this possibility, randomization remains the most trustworthy and acceptable method of equalizing groups. Unusual or deviant assignments such as this one are rare, and the likelihood of obtaining grossly unequal groups is reduced as the number of subjects increases.

Students often wonder why the researcher does not consciously control those subject characteristics that are likely to affect the experimental outcome. The procedure that is sometimes used to accomplish this is known as *matching*. For example, if matching were used in the hypothetical study described above, the researcher might want to ensure that if there were one married, 38-year-old woman with six children in the "counsel" group, there would be a married, 38-year-old woman with six children in the control group as well. There are two serious problems with the matching approach, however. First of all, in order to match we must know what the characteristics that are likely to affect the dependent variable *are*. This knowledge is not always available. Secondly, even if we knew the relevant traits, the complications of matching on more than three or four characteristics are prohibitive. With random assignment, on the other hand, *all* possible distinguishing characteristics—age, sex, intelligence, blood type, religious affiliation, and so on—are likely to be equally distributed in all groups. Over the long run, the groups tend to be counterbalanced with respect to an infinite number of biological, psychological, or environmental traits.

To demonstrate how random assignment is actually performed, we will turn to another example. Suppose we have 15 children who are about to have a tonsillectomy and we are interested in testing the effectiveness of two alternative nursing interventions on the child's level of preoperative anxiety. One intervention might focus on structured information regarding the activities of the surgical team (Procedural Information); the other might focus on structured information regarding what the child will feel (Sensation Information). A third group will receive no special intervention. Five children will be in each of the three groups. Since there are three groups, we can no longer use the flip of a coin to decide the group to which an individual will be assigned. One possibility would be to write the names of the individuals on slips of paper, put the slips into a hat, and then draw names. The first five individuals whose names were drawn would be assigned to Group I, the second five would be assigned to Group II, and the remaining five would be assigned to Group III.

Pulling names from a hat involves considerable work, especially if there are many subjects. Researchers typically use a table of random numbers to facilitate the randomization process. A portion of such a table is reproduced in Table 8-1. A random number table is set up by using the digits from 0 to 9 in such a way that each number is equally likely to follow any other. These tables are often generated by computers. Going in any direction from any point in the table produces a random sequence.

To return to the example at hand, we would number the fifteen individuals from 1 to 15, as shown in the second column of Table 8-2 and then draw numbers between 1 and 15 from the random number table. A simple procedure for finding a starting point is to close your eyes and let your finger fall at some point on the table. For the sake of following the example, let us assume that we have done this and that the starting point is at number 52 as circled on Table 8-1. We can now move from that point in any direction on the table. Our task is to select the first five numbers that fall between 01 and 15. Let us move from the starting point to the right, looking at two-digit combinations to be sure to get numbers from 10 to 15. The next number to the right of 52 is 06. The person

Table 8-1
Small table of random digits

46 85 05 23 26	34 67 75 83 00	74 91 06 43 45
69 24 89 34 60	45 30 50 75 21	61 31 83 18 55
14 01 33 17 92	59 74 76 72 77	76 50 33 45 13
56 30 38 73 15	16 (52) 06 96 76	11 65 49 98 93
81 30 44 85 85	68 65 22 73 76	92 85 25 58 66
70 28 42 43 26	79 37 59 52 20	01 15 96 32 67
90 41 59 36 14	33 52 12 66 65	55 82 34 76 41
39 90 40 21 15	59 58 94 90 67	66 82 14 15 75
88 15 20 00 80	20 55 49 14 09	96 27 74 82 57
45 13 46 35 45	59 40 47 20 59	43 94 75 16 80
70 01 41 50 21	41 29 06 73 12	71 85 71 59 57
37 23 93 32 95	05 87 00 11 19	92 78 42 63 40
18 63 73 75 09	82 44 49 90 05	04 92 17 37 01
05 32 78 21 62	20 24 78 17 59	45 19 72 53 32
95 09 66 79 46	48 46 08 55 58	15 19 11 87 82
43 25 38 41 45	60 83 32 59 83	01 29 14 13 49
80 85 40 92 79	43 52 90 63 18	38 38 47 47 61
80 08 87 70 74	88 72 25 67 36	66 16 44 94 31
80 89 01 80 02	94 81 33 19 00	54 15 58 34 36
93 12 81 84 64	74 45 79 05 61	72 84 81 18 34
82 47 42 55 93	48 54 53 52 47	18 61 91 36 74
53 34 24 42 76	75 12 21 17 24	74 62 77 37 07
82 64 12 28 20	92 90 41 31 41	32 39 21 97 63
13 57 41 72 00	69 90 26 37 42	78 46 42 25 01
29 59 38 86 27	94 97 21 15 98	62 09 53 67 87
86 88 75 50 87	19 15 20 00 23	12 30 28 07 83
44 98 91 68 22	36 02 40 08 67	76 37 84 16 05
93 39 94 55 47	94 45 87 42 84	05 04 14 98 07
52 16 29 02 86	54 15 83 42 43	46 97 83 54 82
04 73 72 10 31	75 05 19 30 29	47 66 56 43 82

Reprinted from *A Million Random Digits with 100,000 Normal Deviates.* New York: The Free Press, 1955. Used with permission of the Rand Corporation, Santa Monica, Cal.

whose number is 06, that is, Nathan O., is assigned to the first group. Moving along in the table, we find that the next number within the range of 01 to 15 is 11. Suzanne T., whose number is 11, is also assigned to Group I. When we get to the end of the row, we move down to the next row, and so forth. To find numbers in the required range, we may have to bypass a good many numbers. The next three numbers we find are 01, 15, and 14. Thus Susan H., Duncan K., and Bill R. are all put in the first group. The next five numbers between 01 and

15 that emerge in the random number table are used to assign five individuals to the second group in the same fashion, as shown in the third column of Table 8-2. The remaining five people are put into the third group. It should be noted that numbers that have already been "used" often reappear in the table before our randomization task is completed. For example, the number 15 appeared four times before the assignment procedure was completed. This is perfectly normal because the numbers are random. After the first time a number ap-

Table 8-2
Example of random assignment procedure

Name of subject	Number	Group assignment
Susan H.	1	I
John P.	2	III
Larry K.	3	III
Edith T.	4	II
Lucia E.	5	II
Nathan O.	6	I
Rose R.	7	III
Gary S.	8	III
Jim M.	9	II
Linda S.	10	III
Suzanne T.	11	I
Vicky P.	12	II
Harlan H.	13	II
Bill R.	14	I
Duncan K.	15	I

pears and is used, subsequent appearances can be ignored.

It might be useful to look at the three groups to see if they are approximately equal with respect to one readily discernible characteristic, that is, the sex of the individual. We started out with eight females and seven males in the total group. The sex breakdown of the three groups is presented in Table 8-3. As this table shows, the randomization procedure did a good job of allocating the two sexes approximately equally across the three groups. We must accept on faith the probability that other characteristics are fairly well distributed in the randomized groups as well.

There is one more step in the randomization process that must be completed before the experiment begins. Note that in the above discussion we did not say that Nathan O., Suzanne T., and the other three individuals in Group I would be assigned to the Procedural Information Group. This is because it is a good experimental strategy to randomly assign groups to experimental treatments, as well as individuals to groups. In fact, a general principle that is useful to remember is to randomize whenever possible. To continue with our example,

we give the Procedural Information, Sensation Information, and Control Condition the numbers 1, 2, and 3, respectively. Finding a new starting point in the random number table, we look for the numbers 1, 2, or 3. This time we can look at one digit at a time, since the range of values we are seeking does not include a two-digit number. Let us say that we start at number 8 in the ninth row of the table, which is indicated by a rectangle. Reading *down* this time, we find the number 1. We, therefore, assign Group I to the Procedural Information condition. Further along in the same column we come to the number 3. Group III, therefore, is assigned to the second condition, Sensation Information, and the remaining group, Group II, is assigned to the Control Condition.

We now have fulfilled all three require-

Table 8-3
Breakdown of the sex composition
of the three groups

	Group I	Group II	Group III
Male	3	2	2
Female	2	3	3

Group	Data Collection	
	Before	After
Experimental—with pretest	X	X
Experimental—without pretest		X
Control—with pretest	X	X
Control—without pretest		X

Figure 8-2. Solomon four-group experimental design.

ments for a true experiment: we have manipulated the situation by devising distinct treatments, we have a control group, and we have randomly assigned subjects to the treatments. If any one of these elements had been missing, we would not have had a true experimental design.

☐
Experimental designs

We have already described two of the most basic designs for experimental research—the posttest only and pretest-posttest designs. Two additional designs of greater complexity are briefly discussed below. Several other designs are described in Chapter 11.

Solomon four-group design

When data are collected both before and after intervention, the pretest (initial) measure sometimes has the potential to distort the results. That is, the posttest measures may be affected not only by the treatment but also by exposure to the pretest. For example, if our intervention was a workshop to improve nurses' attitudes toward the mentally ill, a pretest attitudinal measure may in itself constitute a sensitizing "treatment" and could obscure an analysis of the workshop's effect. Such a situation might call for the *Solomon four-*

group design. In this design there are two experimental groups and two control groups. One experimental group and one control group would be administered the pretest and the other groups would not, thereby allowing the effects of the pretest measure and intervention to be segregated. Figure 8-2 illustrates the Solomon four-group design.

Factorial design

We have to this point considered designs in which the experimenter systematically varies or manipulates only one independent variable at a time. Modern statistical and research design procedures have made it possible to manipulate two or more variables at a time. Suppose that we are interested in comparing two therapeutic strategies for premature infants: one method involves tactile stimulation and the second approach involves auditory stimulation. At the same time, however, we are interested in learning if the daily amount of stimulation is related to the progress of the infant. The dependent variables for this study will be various measures of infant development, such as weight gain, cardiac responsiveness, and so forth. Figure 8-3 illustrates the structure of this experiment.

This type of study, which is known as a *factorial experiment,* offers a number of advantages to the researcher. In effect, factorial designs permit the testing of three hypotheses in a single experiment. In the present example the three research questions being addressed are as follows:

1. Does auditory stimulation have a more beneficial effect on the development of premature infants than tactile stimulation?
2. Is the duration of stimulation (independent of modality) related to infant development?
3. Is auditory stimulation most effective when linked to a certain "dose" and tac-

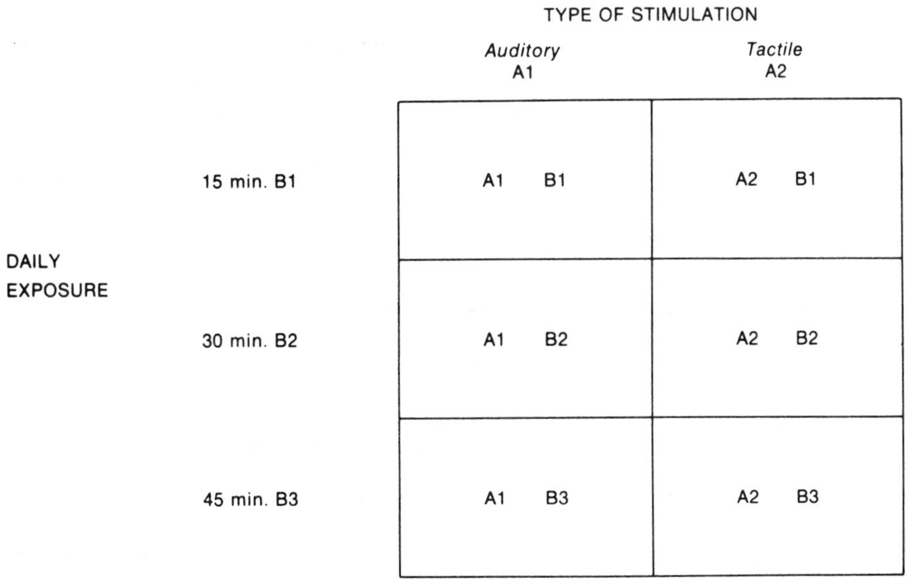

TYPE OF STIMULATION

	Auditory A1	Tactile A2
15 min. B1	A1 B1	A2 B1
30 min. B2	A1 B2	A2 B2
45 min. B3	A1 B3	A2 B3

DAILY EXPOSURE

Figure 8-3. Schematic diagram of a factorial experiment.

tile stimulation most effective when coupled with a different dose?

This third question demonstrates a major strength of factorial designs: they permit us to evaluate not only *main effects* (effects resulting from experimentally manipulated variables, as exemplified in questions 1 and 2) but also *interaction effects* (effects resulting from combining the treatment methods). We may feel that it is not sufficient to say that auditory stimulation is preferable to tactile stimulation (or vice versa) and that 45 minutes of stimulation per day is more effective than 15 minutes per day. Rather, it is how these two variables interact (how they behave in combination) that is of interest. Our results may indicate that 15 minutes of tactile stimulation and 45 minutes of auditory stimulation are the most beneficial treatments. We could not have obtained these results by conducting two separate experiments that manipulated only one independent variable and held the second one constant.

In factorial experiments such as the ones being discussed here, subjects would be assigned at random to a combination of conditions. In the example that Figure 8-3 illustrates, the premature infants would be assigned randomly to one of the six cells. The term *cell* is used in experimental research to refer to a treatment condition; it is represented in a schematic diagram as a box (cell) in the design.

Figure 8-3 can also be used to define some design terminology frequently encountered in the research literature. The two independent variables in a factorial design are referred to as the *factors*. The "type of stimulation" variable is factor A and the "amount of daily exposure" variable is factor B. Each factor must have two or more *levels* (if there were only one level, the factor would not be a variable). Level one of factor A is auditory and level two of factor A is tactile. When describing the dimensions of the design, researchers refer to the number of levels. The design in Figure 8-3 would be described as a 2 × 3 design: two levels in factor A times three levels in factor B. If a third source of stimulation, such as visual stimulation, were added, and if a daily dosage of 60 minutes were also added, the design would be referred to as a 3 × 4 design.

Factorial experiments can be performed with three or more independent variables (factors). However, designs with more than four factors are rare, because the analysis becomes complex and because the number of subjects required would be prohibitive.

☐
Advantages and disadvantages of the experimental approach

Earlier in this chapter we said that controlled experiments represent the ideal of science. In this section, we will explore the reasons why experimental methods are held in high esteem. We will also examine some of the limitations of the experimental approach.

Experimental strengths

True experiments are the most powerful method available to scientists for testing hypotheses of cause-and-effect relationships between variables. Because of its special controlling properties, the scientific experiment offers greater corroboration than any other research approach that, *if* the independent variable (for example, diet, drug dosage, teaching approach) is manipulated in a certain way, *then* certain consequences in the dependent variable (weight loss, recovery of health, learning) may be expected to ensue. This "if-then" type of relationship is important to nursing and medical researchers because of its implications for prediction and control. The great strength of experiments, then, lies in the confidence with which causal relationships can be inferred.

Because the concept of causality is a controversial one, it is appropriate to briefly present

our point of view. Some scholars take the position that the notion of causality among phenomena is untenable, on both metaphysical and empirical grounds. We would agree, as most scientists would, that causal laws can never be proved. Nevertheless, many scientists would support the assertion that "Science was, is, and always will be, concerned ultimately with the causal genus of order" (Harre, 1970, p. 103). We will continue to use the concept of causality in this book in the sense suggested by Selltiz, Wrightsman, and Cook (1976). These authors avoid the issue of metaphysical causes and note that causation is instead a construct with useful properties for scientists: "Causes, like stories, are not discovered; they are invented. A causal sequence is a perspective we place on the world. It is proper, then, to speak of a causal hypothesis and develop criteria for testing the adequacy of the formulation" (1976, p. 114). This view does not invoke mystical "forces" or "impulses" or notions of fate as a way of explaining phenomena. Here, causation between two variables only implies that when variable X occurs, there is a likelihood that variable Y will result.

Paul Lazarsfeld, a sociologist, has identified three criteria for causality (1955). The first criterion is temporal: a cause must precede an effect in time. If we were testing the hypothesis that saccharin causes bladder cancer, it would obviously be necessary to demonstrate that the subjects had not developed cancer prior to exposure to saccharin. The second requirement is that there be an empirical relationship between the presumed cause and the presumed effect. In the saccharin/cancer example, the researchers would have to demonstrate an association between the ingestion of saccharin and the presence of a carcinoma. The final criterion in a causal relationship is that the relationship cannot be explained as being due to the influence of a third variable. Suppose, for instance, that people who use saccharin tend also to drink more coffee than nonusers of saccharin. There is, thus, a possibility that any empirical relationship between saccharin use and bladder cancer in humans reflects an underlying causal relationship between a substance in coffee and bladder cancer. It is particularly because of this third criterion that the experimental approach is so strong. Through the controls imposed by manipulation, comparison, and randomization, alternative explanations to a causal interpretation can often be ruled out or discredited.

Experimental weaknesses

Despite the overwhelming advantages of experimental research, this approach has several limitations. First of all, there are a number of interesting variables that are simply not amenable to experimental manipulation. A large number of human characteristics, such as sex, metabolism or intelligence, or environmental characteristics, such as weather, cannot be experimentally controlled. For example, we cannot randomly confer upon infants their weight at birth in order to observe the effect of birth weight on subsequent morbidity.

A second, but related, limitation is that there are many variables that could technically be manipulated except that ethical considerations prohibit such manipulation. For example, to date there have not been any *experiments* using human subjects to study the effect of cigarette smoking on lung cancer. Such an experiment would require us to randomly assign individuals to a smoking or nonsmoking group. Those in the first group would be required to smoke, while those in the second group would be forbidden from smoking. Experimentation with humans, therefore, is subject to a number of ethical constraints, some of which were discussed more fully in Chapter 2.

In many situations experimentation may not be feasible simply because it is impractical. This often will be the case in hospital settings.

It may, for instance, be impossible in the real world to secure the necessary cooperation to conduct an experiment from administrators or other key people. Cooperation may be withheld for many reasons, from a desire to avoid disruptions to a basic suspicion and uneasiness about the concept of experimentation.

A weakness of experiments that is sometimes mentioned is their artificiality. Part of the difficulty lies in the requirement for randomization and then equal treatment within groups. In ordinary life, the way in which we interact with people is not random. For example, within the nursing field certain aspects of the patient—his or her age, physical attractiveness, personality, or severity of illness—will cause us to modify our behavior and, hence, our care. The differences may be extremely subtle, but they undoubtedly are not random. Another aspect of experiments that is considered artificial by phenomenologists is the focus on only a handful of variables, while attempting to hold all else constant. This requirement is criticized as being reductionist and as artificially constraining human experience.

Another problem with experiments is the *"Hawthorne effect,"* which is a kind of Placebo Effect. The term is derived from a series of experiments conducted at the Hawthorne plant of the Western Electric Corporation in which various environmental conditions such as light and working hours were varied to determine their effect on worker productivity. Regardless of what change was introduced, that is, whether the light was made better or worse, productivity increased. Thus, it seems that the knowledge of being included in a study may be sufficient to cause people to change their behavior, thereby obscuring the effect of the variable of interest. In a hospital situation the researcher might have to contend with a double Hawthorne effect. For example, if an experiment to investigate the effect of a new postoperative patient routine were conducted, nurses and hospital staff, as well as patients, might be aware of their participation in a study, and both groups could alter their actions accordingly. It is precisely for this reason that *double-blind experiments,* in which neither the subjects nor those who administer the treatment know who is in the experimental or control group, are so powerful. Unfortunately, the double-blind approach is not feasible for some types of nursing research since nursing interventions are harder to disguise than medications.

In sum, despite the clear-cut superiority of experiments in terms of their ability to test research hypotheses, they are subject to a number of limitations that make them difficult to apply to many real-world problems. Nevertheless, the fact that experimental conditions are difficult to establish does not mean that all attempts to achieve them should be abandoned. True experiments probably are possible in many situations in which nonexperimental methods are used.

□
Research example of an experiment

Geden and her colleagues (1985) were interested in examining which aspects of the Lamaze method of childbirth preparation are most effective as pain-coping strategies. Three components of Lamaze training were of special interest: Information, Breathing Techniques, and Relaxation Training. Because Lamaze-type preparation is so widely accepted as beneficial, the investigator recognized the potential ethical problem of randomly assigning women in labor to different components of the preparation, while denying them other components. Therefore, she used as subjects 80 nulliparous female undergraduates who were exposed to a laboratory pain stimulus that has been shown to be a good analogue of labor pain. The 80 subjects were randomly assigned to one of eight treatment conditions

representing all possible combinations of the three major components of Lamaze preparation. That is, some subjects received Information alone; others received Information plus Breathing Techniques, and so on. One of the eight groups received no intervention. All subjects were exposed to a one-hour session involving twenty 80-second exposures to a pain stimulus, patterned to resemble labor contractions. The effectiveness of the various components in mediating pain was assessed by obtaining measures of the subjects' systolic and diastolic blood pressure, frontalis EMG, heart rate, and self-reported pain. The findings suggested that the Relaxation Training is the most therapeutically active component of the Lamaze treatment.

The experimental nature of this study should be obvious. The investigators manipulated the independent variable (the nature of the pain-coping strategy), had experimental and control groups, and randomly assigned subjects to groups. The fact that they were able to provide both the interventions and the pain stimulus in a laboratory setting ensured maximal control over the research conditions. Their conclusions were strengthened by having used multiple dependent variables that complemented each other.

□
The quasi-experimental approach

Research that uses a quasi-experimental design often looks very much like an experiment. Quasi-experiments, like true experiments, involve the manipulation of an independent variable, that is, the institution of an experimental treatment. However, quasi-experimental designs lack at least one of the other two properties that characterize true experiments, randomization or a control group.

At the end of this chapter we discuss several specific problems associated with quasi-experiments. At this point it is sufficient to say

R = Randomization	R	O_1	X	O_2
O = Observation or measurement				
X = Treatment or intervention	R	O_1		O_2

Figure 8-4. Symbolic representation of a pretest-posttest experimental design.

that the basic difficulty with the quasi-experimental approach is its weakness, relative to experiments, in allowing us to make causal inferences. We want to know if the experimental treatment does, in fact, cause the effect we observe in the dependent variable. Does our Sensation Information condition result in reduced anxiety in our group of subjects or was the anxiety reduction due to some other factor or combination of factors? Experimental evidence for cause-and-effect relationships is more convincing than findings from quasi-experiments.

Perhaps the problems inherent in quasi-experiments will become clear if we present a few hypothetical examples. Before doing this, however, it will be useful to introduce some notation that will facilitate our discussion.* Figure 8-4 presents a symbolic representation of a pretest-posttest experimental design, identical to the design shown in Figure 8-1. According to the notation used in Figure 8-4, R means that there has been a random assignment to separate treatment groups. An O represents an observation — that is, the collection of data on the dependent variable — and the X stands for the exposure of a group to an experimental treatment. Thus the top line in Figure 8-4 represents the experimental group that has had subjects randomly assigned to it (R), has had both a pretreatment test (O_1) and a post-treatment test (O_2), and has been exposed to the experimental treatment of interest (X). The second row in the figure represents the control group, which differs from the experimental group only by the absence of exposure

* The notation, as well as most of the concepts in this section, are derived from Campbell and Stanley's (1963) classic monograph.

to the experimental treatment. We are now equipped to examine a few quasi-experimental designs.

Nonequivalent control group design

Suppose that we wished to study the effect of introducing the problem-oriented method of charting on nursing staff morale. The system is to be implemented in a 600-bed hospital in a large metropolitan area. Because we anticipate that there might be staff dissatisfaction problems, at least initially, we arrange to conduct a study. There are a number of alternative strategies available in designing the investigation. It will not, however, be possible to conduct an experiment. Hospital staff cannot be randomly assigned to different treatment groups because the new system will affect everyone. Therefore, we decide to find another hospital with similar characteristics (size, geographic location, and the like) that is not instituting the problem-oriented method of charting. We also decide to collect *baseline data* by administering a staff morale questionnaire in both hospitals prior to any change (the pretest). Data are again collected after the system is installed in the experimental hospital (the posttest).

Figure 8-5 depicts this hypothetical study symbolically. The top row is our experimental (problem-oriented charting) hospital, and the second row is the hospital using traditional methods. A comparison of this diagram with the one in Figure 8-4 shows their close resemblance to one another. They are, in fact, identical except that subjects have not been randomly assigned to treatment groups in the second diagram. The design in Figure 8-5 is

$$O_1 \qquad\qquad X \qquad\qquad O_2$$
$$O_1 \qquad\qquad\qquad\qquad O_2$$

Figure 8-5. Nonequivalent control group pretest-posttest design (quasi-experimental).

$$X \qquad\qquad O$$
$$\qquad\qquad O$$

Figure 8-6. Nonequivalent control group posttest only design (pre-experimental).

the weaker of the two because *it can no longer be assumed that the experimental and comparison groups* are equal.* Because of the inability to randomize subjects, our study is quasi-experimental rather than being truly experimental. The design is, nevertheless, a very strong one because the collection of pretest data allows us to determine whether the groups were initially similar in terms of their morale. If the morale of the two groups was very different at the start, our interpretation of the posttest data would be difficult, although there are statistical procedures that help. If the comparison and experimental groups responded similarly, on the average, on their pretest questionnaire, we could be relatively confident that any posttest differences in self-reported morale were the result of the experimental treatment.

Let us pursue this same example a bit further. Suppose we had not thought to or had been unable to collect pretest data before the new method of charting was introduced. The resulting study could be diagrammed to show the scheme in Figure 8-6. This design, which is not uncommon, has a flaw that is difficult to remedy. We have no basis on which to judge the initial equivalence of the two nursing staffs. If we find that the morale of the experimental hospital staff is much lower than that of the control hospital staff, can we conclude that the new method of charting *caused* a decline in staff morale? There could be several alternative explanations for the posttest differences. Campbell and Stanley (1963), in fact, would

* In quasi-experiments, the term "comparison group" is generally used in lieu of "control group" to refer to the group against which outcomes in the treatment group will be evaluated.

call the design shown in Figure 8-6 pre-experimental rather than quasi-experimental because of its essentially irreconcilable weaknesses. Thus, while quasi-experiments lack some of the controlling properties inherent in true experiments, the hallmark of the quasi-experimental approach is the effort to introduce other controls to compensate for the absence of either the randomization or control group component.

Time series design

The designs reviewed in the previous section illustrate studies in which a clearly identified control group was used but randomization was not. The designs we will examine here have neither a control group nor randomization. In some cases where both characteristics are absent there are inherent weaknesses that seriously jeopardize the validity of the findings. However, there are several designs that offer the researcher some measure of protection against these problems.

Let us suppose that a hospital decides to adopt a requirement that all its nurses accrue a certain number of continuing education units before being considered for a promotion or raise. The nursing administrators want to assess some of the positive and negative consequences of this mandate. Some of the indicators they might examine include turnover rate, absentee rate, qualifications of new employee applicants, number of raises and promotions awarded, and so on. For the purposes of this example, let us assume that there is no other comparable hospital that could reasonably serve as a comparison for this study. In such a case, the only kind of comparison that could

$$O_1 \qquad\qquad X \qquad\qquad O_2$$

Figure 8-7. One group pretest-posttest design (pre-experimental).

be made is a before-after contrast. If the requirement were inaugurated in January, one could compare the turnover rate, for example, for the three-month period prior to the new rule with the turnover rate for the subsequent three-month period. The schematic representation for such a study is shown in Figure 8-7.

Although this design seems logical and straightforward, there actually are numerous problems with it. What if either of the three-month periods is atypical, apart from any regulation? What about the effects of any other hospital rules inaugurated during the same period? What about the effects of external factors that influence employment, such as parking facilities, employee benefits at other nearby hospitals, the availability of child care facilities, and the like? The design in question offers no way of controlling any of these problems. This design is also preexperimental because it fails to control for so many possible extraneous factors.

A design that can come to our assistance in this case is known as the *time series design* and is diagrammed in Figure 8-8. The basic notion underlying the time series design is the collection of information over an extended time period and the introduction of an experimental treatment during the course of the data collection period. In the figure, O_1 through O_4 represent four separate instances of observation or data collection on a dependent variable prior to treatment; X represents the treatment (the introduction of the independent variable); and O_5 through O_8 represent four posttreatment observations. In our present exam-

ple, O_1 might be the number of nurses who left the hospital in January through March in the year prior to the new continuing education rule, O_2 the number of resignations in April through June, and so forth. After the rule is implemented, data on turnover are similarly collected for four consecutive three-month periods, giving us observations O_5 through O_8.

Even though the time series design does not eliminate all of the problems of interpreting changes in turnover rate, the extended time perspective immensely strengthens our ability to attribute any change to our experimental manipulation, which in this case is the continuing education requirement. Figure 8-9 attempts to demonstrate why this is so. The two diagrams (A and B) in this figure show two possible outcome patterns for the eight measures of nurse turnover. The dotted line in the center represents the time at which the continuing education rule was implemented. Both A and B reflect a feature that is common to most time series studies, and this is the fluctuation from one "observation" or measurement to another. These fluctuations are, of course, perfectly normal. One would not expect that, if 48 nurses resigned from a hospital in 1 year, the resignations would be spaced evenly during the course of the year with exactly four resignations per month. It is precisely because of these fluctuations that the design shown in Figure 8-7, with only one observation before and after the experimental treatment, is so weak.

Let us compare the kind of interpretations that can be made for the outcomes reflected in A and B of Figure 8-9. In both cases, the number of resignations increases between O_4 and O_5, that is, immediately after the introduction of the continuing education requirement. In

$$O_1 \qquad O_2 \qquad O_3 \qquad O_4 \qquad X \qquad O_5 \qquad O_6 \qquad O_7 \qquad O_8$$

Figure 8-8. Time series design (quasi-experimental).

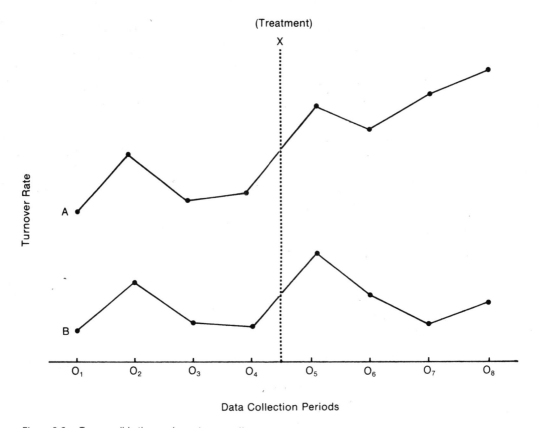

Figure 8-9. *Two possible time series outcome patterns.*

B, however, the number of resignations fall at O_6 and continues to decrease at O_7. The increase at O_5, therefore, looks very similar to other apparently haphazard fluctuations in the turnover rate at other periods. Therefore, it probably would be erroneous to conclude that the treatment had had an effect on resignations. In A, on the other hand, the number of resignations increases at O_5 and remains relatively high for all subsequent periods of data collection. It is true, of course, that there may be other explanations for a change in turnover rate from one year to the next. The time series design, however, does permit us to rule out the possibility that the data reflect an unstable measurement of resignations made at only two points in time. If we had used the design in

Figure 8-7 to study this problem, it would have been analogous to obtaining the measurements at O_4 and O_5 of Figure 8-9 only. The outcomes in both A and B of this figure look quite similar at these two points in time. Yet, as we have seen, the use of a broader time perspective leads us to draw very different conclusions about the nature of the changes from one pattern of outcomes to the next.

□
Threats to internal validity

We have examined several examples of quasi-experimental designs in order to establish some idea of the kinds of research that utilize such designs, as well as to illustrate some of the limitations of this approach. It is beyond the scope of this introductory text to acquaint the reader with the numerous quasi-experimental designs that have been developed. It is sufficient at this point to recognize that quasi-experiments are studies in which the investigator introduces an experimental treatment but is unable to either randomize or secure a control group. Unlike the very weak preexperimental designs, however, quasi-experiments include some type of control, such as pretests or the collection of data over time, that enhances the interpretative process.

It should be clear at this point, nonetheless, that the kinds of cause-and-effect inferences that we often seek in conducting scientific research cannot be made as easily with quasi-experiments as they can with true experiments. Campbell and Stanley (1963) have provided us with a very useful framework with which to evaluate various research designs. These authors use the term *internal validity* to refer to the extent to which it is possible to make an inference that the experimental manipulation resulted in any observed differences. True experiments possess a high degree of internal validity because the use of control procedures (comparison groups and randomization) enables the researcher to rule out most alternative explanations for the results. With quasi-experiments the investigator must always contend with competing explanations for the obtained results. These competing explanations, referred to as *threats to internal validity*, have been grouped into several classes, a few of which will be examined here.

History

The threat of *history* refers to the occurrence of events external to the treatment that take place concurrently with the treatment and that can affect the dependent variables. In the study used to illustrate the time series design, for example, let us suppose that at about the same time the continuing education rule was put into effect, a nurse in the hospital was sued for malpractice. The lawsuit might bring to the nurses' attention a host of problems concerning their legal liability and the method used by the hospital in handling these problems. Our dependent variable in this case, turnover rate, is now subject to the influence of (at least) two forces, and it becomes impossible for us to "unconfound" the two effects. In a true experiment, history generally is not a threat to the internal validity of a study because we can often assume that external events are as likely to affect one group as another. When this is the case, any differences in the groups that emerge at the end of the study represent effects over and above those created by external factors.

Selection

The term *selection* encompasses biases resulting from pretreatment differences between experimental and control groups. When individuals are not assigned randomly to groups, we must always be aware of the possibility that the groups are not equivalent. They may differ, in fact, in ways that are quite subtle and difficult to detect. If the groups are nonequivalent, the researcher is faced with the possibility that any post-treatment differences are due to initial differences rather than to the effect of the experimental treatment. The problem of selection is clearly reduced when pretreatment data are collected, but the problem does not disappear altogether. The selection "threat" is a very common one and may be especially problematic if subjects are recruited into groups on a volunteer basis.

Maturation

In a research context, *maturation* refers to processes occurring within the subjects during the course of the study as a result of time rather than as a result of the treatment, such as developmental growth, fatigue, and the like. To take an example, if we wanted to evaluate the effects of a special sensorimotor development program for developmentally retarded children, we would have to take into account the fact that progress does take place in these children even without special assistance. A design such as the one diagrammed in Figure 8-7 would be highly susceptible to this threat to internal validity.

There are many areas of nursing research in which maturation would be a relevant consideration. Remember that the term here does not refer to aging or developmental changes exclusively but, rather, to any kind of change that occurs with the individual as a function of time. Thus, wound-healing, postoperative recovery, and many other bodily changes that can occur with little or no nursing intervention must be considered as an explanation for post-treatment results that rivals an explanation based on the experimental manipulation.

Testing

The effects of taking a pretest upon the scores of a posttest are known as *testing* effects. It has been documented in numerous studies, particularly in those dealing with opinions and attitudes, that the mere act of collecting information from people changes them. Let us say that we administer to a group of nursing students a questionnaire dealing with their attitudes toward euthanasia. We then proceed to acquaint the students with various arguments that have been made for and against euthanasia, outcomes of court cases, and the like. At the end of instruction we give them the same attitude measure as before and observe whether or not their attitudes have changed as a function of the instruction. The design is the preexperimental scheme shown in Figure 8-7. The problem here is that the first administration of the questionnaire might sensitize the students to issues that they had not contemplated before. The sensitization may, in fact, result in attitude changes whether or not instruction follows. If a comparison group is not used in the study, it becomes impossible to segregate the effects of the experimental treatment (the instruction) from the effects of testing, history, maturation, and so forth. In true experiments, testing may not be a problem because its effects would be expected to be approximately equal in all groups, but the Solomon four-group design could be used if the researcher wanted to segregate the effects of the intervention from that of the pretest. Sensitization, or testing, problems are typically much more likely to occur when we are exposing the subjects to controversial or novel material in the pretest.

Mortality

Mortality refers to the differential loss of subjects from comparison groups. The loss of subjects during the course of a study, often referred to as *attrition,* may differ from one group to another because of a priori differences in interest, motivation, and the like. For example, in our illustration of the nonequivalent control group design (Figure 8-5), we used the hypothetical case of assessing the morale of the nursing personnel from two different hospitals, one of which was initiating the problem-oriented method of charting. The dependent variable here, it may be recalled, was a questionnaire assessing nursing staff satisfaction. The comparison group, which may have no particular commitment to the study, may be reluctant to complete a posttest questionnaire. Those who do fill it out may be unrepresentative of the group as a whole—they may be those who are most enthusiastic about their work environment, for example. Thus, on the average, it might appear that the morale of the control hospital improved, but this improvement might only be an artifact of the "mortality" of a biased segment of this group. In clinical nursing studies, the problem of attrition may be especially acute because of patient discharge and death.

□
Advantages and disadvantages of the quasi-experimental approach

The great strength of quasi-experiments lies in their practicality, feasibility, and, to a certain extent, their generalizability. In the "real world" it is often quite impractical, if not impossible, to conduct true experiments. A good deal of the research that is of interest to nurses occurs in natural settings. Frequently, it is difficult to deliver an innovative treatment to only half of a group, and randomization may be even more unmanageable. The inability to randomize, or even to secure a control group, need not force a researcher to abandon all hopes of conducting an investigation. Quasi-experimental designs are research plans that introduce some controls over potential threats to internal validity when full experimental control is lacking.

However, it is precisely because the control inherent in true experiments *is* absent in quasi-experiments that the researcher needs to be acquainted with the weaknesses of this approach. The threats to internal validity discussed in the previous section may be thought of as "rival hypotheses," competing with the experimental manipulation as explanations for observed results. Take as an example the case in which we administer certain medications to a group of babies whose mothers are heroin addicts. Suppose we are interested in whether this treatment will result in a weight gain in these typically low-weight babies. If we use no comparison group or we utilize a nonequivalent control group and then observe a weight gain, we must ask ourselves the question: Is it *plausible* that some other external factor caused or influenced the gain (the "his-

tory" threat)? Is it *plausible* that selection influenced the gain? How about the threat of maturation? If we answer "yes" to any of these questions, then the inferences we can make about the effect of the experimental treatment are weakened considerably. The plausibility of any one threat cannot, of course, be answered unequivocally. It is generally a situation in which judgment must be exercised. It is because quasi-experiments ultimately depend in part on human judgment rather than on more objective criteria that the validity of cause-and-effect inferences must be challenged. We must hasten to add that the quality of a study is not necessarily a function of its design. There are many excellent quasi-experimental investigations, as well as very poor experiments.

□
Research example of a quasi-experiment

Osguthorpe and her colleagues (1983) tested the effectiveness of alternative methods of increasing medication knowledge among psychiatric patients. These investigators developed four alternative treatment conditions relating to how patients were instructed about their medications: (1) a Drug Information Sheet condition; (2) a Videotaped Nurse Explanation condition; (3) a combined Drug Information Sheet/Videotaped Nurse Explanation condition; and (4) a Control condition (usual ward practices). Because the study took place in a psychiatric hospital, it was impractical to randomly assign patients to these four conditions. Instead, the investigators randomly assigned general psychiatric wards to conditions. Strictly speaking, even though the investigators used a random procedure to assign the wards to the treatment groups, this design is not experimental. This is because patients might have been assigned to different wards by some nonrandom procedure in the first place. Therefore, the groups could not be assumed to be equivalent at the beginning of the study.

In such a design, the major threat to the internal validity of the research is selectivity. Osguthorpe and her associates recognized this potential problem and collected information about the subjects' medication knowledge (the dependent variable) both prior to the intervention (the alternative teaching strategies) and after its completion. The analyses took the preintervention test scores into account through the computation of *change scores.* That is, the investigators analyzed how much *improvement* in scores of the four groups had occurred following the intervention, rather than simply comparing the groups' final test scores. This type of analysis has the effect of removing any preintervention differences among the groups, thereby minimizing selectivity biases. The results of the study failed to support the hypothesis that the patients would be better informed using teaching methods other than the normal ward procedures.

☐
Summary

In this chapter we have examined two important types of research that nurse researchers are increasingly using: experiments and quasi-experiments. True experiments are characterized by three fundamental properties. *Manipulation* involves doing something to or acting upon at least some of the subjects in a research study. The experimenter manipulates, or varies, the independent variable (often referred to as the experimental *treatment* or *intervention*) to see if the manipulation has an effect on the dependent variable or variables of interest. True experiments always require the utilization of a *control group,* whose performance on the dependent measures is used as a basis for assessing the performance of the experimental group on the same measures.

The third requirement for an experiment is that subjects be assigned to control and experimental groups by a process known as *randomization.* The random assignment procedure can be accomplished by any method that allows every subject an equal chance of being included in any group. In the chapter we referred to several such methods, including flipping a coin, drawing names from a hat, and using a *table of random numbers.* Randomization does not guarantee that all groups will be equal, but this technique is the most reliable method for equating groups on all possible characteristics that could affect the outcome of the study.

The most basic experimental design is the *after-only* or *posttest-only* design, which involves collecting data from subjects after the experimental treatment has been introduced. When data are also collected prior to treatment, the design is a *before-after* or *pretest-posttest* design. If pretest sensitization might obscure the effect of the treatment, a *Solomon four-group design* might be needed. When a researcher manipulates more than one variable at a time, the design is known as a *factorial experiment.* Such a design is efficient in that it permits two simultaneous experiments with one pool of subjects. Furthermore, with factorial designs we can test both *main effects* (effects resulting from the experimentally manipulated variables) and *interaction effects* (effects resulting from combining the treatments). In factorial designs each independent variable is referred to as a *factor* and each factor consists of two or more *levels* of the treatment.

True experiments are considered the ideal of science because they provide the most rigorous tests of our research hypotheses. We often want to know if our experimental treatment *causes* an observed outcome. Experiments come closer than any other type of research approach to meeting the criteria for inferring causal relationships. On the other hand, there are many situations in which an experimental design is not possible, owing to ethical or practical considerations. Experiments have also been criticized because of their artificiality.

Quasi-experiments involve manipulation but lack a comparison group or randomization. Quasi-experimental designs are designs in which efforts are made to introduce controls into the study in order to compensate in part for the absence of one or both of these important characteristics. By contrast, *preexperimental designs* have no such safeguards and, therefore, are subject to ambiguity and multiple interpretations of results.

Two specific quasi-experimental designs were presented. The *nonequivalent control group design* involves the use of a control group that is not designated by a randomization procedure. The problem with the use of such a comparison group is the possibility that the groups are initially different in ways that will affect the research outcomes, and so the collection of pretreatment data becomes an important means of assessing their initial equivalence. In studies in which there is no control group, a method for overcoming some of the difficulties in the interpretation of results is the collection of information over a period of time before and after the treatment is instituted. Such a study is known as the *time series design.*

In evaluating the results of quasi-experiments, it is useful to ask whether it is plausible that factors other than the experimental treatment caused or affected the obtained outcomes. A number of plausible *rival hypotheses* known as *threats to the internal validity* of a study were discussed. These threats include *history, selection, maturation, differential mortality,* and *testing* or pretest sensitization. Despite some of the problems inherent in quasi-experimental designs, they are often more practical in the nursing field than the more rigorous experimental designs and, therefore, merit increased attention by nursing researchers.

□
Study suggestions

1. A researcher is interested in studying the effect of sensitivity training for nurses on their behavior in crisis intervention situations. Describe how you would set up an experiment to investigate this problem.

2. Using the same situation described in Stiudy Suggestion 1, describe two quasi- or preexperimental designs that could be used to study the same problem. Discuss what the weaknesses of each would be in terms of threats to the internal validity of the study.

3. Assume that you have ten individuals — Z, Y, X, W, V, U, T, S, R, and Q — who are going to participate in an experiment you are conducting. Using a table of random numbers, assign five individuals to Group I and five to Group II. Then randomly assign the groups to an experimental or control treatment.

4. Suppose that you were interested in testing the hypothesis that systematic relaxation procedures taught by nurses to presurgical patients would reduce stress. Describe what you might do to test this hypothesis on an experimental and quasi-experimental basis. Compare the kinds of conclusions you could make with each approach.

5. In the section on randomization in this chapter, it was noted that the probability of obtaining deviant or nonequivalent groups via random assignment increases as the number of subjects in the experiment decreases. Why do you think this might be so?

6. In the hypothetical example of the hospital administration that wanted to study the effect of a new continuing education requirement on its nursing staff, preexperimental and quasi-experimental designs were discussed. What might some of the problems be in trying to study this problem experimentally?

7. Using the notation presented in Figures 8-4

to 8-8, diagram a few of the research examples described in the text that are not already diagrammed.

☐
Suggested readings

Methodological references

Battle, A.O. (1964). Quasi-experimental research designs in nursing. *Nursing Outlook, 12,* 30–32.

Campbell, D.T. & Stanley, J.C. (1963). *Experimental and quasi-experimental designs for research.* Chicago: Rand McNally Publishing Co.

Cook, T.D. & Campbell, D.T. (1979). *Quasi-experimental design and analysis issues for field settings.* Chicago: Rand McNally Publishing Co.

Harre, R. (1970). *The principles of scientific thinking.* Chicago: University of Chicago Press.

Hulicka, I.M. & Hulicka, K. (1962). To design experimental research. *American Journal of Nursing, 62,* 100–103.

Kerlinger, F.N. (1973). *Foundations of behavioral research* (2nd ed.). New York: Holt, Rinehart and Winston. (Chapters 18 & 19).

Lazarsfeld, P. (1955). *Survey design and analysis* (Foreword in H. Hyman). New York: The Free Press.

Levine, E. (1960). Experimental designs in nursing research. *Nursing Research, 9,* 203–212.

Selltiz, C., Wrightsman, L.S. (1976). *Research methods in social relations* (3rd ed.). New York: Holt, Rinehart and Winston. (Chapter 5).

Waltz, C. & Bausell, R.B. (1981). *Nursing research: Design, statistics and computer analysis.* Philadelphia: F.A. Davis. (Chapter 9).

Wilson, H.S. (1985). *Research in nursing.* Menlo Park, CA: Addison-Wesley. (Chapter 6).

Substantive references

Research utilizing experimental designs

Anderson, C.J. (1981). Enhancing reciprocity between mother and neonate. *Nursing Research, 30,* 89–93.

Andrews, C.M. & Andrews, E.C. (1983). Nursing, maternal postures, and fetal position. *Nursing Research, 32,* 336–341.

Cannon, K., Mitchell, K.A. & Fabian, T.C. (1985). Prospective randomized evaluation of two

methods of drawing coagulation studies from heparinized arterial lines. *Heart & Lung, 14,* 392–395.

Geden, E. *et al.* (1985). Self-report and psychophysiological effects of Lamaze preparation: An analogue of labor pain. *Research in Nursing and Health, 8,* 155–165.

Goldberg, W.G. & Fitzpatrick, J.J. (1980). Movement therapy with the aged. *Nursing Research, 29,* 339–346.

Jacobs, M.K., McCance, K.L. & Stewart, M.L. (1986). Leg volume changes with EPIC and posturing in dependent pregnancy edema. *Nursing Research, 35,* 86–89.

Kurzuk-Howard, G., Simpson, L., & Palmieri, A. (1985). Decubitus ulcer care: A comparative study. *Western Journal of Nursing Research, 7,* 58–74.

Sime, A.M. & Libera, M.B. (1985). Sensation information, self-instruction and responses to dental surgery. *Research in Nursing and Health, 8,* 41–47.

Research utilizing quasi-experimental or pre-experimental designs

Constantino, R.E. (1981). Bereavement crisis intervention for widows in grief and mourning. *Nursing Research, 30,* 351–353.

Mills, M.E., Arnold, B., & Wood, C.M. (1983). Core-12: A controlled study of the impact of 12-hour scheduling. *Nursing Research, 32,* 356–361.

Mitchell, P.H., Ozuna, J., & Lipe, H.P. (1981). Moving the patient in bed: Effects on intracranial pressure. *Nursing Research, 30,* 212–218.

Osguthorpe, N., Roper, J., & Saunders, J. (1983). The effect of teaching on medication knowledge. *Western Journal of Nursing Research, 5,* 205–215.

Parson, L.C., Peard, A.L.S., & Page, M.C. (1985). The effect of hygiene interventions on the cerebrovascular status of severe closed head injured persons. *Research in Nursing and Health, 8,* 173–181.

Pender, N.J. (1985). Effects of progressive muscle relaxation training on anxiety and health locus of control among hypertensive adults. *Research in Nursing and Health, 8,* 67–72.

Santopietro, M.S. (1980). Effectiveness of a self-instructional module in human sexuality counseling. *Nursing Research, 29,* 14–19.

Chapter 9
□
Nonexperimental research

When a researcher is in a position to introduce a "treatment," the effects of which he or she is interested in assessing, we say that the independent variable is being controlled or manipulated by the investigator. We noted in the last chapter that manipulation is a key element in true experiments, and in quasi-and preexperimental designs as well. When experimentation or quasi-experimentation is possible, these approaches are generally the most highly effective methods for testing hypotheses concerning causal relationships among variables.

There are, nevertheless, a number of research problems that, for one or more reasons, do not lend themselves to an experimental or even quasi-experimental design. Let us say, for example, that we are interested in studying the effect of widowhood on physical and psychological functioning. We could use as our dependent variables an existing psychological diagnostic instrument, such as the Minnesota Multiphasic Personality Inventory, as well as physiological and medical measures such as blood pressure, number of medications consumed, and self-reports on eating and sleeping patterns. Our independent variable is widowhood versus nonwidowhood. Clearly, researchers would be unable to manipulate widowhood. Spouses become widows or widowers by a process that is neither random nor subject to research control. Thus, the investigator must proceed by taking two groups as they naturally occur (those who are widowed and those who are not) and comparing them in terms of psychological and physical well-being.

There are essentially two broad classes of nonexperimental research. One, as in the widowhood example above, is referred to as *ex*

```
GROUP A      X                O       Non-equivalent control group
             ─────────────────        (pre-experimental) design
GROUP B                       O

GROUP A                       O
             ─────────────────        Ex post facto design
GROUP B                       O
```

Figure 9-1. *Schematic diagram comparing non-equivalent control group and ex post facto designs.*

post facto research. The literal translation of the Latin term ex post facto is "from after the fact." This expression is meant to indicate that the research in question has been conducted *after* the variations in the independent variable have occurred in the natural course of events.

The second broad class of nonexperimental research is pure descriptive research. Descriptive studies are not concerned with relationships among variables. Their purpose is to observe, describe, and document aspects of a situation. Because the intent of such research is not to explain or to understand the underlying causes of the variables of interest, experimental designs are not required. Since the bulk of nonexperimental research is ex post facto in nature, most of this chapter focuses on the characteristics of ex post facto research.

Ex post facto studies often share a number of structural and design characteristics with experimental, quasi-experimental, and pre-experimental research. If we use the notation scheme outlined in the previous chapter to symbolically represent the hypothetical widowhood study, we find that it bears a strong resemblance to the nonequivalent control group posttest only design discussed earlier. Both designs are presented in Figure 9-1. As these diagrams show, the pre-experimental design is distinguished from the ex post facto study only by the presence of an X, the manipulation of some experimental treatment by the researcher in the former design.

The basic purpose of ex post facto research is essentially the same as experimental re-

search: to determine the relationships among variables. The most important distinction between the two is the difficulty of inferring *causal* relationships in ex post facto studies because of the lack of manipulative control of the independent variables. In experiments, it will be remembered, the investigator makes a prediction that a deliberate variation in X, the independent variable, will result in the occurrence of some event or behavior, Y (the dependent variable). For example, the prediction is made that, if some medication is administered, then patient improvement will ensue. The experimenter has direct control over the "X": the experimental treatment can be administered to some and withheld from others, and subjects can be randomly assigned to the experimental groups.

In ex post facto research, on the other hand, the investigator does not have control of the independent variables because they have already occurred. The examination of independent variables—the presumed causative factors—is done retrospectively. Because of this fact, attempts to draw any cause-and-effect conclusions may be unwarranted. Of course, even experimentation is not sufficient to *prove* a causal relationship, but the experimenters can place considerably more confidence in their inferences than can researchers using an ex post facto approach.

Some types of ex post facto research are referred to as correlational research.* The pre-

* The use of the terms "ex post facto" and "correlational" is not entirely consistent in the literature on research methods. Some authors appear to use ex post facto to refer

cise meaning of this latter term will become clearer when we have covered some statistical concepts. Basically, a correlation is an index of the extent to which two variables are interrelated. Thus, we might hypothesize that there is a correlation between the number of cigarettes smoked and the incidence of lung cancer. The inference we would like to make based on observed relationships is that cigarette smoking *causes* cancer. This kind of inference is a fallacy that has been called *post hoc ergo propter* ("after this, therefore caused by this"). The fallacy lies in the assumption that one thing has caused another merely because it occurred chronologically before the other. To illustrate here why such cause-and-effect conclusion might not be warranted let us assume that there is a preponderance of cigarette smokers in urban areas, while people living in rural areas are largely nonsmokers. Let us further assume that bronchogenic carcinoma is actually caused by the poor environmental conditions typically associated with cities and industrial areas. We would, therefore, be incorrect in concluding that cigarette smoking had caused lung cancer, despite the strong relationship that might be shown to exist between the two variables. This is because there is *also* a strong relationship between cigarette smoking and the "real" causative agent, living in a polluted environment. Of course, the cigarette-lung cancer studies have in real life been replicated in so many different places with so many different groups of people that causal inferences are increas-

ingly justified. This hypothetical example has been used here to illustrate a famous research dictum: Correlation does not prove causation. That is, the mere existence of a relationship — even a strong one — between two variables is not enough to warrant the conclusion that one variable has caused the other.

□ Reasons for conducting nonexperimental research

Many of the research studies in which human beings are involved are nonexperimental in nature. This is certainly true of a large number of nursing research investigations. A brief look at the reasons that researchers conduct nonexperimental research should provide the reader with a better understanding of the value of such investigations and the problems associated with them.

Independent variable inherently not manipulable

There are a vast number of characteristics associated with individuals and institutions that are inherently not subject to experimental control. For instance, blood type, personality, medical diagnosis, and allergic reactions are examples of human characteristics that individuals bring with them to the research situation. It should be clear that the effects of these characteristics on some phenomenon of interest cannot be studied experimentally. We simply cannot, for example, randomly confer upon incoming hospital patients various diagnoses in order to study the effect of the diagnosis upon preoperative anxiety. Nevertheless, the relationship between these attribute variables, as they are sometimes called, and a whole range of criterion variables is quite often of considerable theoretical or practical interest. Does a person's cultural background affect his or her health beliefs? Does a patient's age affect the incidence of decubitus ulcer?

all nonexperimental research that examines relationships among variables (Kerlinger, 1973); others use the term correlational for this purpose (Crano and Brewer, 1973). Still other researchers prefer to make a distinction between whether the intent of the study is causal and comparative (ex post facto) or merely descriptive of relationships (correlational) (Ary, et al., 1979). In general, the terms will be used roughly equivalently in this chapter to designate studies of relationships among independent variables when the variable is not under the researcher's control.

What are the psychological effects of multiple episodes of ventricular fibrillation? Such questions cannot be answered using experimental procedures.

Ethical constraints on manipulation

In nursing research, as in other fields where human behavior is of primary interest, there are numerous variables that could technically be manipulated but which should not be manipulated for ethical reasons. One example we have already discussed is the number of cigarettes smoked per day by humans. If the nature of the independent variable is such that its manipulation could cause physical or mental harm to subjects, then that variable should not be controlled experimentally. For example, if we were interested in studying the effect of prenatal care on infant mortality, it would be considered unethical to provide such care to one group of pregnant women while totally depriving a second group.

Unfortunately, it is not always entirely clear where the ethical line must be drawn. Experimental drug studies have sometimes been criticized on the grounds that any presumed cure should be administered to all individuals in need of treatment. Others object to the use of deception which the administration of placebos often implies. We must urge researchers to consult with colleagues or specially formed ethical committees before engaging in any experiment that involves questionable procedures.

Although true experiments are the ideal of science, there are numerous high quality and useful nonexperimental studies. In the hypothetical example of prenatal care mentioned earlier, it might be possible to locate a naturally occurring group of mothers-to-be who have not received such care. The birth outcomes of these women could then be compared with those of a group of women who had received prenatal care.

The problem, of course, is that the two groups of women might be expected to differ in terms of a number of other characteristics such as age, education, nutrition, and health, any of which individually or in combination could have an impact on infant mortality independent of the absence or presence of care prior to the child's birth. Thus, even if it could be shown that the infants of women who had received prenatal care were less likely to die than the infants of women who had not been exposed to such care, conclusions about the causal effects of prenatal care would be difficult to draw.

Practical constraints on manipulation

There are many research situations in which it is simply not practical or even desirable to conduct a true experiment. Such constraints might involve insufficient time, lack of cooperation, or lack of adequate funds. For instance, let us suppose that we were interested in studying the effect of hospital noise levels on patient well-being and recovery. Certain areas of the hospital might be particularly noisy while other areas might be much quieter. Let us say that we have categorized all the rooms as either "above average" or "below average" in terms of noise intensity. Technically, it might be possible to randomly assign incoming patients to rooms, but this would typically be rather impractical. We must be content in this situation to perform an ex post facto study. We would collect information on patient well-being—number of hours slept, blood pressure, need for medications and so on—and compare groups exposed to the two different noise conditions on these various indices. Of course, we would want to control for a number of other variables that might confound our results. For example, we might want to restrict our study to patients with certain kinds of diagnoses, or to rooms of a particular type, such as semiprivate.

Research perspective on manipulation

Phenomenologically based studies seek to capture what people think, feel, and behave in their naturalistic environments. Because of this goal, researchers conducting qualitative studies want as little disturbance as possible to the people or groups they are studying. Manipulation is neither attempted nor considered desirable; the emphasis is on the natural every day world of human beings. Thus, although phenomenological researchers often focus on concepts that could be manipulated or could be affected by manipulation (e.g. dependency, coping, decision-making), they reject manipulation as a technique for studying certain problems.

□
Types of nonexperimental research

It is hoped the preceding discussion has provided the reader with a basic understanding of the kinds of situations that might rule out the use of experimental designs to answer our research questions. In this section we will take a brief look at various nonexperimental studies. This discussion is not intended to be an exhaustive coverage of typology; a neat classification scheme does not, in fact, exist. The intent here, rather, is to acquaint the reader with some terms that frequently arise in a research context.

Retrospective studies

Retrospective* studies are ex post facto investigations in which some phenomenon existing in the present is linked to other phenomena

---

* The term retrospective is also used in another context in research methods to refer to questions that ask respondents to recall and narrate experiences, thoughts, feelings, and so forth that occurred in the past.

---

occurring in the past. That is, the investigator is interested in some "effect" and attempts to shed light upon the factors that have caused it. Many epidemiological studies are retrospective in nature, and this approach has been used by medical researchers for over a century. In the nineteenth century, for example, Snow studied the relationship between the distribution of deaths from cholera on the one hand and the source of drinking water on the other.

In nursing research, as in medical research, retrospective studies are quite prevalent. Patient well-being, recovery, or satisfaction are phenomena that have been linked retrospectively to different nursing interventions or modes of treatment. Many studies in the field of nursing education have also been of this type. To illustrate the concept of retrospection more concretely, let us take as an example the case of a nursing school that is trying to understand the factors that cause certain students to drop out of its baccalaureate program while other students continue until graduation. The researcher's problem is to try to identify and disentangle the independent variables (such as motivation, academic ability, financial problems, personality traits, and so on) that have "caused" some students to leave the program before completion.

In a sense, this kind of ex post facto study can be viewed as the converse of true experiments. In experiments the researcher creates the "cause" by directly manipulating the independent variable and then observes the effect of the manipulation on some dependent variable. In contrast, in a retrospective study the investigator begins with a description of some situation and attempts to identify the previously occurring causative factors. Retrospective studies are considerably weaker than experiments in their ability to shed light on causal relationships. Findings from a single retrospective study are rarely convincing and, thus, often require confirmatory research efforts.

Prospective studies

A nonexperimental prospective study starts with an examination of presumed causes and then goes forward in time to the presumed effect. For example, a researcher might want to test the hypothesis that the incidence of rubella during pregnancy is related to malformations in the offspring. To test this hypothesis prospectively, the investigator would begin with a sample of pregnant women, some of whom have contracted the disease during their pregnancy while others have not. The subsequent occurrence of congenital anomalies would be observed. The researcher would then be in a position to test whether women who had contracted the disease during pregnancy were more likely to bear malformed babies than women who did not have rubella.

Prospective studies are often more costly than retrospective studies and perhaps are less common for this reason. Prospective research often requires large samples, particularly if the dependent variable of interest is rare. For example, in prospective studies of the antecedents of heroin addiction, a very large sample would be required initially in order to yield a sufficient number of heroin addicts. Another difficulty with prospective studies is that a substantial follow-up period may be necessary before the phenomenon or effect under investigation manifests itself, as is the case in prospective studies of cigarette smoking/lung cancer.

Despite these problems, prospective studies are considerably stronger than retrospective studies. For one thing, any ambiguity concerning the temporal sequence of phenomena usually is resolved in prospective research. In addition, samples are more likely to be representative, and investigators may be in a position to impose numerous controls to rule out competing explanations for observed effects. Despite these advantages, causal inferences cannot be made with the same degree of confidence in prospective correlational studies as

in the case of experiments. Without the ability to manipulate the independent variable and randomly assign individuals to different conditions, there is no way to equate groups on all relevant factors. Because of this fact, alternative "causes" or antecedents may compete with those which the researcher has hypothesized.

Prediction studies

There are many practical situations in which it is useful to make a forecast about how people will perform or behave. Predictive research is often used to facilitate decision-making about individuals, such as in the selection of individuals for programs or special treatment. For example, let us suppose that a university nursing school has just begun a master's level program in nursing research and that 20 students are admitted to the program during its first year of operation. These first 20 students have been selected from an applicant pool of about 100 individuals and the principal criteria for selection were undergraduate grades and recommendations. However, there are also numerous other pieces of information available about each new student, such as Graduate Record Examination (GRE) test scores, Miller Analogies test scores, and rank in class. At the end of the first year we find that the 20 students varied considerably in their course performance. In order to reduce the probability of admitting students who will fare poorly in the new program, a study can be conducted to examine the relationship between various antecedent factors and the grade-point average of the first group of students. It might be found, for example, that the scores on the quantitative section of the GRE test were more strongly related to performance in the new program than any other piece of information. So far, then, the study has been completely retrospective. That is, the aim has been to identify some preexisting characteristic of the individual that bears a strong relationship to the dependent variable of interest, grade-point average in the master's level program. However, once this relationship is determined, it becomes possible to make some predictions about the kind of students who are likely to succeed in future years. The fundamental feature of prediction studies is the examination of relationships among variables in one group in order to make predictions about the behavior of another similar group.

Descriptive correlational studies

Although there is considerable stress in scientific research on understanding what "causes" behaviors, conditions, and situations, we can often do little more than describe existing relationships without fully comprehending the complex causal pathways that exist. Thus, many of our research problems are often cast in noncausal terms. We ask, for example, are men more likely than women to become alcoholics, not whether or not a particular configuration of sex chromosomes has caused a predisposition for alcohol.

As in the case of other types of ex post facto research, the investigator engaged in a descriptive correlational study has no control over the independent variables. That is, there is no experimental manipulation or random assignment to groups. Unlike other types of ex post facto studies, however — studies such as the cigarette smoking/lung cancer investigations — the aim of descriptive correlational is to describe the relationship among variables rather than to infer cause-and-effect relationships.

Consider the following example. Suppose we have hypothesized that patients' adherence to prescribed hypertensive medication (as measured by changes in blood pressure readings) is related to type of profession. We may find, for example, that lawyers have greater adherence to a medication regime than members of other professions. Given the existence of this relationship, is it meaningful

or reasonable to say that the type of profession *caused* adherence? Clearly it is not. Yet the knowledge of a relationship is interesting and could lead to practical applications (such as an examination of the constraints to adherence among professionals other than lawyers). In other words, descriptive correlational research is often quite useful in its own right and sometimes lays the groundwork for further, more rigorous research.

Univariate descriptive studies

The purpose of descriptive studies is to obtain information about the current status of phenomena of interest. We use the term "univariate" here to distinguish descriptive correlational studies from those studies that intend simply to describe what exists in terms of frequency of occurrence (or its presence versus absence) rather than to describe the relationship between variables. For example, an investigator may wish to determine the percentage of teenage mothers whose babies are premature.

Univariate descriptive studies are not necessarily focused on only one variable. For example, a researcher might be interested in women's experience during menopause. The investigation might describe the frequency with which various symptoms are reported, the average age at menopause, the percentage of women seeking formal health care, and the percentage of women using medications to alleviate symptoms. There are multiple variables in this study, but the purpose is to describe the status of each, and not to relate them to one another.

☐
Strengths and weaknesses of ex post facto/correlational research

The quality of a study is not necessarily related to its approach: there are many excellent nonexperimental studies as well as flawed experi-

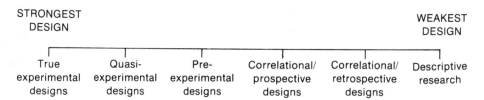

STRONGEST
DESIGN

WEAKEST
DESIGN

| True experimental designs | Quasi- experimental designs | Pre- experimental designs | Correlational/ prospective designs | Correlational/ retrospective designs | Descriptive research |

Figure 9-2. Continuum of research designs with respect to elucidating causal relationships.

ments. Nevertheless, there is a continuum of design types in terms of capacity to reveal causal relationships. True experimental designs are at one end of that continuum, and univariate descriptive research is at the other, as shown in Figure 9-2. While it should be obvious why descriptive studies are weak in this regard, the discussion below examines the limitations of the ex post facto approach.

Weaknesses of ex post facto/ correlational research

Kerlinger (1973) has noted three major problems associated with ex post facto research: (1) the inability to actively manipulate the independent variables of interest, (2) the inability to randomly assign individuals to experimental treatments, and (3) the possibility of faulty interpretation of study results.

In ex post facto studies the researcher works with preexisting groups that have not formed by a random process but, rather, by what might be termed a self-selecting process. Kerlinger (1973) has offered the following description of self-selection: "Self-selection occurs when the members of the groups being studied are in the groups, in part, because they differentially possess traits or characteristics extraneous to the research problem, characteristics that possibly influence or are otherwise related to the variables of the research problem" (p. 381). It may be recalled from the previous chapter that selection constitutes one of the threats to the internal validity of a study. In correlational research the researchers cannot assume that the groups being studied were similar at the beginning of the investigation. Because of this fact, preexisting differences may be a plausible alternative explanation for any observed differences on the dependent variable of interest.

As an illustration of this problem, let us take a hypothetical study in which the researcher is interested in examining the relationship between type of nursing program (the independent variable) and job satisfaction after graduation. If the investigator finds that diploma school graduates are more satisfied with their work than baccalaureate graduates one year after graduation, the conclusion that the diploma school program provides better preparation for actual work situations and, hence, leads to increased satisfaction may or may not be accurate. The students in the two programs were undoubtedly different to begin with in terms of a number of important characteristics such as social class, personality, career goals, and so forth. In other words, students self-selected themselves into one of the two programs and it may be the selection traits themselves that resulted in different job expectations and satisfactions.

A large part of the difficulty of interpreting correlational findings stems from the fact that in the real world behaviors, states, attitudes, and characteristics are interrelated (correlated) in complex ways. An example might help to make this clear. Let us suppose we were interested in studying the differences be-

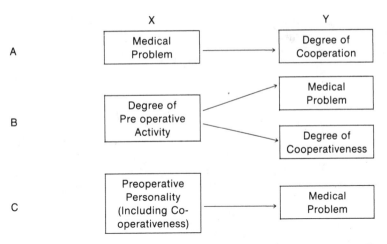

Figure 9-3.   *Three possible explanations for relationship between medical diagnosis and degree of cooperativeness in patients. Arrows show direction of influence; variable X is presumed to "cause" variable Y.*

tween the postoperative convalescent behavior of patients who had undergone surgery for two different medical problems — hernia and ulcers. Our independent variable in this hypothetical study is the type of medical problem. We might use as our measures of the dependent variable (postoperative convalescent behavior) one or more of the following: ratings of nurses on the degree of cooperativeness of the patient, number of times the patient calls the nurse for help, the patient's self ratings of distress, and the number of medications required to induce sleep or alleviate pain. Let us say that we find that the hernia patients receive a significantly lower rating by the nurses on degree of cooperation than the ulcer patients. We could interpret this finding to mean that particular medical problems and their accompanying surgical treatment produce different patterns of cooperative behavior in individuals. This relationship is diagrammed in Figure 9-3,A. Note that, even with this interpretation, it is essentially impossible to separate the effects of (1) the type of medical problem and (2) type of surgical procedure, since one necessarily follows the other.

For the sake of this discussion, let us examine some alternative explanations for the findings. Perhaps there is a third variable that influences *both* the degree of convalescent cooperativeness and the type of medical ailment, such as the degree of physical activity to which an individual is accustomed. That is, it may be possible that hernia patients are usually engaged in a greater degree of physical activity than are ulcer patients, and this fact may be one of the causes of both the diagnosis and the inability to cope properly with the sedentary hospital routine. This set of relationships is diagrammed in Figure 9-3,B.

A third possibility may be *reversed* causality, as shown in Figure 9-3,C. Willingness to cooperate in general may be thought of as one aspect of a person's personality and it is possible that the dynamics of a person's psychological makeup will result in the manifestation of different medical problems. In this interpretation, it is the person's disposition that causes the diagnosis and not the other way around.

Undoubtedly, the reader will be able to invent other alternatives. The point is that interpretations of ex post facto results should generally be considered tentative, particularly if the research has no theoretical basis.

Strengths of ex post facto/ correlational research

In an earlier section of this chapter we discussed various constraints that limit the possibility of applying an experimentation approach to some research problems. Ex post facto and correlational research will continue to play a crucial role in nursing, medical, and social science research precisely because many of the interesting problems to be solved in those fields are not amenable to experimentation.

Despite our emphasis on causality in relationships, it has already been noted that in some kinds of research, such as predictive or descriptive research, a full understanding of causal networks may not be important. Furthermore, if the study is testing a hypothesis that has been deduced from an established theory, determining the direction of causation may be relatively straightforward.

Correlational research is often an efficient and effective means of collecting a large amount of data about a problem area. For example, it would be possible to collect extensive information about the health histories and eating habits of a large number of individuals. Researchers could then examine which health problems are correlated with which diets. By doing this, a large number of interrelationships could be discovered in a relatively short amount of time. By contrast, an experimenter usually looks at only a few variables at a time. For example, one experiment might be devoted to manipulating foods high in cholesterol to observe the effects on certain medical symptoms, while another experiment could manipulate saccharin consumption, and so forth.

Finally, ex post facto research is often strong in realism and, therefore, has an intrinsic appeal for the solution of many practical problems. Unlike many experimental studies, ex post facto research is seldom criticized for its artificiality.

☐
Research examples

We have used a number of hypothetical problems to help explain many of the points made in this chapter. We conclude with a discussion of two actual studies.

Example: two-group ex post facto study

Shannahan and Cottrell (1985) conducted a study to investigate the effect of delivering a baby in a birth chair as opposed to on a traditional delivery table. They hypothesized that women who deliver in a birth chair would have shorter second-stage labor, better fetal outcome, but greater blood loss than women delivering more traditionally. In this study, the independent variable (type of delivery) was not manipulated by the investigators; the data were collected after the fact, in this case after the woman had made the decision as to which type of delivery she would use. Data on the dependent variables (the childbirth outcomes) were collected through a chart review of 60 primiparous women who had a normal pregnancy and spontaneous onset of labor. Half the sample had delivered in a birth chair and the remaining half had delivered on a delivery table.

The results of the study failed to support the first two hypotheses. The women in the two groups were not significantly different with regard to the average length of second stage labor. Furthermore, the Apgar scores of the infants of mothers in the two groups were nearly identical. However, there was evidence that maternal blood loss was greater among the birth-chair mothers than among the delivery-table mothers, which supported the third hypothesis.

Because this study was nonexperimental, the investigators had no control over whether a woman would use the birth chair or the delivery table. The investigators introduced some controls to minimize selectivity biases—for example, they ensured that only women with normal pregnancies and those with spontaneous, vaginal deliveries were included in the sample. They also noted that the two groups were similar in terms of marital status, number of pregnancies, ethnic origin, and length of pregnancy. Nevertheless, it is difficult to interpret the results of this study because it is not clear that the two groups of women were identical in every respect *except* for mode of delivery. In fact, there is some indication that the groups *did* have predelivery differences. The hemogram test results revealed that the birth chair group had higher hemoglobin and hematocrit values than the delivery table group at the time of admission. Because the predelivery equivalence of the two groups cannot be ascertained, it is difficult to conclude with confidence that the results of the study reflect the effects (or noneffects) of the mode of delivery or the effects of other characteristics of the study sample.

Example: descriptive/correlational study

McKeever and Galloway (1984) were interested in the effects of nongynecological surgery on menstrual cycle alterations among adolescent and adult surgical patients. Portions of the study were purely descriptive, in keeping with the fact that little information was available concerning the incidence of menstrual cycle alterations following surgery. For example, the investigators wanted to answer the basic question of whether the menstrual cycle length was, in fact, affected by surgery performed under general anesthesia. In addition, they sought information about how a number of variables were interrelated. For example, one of the research questions was whether there is a relationship between the menstrual cycle phase at the time of surgery and the onset of the first postoperative menses. They also examined whether the patients' perceptions of stress during hospitalization was related to postoperative menstrual cycle alterations.

Data for this investigation were obtained from a sample of 77 women aged 12 to 45, all of whom reported having had regular menstrual cycles prior to hospitalization. The subjects were interviewed within 72 hours of surgery and again six weeks later. The results revealed that the majority of women in the sample experienced a postoperative menstrual cycle length alteration, although the alteration was found to be unrelated to menstrual phase at the time of surgery. The women who experienced no alterations were those who encountered relatively low levels of both physiological and psychological stress. High stress was especially likely to be associated with an early onset of menses.

This study is clearly nonexperimental in nature. The investigators did not manipulate any variables. Unlike the preceding example, this research studied variables that are inherently nonmanipulable. That is, the investigators could not manipulate the phase of the patients' menstrual cycle at the time of surgery nor their perceived level of stress during hospitalization. The investigators acknowledged that the results of their study were open to various interpretations, and concluded that the "effects of environmental, social, and psychological stressors on the menstrual cycle should be explored further" (p. 45).

□
Summary

Nonexperimental research includes two broad categories: descriptive research and ex post facto/correlational research. *Descriptive research* is designed to summarize the status of some phenomena of interest as they currently exist. *Ex post facto* or *correlational studies* are research investigations designed to examine the relationships among variables. Unlike experimental or quasi-experimental studies, however, ex post facto research lacks active manipulation of the independent variable. Because the investigation of the independent variable is done retrospectively—that is, after it has occurred in the natural course of events—it becomes difficult to draw cause-and-effect conclusions. It is for this reason that, methodologically speaking, experimental studies are considered more rigorous.

There are basically three types of constraints that preclude experimentation and, therefore, make a nonexperimental approach useful or necessary. A number of independent variables, such as height, sex, and race, are human characteristics that are not amenable to control and randomization. Other independent variables are technically manipulable but are ethically inappropriate for experimental purposes with human subjects, as in the case of number of cigarettes smoked or levels of vitamins ingested. Finally, it may often be impractical or impossible to manipulate variables owing to insufficient time, inconvenience, or prior manifestation of the phenomena of interest. In addition to these constraints, researchers sometimes deliberately choose not to manipulate variables in order to get a more realistic understanding of some phenomena as they operate in naturalistic settings.

A number of special types of nonexperimental studies were briefly described in this chapter. *Retrospective studies* are investigations in which the researcher observes the manifestation of some phenomenon (the dependent variable) and tries to identify its antecedents or causes (the independent variable). *Prospective studies* start with an observation of presumed causes and then go forward in time to observe the consequences. Prospective research is typically initiated after evidence of important relationships are suggested by retrospective investigations. *Prediction studies* use retrospective information about the relationships among variables in one group to make a forecast about the outcomes of another similar group. *Descriptive correlational studies* are less concerned with determining cause-and-effect relationships than with a description of how one phenomenon is related to another. *Univariate descriptive research* provides information on the occurrence, frequency of occurrence, or average value of the variables of interest without examining how variables are interrelated.

The primary weakness of ex post facto and correlational research is that the researcher lacks experimental control, both in terms of inability to manipulate the independent variable and inability to randomly assign subjects to treatment groups. The problem of *self-selection* into groups is associated with the inability to randomize. Because of this lack of control, ex post facto and correlational research are more likely to run the risk of erroneous interpretation of results than experimental research.

On the other hand, since experimentation is often unfeasible or impractical in many research situations, ex post facto and correlational studies are considered very important. Correlational research is generally an efficient and useful method of collecting a large amount of data in a relatively short period of time. Finally, ex post facto studies are typically strong in terms of their realism. Because they tend to lack the artificiality that frequently accompanies laboratory experiments, their results are more likely to be generalizable to other realistic settings.

☐
Study suggestions

1. A nurse researcher is interested in studying the success of several different approaches

to feeding patients with dysphagia. Can the researcher use an ex post facto design to examine this problem? Why or why not? Could an experimental or quasi-experimental approach be used? How?

2. A nurse researcher is planning to investigate the relationship between the social class of hospitalized children and the frequency and content of children-initiated communications with the nursing staff. Which is the independent and which is the dependent variable? Would you classify this research as basically experimental or correlational, or could both approaches be used?

3. In the example in the chapter involving hernia and ulcer patients, three interpretations of the results were advanced. Describe one or two other possibilities.

4. Classify the following list of potential independent variables in terms of whether it would be impossible, unethical, or impractical to manipulate the variable and, hence, to conduct an experiment: psychiatric disorder, method of contraception, individual's weight, preoperative anxiety in patients, body temperature, method of asthma therapy, white blood cell count, heroin addiction, membership in a professional nursing association, marital status.

5. Design a hypothetical descriptive study in some setting of interest. What kind of variables would you be interested in examining?

6. Read one of the studies listed under "Substantive References." Identify the independent and dependent variables. Could the study have used an experimental or quasi-experimental design? Why or why not? Diagram (if appropriate) the directionality of the cause-effect relationship as shown in Figure 9-3. Can you offer an alternative explanation?

7. In the section on prospective studies, an example relating to rubella and congenital anomalies was cited. How could such a problem be studied retrospectively? Would an experimental approach with humans be possible? Why or why not?

Suggested readings

Methodological references

Ary, D., Jacobs, L.C. & Razavich, A. (1979). *Introduction to research in education* (2nd ed.). New York: Holt, Rinehart and Winston. (Chapters 3 & 4).

Burdette, W.J. & Gehan, E.A. (1970). *Planning and analysis of clinical studies.* Springfield, IL: Charles C Thomas. (Chapters 3 & 4).

Crano, W.D. & Brewer, M.B. (1973). *Principles of research in social psychology.* New York: McGraw-Hill. (Chapter 5).

Kerlinger, F. (1973). *Foundations of behavioral research* (2nd ed.). New York: Holt, Rinehart and Winston. (Chapter 22).

Waltz, C. & Bausell, R.B. (1981). *Nursing research: Design, statistics, and computer analysis.* Philadelphia: F.A. Davis.

Substantive references

Barkauskas, V.H., Chen, S.C. & Chen, E.H. (1985). Health problems encountered by nurse practitioners and physicians in family practice clinics. *Western Journal of Nursing Research, 7,* 101–115.

Blackburn, S. & Lowen, L. (1986). Impact of an infant's premature birth on the grandparents and parents. *Journal of Obstetric, Gynecologic, and Neonatal Nursing, 15,* 173–178.

Cogan, R. & Edmunds, E.P. (1980). Pronominalization: A linguistic facet of the maternal–paternal sensitive period. *Nursing Research, 29,* 225–227.

Cox, C.L., Sullivan, J.A., & Roghmann, K.J. (1984). A conceptual explanation of risk-reduction behavior and intervention development. *Nursing Research, 33,* 168–173.

Dawson, C. (1985). Hypertension, perceived clinician empathy, and patient self-disclosure. *Research in Nursing and Health, 8,* 191–198.

McKeever, P. & Galloway, S.C. (1984). Effects of Nongynecological surgery on the menstrual cycle. *Nursing Research, 33,* 42–46.

Saltzer, E.B. & Golden, M.P. (1985). Obesity in lower and middle socioeconomic status mothers and their children. *Research in Nursing and Health, 8,* 147–153.

Shannahan, M.D. & Cottrell, B.H. (1985). Effect of the birth chair on duration of second stage labor, fetal outcome and maternal blood loss. *Nursing Research, 34,* 89–92.

Tilden, V.P. (1984). The relation of selected psychosocial variables to single status of adult women during pregnancy. *Nursing Research, 33,* 102–107.

Williams, M.A., *et al.* (1985). Predictors of acute confusional states in hospitalized elderly patients. *Research in Nursing and Health, 8,* 31–40.

Wineman, N.M. (1980). Obesity: Locus of control, body image, weight loss, and age-at-onset. *Nursing Research, 29,* 231–237.

Chapter 10
☐
Some additional
types of research

In the preceding two chapters we explored different kinds of research in terms of one dimension: the tightness of the controls introduced by the investigator for the purpose of inferring cause-and-effect relationships. All research studies can be categorized as either experimental, quasi-/preexperimental, or nonexperimental in design.

The discussion of experimental versus nonexperimental research, although useful in introducing some concepts of research design, nevertheless fails to provide the beginning researcher with a sense of the full range of purposes of nursing research. This chapter is devoted to examining some additional types of research not already discussed in previous chapters: survey research, evaluation research, needs assessments, historical research, case studies, field studies, secondary analyses, methodological research, and meta-analysis. It should be noted that these nine types of research are not necessarily linked to a specific type of research design, as shown in Figure 10-1.

☐
Survey research

A survey is designed to obtain information from populations regarding the prevalence, distribution, and interrelations of variables within those populations. The dicennial census of the U.S. population is one example of a survey. Political opinion polls, such as those conducted by Gallup or Harris, are other examples. Although the distinction between a *population* and a *sample* was pointed out in Chapter 3, it is useful to repeat it here. The term *population* refers to the entire set of indi-

	Experimental	Quasi-Experimental	Correlational/Ex Post Facto	Descriptive
Survey Research			X	X
Evaluation Research	X	X	X	X
Needs Assessments			X	X
Historical			X	X
Case Study		X	X	X
Field Study			X	X
Secondary Analysis			X	X
Methodological	X	X	X	X
Meta-Analysis			X	X

Figure 10-1. *Possible designs for various types of research.*

viduals (or objects) having a common characteristic. For example, all registered nurses in the United States constitute one population, while all parents of physically handicapped children constitute another. Any subset of the larger population is called a *sample.* When surveys study samples, as they usually do, they are often referred to as *sample surveys* (as opposed to a *census,* which covers the entire population).

The term *survey* can be used to designate any research activity in which the investigator gathers data from a portion of a population for the purpose of examining the characteristics, opinions, or intentions of that population. For example, a researcher could do a survey of blood types by analyzing blood samples from a population of Red Cross donors. However, in practice the term survey generally refers to studies in which information is obtained from a sample of individuals by means of self-report—that is, the sample responds to a series of questions posed by the investigator.

The content of survey research

The content of a self-report survey is essentially limited only by the extent to which respondents are willing to report on the topic. Any information that can reliably be obtained by directly asking a person for that information is acceptable for inclusion in a survey.

Often, a survey focuses on what people do: how or what they eat, how they care for their health needs, their compliance in taking medications, what kinds of family-planning behaviors they engage in, what their sleeping patterns are, and so forth. In some instances, particularly in political surveys, the emphasis is on what people plan to do—how they plan to vote, for example. Surveys also collect information on people's knowledge, opinions, attitudes, and values. For example, we might be interested in learning about the public's knowledge of and attitude toward health-maintenance organizations. Another example would be a survey of nurses' opinions about proposed legislation to limit the activities of nurse practitioners.

Almost invariably, survey researchers ask respondents for information about their personal background or situation. Most surveys secure data on many of the following characteristics: age, sex, nationality (or ethnicity), marital status, education, religion, political preference, occupation, income, father's and mother's education, race, and family size. Demographic characteristics such as these are rarely the focus of any survey except in the case of a national census. There are, however, two important reasons for collecting background data. First of all, personal characteristics such as age, education, and sex have been shown time and again to be related to a person's behavior and attitudes. These variables, in other words, often play a valuable explanatory role. The second reason for collecting this information is to enable the researcher to compare characteristics of the sample with those of the population. If it is known, for instance, that the population under examination comprised about 50% men and 50% women, one might have reason to question the validity of conclusions based on the survey of a sample in which 85% of the respondents were women.

Types of survey techniques

Survey data can be collected in a number of ways. The three most common methods are face-to-face interviews, telephone interviews, and mailed questionnaires.

The most powerful method of securing survey information is through *personal interviews,* the method in which interviewers meet with individuals in a face-to-face situation and secure information from them. In most cases the interviewer will use a carefully developed set of questions, referred to as an *interview schedule.* The length of time needed for a personal interview varies considerably from study to study and from respondent to respondent. Some interviews may be completed in a matter of minutes, while others may take, literally, hours to complete. Generally, personal interviews are rather costly. They require considerable planning and interviewer training in order to be successful; they also tend to involve a lot of personnel time. Nevertheless, personal interviews are regarded as the most useful method of collecting survey data because of the depth and quality of the information they yield. Furthermore, personal interviews usually result in a high number of "returns." That is to say, relatively few people refuse to be interviewed in person.

Telephone interviews are a less costly, but less effective, method of gathering survey information. Whenever detailed information is needed from respondents, a personal interview is usually preferable. When the interviewer is unknown, respondents may be uncooperative and unresponsive in a telephone situation. Telephone interviews inherently lack the ability to build rapport, which is a feature of face-to-face interviews. However, telephoning can be a convenient method of collecting a lot of information quickly if the interview is short, specific, and not too personal.

Questionnaires differ from interviews primarily in that they are self-administered. That is, the respondent reads the questions on the schedule and gives an answer in writing. A person associated with the survey may or may not be present at the time the questionnaire is completed to answer questions that arise. Because of this fact, and because respondents differ considerably in their reading levels and in their ability to communicate in writing, questionnaires are *not* merely a printed form of an interview schedule. Great care must be taken in the development of a questionnaire to word questions clearly, simply, and unambiguously. The most common way of distributing questionnaires is through the mail. Compared with personal interviews, the cost of a mailed questionnaire is quite low, especially if the population is spread over a wide geographical area.

Advantages and disadvantages of surveys

The greatest advantage of survey research is its flexibility and broadness of scope. It can be applied to many populations, it can focus on a wide range of topics, and its information can be used for many purposes. Good surveys can be much more costly than experiments, but when one considers the amount of information obtained in the course of normal surveys, they are not uneconomical.

There are, however, a number of limitations

of survey research that should be considered. First of all, the information obtained in most surveys tends to be relatively superficial. Interviews and questionnaires rarely probe very deeply into such complexities as contradictions of human behavior and feelings. Survey research is better suited to extensive rather than intensive analysis.

A second drawback of survey research is one we mentioned previously in connection with ex post facto research, and that is that survey data do not permit the researcher to have much confidence in inferring cause-and-effect relationships. Survey researchers have no control over independent variables (that is, they do not manipulate any variables).

Another difficulty with survey research is that it is very demanding of personnel time and other resources. In a large survey literally dozens of workers may be required to complete the study. Although smaller survey studies can often be successfully completed by a small group of researchers, even localized surveys generally require a considerable investment of time and energy and rarely result in any findings before months of effort.

Survey research example

O'Rourke (1983) investigated whether women's subjective appraisal of their overall psychological well-being is related to the presence of menstrual and nonmenstrual symptoms, and to women's background characteristics. O'Rourke addressed this problem through a survey of 633 healthy, menstruating women between the ages of 21 and 44. The sample was drawn from employees of a large metropolitan university health science campus. Each subject was asked to complete a questionnaire, which was distributed to the sample through the campus mail.

The questionnaire gathered varied types of information. The instrument included questions about the subjects' health history; ques-

tions about their personal background characteristics (i.e., age, income, ethnicity); a standardized set of questions designed to measure psychological well-being; a standardized set of questions to assess the presence and severity of menstrual symptoms; and additional questions about coping strategies for the management of symptoms.

The results indicated that variations in the women's self-reported psychological well-being (the dependent variable) were related to many of the independent variables. For example, older subjects and those with higher incomes reported higher levels of well-being than younger subjects and those with lower incomes. Also, subjects who perceived that they were healthy also tended to have high well-being scores. Above and beyond these influences, it was found that the number, type, and severity of symptoms was strongly related to the subjects' psychological well-being, but the source of the symptoms (menstrual *versus* nonmenstrual) was not. The author concluded that "although women might experience specific menstrual symptoms that are distressful, this experience did not negatively affect the overall assessment of their psychological state" (p. 291).

☐ Evaluation research

Evaluative research is an "applied" form of research. Basically, evaluation research involves finding out how well a program, practice, procedure, or policy* is working. Its goal is to assess or evaluate the success of a program. In other words, evaluative research deals with the question of how well the program is meeting its objectives. In nursing practice, nursing administration, and nursing

---

* We will, for the most part, use the term "program" throughout our discussion, but the reader should be aware that this term is meant to include practices, procedures, and policies as well.

education there is obviously a need to sit back and pose such questions as: How are we doing? Are we accomplishing our goals? For example, a clinical nurse may want to evaluate the effectiveness of structured as opposed to casual observations of patients in the development of nursing care plans. A nursing administrator may want to assess the success of certain hospital policies and practices with respect to nurses' performance and job satisfaction. A nursing educator may want information concerning the effectiveness of an autotutorial approach in teaching nursing students how to administer subcutaneous injections. Evaluation research has an important role to play both in localized settings and in programs at the national level.

In each of these examples, the research objective is utilitarian. The purpose of the evaluation is to answer the practical questions of people who must make decisions: Should the program be continued? Do current practices need to be modified or should they be abandoned altogether? When programs are found to be only partially effective, evaluation research can often provide directions for making improvements.

Evaluation research approaches

There are various schools of thought concerning the conduct of evaluation research. In this section we will examine briefly two that are, in a sense, at opposite ends of the spectrum. There are other evaluation models that fall between these extremes, and the reader interested in pursuing evaluation research might want to consult the references at the end of this chapter.

The traditional strategy for the conduct of evaluation research consists of four broad phases: (1) determining the objectives of the program, (2) developing a means of measuring the attainment of those objectives, (3) collecting the data, and (4) interpreting the data

vis-à-vis the objectives. These steps sound rather straightforward—much like the steps in most research studies. Often, the most difficult task is to spell out in detail the goals of a program or practice. Typically, there are numerous objectives of a program, and these objectives may be vague. For example, the principal goal of many nursing practices is the improvement of patient care. This aim, though laudable, is so vague as to be almost meaningless in terms of evaluating its realization. What exactly do we *mean* by improving patient care? How will we know if we have succeeded?

The term *behavioral objective,* frequently referred to in evaluation research literature, is a concept that has evolved as a means of coping with the broadness and fuzziness of program goals. A behavioral objective is the intended outcome of a program stated in terms of the behavior of the individuals at whom the program is aimed. Thus, the goal of "improved patient care" might in one instance translate as "the patient will learn how to cough productively following surgery" or in another as "the patient will walk the length of the corridor within five days after surgery." Note that behavioral objectives always focus on the behavior of the *beneficiaries,* rather than the *agents,* of the program. In the examples above, the objectives were worded to reflect the intended behavioral outcome of the *patient*—not the behavior of the nurse. It would be inappropriate, for example, to use the objective "the nurse will teach the patient to measure his heart rate by counting his radial pulse for a full minute." The emphasis on behavioral objectives can be taken to extremes. There are many times when our interest centers on psychological dimensions such as morale or an emotion (for example, fear) that do not always manifest themselves in behavioral terms. But the evaluator who tries to formulate program goals in terms of behavioral objectives will almost always find that the goals are less vague and diffuse than they might otherwise have been.

Once the program goals have been delineated, the evaluation using a traditional approach can be designed much like other research studies. An evaluation can use either an experimental design (with subjects randomly assigned to either the program being evaluated or to a control group), a quasi-experimental design, or a nonexperimental design. The final step in the classical evaluation model is to analyze the data in such a way that some decisions can be made about the program or practice under consideration, or some action can be taken to make the program more effective.

In recent years, the traditional model of evaluators has been criticized by a number of writers for a certain narrowness of conceptualization. One alternative evaluation model is the so-called goal-free approach. Proponents of this model argue that programs may have a number of consequences besides accomplishing the official objectives of the program and that the classical model is handicapped by its inability to investigate these other effects. According to advocates of goal-free evaluation, the mere knowledge of the program objectives has the potential of biasing the evaluator by suggesting the areas of the program that should be researched.

Thus, goal-free evaluation represents an attempt to evaluate the outcomes of a program in the absence of information about *intended* outcomes. The job of the evaluator—a very demanding one—is basically that of describing the repercussions of a program or practice on various components of the overall system. A goal-free evaluation of a procedure to reduce preoperative anxiety, for example, might assess the impact of the procedure not only on patients but also on other individuals such as staff, administrators, and visitors of the patients *and* on other procedures, policies, or costs. The goal-free evaluation model is, in many respects, congruent with the medical model of patient evaluation, with its concern for monitoring possible side-effects of a treatment.

The goal-free model might often be a profitable approach, and certainly leaves more room for creativity on the part of the evaluator. In many cases, however, the model may not be practical, from two points of view. First of all, there are seldom unlimited resources (personnel, time, or money) for the conduct of an evaluation. Decision-makers may need to know, quite simply, whether objectives are being met so that immediate decisions can be made. Secondly, precisely because goal-free evaluation allows for creativity, the quality of the data depends to a great extent on the ingenuity of the evaluator. Without an understanding of the program goals, the evaluator has no guidelines or structure within which to operate. In the final analysis, the choice of a model will depend, to a large extent, on the informational needs of the decision-maker and on the position of the evaluator within the organization.

Formative and summative research

Formative evaluation refers to the ongoing process of providing evaluative feedback in the course of developing a program or policy. For example, if the nursing faculty were interested in devising a curriculum to teach research methods to undergraduate nursing students, they could benefit from a system of evaluating new material as it was being developed and presented so that modifications could be made. The aim of formative evaluation, then, is to provide information about improving the content, structure, or agents of a program. Formative evaluation often employs rather ''loose'' methods. That is, suggestions for improvement can come from unstructured discussions with relevant individuals, from informal observations of the program in operation, from an armchair analysis of materials and objectives and so forth. This is not to say that a more rigorous approach is inappropriate. For example, in the research curriculum example mentioned, formal feedback might be gathered by testing students on their understanding of the course materials. However, the focus of formative evaluation is on a careful monitoring of a program as it evolves.

Summative evaluation, on the other hand, assesses the worth of a program after it is already in operation. The aim of such evaluation is not to improve a program or practice, but, rather, to help people decide whether it should be discarded, replaced, modified, or continued. Let us say that a group-oriented approach to teaching postoperative breathing and coughing exercises to preoperative patients has been developed in a hospital, and a true experimental design was adopted to test the effectiveness of the new approach. Presurgical patients would be randomly assigned to an experimental (group-teaching) condition or a control condition (individual teaching). The effectiveness of the new intervention could then be evaluated by comparing postoperative outcomes on preestablished criteria (for example, length of hospital stay or physiological measures such as vital capacity, arterial blood gas levels, or presence of respiratory infection) for the two conditions. If there were no differences between the two procedures, decisions concerning which approach to adopt would probably be based on other conditions such as administrative ease, costs, or personnel utilization.

There are many cases in which summative evaluation may not be applicable simply because the program or practice is constantly fluid and open to change and improvement. In such cases the information provided by formative evaluation may play a continuingly important role.

Obstacles and problems in evaluation research

All research projects encounter difficulties that are, usually, unanticipated. Evaluation researchers often come up against several obstacles that can be foreseen because they emerge so frequently. We will briefly review several of the most recurrent problem areas in the hope that advanced planning may help to alleviate the difficulties.

First of all, evaluation research can be threatening to individuals. Even when the focus of an evaluation is on a nontangible entity, such as a program, procedure, policy, or the like, it is *people* who developed the entity and are implementing it. People tend to think that they, or their work, are being evaluated and may in some cases feel that their job or reputation is at stake. Evaluation researchers, thus, need to have more than methodological skills: they need to be diplomats, adept in interpersonal dealings with people. If the persons operating a program are defensive and noncooperative, the evaluation could be unproductive.

Even when program staff are not on the defensive, they can be reluctant to cooperate for other reasons. If they are convinced about the merit of the program or policy that is being evaluated, they may not see the need for more objective information. They may believe that their time is better spent in providing services to people than in helping a researcher evaluate the adequacy of their services.

Yet another difficulty that many evaluation researchers encounter is the problem of ascertaining the goals of the program. In the classical approach to evaluating a program, the evaluator must have a clear idea of what the program is attempting to accomplish. When a program or practice has a simple goal, the evaluator need only develop some method of measuring its attainment. More often, however, the objectives of a program are multiple and diffuse; in many cases the goals refer to behaviors or conditions in the distant future.

A program with multiple goals can be problematic from another point of view. What happens—as is often the case with broadly aimed programs—when some of the objectives are satisfied but others are not? Should the program be continued anyway, or should it be discarded? If modifications are needed, how will an evaluator know the full implications of the recommended changes on the goals that were already being met?

A problem related to the complexity of the goals is the question of the complexity of the program itself. Suppose we were to evaluate a hospital program whose principal aim was to encourage nurses to enroll in continuing education courses. In this case the goal is relatively straightforward and easily measured. But if the program itself involves a number of components it will be difficult to determine what accounts for its success (or failure). Because decision-makers are generally concerned with the costs of their programs and practices, it is often useful to understand which components have the greatest impact, but this can be quite difficult for an evaluator to determine.

This list of barriers or obstacles to conducting effective evaluation is not intended to discourage researchers but rather to alert persons about to embark on such endeavors to the more frequent evaluation problems. Difficulties arise in all research projects — permissions can be delayed, telephones malfunction, research personnel become ill, and so forth. In evaluation research, however, the researcher must often contend with a characteristic set of problems that are organizational, interpersonal, or political in nature. The wise person will enter an evaluation project with eyes wide open, aware of the obstacles that may arise, yet sensitive to the genuine contribution that evaluations can make to program functioning and to the improvement of health care.

Example of evaluation research

Mills and her colleagues (1985) evaluated the effectiveness of an inpatient cardiac education program. The group education program was implemented because of the large number of patients being treated at the hospital (the Little Rock Veterans Administration Medical Center) with a diagnosis of ischemic heart disease. The patient education program consisted of five 1-hour classes. The objectives of the program were to increase patients' knowledge in specific areas and to increase postdischarge compliance with a prescribed treatment plan. A number of behavioral objectives were developed. For example, one of the objectives for the first of the five classes was as follows: The patient will be able to describe what happens to the heart muscle when a person has a heart attack.

A total of 277 patients participated in the study. A 23-item multiple-choice test of knowledge was administered to subjects prior to the treatment (the five classes) and then upon completion of the course. Four weeks after discharge from the program, participants were again contacted and asked to complete a behavior assessment (compliance) questionnaire. The results revealed that there were significant gains in knowledge, as measured by the test, after the patients completed the education program. The design for this portion of the study can best be described as preexperimental, because there was no control group of subjects who were *not* exposed to the intervention. However, the investigators did incorporate a design element that gives us greater confidence that the increase of knowledge did not reflect a "testing" effect. Some subjects were randomly assigned to a group that did not receive an initial test of knowledge. There were no differences between the two groups in terms of their posttreatment test scores, so it seems reasonable to conclude that the knowledge gain reflects the influence of the program.

A further analysis indicated that the greater the number of classes a patient attended and the higher the posttest knowledge scores, the higher the compliance with the prescribed treatment plan. Unfortunately, the findings do not allow us to conclude that compliance can be increased by increasing a patient's exposure to an educational program. More highly motivated patients were probably more likely to attend more classes; therefore, it is plausible that self-selection factors influenced the relationship between class attendance and compliance scores.

□
Needs assessments

Like evaluation research, a needs assessment represents an effort to provide a decision-maker with information for action. As the name implies, a needs assessment is a study in which a researcher collects data for estimating the needs of a group, community, or organization. In other words, a needs assessment provides informational input in a planning process.

A needs assessment generally is undertaken by agencies or groups that have a service component. Nursing educators may wish to assess the needs of their clients (students); hospital staff members may wish to learn the needs of those they serve (patients); a mental health outreach clinic may wish to gather information on the needs of some target population (for example, adolescents in the community). Because resources are seldom limitless, information that can help in establishing priorities is almost always valuable. Needs assessments are useful in this capacity not only when a program or policy becomes established but also after the program is in operation. Organizations and communities are dynamic entities whose needs are almost always in transition. A program whose objectives are structured to meet the needs of the group at one point may find that it becomes ineffective because the objectives are no longer meaningful. Thus, while an evaluation might seek to ascertain if a program is attaining its objectives, the aim of needs assessments is to determine if the objectives of a program are meeting the needs of the individuals who are supposed to benefit from it.

Needs assessment approaches

The methods of a needs assessment may vary considerably in complexity, cost, and length of time required to perform the study. The various approaches noted here are not necessarily mutually exclusive. Several methods often are used quite profitably to supplement one another in a single study. The *key informant approach,* as the name implies, collects information concerning the needs of a group from key individuals who are presumed to be in a position to know those needs. These key informants could be community leaders, prominent health-care workers, agency directors, or other knowledgeable individuals. Questionnaires or interviews are generally used to collect the data.

A second method is the *survey* approach in which data are collected from a sample from the target group whose needs are being assessed. In a survey there would be no attempt to question only persons who are in positions of authority or who are knowledgeable. Any member of the group or community could be asked to give his or her viewpoint.

Another alternative is to use an *indicators* approach, which relies on inferences made from statistics available in existing reports or records. For example, a nurse-managed clinic that is interested in analyzing the needs of its clients could examine over a five-year period the number of appointments that were kept, the employment rate of its clients, the changes in risk appraisal status, methods of payment, and so forth. The indicators approach is very flexible and may also be quite economical because the data are generally available but need organization and interpretation.

The final phase of a needs assessment almost always involves the development of recommendations. These recommendations for action typically involve the delineation of priorities as revealed by the findings, but the suggestions are rarely totally objective. The role of the researcher conducting a needs assessment is often that of making judgments about priorities in light of considerations such as costs and feasibility and in advising on means by which the most highly prioritized needs can be serviced.

Example of a needs assessment

A study designed to assess the health needs of elderly residents living in high-rise apartments was conducted by Hain and Chen (1976). These researchers identified the lack of existing information concerning the health needs of the noninstitutionalized elderly and the barriers to adequate health care as a potentially serious problem. They set out to document such needs and barriers by utilizing a survey approach.

The participants in this study were residents aged 65 or older who lived in two high-rise apartments in Pennsylvania for at least six months. The final sample included 128 residents, ranging in age from 65 to over 85. The data were collected by means of an interview, in which twenty questions were read from a prepared interview schedule. The questions covered such topics as access to medical care, health condition, physical functioning, transportation to health facilities, and cost of health care.

After developing composite indicators for health condition, the researchers determined that 24.3 percent of the elderly surveyed were not well. Thirty-two percent of the sample were classified as having problems with physical functioning, and females living alone were significantly more likely to have physical difficulties than males living alone or couples. Another finding was that approximately 12 percent of the elderly questioned had no access to medical care. Based on these results, the in-

vestigators were able to develop a series of recommendations for meeting the health needs of such noninstitutionalized older persons. These recommendations included the implementation of health education, screening, and monitoring programs and the utilization of visiting nurse practitioners and home health aides.

This needs assessment, which chose a survey rather than a key informant approach, enabled the investigators to document specific needs and, further, to identify subgroups that were in particular need of certain services. By conducting such a study the researchers were able to lay the foundation for rational planning and decision-making. Clearly, the purpose for performing an investigtion of this type — whether the topic is health needs of a client group, the educational needs of nurses, or the organizational needs of administrators — is to collect data that will provide a basis for action.

□

Historical research

Historical research is the systematic collection and critical evaluation of data relating to past occurrences. Generally, historical research is undertaken in order to test hypotheses or to answer questions concerning causes, effects, or trends relating to past events that may shed light on present behaviors or practices. An understanding of contemporary nursing theories, practices, or issues can often be enhanced by an investigation of a defined segment of the past. Particularly in this time when nurses are working to define and extend their professional roles, a knowledge of the roots of nursing has the capacity to put nursing theories and procedures into an appropriate context. For example, the struggles experienced by several states in enacting new laws that recognize nurses as independent practitioners had their roots in the "handmaiden to the physician" attitude so long accepted by physicians, nurses, and society at large.

The steps involved in performing historical research actually are quite similar to those for other types of research: a problem area is defined, hypotheses or specific questions are developed, data are collected according to a systematic framework, data are analyzed, and findings are interpreted. Historical research differs from other types of research, however, in two important respects. First, considerable effort is usually required to identify data sources on events, situations, and human behavior occurring in the past. Second, since the researcher has no control over the quality of data available, another research task involves the critical evaluation of gathered information.

Historical research is inherently nonexperimental. The researcher can neither manipulate nor control the variables, nor is there any possibility of random assignment. In fact, the historical researcher must cope with a number of handicaps. In ex post facto or survey research the investigator may not be able to manipulate variables but usually there are opportunities to construct or select the data collection tool. Historians, however, have no control over the documents, records, or artifacts available for study. The historian is at a similar disadvantage with regard to sampling. Only surviving records can be consulted, and these records may contain a number of biases.

Formulation of the problem and hypotheses

Like other forms of research, it is important for the historian to formulate a feasible, well-articulated problem area to explore. It is easy for a historical problem to become unmanageable because there is less closure than in a study that creates new data. That is, the historian may lack a definitive end-point at which the data can be said to have been collected. On the other hand, a unique problem in historical research is the possibility that a sufficient quantity of data (of adequate quality) will be unavailable. Thus, the historical researcher should be familiar enough with the problem area to choose a well-defined topic that can be studied in depth and for which there are at least enough data to permit a test of some hypotheses or provide answers to specific questions.

The student should be careful not to confuse historical research with a review of the literature, although a literature review will undoubtedly be an early step in the research process. The purpose of historical research should be to explain the present or to anticipate future events; it is not merely to find out what is already known about an issue and to paraphrase it. Like other types of research, historical inquiry has as its goal the discovery of new knowledge.

One important difference between historical research and a literature review is that a historical researcher is often guided in the collection of information by the formulation of specific hypotheses or questions. The hypotheses represent attempts at explaining and interpreting the conditions, events, or phenomena under investigation. Hypotheses in historical research are not usually tested in a statistical sense. They are, generally, broadly stated conjectures about relationships among historical events, trends, and phenomena. For example, it might be hypothesized that a relationship exists between the presence or absence of war on the one hand and the amount of scientific nursing knowledge generated on the other. This hypothesis could be tested by analyzing research trends in nursing during the twentieth century.

Collection of historical data

Data for historical research are usually in the form of written records of the past: periodicals, diaries, books, letters, newspapers, minutes of meetings, legal documents, and so forth. However, a number of nonwritten materials may also be of interest. For example, physical remains and objects are potential sources of information. Visual materials such as photographs, films, and drawings are forms of data, as are audio materials such as records, tapes, and so forth. It is evident that many of these materials may be difficult to obtain and even written materials will not always be conveniently indexed by subject, author, or title. The identification of appropriate historical materials may require a considerable amount of time, effort, and detective work. Fortunately, there exist several archives of historical nursing documents, such as the collections at several universities (Columbia, Radcliffe, Boston University, Johns Hopkins) as well as collections at the National Library of Medicine, the Nursing Museum in Philadelphia, the American Journal of Nursing Company, and the National League for Nursing.

If the event or phenomenon of interest occurred in the recent past, it may be possible to identify living persons who participated in or witnessed the event or who personally knew a historical figure. When this is the case, interviews with such persons contribute another form of data.

Historical materials generally are classified as either primary or secondary sources. A *primary source* is first-hand information, such as original documents, relics, or artifacts. Examples are Louisa May Alcott's book *Hospital Sketches,* minutes of early ANA meetings, hospital records, and so forth. Primary sources represent the most direct link with historical events or situations: only the narrator (in the case of written materials) intrudes between original events and the historian.

Secondary sources are second- or third-hand accounts of historical events or experiences. For example, textbooks, encyclopedias, or other reference books are generally secondary sources. Secondary sources, in other words, are discussions of events written by individuals who are summarizing or interpreting primary source materials. Primary sources should be used whenever possible in historical research. The further removed from the historical event the information is, the less reliable, objective, and comprehensive the data are likely to be. Of course, primary sources generally are more difficult to locate and use, but historical research that relies exclusively or heavily on secondary materials is bound to have numerous limitations.

Evaluation of historical data

Historical evidence usually is subjected to two types of evaluation, which historians refer to as external and internal criticism. *External criticism* is concerned basically with the authenticity and genuineness of the data. For example, a nursing historian might have a diary presumed to be written by Dorothea Dix. External criticism would involve asking such questions as: Is this the handwriting of Ms. Dix? Is the paper on which the diary is written of the right age? Are the writing style and ideas expressed consistent with her other writings?

There are various scientific techniques available to determine the age of materials, such as x-ray and radioactive procedures. But other flaws may be less easy to detect. For example, there is the possibility that material of interest may have been written by a ghost writer—that is, by someone other than the person in whom we are really interested. There is also the potential problem of mechanical errors associated with transcriptions, translations, or typed versions of historical materials. Furthermore, even if a document or object is original, it is possible that alterations were made at a later point. There may be no way to prove the authenticity of historical materials. If the researcher finds any reason to question the genuineness of the documents or objects, however, great caution should be exercised in their use.

Internal criticism of historical data refers to the evaluation of the worth of the evidence. The focus of internal criticism is not so much on the physical aspects of the materials but rather on their content. An important issue here is the accuracy or truth of the data. For example, the historian must question whether a writer's representations of historical events are unbiased. It may also be appropriate to ask if the author of a document was in a position to make a valid report of an event or occurrence, or whether the writer was competent as a recorder of fact. Evidence bearing on the accuracy of historical data might include one of the following: (1) comparisons with other people's accounts of the same event to determine the degree of agreement; (2) knowledge of the time at which the document was produced (reports of events or situations tend to be more accurate if they are written immediately following the event, such as in diaries or minutes of a meeting); (3) knowledge of the point of view or biases of the writer; and (4) knowledge of the degree of competence of the writer to record events authoritatively and accurately.

Data synthesis and analysis

After evaluating the authenticity and accuracy of historical data, the researcher must begin to pull the materials together, to analyze them, and to test the research hypotheses. Data that have passed the tests of internal and external criticism are not uniformly useful: the relative value of the various sources must be weighed. The historian must be extremely careful at this point because the analysis of historical information involves logical processes rather than statistical ones and, therefore, the possibility of subjectivity arises. That is to say, the researcher must take care not to disregard evidence that either contradicts or fails to support

the hypotheses. In essence, the final steps of historical research involve a considerable amount of decision-making. The entire mass of evidence must be organized and weighed, and problems about inconsistencies must be resolved. Judgments have to be made, but they should be made in as objective a manner as possible.

Once the data have been organized, analyzed, and synthesized, conclusions and interpretations need to be formulated. The historian, to a greater degree than other researchers, must be cautious in generalizing the results of the research because events can never be duplicated exactly.

Example of historical research

Regan (1976) conducted a historical research study concerning the role of the school nurse in American society. The study focused on medical, nursing, educational, and societal factors that influenced the development of the role since its inception in 1902 in New York City.

Data concerning the concepts of role status, role expectations, role discrepancies, and reference groups were gathered from nursing, educational, and medical sources. The data were grouped into four sequential time periods: 1902 to 1923, 1924 to 1949, 1950 to 1969, and the 1970s. A major goal of the study was to use information concerning the first three time periods as a basis for forecasting and recommending future directions for the school nurse's role.

The primary sources used for collecting data included original manuscripts, addresses made by nursing or school health personnel, letters written by nurses or school health personnel, and memoirs. Secondary sources included both published and unpublished reports of studies from school health, nursing, medical, and educational associations as well as textbooks and journal articles.

The analysis and synthesis of the collected data revealed that the status of the role and the kinds of behaviors expected of the school nurses by various reference groups were determined to a large extent by society's and education's perceptions of health needs during the various time periods. For example, one of the trends that occurred during the 1950 to 1969 period was emphasis on coordination in planning health programs. Regan noted that collaborative efforts between nurses and other school personnel enhanced the status of the school nurse role.

□
Case studies

Case studies are in-depth investigations of an individual, group, institution, or other social unit. The researcher conducting a case study attempts to analyze and understand the variables that are important to the history, development, or care of the subject or the subject's problems. As befits an intensive analysis, the focus of case studies is typically on determining the dynamics of *why* the subject of the investigation thinks, behaves, or develops in a particular manner, rather than *what* his or her status, progress, actions, or thoughts are. It is not unusual for probing research of this type to require a rather detailed study over a considerable time period. Data are often collected that relate not only to the subject's present state but also to past experiences and situational and environmental factors relevant to the problem being examined.

The functions of case studies

Case studies are a useful way to explore phenomena that have not been rigorously researched. For example, as new reproductive technologies have emerged (such as *in vitro* fertilization) several case studies have reported on the experiences of the couple undergoing treatment, laying the groundwork for more extensive research.

The information obtained in case studies can be extremely useful in the production of hypotheses to be tested more rigorously in subsequent research. Indeed, many writers consider this the most obvious and direct scientific function of case materials. For example, Freud's case studies of clients with personality disorders and problems led him to formulate an elaborate theoretical system. Although Freud did not test the hypotheses implied by his theories, some of the relationships suggested by his work have been studied more systematically by subsequent investigators. The intensive probing that characterizes case studies often leads to insights concerning previously unsuspected relationships. Furthermore, in-depth case studies may serve the very important role of clarifying concepts and variables or of elucidating ways to measure them.

Case studies sometimes are used in conjunction with more quantitatively oriented research to serve in an illustrative capacity. Research reports that are filled with extensive statistical information often fail to convey some of the richness of the real-life subject matter. Case materials presented in such a context can be extremely effective in elucidating certain points or in imparting a more realistic impression to data that might otherwise appear far removed from practical concerns.

It is usually unwise to make predictions or generalizations to a broader population based upon case study data. However, it may be perfectly reasonable to predict the future behavior of an individual who is the subject of the case study based on events or relationships experienced by the person in the past. In this limited sense, hypothesis testing is an appropriate activity for case studies.

Case study methods

Unlike many of the types of research we have discussed in earlier chapters, there is no clear-cut, specified technique associated with case studies. The first step, as one might expect, is to delineate the problem area to be studied. This is seldom difficult in case studies because the majority of such studies seem to arise from attempts to solve a specific practical problem, as often happens in nursing situations. Once the problem area and the case or cases to be studied have been identified, the researcher must develop a data collection plan.

There is considerable freedom in selecting or devising a way to gather data for case studies. Virtually all the data-collecting methods available in research are amenable to use in a case study: questionnaires and interviews, observation schemes, rating devices, physiological measures, personal documents such as diaries or letters, statistical records, and so forth. The researcher may select one of these techniques or may combine several.

Finally, the data collected must be analyzed and interpreted. Because the investigator becomes well acquainted with the subject, and because there are no controls or comparisons to put the data into broader perspective, there is always a risk of subjectivity or bias in performing case studies. It is wise to be conservative in interpreting case study data.

Some case studies involve the administration of a treatment and an analysis of ensuing consequences on the individual. Such studies are sometimes referred to as *single-subject experiments.* For example, suppose we were interested in examining the effect of a therapeutic approach on the behavior of an autistic child. We would begin by isolating one or more specific behaviors as a measure of the child's status, as for example, the child's ability to play quietly without becoming violent or the child's willingness to take medications. Before instituting any treatment (therapy), we would record the child's behavior on the criterion measures for a short period of time. These data generally are referred to as *baseline data.* Once therapy begins, the criterion measures would be carefully monitored and recorded either until the desired behavior patterns were obtained or for a specified period of time. The

appearance of desirable behavior (or the disappearance of undesirable behavior) after the institution of a therapeutic treatment is not usually sufficient evidence that the treatment was effective. In this particular example, other events or circumstances in the child's life could be responsible for improved behavior. For this reason, two additional phases of data collection are recommended. The *reversal phase* is the period in which the treatment is withheld. If there is subsequent deterioration in the subject's behavior pattern, the researcher will have more confidence that it is the treatment, rather than extraneous factors, that is producing the desired effect. Finally, treatment is reinstituted, and further measurements of the criterion variable are made. Figure 10-2 presents some "ideal" hypothetical data for the example of the autistic child's play behavior. These data are ideal in the sense that they provide rather clear-cut evidence of the treatment's efficacy. Most actual data are often less conclusive.

Strengths and weaknesses of case studies

Unquestionably the greatest advantage of case studies is the depth that is possible when a limited number of individuals, institutions, or groups is being investigated. A common complaint leveled at other types of research is that the data tend to be rather superficial. Case studies provide the researcher with the opportunity of having an intimate knowledge of the subject's condition, thoughts, feelings, actions (past and present), intentions, and environment.

On the other hand, this same strength is a potential weakness, because the familiarity of the researcher with the subject makes objectivity more difficult. Objectivity may be particularly problematic if the data are collected by observational techniques for which the researcher is the main (or only) observer.

Perhaps the most serious disadvantage of

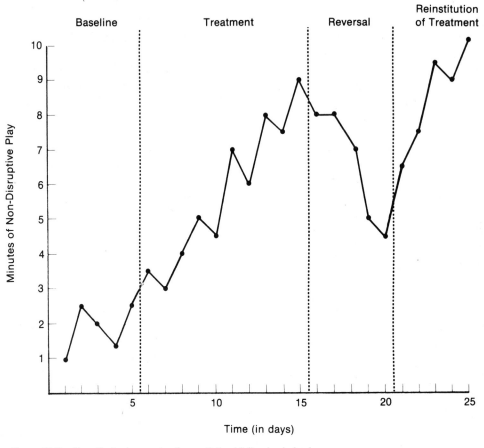

Figure 10-2. *Hypothetical example of an autistic child's play behavior.*

the case study method is its lack of generaliz-ability. That is, if the researcher reveals the existence of important relationships, it would be difficult to argue that the same relation-ships would manifest themselves in other sub-jects. Inasmuch as case studies cannot be counted upon to produce valid generaliza-tions, their usefulness as an approach to test-ing hypotheses is severely limited.

Example of a case study

Baltes and Zerbe (1976) conducted a case study on an elderly woman living in a nursing home who, although physically able, was not feeding herself. The researchers hypothesized that a change in environmental conditions would result in a change in the subject's self-feeding behaviors.

The investigators observed and recorded the subject's eating behavior during breakfast, dinner, and supper for 1 week before begin-ning any treatment. The treatment consisted of prompting the subject to feed herself by giving verbal instructions, placing the spoon in the subject's hand, and progressively raising it to her mouth. As soon as the subject responded to any stage of the treatment, reinforcement of the positive self-feeding behavior occurred by providing flowers, music, and liquids. Nonself-feeding behaviors of the subject resulted in removal of the flowers, stopping the music, and turning the investigator's back to the subject. As soon as the lady began to feed herself, the positive reinforcers returned.

The results of the study supported the hypothesis that changes in environmental conditions resulted in a change in the subject's self-feeding behavior. The presence of flowers, music, and social interaction enhanced self-feeding. Return to the environmental conditions existing prior to the study produced a decline in self-feeding behavior.

This case study involved the administration of a treatment. Baseline data were collected prior to instituting the treatment. Once the subject began to feed herself in a consistent fashion, the treatment was withheld, or the reversal phase implemented. As the subject's self-feeding behavior declined during the reversal phase, the investigators gained more confidence that the change in self-feeding behavior resulted from the treatment. The treatment was not reinstituted in this study because the subject died.

□
Field studies

Qualitative research that aims at describing and exploring phenomena in naturalistic settings is frequently referred to as field research. *Field studies* are investigations that are done "in the field," in such social settings as hospitals, clinics, intensive care units, nursing homes, housing projects, and so on. The purpose of field studies is to examine in an in-depth fashion the practices, behaviors, beliefs, and attitudes of individuals or groups as they normally function in real life. Like case studies, field studies are often intensive rather than extensive, and data are collected in a variety of ways. However, case studies do not always involve the collection of data "in the field," and case study data might in some cases be very structured, quantitative information. In field studies, the researcher, by definition, engages in field work (i.e., goes out to the setting where the subjects normally operate). The data that are collected are usually narrative materials, based on researcher observation, conversations with subjects, or available documents. The aim of the field researcher is to "get close" to the people under study in order to really understand a problem or situation from their perspective.

Anthropologists have engaged in field research for decades in their efforts to understand the functioning of human cultures. Nurse researchers, because of their interest in nurse-patient-environment interactions, are becoming increasingly interested in field research. Examples of the kinds of nursing problems that could fruitfully be addressed through field research include the following: What are the health-care needs of the homeless, and what are the barriers to providing that care? What environmental conditions and stresses lead to dysfunctional parenting and child abuse? What types of interpersonal style characterize hospitalized psychiatric patients?

Characteristics of field research

In traditional scientific research, a heavy emphasis is placed on control and objectivity. In field research, the researcher continually uses subjective judgments about whom to interview, what to observe, what questions to ask, and so on. In field research, the main instrument of data collection *is* the researcher, rather than technical apparatus or formal written tools.

Typically, data collection and analysis are ongoing, simultaneous activities in the field. The analysis of information often leads the investigator to pursue new avenues of inquiry. In traditional approaches, data to be collected are prespecified and generally remain unanalyzed until all the data are "in."

Field research is typically less linear than other types of research. That is, the steps do not follow a linear progression such as that suggested in Chapter 3. The field researcher may begin with only a general problem area or hypothesis to be explored. Or, hypotheses may be generated in the course of data collection/analysis and pursued more rigorously in subsequent data collection. Field researchers try to remain open and flexible about the research process in the hope that such flexibility will allow them to pursue the realities of the subjects' experience as that experience is lived.

Conducting field research

Wilson (1985) has identified the five following stages of field research:

- Stage I: Identifying the setting in which the fieldwork will take place and assessing the appropriateness of the setting for the problem of interest.
- Stage II: Gaining access to the people or groups to be studied.
- Stage III: Assuming an appropriate role in the social setting on a participant-observer continuum (appropriate in terms of research aims and/or the demands/constraints of those under study).
- Stage IV: Collecting, recording, analyzing, and interpreting data.
- Stage V: Leaving the field.

Appraisal of field research

Field studies are strong on realism because they are done in natural settings without structure or controls imposed by the researcher. Because of the in-depth and flexible nature of field studies, they often provide a depth of understanding of social phenomena that is unattainable with more traditional methods of scientific research. For example, Norris' (1975)

in-depth study of restlessness led to a careful delineation of the meaning of this phenomena and a description of its precursors.

Some of the very elements that make field research strong are potential problem areas. During data collection and analysis, the researcher is so thoroughly immersed in the phenomenon that the risk of bias becomes great. Perhaps the most problematic aspect of field research, however, is the difficulty with which investigators describe how they have arrived at their conclusions. Field research can almost never be replicated because the methods evolve *in situ*. It is often difficult to evaluate whether two independent field researchers would come to different conclusions based on the same investigation. Because of these problems, field research is sometimes characterized by hard-line scientists as "soft" and "fuzzy."

Example of a field study

Madeleine Leininger has been a leader in an area she calls *ethnonursing research,* which she defines as "the study and analysis of the local or indigenous people's viewpoints, beliefs, and practices about nursing care behavior and processes of designated cultures" (Leininger, 1985, p. 38). One of the many field studies she has conducted focused on blacks and whites living in a rural community in central Alabama (Leininger, 1985, pp. 195–216). The purpose of the research was to systematically study the care and health values, beliefs, attitudes, and general lifeways of these two cultural groups. Among the many research questions addressed by her research were the following: "What is the general lifeway of the Black and White villagers, especially related to care and health cultural expressions?" and "What are the perceived differences and similarities between the rural folk and the urban professional health care practices?" (p. 196).

To address these research questions, Leininger spent ten months in the field, intensively studying a community of under 3000 people that she called Friendly Village and, for the purposes of "reflective comparison," a similar community called Pecan Village. During the ten months of her fieldwork, Leininger observed the living habits and customs of the residents of these communities, participated in some of their lifeways, and interviewed about 90 Friendly Villagers. Sixty of them were selected for in-depth observation and interviewing.

Through such intensive study, the investigator was able to gain rich information about how people in this culture felt about health and health care, and about how those beliefs influenced their health behavior. Only a few examples of the kinds of in-depth insights she derived from her research can be presented here. For example, a dominant theme that emerged in connection with the meaning of health to the villagers was that "health means being able to do your work in the home, church, and community" (p. 204). Leininger also learned the strength of the villagers' perceived linkage between health and religion. From the villagers' viewpoint, it made no sense to speak of health without considering spiritual health as a total process of living; health in that community was associated with living properly by the Bible and doing what God teaches. A full understanding of such beliefs would clearly be important to the provision of culturally acceptable health care in such communities.

□
Secondary analysis

The types of research reviewed thus far have an important characteristic in common, and that is that the investigator must collect or organize new data. This section deals with research projects that use previously gathered data.

The amount of research conducted every year in such fields as nursing, medicine, public health, nutrition, the life sciences, and the social sciences is overwhelming. In a typical research project, more data are collected than the investigator actually analyzes. Even when the initial researcher does utilize all of the data, he or she does not typically exhaust the possibilities of examining the relationships among the variables. This is particularly true of large-scale data sets, such as the ones collected by the National Center for Health Statistics, but may be true of smaller research projects as well. It is, therefore, becoming increasingly common for researchers to use available data to test their research hypotheses. This type of research activity, referred to as *secondary analysis,* is extremely valuable because it is efficient and economical.

Secondary analysis approaches

Let us explore some of the possibilities of secondary analysis by considering a hypothetical example. Suppose that an investigator is interested in exploring staff attitudes toward mental illness and modes of patient treatment in psychiatric hospitals, and the relationship between these attitudes and a variety of patient outcomes (for example, number of patients released on trial visits, number of hours of restraint or seclusion, number of unauthorized absences of the patients, and so forth). Let us assume that the researcher has collected the attitudinal information from several hundred staff members in five hospitals by means of a questionnaire, which also included a number of background information questions about each staff person, such as a position, number of years of experience, age, education, sex, and so forth. The original research study, however, does not make use of this background information, because the focus of the investigation is on hospital units, not on individual staff members. Thus, the original investigator may find that in hospital units where the staff as a whole tended to view patients unfavorably and tended to interpret hospital rules in an authoritarian manner, there also tended to be fewer patients released on trial visits, a greater number of patient elopements, and a higher number of hours during which patients were secluded or restrained.

At this point, the researcher has tested the hypotheses that guided the initial study, yet has left unanalyzed a considerable amount of data. A nurse researcher might hypothesize that an authoritarian attitude toward mentally ill patients among the nursing staff would be related to the nurse's age, educational background, status in the nursing hierarchy, and other background characteristics. The information collected in the original study could provide the nurse researcher with an excellent opportunity for testing the new hypotheses. In such a situation, the unit of analysis would be individual staff members and would be restricted only to nursing personnel. This secondary analysis would ignore the data relating to patient outcomes, because they are not relevant to the hypotheses of the new investigation.

This example illustrates a number of avenues for secondary analyses. First of all, as already noted, variables that are unanalyzed in an initial investigation are prime targets for further research. Furthermore, different relationships among variables can be explored in later uses of the data. In the example discussed above, the attitudinal variables that were the independent variables in the primary analysis became the dependent variables in the secondary analysis. That is, the initial analysis used the staff attitudes to "explain" patient outcomes; the secondary analysis used background characteristics to "explain" nursing staff attitudes.

The example shows two other approaches adopted in secondary analyses. Whereas the

initial researcher utilized data from all subjects, the investigator in the later project was interested in only a subsample, the nursing personnel. It is frequently the case that secondary analysis concentrates on a particular subgroup rather than on the entire sample. A study that examined nursing students' withdrawal from a nursing program might generate data useful for further research on the needs and problems of minority nursing dropouts. An investigation of health habits and health-related behaviors in urban areas could produce information of interest to a researcher concerned with pica practice among urban children.

Another possibility for secondary analysis illustrated by the above example is a change in the *unit of analysis*. In this example the original research was concerned with aggregate data, that is, with the data from several individuals collapsed (averaged) within a bigger unit —the hospital ward. The researcher could have used an even larger unit—the hospital as a whole. The secondary analysis used the most basic element (individual responses) as the unit of analysis.

It should also be pointed out that secondary analysis can be particularly powerful if it is possible to obtain two or more data sets with comparable variables. If similar relationships between variables are revealed in different samples or populations, the researcher can be much more confident that the results are generalizable to other groups. Secondary analyses of data sets that complement each other in this way can be particularly valuable in formulating general propositions or theories.

Sources of data for secondary analysis

In recent years a number of groups such as university institutes and federal agencies have been attempting to organize data and make them available to researchers for secondary analysis. The policies regulating the public use of data vary from one organization to another, but it is not unusual for data to be provided to an interested researcher at about the costs for duplication plus handling. Thus, in some cases in which the gathering of the data involved an expenditure of thousands of dollars, reproduced materials may be supplied for less than one percent of the initial costs.

Secondary analysis of large-scale data sets is becoming increasingly feasible by the development of data libraries, such as the International Data Library and Reference Service at the University of California (Berkeley) or the Roper Public Opinion Research Center at Williams College. There are also a number of groups, in some cases funded by the National Science Foundation, that are attempting to inventory and catalogue the data libraries, such as the Council of Social Science Data Archives in New York City. The federal government sometimes sponsors the establishment of data archives on health-related topics. For example, the Office of Population Affairs sponsors the Data Archive on Adolescent Pregnancy Prevention.

Small-scale, localized studies are unlikely to be included in data libraries. Nevertheless, the research community often cooperates in supplying data for secondary analysis to other researchers. Thus, an investigator may learn of existing data that are suitable for his or her research needs in a journal article, report, or a presentation at a professional conference or from colleagues. In such an event it may well be worth exploring the possibility of borrowing the data or of engaging in a collaborative research activity.

Strengths and weaknesses of secondary analysis

The use of available data makes it possible for the researcher to bypass time-consuming and costly steps in the research process. Investigators engaged in secondary analysis can typically proceed directly from the formulation of research hypotheses to a testing of those hypotheses. There is no need to obtain a sample, design an instrument, or gather the data. Thus, the greatest advantage of secondary analysis is its expediency.

On the other hand, there are numerous disadvantages in working with existing data. If an investigator does not play a role in collecting the data, the chances are pretty high that the data set will be deficient or problematic in one or more ways, such as in the sample used, the variables measured, and so forth. The researcher may continuously face "if only" problems: if only they had asked a question about X, or if only they had included Y in their sample. Furthermore, one always takes a risk of obtaining data that are inaccurate or erroneous. Errors can enter into the research endeavor at a number of phases; the interviewers may have been inexperienced, clerical errors can be made, questionnaires can be lost, and so forth. This is not to say that errors do not arise in one's own project, but at least with self-collected data the problem areas are more likely to be known. It is usually easier, in any event, to work with one's own mistakes than with someone else's. Finally, it may be difficult, if not impossible, to find data relevant to a research area of interest.

Example of a secondary analysis

For over a decade, the U.S. Department of Education has sponsored large-scale surveys of high school students for the purpose of understanding how educational variables later affect the life outcomes of students. The first of these surveys involved some 19,000 male and female seniors selected from a national sample of high schools in 1971–1972. The study, referred to as the National Longitudinal Study of the Class of 1972, or NLS, has subsequently obtained follow-up data from the same students in 1973, 1974, 1976, and 1979.

Dunkelberger and Aadland (1984) made use of this publicly available data set to examine patterns of attainment of nursing careers.

From the thousands of participants in the NLS survey, the investigators selected three subgroups for secondary analysis: (1) those who expected to become nurses while they were in high school and went on to do so; (2) those who expected to become nurses while in high school but failed to do so; and (3) those who did not expect a nursing career but went on to become nurses. A total of 768 subjects in the NLS sample fell into one of these categories.

The investigator's analyses revealed that only 34 percent of those who planned to become nurses actually did so. Background variables were found to be related to nonattainment of a nursing career goal. Those who failed to become nurses despite their early interest were more often from low socioeconomic backgrounds and were more often nonwhite than those in the other two groups. However, among the subjects who did ultimately become nurses, few characteristics distinguished those who had articulated their goals in high school from those who had not.

This study capitalized on available data to answer questions about patterns of pursuing a nursing career. Such data, involving a survey of a national sample of students over a 7-year period, would have been prohibitively expensive if the investigators had had to collect the information themselves.

☐
Meta-analysis

Chapter 5 described the function of a literature review as a preliminary step in a research project. However, there is a growing recognition of the fact that the careful integration of knowledge on a topic in itself constitutes an important scholarly endeavor that can contribute new knowledge.

The procedure known as *meta-analysis* represents an application of statistical procedures to findings from research reports. In essence, meta-analysis regards the findings from one study as a data point. The findings from multiple studies on the same topic can, therefore, be combined to yield a set of data that can be analyzed in a manner similar to that of data obtained from individual subjects.

Meta-analysis procedures

The earliest form of nonnarrative research integration used what has been referred to as the "voting method." This procedure involves tallying the outcomes of previous studies to determine what outcome has received the greatest empirical support. For example, suppose we were reviewing studies that investigated whether exposing low-birthweight infants to auditory stimulation resulted in improved behavioral development compared to infants with no special treatment. There are three possible outcomes: a gain for infants exposed to auditory stimulation, a gain for those not exposed, and no group difference. An analysis using the voting method would involve counting which of these three outcomes was obtained most frequently in studies performed to date.

The voting method has since been superseded by methods of considerable sophistication and complexity. Because beginning researchers may have no statistical background, a discussion of actual statistical procedures cannot be included here. Suffice it to say that these methods, described in detail by Glass and his colleagues (1981), generally involve the calculation of an index known as the *effect size,* which quantifies how different two groups are with respect to the dependent variable. The effect size statistic is computed in such a way that it is independent of the method of measuring the dependent variable. For example, Falbo and Polit (1985) compared the effect of being raised with and without siblings on a child's development. In studying the intellectual development of only children and siblings, the results of studies using a variety of measures of intellectual ability (SAT scores, Wechsler IQ scores, Raven Progressive Matrices scores, and so on) were combined.

Because the effect size statistic is a numerical value, it is possible to perform analyses focusing on the relationship between the effect size and other variables. In other words, it is possible to test hypotheses concerning variations in the effect size. For example, in the study mentioned above, Falbo and Polit (1985) found that, across numerous studies, only children scored higher on tests of ability than children raised with siblings. However, the difference was especially pronounced among younger children and diminished in magnitude with older subjects. Thus, meta-analysis permitted an examination of the relationship between age and only/nononly differences in ability.

Advantages and disadvantages of meta-analysis

Traditional narrative reviews of the literature are handicapped by several factors not characteristic of meta-analysis. The first is that if the number of studies on a specific topic is large and if the results are inconsistent, then it is difficult to draw conclusions. The second is that narrative reviews are often subject to potential biases. The researcher may unwittingly give more weight to findings that are congruent with his or her own viewpoints. Finally, in narrative reviews it is seldom possible to examine relationships between the findings and other study variables. Thus, meta-analytic procedures provide a convenient and objective method of integrating a large body of findings and of observing patterns and relationships that might otherwise have gone undetected. Furthermore, meta-analysis provides information about the magnitude of differences and relationships. Meta-analysis can thus serve as an important scholarly tool in

theory development and in pointing the way for new areas of research.

Meta analysis has also been criticized on a number of grounds. One issue has been called the "fruit problem"—that is, the possibility of combining studies that conceptually do not belong with each other (apples and oranges). Another issue is that there is generally a bias in the studies appearing in published sources. Studies in which no differences or no relationships have been found are less likely to be published and, therefore, less likely to be included in the meta-analysis. It should be noted that narrative literature reviews are subject to the same two problems, but these problems may take on added significance in a meta-analysis because the quantitative results make the conclusions seem more concrete and absolute. Another problem is that a research report could provide general information about the study's findings but might not include sufficient quantitative information for computing an effect size. Despite these potential problems, careful and thorough meta-analyses represent an important advancement to the scientific community.

Example of a meta-analysis

Devine and Cook (1983) performed a meta-analysis of 49 studies that investigated the effect of psychoeducational interventions on patients' length of postsurgical hospital stay. Their research examined whether interventions such as teaching skills to reduce pain, providing psychological support, and providing information about the surgical procedures were associated with reductions in hospital stay. Their analyses also involved the testing of several hypotheses. For example, because the average hospital stay has declined over time, the question of whether the effects (if any) of interventions have remained stable over time or were subject to "floor effects" (i.e., perhaps the lower limit of length of patient stay has been reached, regardless of psychoeducational interventions) was raised.

Devine and Cook did a thorough review of both published and unpublished sources. Their analysis revealed that across the 49 studies interventions reduced hospital stay by about 1.25 days. This reduction was not found to depend on whether the study was published or unpublished or on whether the discharging physician was aware of the patients' experimental condition. They also found that the beneficial effects of the psychoeducational intervention became smaller over time.

This research provided not only a summary of the effectiveness of the interventions but also an estimate of the magnitude of the effect. Furthermore, Devine and Cook were able to address several questions about variations in the effect over time and across studies with different methods. Their review provided considerably more information than could have been obtained with more traditional methods of review.

☐
Methodological research

We will conclude this chapter with a brief discussion of research whose central aim is to make a contribution to the methods used in performing research. Methodological research refers to controlled investigations of the ways of obtaining, organizing, and analyzing data. Methodological studies address the development, validation, and evaluation of research tools or techniques. There has been an increasing interest in methodological research by nurse researchers in recent years. This is not surprising in light of growing demands for sound and reliable measures and for sophisticated procedures for obtaining and analyzing data.

The methodological researcher may, to take an example, concentrate on the development of an instrument that accurately measures patients' satisfaction with nursing care. The researcher in such a case is not interested in the level of patient satisfaction, nor in how such satisfaction relates to characteristics of the nurses, the hospital, or the patients. The goal of the researcher is to develop an effective, serviceable, and trustworthy instrument that can be used by other researchers, and to evaluate his or her success in accomplishing this goal.

Another example of methodological research would be a study that investigated procedures for preventing low response to questionnaires. The investigator might use a true experimental design in which subjects might be randomly assigned to one of three types of cover letters accompanying the questionnaire: a simple cover letter requesting cooperation, written by the investigator; a cover letter written on the official stationery of some important and prominent person, such as the head of a state licensing board for nurses; and a cover letter that promised the prospective participant a reward (monetary or otherwise) for cooperating in the study.

Methodological research may seem less exciting and less rewarding than substantive research, but it is virtually impossible to conduct outstanding and meaningful research on a substantive topic with inadequate research tools. Studies of a methodological nature are indispensable in any scientific discipline, and perhaps especially so when a field is relatively new and deals with highly complex, intangible phenomena such as human behavior or welfare, as is the case in nursing research.

Examples of methodological research

In 1981, an entire issue of the journal *Nursing Research* was devoted to methodological research — specifically, to studies designed to develop, improve, or evaluate measuring tools for nursing research. For example, Mishel (1981) discussed the development of a conceptual model for understanding the role of "uncertainty in illness" as an important determinant of patients' experiences in illness, treatment, and hospitalization. Based on the model, a 30-item test was developed, the Mishel Uncertainty in Illness Scale (MUIS). The report described the procedures the author used in three separate validation studies to evaluate the utility of the new instrument. The author concluded that "the MUIS appears to be a useful instrument for investigating the role of uncertainty in illness and recovery" (p. 263).

Another example from the same issue of *Nursing Research* is that of Brandt and Weinert (1981), who described the development of the Personal Resource Questionnaire, or PRQ, an instrument designed to measure the availability and intensity of a person's social supports. The focus of the report was on methodological considerations; that is, the authors described the steps that were taken to develop, refine, and evaluate the worth of the PRQ.

Careful methodological research has as its ultimate goal the improvement of the quality of research with a more substantive focus. The two instruments described above have subsequently been used in other research studies. For example, Brandt (1984) used the PRQ to examine whether mothers of children with a developmental delay varied their discipline in relation to the amount of social support available to them. Mishel (1984) also reported the results of a study in which the MUIS was used to investigate perceived uncertainty and stress in illness.

□
Summary

Survey research is the branch of research that examines the characteristics, behaviors, attitudes, and intentions of a group of people by asking individuals belonging to that group (typically only a subset) to answer a series of questions. Survey research is an extremely flexible research approach and, therefore, is quite diversified with respect to populations studied, scope, content, and purpose. The most powerful method of collecting survey information is the *personal interview* in which interviewers meet with participants in a face-to-face situation and question them directly. This method has the advantage of encouraging cooperation, which results in higher response rates and a better quality of data. *Telephone interviews* have grown in popularity in recent years but, while this approach is convenient and economical, it is not recommended when the interview is long or detailed or when the questions are sensitive or highly personal. *Questionnaires* are self-administered; that is, questions are read by the respondent, who then gives a written response. Questionnaires are often distributed through the mails, but because of the generally low response rates of mailed surveys, some type of personal contact generally is recommended.

Evaluation research is the process of collecting and analyzing information relating to the functioning of a program, policy, or procedure to assist decision-makers in choosing a course of action. Evaluations are undertaken with the aim of providing answers to questions about the effectiveness of the practice under consideration. Various models or approaches to the conduct of evaluation research have been developed. The *classical approach* begins with a determination of the goals of the program. Goals are typically phrased in the form of *behavioral objectives,* which delineate the intended outcomes of a program in terms of the behaviors of the program's beneficiaries. The research task is then one of establishing the degree of congruence between program objective and actual outcomes. The *goal-free approach* does not begin with an analysis of intended outcomes of the program. Proponents of the goal-free model argue that the evaluator should assess actual effects and achievements rather than intentions and, further, that knowledge of program goals interferes with an unbiased evaluation of the outcomes of a program.

Evaluation research can be categorized relative to its role. *Formative evaluation* refers to the collection and analysis of data relating to program outcomes as the program is evolving. The function of formative evaluation is to provide immediate feedback to program developers so that modifications can be adopted before procedures become too rigid. *Summative evaluation,* on the other hand, refers to an assessment of the worth of a program or practice that is already functioning.

Needs assessments are another type of applied research aimed at providing useful information for planners and decision-makers. A needs assessment is an investigation of the needs of a group, community, or organization for certain types of services or policies. Because organizations and groups are almost constantly in transition and because their needs may change through time, needs assessments can serve a useful purpose both before *and* after a service program is in operation. Several techniques or approaches are used in the conduct of needs assessments, notably the *key informant, survey,* or *indicator* approaches.

Historical research is the systematic attempt to establish facts and relationships concerning past events. The historical researcher utilizes the scientific method insofar as possible to answer questions or test hypotheses by objectively evaluating and interpreting available historical evidence. Historiographers are at a disadvantage from a research point of view in that they can neither manipulate nor randomize anything, nor have they much control over the quality and quantity of their data. The data are usually in the form of written records from the past (such as letters, diaries, or legal documents), but physical artifacts and audio or visual materials represent another potential source of information. Historical data are normally subjected to two forms of evaluation: *external criticism,* which is concerned with the authenticity of the source, and *internal criticism,* which assesses the worth of the evidence. Historical research is extremely valuable in nursing at this time when the profession is striving to understand and conceptualize the practice and process of nursing.

Case studies are intensive investigations of a single entity or a small number of entities. Typically, that entity is a human being, but groups, organizations, families, or communities may sometimes be the focus of concern. In a case study the investigator examines the individual in depth by probing into the history or development of the subject with respect to the characteristics or behaviors of interest. Case studies can be quite valuable in the production of hypotheses or the demonstration of some clinical approach that could be subjected to more rigorous testing. When an intervention is being demonstrated or assessed, it may be possible to conduct a *single subject experiment.* Such studies generally involve collecting data over an extended time period and, when possible, to subdivide the time frame into *baseline, treatment, reversal,* and *reinstitution* phases. The case study offers the potential of great depth but runs the risk of subjectivity and severely limited generalizability.

Field studies are in-depth studies of people or groups conducted in naturalistic settings. The aim of the researcher is to "get close" to some phenomenon as it evolves in real life (i.e., to obtain first-hand information about how people think, act, and feel relative to the phenomenon of interest). Field research generally involves the simultaneous collection and analysis of narrative, qualitative materials.

Secondary analysis refers to research projects in which the investigator analyzes previously collected data. Research studies typically produce more data than can be analyzed at one time, and, hence, existing data sets offer an economical and efficient means of testing hypotheses. Four possible approaches to secondary analysis were explored:

the secondary investigator may examine unanalyzed variables, test unexplored relationships, focus on a particular subsample, or change the unit of analysis. The use of existing data offers the potential of saving time and resources, but the secondary analyst pays for this efficiency by the inability to gather *exactly* the kinds of data he or she needs and by the possibility of working with inaccurate or problematic data sets.

Meta-analysis is a method of integrating the findings of prior research using statistical procedures. Meta-analyses typically involve the calculation of an *effect size* that quantifies relationships and differences between groups. Effect sizes from numerous studies can then be averaged to provide a numerical estimate of the magnitude of relationships; effect size variations can also be studied in relation to sample characteristics and study approaches. Although meta-analytic procedures are subject to some constraints and problems, they represent an important avenue of integration and theory development.

In *methodological research,* the investigator is concerned with the development, validation, and assessment of methodological tools or strategies. The researcher conducting a methodological study focuses primarily on increasing knowledge with respect to the methods used in performing scientific research rather than contributing to some substantive area. In nursing research, methodological studies are playing an increasingly important role in refining and improving the techniques for analyzing nursing problems. In particular, considerable attention is being paid to the development and evaluation of accurate and meaningful measuring tools.

□
Study suggestions

1. Read one of the studies listed under "Substantive References: Survey Research." Ascertain the type of questions (background information, behavioral data, etc.) asked in the survey.

2. Suppose you were interested in studying the attitude of nurses toward caring for patients with Autoimmune Deficiency Syndrome (AIDS). Would you use a personal interview, telephone interview, or questionnaire to collect your data? Why?

3. An investigator is conducting a survey of job satisfaction among nurses and is also examining such variables as age, shift, educational preparation, and marital status. Specify the independent and dependent variables.

4. Are the problems that survey researchers address usually amenable to experimentation? Why or why not?

5. A nurse researcher is developing a study to evaluate the effectiveness of a program that uses nurse practitioners to manage common respiratory infections. Suggest a design for a summative evaluation.

6. A psychiatric nurse therapist working with emotionally disturbed children is interested in evaluating a program of play therapy. Explain how you might proceed if you were to use (a) the classical evaluation model and (b) a goal-free approach. Which approach do you think would be more useful, and why?

7. For each of the following practices or procedures derive one or more hypothetical objectives and state them as *behavioral* objectives:
   a. a crisis intervention program for drug abusers
   b. procedures to educate primaparas with respect to breast feeding of their infants
   c. a program to interest nursing students in working with elderly people
   d. an instructional unit to teach student nurses how to administer subcutaneous injections

8. Explain how you would use the key informant, survey, and indicator approaches to

assess the need to teach Spanish to nurses in a given community.

9. Identify a problem for study using the historical research approach. Formulate hypotheses. What might serve as primary sources for the data? How would you check the data for internal criticism?

10. Suppose you are interested in conducting a case study on sleep promotion. What kinds of baseline data would you need to collect? What might your treatment be? What ethical considerations are involved in withdrawing the treatment?

11. Read the secondary analysis study by Munro (1983) listed in the "Substantive References." Develop some hypotheses that could be tested using the same data set.

12. Read one of the reports listed under meta-analysis in the list of substantive references below. Identify the conclusions reached by the researchers that would not have been possible in a narrative literature review.

13. Read the methodological study by Hymovich (1983) in *Nursing Research*. Design at least one substantive study that would use her measure of parental coping with chronic childhood disorders as the dependent (criterion) variable.

☐
Study readings

Methodological references

Backstrom, C.H. & Hursh, G.D. (1981). *Survey research* (2nd ed.). Evanston, IL: Northwestern University Press.

Barlow, D.H. & Hersen, M. (1973). Single-case experimental designs. *Archives of General Psychiatry, 29,* 319–325.

Boruck, R.F. (1978). *Secondary analysis.* San Francisco: Josey-Bass.

Christy, T.E. (1975). The methodology of historical research. *Nursing Research, 24,* 189–192.

Foreman, P.B. (1971). The theory of case studies. In B.J. Franklin & H.W. Osborne (Eds.), *Research methods: Issues and insights.* Belmont, CA: Wadsworth. (pp. 187–205).

Fowler, F.J. (1984). *Survey research methods.* Beverly Hills, CA: Sage.

Guba, E.G. & Lincoln, Y.S. (1981). *Effective evaluation: Improving the usefulness of evaluation results through responsive and naturalistic approaches.* San Francisco: Josey Bass.

Glass, G.V., McGaw, B., & Smith, M.L. (1981). *Meta-analysis of social research.* Beverly Hills: Sage.

Holm, K. (1983). Single subject research. *Nursing Research, 32,* 253–255.

Hyman, H.H. (1972). *Secondary analysis of sample survey: Principles, procedures and potentialities.* New York: John Wiley and Sons.

Kiecolt, K.J. & Nathan, L.E. (1985). *Secondary analysis of survey data.* Beverly Hills, CA: Sage.

Leininger, M. (Ed.) (1985). *Qualitative research methods in nursing.* New York: Grune & Stration.

McCain, N.L., Smith, M.C. & Abraham, I.L. (1986). Meta-analysis nursing interventions. *Western Journal of Nursing Research, 8,* 155–167.

McKinlay, J.B. (1973). *Research methods in health care.* New York: Prodist.

Notter, L.E. (1972). The case for historical research in nursing. *Nursing Research, 21,* 483.

Rosenthal, R. (1984). *Meta-analytic procedures for social research.* Beverly Hills, CA: Sage.

Rossi, P.H. & Freeman, H.E. (1979). *Evaluation: A systematic approach.* Beverly Hills: Sage.

Rossi, P.H. (1984). *Handbook of survey research.* New York: Academic Press.

Schatzman, L. & Strauss, A. (1982). *Field research: Strategies for a natural sociology* (2nd ed.). Englewood Cliffs, NJ: Prentice-Hall.

Schulberg, H.C. & Baker, F. (1979). *Program evaluation in the health fields* (Vol. II). New York: Human Sciences Press.

Shields, M. (1974). An evaluation model for service programs. *Nursing Outlook, 22,* 448–451.

Stewart, D.W. (1984). *Secondary research: Information services and methods.* Beverly Hills, CA: Sage.

Warheit, G.J., Bell, R.A., & Schwab, J.J. (1975). *Planning for change: Needs assessment ap-*

proaches. Washington: National Institute for Mental Health.

Wilson, H.S. (1985). *Research in nursing.* Menlo Park, CA: Addison-Wesley. (Chapter 13).

Yin, R.K. (1984). *Case study research.* Beverly Hills, CA: Sage.

Substantive References

Survey Research

Brimmer, P.F. *et al.* (1983). Nurses with doctoral degrees: Education and employment characteristics. *Research in Nursing and Health, 6,* 157–166.

Deets, C. & Froebe, D.J. (1984). Incentives for nurse employment. *Nursing Research, 33,* 242–246.

O'Rourke, M.W. (1983). Subjective appraisal of psychological well-being and self-reports of menstrual and nonmenstrual symptomatology in employed women. *Nursing Research, 32,* 288–292.

Shamansky, S.L., Schilling, L., & Holbrook. T.L. (1985). Determining the market for nurse practitioner services. *Nursing Research, 34,* 242–247.

Yeager, S.J. & Kline, M. (1983). Professional association membership of nurses. *Research in Nursing and Health, 6,* 45–52.

Evaluations and Needs Assessments

Dixon, J. (1984). Effect of nursing interventions on nutritional and performance status in cancer patients. *Nursing Research, 33,* 330–335.

Frank, P. (1979). A survey of health needs of older adults in North West Johnson County, Iowa. *Nursing Research, 28,* 360–368.

Hain, M.J. & Chen, S.C. (1976). Health needs of the elderly. *Nursing Research, 25,* 433–439.

Jako, K.L. (1980). Defining and measuring student success: A three-dimensional approach. *Western Journal of Nursing Research, 2,* 477–481.

Mills, G. *et al.* (1985). An evaluation of an inpatient cardiac patient/family education program. *Heart & Lung, 14,* 400–406.

Ventura, M.R. *et al.* (1984). Effectiveness of health promotion interventions. *Nursing Research, 33,* 162–167.

Historical research

Baer, E.D. (1985). Nursing's divided house—an historical view. *Nursing Research, 34,* 32–38.

Buhler-Wilkerson, K. (1985). Public health nursing: In sickness or in health? *American Journal of Public Health, 75,* 1155–1161.

Church, O.M. (1985). Emergence of training programs for asylum nursing at the turn of the century. *Advances in Nursing Science, 7,* 35–46.

Regan, P.A. (1976). Historical study of the school nurse role. *Journal of School Health, 46,* 518–521.

Silverstein, N.G. (1985). Lillian Wald at Henry Street, 1893–1895. *Advances in Nursing Science, 7,* 1–12.

Wheeler, C.E. (1985). *The American Journal of Nursing* and the socialization of a profession, 1900–1920. *Advances in Nursing Science, 7,* 20–34.

Case studies

Anderson, J.M. (1985). Perspectives on the health of immigrant women: A feminist analysis. *Advances in Nursing Science, 8,* 61–76.

Baltes, M.M. & Zerbe, M.B. (1976). Reestablishing self-feeding in a nursing home resident. *Nursing Research, 25,* 24–26.

Peterson, B.H. (1985). A qualitative clinical account and analysis of a care situation. In M.M. Leininger (Ed.). *Qualitative Research Methods in Nursing.* New York: Grune & Stratton.

Wilson, H.S. (1982). *Deinstitutionalized residential care for the mentally disordered: The Soteria House approach.* New York: Grune & Stratton.

Field studies

Brink, P.J. (1984). Value orientations as an assessment tool in cultural diversity. *Nursing Research, 33,* 198–203.

Dougherty, M.C., Courage, M.M., & Schilling, L.S. (1985). Ethnographic nursing research in a black community. In M.M. Leininger (Ed.), *Qualitative Research Methods in Nursing.* New York: Grune & Stratton.

Leininger, M.M. (1985). Southern rural black and white American lifeways with a focus on care and health phenomena. In M.M. Leininger (Ed.).

Qualitative Research Methods in Nursing, New York: Grune & Stratton.

Norris, C.M. (1985). Restlessness: A nursing phenomenon in search of a meaning. *Nursing Outlook, 23,* 103–107.

Secondary analysis

Cohen, M.Z. & Loomis, M.E. (1985). Linguistic analysis of questionnaire responses: Methods of coping with work stress. *Western Journal of Nursing Research, 7,* 357–366.

Dunkelberger, J.E. & Aadland, S.C. (1984). Expectation and attainment of nursing careers. *Nursing Research, 33,* 235–240.

Greenleaf, N.P. (1983). Labor force participation among registered nurses and women in comparable occupations. *Nursing Research, 32,* 306–322.

Munro, B.H. (1980). Dropouts from nursing education: Path analysis of a national sample. *Nursing Research, 29,* 371–377.

Munro, B.H. (1983). Job satisfaction among recent graduates of schools of nursing. *Nursing Research, 32,* 350–361.

Meta-analysis

Devine, E.C. & Cook, T.D. (1983). A meta-analytic analysis of effects of psychoeducational interventions on length of post-surgical hospital stay. *Nursing Research, 32,* 267–274.

Falbo, T. & Polit, D. (1985). A meta-analysis of the only child literature. *Pediatric Nursing, 11,* 356–360.

Okun, M.A. *et al.* (1984). Health and subjective well-being: A meta-analysis. *International Journal of Aging and Human Development, 19,* 111–132.

Ottenbacher, K.J. & Petersen, P. (1983). The efficacy of vestibular stimulation as a form of specific sensory enrichment. *Clinical Pediatrics, 23,* 428–433.

Straw, R.B. (1983). Deinstitutionalization in mental health: A meta-analysis. In R.J. Light (Ed.). *Evaluation Studies Review Annual,* (Vol. 8). Beverly Hills: Sage.

Methodological research

Blank, D.M. (1985). Development of the infant tenderness scale. *Nursing Research, 34,* 211–216.

Brandt, P.A. & Weinert, C. (1981). The PRQ—A social support measure. *Nursing Research, 30,* 277–280.

Cox, C.L. (1985). The Health Self-Determination Index. *Nursing Research, 34,* 177–183.

Goodwin, L., Prescott, P., Jacox, A., & Collor, M. (1981). The Nurse Practitioner Rating Form Part II: Methodological development. *Nursing Research, 30,* 270–276.

Hester, N.O. (1984). Child's health self-concept scale: Its development and psychometric properties. *Advances in Nursing Science, 7,* 45–55.

Hymovich, D. (1983). The chronicity impact and coping instrument: Parent questionnaire. *Nursing Research, 32,* 275–281.

Mishel, M.H. (1981). The measurement of uncertainty in illness. *Nursing research, 30,* 258–263.

Woods, N.F., Most, A., & Dery, G.K. (1982). Estimating premenstrual distress: A comparison of two methods. *Research in Nursing and Health, 5,* 81–92.

Chapter 11
□
Principles of research design

Chapters 8 through 10 have introduced the reader to a wide variety of research approaches, but relatively little attention has been paid to a consideration of how the investigator would go about designing the study. Because many of the issues relating to research design are common to several types of research, it was considered preferable to deal with these issues in a single chapter. The principal aim of this chapter is to introduce design techniques that strengthen the quality of research studies or enhance the interpretability of their findings.

□
Techniques of research control

Basically, the central purpose of scientific research design is to maximize the amount of control that an investigator has over the research situation and variables. As discussed in Chapter 3, the researcher needs to control extraneous variables in order to determine the true nature of the relationships between the independent and dependent variables under investigation. Extraneous variables, it will be recalled, are variables that have an irrelevant association with the dependent variable and that can confound the testing of the research hypothesis. There are two basic types of extraneous variables: (1) those that are intrinsic to the subjects of the study and (2) those that are external factors stemming from the research situation. It should be noted that many of the control techniques outlined in this chapter are not normally invoked in field studies, where the aim is for the research setting to be as natural as possible.

Controlling external factors

In scientific research, steps usually are taken to minimize situational contaminants. The researcher should seek to make the conditions under which the data are collected as similar as possible for every participant in the study. The control that a researcher imposes on a study by attempting to maintain constancy in the research conditions probably represents one of the earliest forms of scientific control.

The environment has been found to exert a powerful influence on people's emotions and behavior. In designing research, therefore, the investigator needs to pay attention to the environmental context within which the study is to be conducted. Control over the environment is most easily achieved in *laboratory experiments* in which all subjects are brought into an environment that the experimenter is in a position to arrange.* Researchers have much less freedom in controlling the environment in studies that occur in natural settings. This does not mean that the researcher should abandon all efforts to make the environments as similar as possible. For example, in conducting a survey in which the information is to be gathered by means of an interview, the researcher should attempt to conduct all interviews in basically the same kind of environment. That is, it would not be desirable to interview some of the respondents in their own homes, some in their place of work, some in the researcher's office, and so forth. In each of these settings the participant normally assumes different roles (wife, husband, parent; employee; client or patient; and so forth) and responses to questions may be influenced to some degree by the role in which the respondent is operating.

* The term "laboratory" typically connotes a setting in which scientific equipment is installed. Here, the term is used in a general sense to refer to a physical location apart from the routine of daily living, which is used by the researcher as the site for the collection of data and where subjects report to participate in the research project.

One of the advantages of conducting a study in an artificial setting such as a laboratory is that the researcher has greater confidence of having control over the independent and extraneous variables. In real-life settings, even when there are randomly assigned groups, the differentiation between groups may be difficult to control. Let us look at another example to see why this is so. Suppose we are planning to teach nursing students a unit on dyspnea, and we have used a lecture-type approach in the past. If we are interested in trying an individualized, autotutorial approach to cover the same material and want to evaluate the effectiveness of this method before adopting it for all students, we might randomly assign students to one of the two methods. Scores on a test covering the content of the unit could be used as the dependent or criterion variable. But now, suppose the students in the two groups talk to one another about their learning experiences. Some of the lecture-group students might go through parts of the programmed text. Perhaps some of the students in the autotutorial group will sit in on some of the lectures. In short, field experiments are often subject to the problem of *contamination of treatments.* In the same study, it would also be difficult to control other variables, such as the time or place in which the learning takes place for the individualized group.

A second external factor that should be controlled is the time factor. Depending on the topic of the study, the criterion variable may be influenced by the time of day or time of year in which the data are collected, or both. It would, in such cases, be important for the researcher to ensure that constancy of times across subjects is maintained. If an investigator were studying fatigue or perceptions of physical well-being, it would probably matter a great deal whether the data were gathered in the morning, afternoon, or evening, or in the summer as opposed to the winter. While time constancy is not always critical, it is often relatively easy for the researcher to control and should, therefore, be sought whenever possible.

Another aspect of maintaining constancy of conditions concerns constancy in the communications to the subjects and in the treatment itself in the case of experiments or quasi-experiments. In most research efforts, participants are informed about the purpose of the study, what use will be made of the data, under whose auspices the study is being conducted, and so forth. This information generally should be prepared ahead of time and the same message should be delivered to all subjects. In most research situations, there should be as little ad libbing as possible. Surveys, for example, almost always make use of a structured interview schedule rather than having the interviewer develop questions in the course of the interview situation.

In studies involving the implementation of a treatment, care should be taken to adhere to the specifications (often referred to as *research protocols*) for that treatment. For example, in experiments to test the effectiveness of a new drug to cure a medical problem, great care would have to be taken to ensure that the subjects in the experimental group received the same chemical substance and the same dosage, that the substance was administered in the same way, and so forth. Some treatments are much "fuzzier" than in the case of administering a drug, as is the case for most nursing interventions. In such a situation, the investigator should spell out in detail the exact behaviors required of the personnel responsible for delivering or administering the treatment.

One of the features that distinguishes nonexperimental research from experimental and quasi-experimental studies is that if the researcher has not manipulated the independent variable, then there is no means of ensuring constancy of conditions. Let us take as an example an ex post facto study that attempts to determine if there is a relationship between a person's knowledge of nutrition and his or her own eating habits. Suppose the investigator finds no relationship between nutritional knowledge and eating patterns. That is, the investigator finds that persons who are well-informed about nutrition are just as likely as uninformed persons to maintain inadequate diets. In this case, however, the researcher has had no control over the source of a person's nutritional knowledge (the independent variable). This knowledge was measured after the fact (post facto), and the conditions under which the information was obtained cannot be assumed to be constant or even similar. The researcher may conclude from the study that it is useless to teach nutrition to people because knowledge has no impact on their eating behavior. It may be, however, that different methods of providing nutritional information vary in their abilitiy to motivate people to alter their nutritional habits. Thus, the ability of the investigator to control or manipulate the independent variable of interest may be extremely important in understanding the relationships between variables.

Controlling intrinsic factors

Characteristics of the participants in a scientific study almost always need to be controlled. The control of intrinsic extraneous variables is especially important when the dependent variable is psychosocial rather than biophysical in nature. That is because psychosocial variables (e.g., stress) are more subject to the influence of individual characteristics (sex, social class, marital status) than biophysical ones (body temperature, heart rate). This section describes six specific ways of controlling extraneous variables associated with subject characteristics.

Randomization
We have already discussed the most effective method of controlling individual extraneous variables, which is randomization. The pri-

mary function of randomization is to secure comparable groups, that is, to equalize the groups with respect to the extraneous variables. A distinct advantage of random assignment, compared with other methods of controlling extraneous variables, is that randomization controls *all* possible sources of extraneous variation, without any conscious decision on the researcher's part about which variables need to be controlled.

Suppose, for example, that we were interested in assessing the effect of a physical training program on cardiovascular functioning among nursing home residents. Characteristics such as the individuals' age, sex, prior occupation, and length of stay in the nursing home could all affect the patients' cardiovascular system, independently of the physical training program. The effects of these other variables are extraneous to the research problem and should be controlled. Through randomization, we could expect that an experimental group (receiving the physical training program) and control group (not receiving the program) would be comparable in terms of these as well as any other factors that influence cardiovascular functioning.

Homogeneity

When randomization is not feasible, there are several other methods of controlling intrinsic subject characteristics that could contaminate the relationships under investigation. The first alternative is to use only subjects who are homogeneous with respect to those variables that are considered extraneous. The extraneous variables, in this case, are not allowed to vary. In the example of the physical training program cited above, if sex were considered to be an important confounding variable, the researcher might wish to use only men (or only women) as subjects. Similarly, if the researcher were concerned about the effects of the subjects' age on cardiovascular functioning, participation in the study could be limited

to those within a specified age range. This method of utilizing a homogeneous subject pool is fairly easy and offers considerable control. However, the limitation of this approach lies in the fact that the research findings can only be generalized to the type of subjects who participated in the study. If the physical training program was found to have beneficial effects on the cardiovascular status of a sample of men aged 65 to 75, its usefulness for improving the cardiovascular status of women in their eighties would be strictly a matter of conjecture.

Blocking

Another approach to controlling extraneous variables is to include them in the design of a study as independent variables. To pursue our example of the physical training program, if sex was thought to be a confounding variable, it could be built into the study design, as shown in Figure 11-1. This procedure would allow us to make an assessment of the impact of our training program on the cardiovascular functioning of both elderly men and women. Furthermore, although the reason for this may not be clear until the reader is familiar with inferential statistics, this approach has the advantage of adding greater precision and enhancing the likelihood of detecting differences between our experimental and control groups.

Let us consider this second approach in greater detail. We will refer to the design shown in Figure 11-1 as a *randomized block design*.* The variable sex, which cannot be manipulated by the researcher, is known as a *blocking variable*. In an experiment to test the

---

* The terminology for this design varies from text to text. Some authors (e.g., Kerlinger, 1973) refer to this as a factorial design; others call it a levels-by-treatment design. We have chosen not to use the term factorial because sex is not under experimental control and, hence, complete randomization is not possible. (See Dayton, 1970 for this use of randomized block design.)

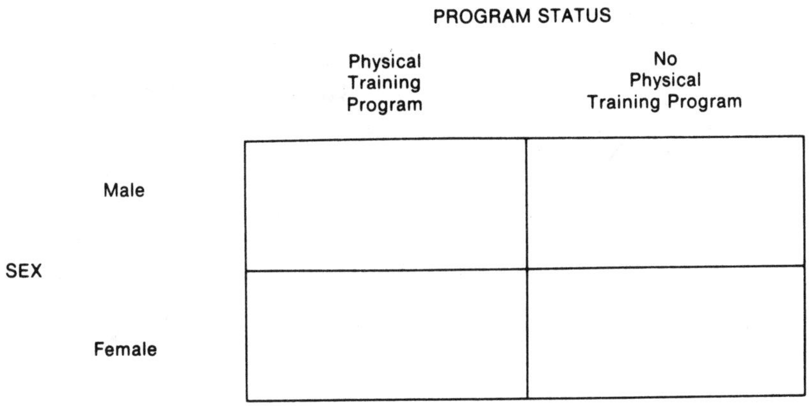

PROGRAM STATUS

Figure 11-1.   Schematic diagram of a randomized block design.

effectiveness of the physical training program, the experimenter obviously could not randomly assign subjects to one of four cells: the sex of the subjects is a "given." But the experimenter can and should randomly assign males and females separately to the experimental and control conditions. Let us say there are forty males and forty females available for the study. The researcher should *not* take the eighty subjects and assign half to the physical training program group and the other half to the "no program" group. Rather, the randomization procedure should be performed separately for the two sexes, thereby guaranteeing twenty subjects in each cell of the four-cell design.

The design can be extended to include more than one blocking variable, as shown in Figure 11-2. Here the age of the subject has been included to control for this second extraneous variable. Once again, the experimenter should randomly assign subjects from each block to either the experimental or control conditions. In other words, half of the men aged 66 to 70 would randomly be assigned to the program, as would half of the men aged 71 to 75, and so forth. While in theory the number of blocks that could be added is unlimited, practical concerns usually dictate a relatively

small number of blocks (and, hence, a small number of extraneous variables that can be controlled). Expansion of the design usually requires that a larger subject pool be used. As a general rule of thumb, a minimum of ten subjects per cell is often recommended. This means that whereas a minimum of 40 subjects would be needed for the design in Figure 11-1, 120 subjects would be needed for the design in Figure 11-2. This suggests that, if a decision is made to introduce extraneous variables into the design of a study, great care should be taken to choose the most relevant subject characteristics.

Strictly speaking, the type of design we have discussed is appropriate only in experimental studies, but in reality it is used quite commonly in quasi-experimental and ex post facto studies as well. If an investigator were studying the effects of a physical training program on cardiovascular functioning after the fact (that is, subjects self-selected themselves into one of the two groups and the researcher had no control over who was included in each group), he or she might want to set up the analysis in such a way that differential effects for men and women would be analyzed. The design structure would look the same as the one presented in Figure 11-1, although the

PROGRAM STATUS

SEX	AGE GROUP	Physical Training Program	No Program
Males	66–70		
	71–75		
	76–80		
Females	66–70		
	71–75		
	76–80		

Figure 11-2. Schematic diagram of a randomized block design.

implications and conclusions that could be drawn from the results would be quite different than if the researcher had been in control of the manipulation and randomization procedures.

Matching

The fourth method of dealing with extraneous variables is known as *matching*. Matching involves using knowledge of subject characteristics to form comparison groups. If a matching procedure were to be adopted for our physical training program example, and age and sex were the extraneous variables of interest, we would need to match two subjects with respect to age and sex in the experimental and control group. If the subjects could be assigned on a random basis, we would actually have a special type of randomized block design with one subject per cell.*

However, matching is usually a post hoc attempt to approximate this experimental blocking design. That is, the researcher may begin with twenty subjects who participate in the training program and then create a control group by matching, one by one, individuals from the general population in terms of age and sex of the experimental subjects. Studies using such a matching procedure to equate two (or more) groups are sometimes referred to as *case-control studies*. This design is very common in epidemiological research.

---

* In this special case the requirement of ten cases per cell is irrelevant because no attempt is made to assess the effects of the extraneous variables on the dependent variable. Matching merely attempts to produce equivalent groups for comparison purposes. The requirement of ten cases per cell relates to the fact that an estimate of an effect of a treatment is unstable (can fluctuate markedly from one individual to the next) when the number of cases is small. But if the researcher is not interested in how, for example, the physical training program affects males versus females, but is interested in securing equivalent groups, matching on a one to one basis and then randomly assigning subjects to conditions is acceptable.

Despite the intuitive appeal of such a design, there are a number of reasons why matching should be avoided if possible. First, in order to match effectively, the researcher must know in advance what the relevant extraneous variables are. Secondly, after two or three variables, it often becomes impossible to match adequately. Let us say we are interested in controlling for the age, sex, race, and length of nursing home stay of the subjects. Thus, if subject number one in the physical training program is a black woman, aged 80, whose length of stay is five years, the researcher must seek another woman with these same characteristics as a control. With more than three variables, the matching procedure becomes extremely cumbersome, if not impossible. For these reasons, matching as a technique for controlling extraneous variables should, in general, be used only when other, more powerful procedures are not feasible, as might be the case for some ex post facto studies.

Analysis of covariance

Yet another method of controlling unwanted variables is through statistical procedures. It is recognized that at this point many readers are unfamiliar with basic statistical procedures, let alone sophisticated techniques such as are being referred to here. Therefore, a detailed description of a powerful statistical control mechanism, known as *analysis of covariance,* will not be attempted. The interested reader with a background in statistics should consult Chapter 22 or a textbook on advanced statistics for fuller coverage of this topic. However, since the possibility of statistical control may mystify readers, we will attempt to explain the underlying principle with a simple illustration.

Returning to the example used throughout this section, suppose we have a group that is undergoing a physical training program and we have another group that is not. The groups represent intact groups (e.g., residents of two

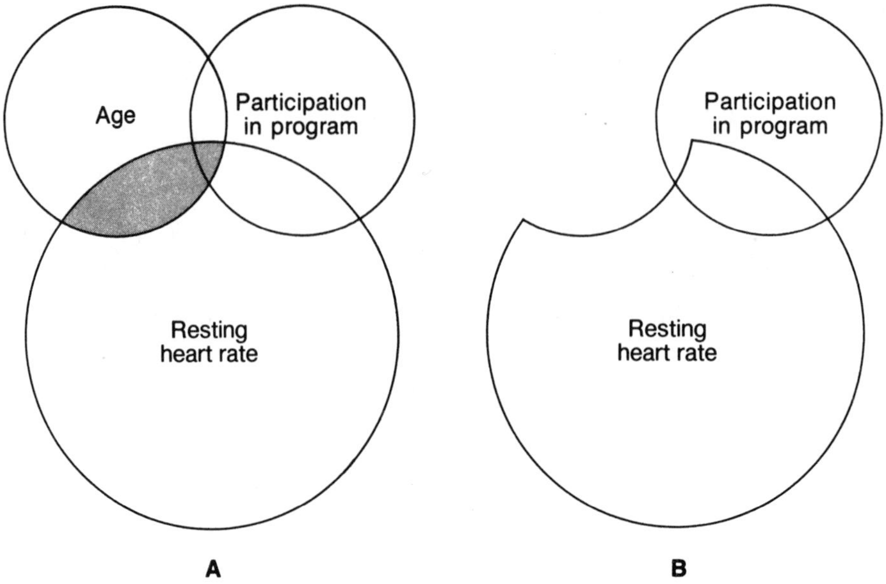

Figure 11-3. Schematic diagram illustrating the principle of analysis of covariance.

different nursing homes), and therefore randomization is not possible. As our measures of cardiovascular functioning, suppose we use maximal oxygen consumption and resting heart rate. As with most things in life, there undoubtedly will be individual differences on these two measures. The research question is "Can some of the individual differences be attributed to a person's participation in the physical training program?" Unfortunately, the individual differences in cardiovascular functioning are also related to other, extraneous characteristics of the subjects, such as age. The large circles in Figure 11-3 may be taken to represent the total variability (extent of individual differences) for both groups on, say, resting heart rate. A certain amount of that total variability can be explained simply by virtue of the subject's age, which is schematized in the figure as the small circle on the left in part A of Figure 11-3. Another part of the variability can be explained by the subject's participation or nonparticipation in the physical training program, represented here as the small circle on

the right. In part A, the fact that the two small circles (age and program participation) overlap tells us that there is a relationship between those two variables. In other words, subjects in the group receiving the physical training program are, on average, either older or younger than members of the comparison group. Therefore, age should be controlled.

Analysis of covariance can accomplish this control function by statistically removing the effect of the extraneous variable on the dependent variable. In our illustration, that portion of heart rate variability that is attributable to age could be removed through the analysis of covariance technique. This is designated in part A of Figure 11-3 by the darkened area in the large circle. Part B illustrates that the final analysis would examine the effect of program participation on heart rate after removing the effect of age. With the variability of heart rate resulting from age controlled, we can have a much more precise estimate of the effect of the training program on heart rate. Note that even after removing the variability resulting from age, there is still individual variability not associated with the program treatment (the bottom half of the large circle). This means that the precision of the study could probably be further enhanced by controlling additional extraneous variables, such as sex, type of previous occupation, and so forth. The analysis of covariance procedure can accommodate multiple extraneous variables. When pretest measures of the dependent variables have been obtained, these are often controlled statistically through analysis of covariance.

Repeated measures

The last technique we will consider uses the subjects themselves as their own controls. In some experiments one group of subjects can be exposed to more than one condition or treatment. This type of design is known as a *repeated measures design.* This design has the advantage of assuring the highest possible degree of equivalence between subjects exposed to different conditions. Suppose that we are interested in studying the relationship between the content of a patient's talk and nurses' listening behavior. We might set up a laboratory experiment rather than a field experiment to control for a host of confounding environmental or situational factors. Let us say that a simulated hospital room is created, and a confederate of the researcher poses as a hospital patient. Our subjects (nurses) enter the room with instructions to perform certain nursing routines. Now suppose that the three types of verbal content we are interested in are conversation relating to (1) physical pain, (2) emotional pain such as fear and loneliness, and (3) general talk about the weather and so forth. The confederate patient would learn three "scripts" relating to these areas and we could then assess the nurses' listening behavior by having them answer questions about what the patient has said. How could we proceed to conduct this study? We *could* start with 30 nurses, and then randomly assign ten to one of the three conditions. Then each group would only be exposed to one of the three scripts. There are, however, a number of extraneous variables that this design would not control, such as the specialty and number of years of experience of the nurses. The randomization procedure would probably control for such differences, but with only ten subjects per condition, it might be possible by chance alone to get a group that overrepresents nurses with, say, a psychiatric specialty. An alternative would be to use a repeated measures design wherein all 30 nurses are exposed to the three scripts. This would clearly guarantee equivalence across conditions, thereby controlling extraneous variables. Furthermore, repeated measures provide the researcher with more data: in the present example we would have ninety pieces of information (thirty subjects by three conditions).

Repeated measures designs often are not appropriate because of the problem of carry-over effects. When subjects are exposed to two different treatments or conditions, they may be influenced in the second condition by their experience in the first condition. Since the two (or more) treatments are not applied simultaneously, the order of the treatment may be important in affecting the subject's performance. The procedure of *counterbalancing* is frequently used in conjunction with repeated measures designs to minimize the impact of ordering effects. In our example of nurses' listening behavior, the order of presentation of the three scripts would be systematically varied so that the attention paid to a given conversation would not depend upon whether it was heard first, second, or third. Table 11-1 illustrates a counterbalanced order of presentation for the first twelve subjects in our hypothetical experiment. In sum, repeated measures can be a useful and efficient design for eliminating extraneous variables, but when carry-over effects from one condition to another are antici-

Table 11-1
Counterbalanced order of presentation
of patient scripts

Subject	First	Second	Third
1	A	B	C
2	B	C	A
3	C	A	B
4	A	C	B
5	C	B	A
6	B	A	C
7	A	B	C
8	B	C	A
9	C	A	B
10	A	C	B
11	C	B	A
12	B	A	C

A—Script dealing with physical pain
B—Script dealing with emotional pain
C—Script dealing with "small talk"

pated, as might be the case in many medical or nursing interventions, other designs will have to be sought.

Evaluation of control methods

Overall, the random assignment of subjects to groups is the most effective approach of managing extraneous variables, because randomization tends to produce a "cancelling out" of individual variation on all possible extraneous variables. Repeated measures designs, though also useful in controlling all possible sources of extraneous variation, cannot be applied to many nursing research problems. The four remaining alternatives to randomization described here have one disadvantage in common: the researcher must know or predict in advance the relevant extraneous variables. In order to select homogeneous samples, develop a blocking design, match, or perform an analysis of covariance, the researcher must make a decision about what variable or variables need to be controlled. This constraint may pose severe limitations on the degree of control that is possible, particularly because the researcher can seldom deal explicitly with

more than two or three extraneous variables at a time.

Although we have repeatedly hailed randomization as the ideal mechanism for controlling extraneous subject characteristics, it is clear that randomization is not always possible. For example, if the independent variable cannot be manipulated, then other techniques must be used. In ex post facto and quasi-experimental studies, the control options available to researchers include homogeneity, blocking, matching, and analysis of covariance.

☐
Internal and external validity

The researcher can be confident in the validity of the results of a study if (1) the obtained findings are due only to the independent variable of interest and (2) the results are generalizable to situations outside of the research setting. These two conditions are referred to as *internal validity* and *external validity*.

Internal validity

The control mechanisms reviewed in the previous section all aimed at improving the internal validity of research studies. If the researcher is not careful in managing extraneous variables and in other ways controlling the design of the study, there may be reason to challenge the conclusion that the subjects' performances on the criterion measure resulted from the effect of the independent variable.

In Chapter 8 we reviewed five "threats" to the internal validity of studies, with particular emphasis on quasi-experiments: history, selection, maturation, testing, and mortality. A good experimental design will normally control for these factors, but it must not be assumed that in a true experiment the researcher need not worry about them. For example, if constancy of conditions is not maintained for experimental and control groups, then history might be a rival explanation for obtained results. Experimental mortality is, in particular, a salient threat in true experiments. If the experimenter does something differently with two or more groups, then subjects may drop out of the study differentially among the comparison groups. This is particularly apt to happen if the experimental treatment is painful, inconvenient, or time consuming or if the control condition is boring and uninvolving to the subjects. When this happens, the subjects remaining in the study may differ from those who left in important ways, thereby nullifying the initial equivalence of the groups.

Researchers engaged in nonexperimental studies should also consider the various competing explanations for the results they obtain. For example, selection is clearly a problem in ex post facto studies and may also pose difficulties in historical research and case studies. When the investigator does not have control over the numerous extraneous variables that can interfere with a straightforward understanding of relationships, great caution should be exercised in interpreting the results and in drawing conclusions from them.

External validity

The term *external validity* refers to the generalizability of the research findings to other settings or samples. Research is almost never conducted with the intention of discovering relationships among variables for one group of people at one point in time. The aim of research is typically to reveal enduring relationships, the understanding of which can be used to improve the human condition. If a nursing intervention under investigation is found to be successful, others will want to adopt the procedure. Therefore, an important question is whether the intervention will "work" in another setting and with different patients. Researchers should routinely ask themselves: to what populations, environments, and conditions can the results of the study be applied?

Strictly speaking, the findings of a study can only be generalized to the population of subjects from which a study sample has been randomly selected. If an investigator were studying the effects of a newly developed therapeutic treatment for heroin addicts, the researcher might begin with a population of addicts in a particular clinic or drug treatment center. From this population, a random sample of drug users could be selected for participation in the study. Individuals from the sample would then be randomly assigned to one of two or more conditions assuming that an experiment were possible. If the results revealed that the new therapeutic treatment was highly effective in reducing recidivism among the sample of addicts, can it be concluded that all addicts in the United States would benefit from the treatment? Unfortunately, no. The population of heroin addicts undergoing treatment in one particular facility may not be representative of all addicts. For example, the facility in question may attract drug users from certain ethnic, socioeconomic, or age groups. Perhaps the new treatment is only effective with individuals from such groups.

Of relevance here is Kempthorne's (1961) distinction between accessible populations and target populations. The *accessible population* is the population of subjects available for a particular study. In our example above, all the heroin addicts in treatment at a particular treatment center would constitute the accessible population. When random procedures have been used to select a sample from an accessible population, there is no difficulty in generalizing the results to that group.

The term *target population* refers to the total group of subjects about whom the investigator is interested and to whom the results could reasonably be generalized. This second type of generalization is considerably more risky than the first and cannot be done with as much confidence as in the case of generalizations to the accessible population. The adequacy and utility of this type of inference hinges very strongly upon the similarity of the characteristics of the two populations. Thus, the researcher must be aware of the characteristics of the accessible population and in turn define the target population to be like the accessible population. In the drug treatment example, the accessible population might consist predominantly of voluntarily admitted white males in their twenties living in New York City. Although we might ideally like to generalize our results to all drug addicts, we would be on much safer ground if we defined our target population as young, urban, white men who present themselves for treatment.

In addition to characteristics of the sample that limit the generalizability of research findings, there are various characteristics of the environment or research situation that affect the study's representativeness and, hence, its external validity. Braucht and Glass (1968) have extended the work of Campbell and Stanley (1963) by presenting a number of threats to the external validity of studies.

1. *The Hawthorne Effect.* Subjects in an experiment may behave in a particular manner largely because they are aware of their participation in a study. If a certain type of behavior or performance is elicited only in a research context, the results cannot be generalized to more natural settings.
2. *Novelty Effects.* When a treatment is new, subjects and research agents alike might alter their behavior in a variety of ways. People may be either enthusiastic or skeptical about new methods of doing things. The results may reflect these reactions to the novelty; once the treatment is more familiar, the same results may fail to appear.
3. *Interaction of History and Treatment Effects.* The results may reflect the impact of the treatment *and* some other events external to the study. When the treatment is implemented again in the absence of the other events, different results may be obtained.
4. *Experimenter Effects.* The performance of the subjects may be affected by characteristics of the researchers. The investigators often have an emotional or intellectual investment in demonstrating that their hypotheses are correct and may unconsciously communicate their expectations to the subjects or they may be somewhat biased in their observations.
5. *Measurement Effects.* In research studies the investigators collect a considerable amount of data, such as pretest information, background data, and so forth. The results may not apply to another group of people who are not also exposed to the same data-collection procedures.

In conclusion, the researcher should strive to design studies that are strong with respect to both internal and external validity. In some instances, however, the requirements for assuring one type of validity may interfere with the possibility of achieving the second. That is, if the researcher exerts a high degree of control over a study in an effort to maximize internal validity, the setting may become highly artificial and pose a threat to the generalizability of the findings to more naturalistic environments. Thus, it is often necessary to reach a compromise by introducing sufficient controls while maintaining some semblance of realism. In this regard the concept of *replication,* or the repeating of a study in a new setting with new subjects, is extremely useful. Much greater confidence can be placed in the findings of a study if it can be demonstrated that the results can be replicated.

☐
Characteristics of good design

The criteria of internal and external validity represent one frame of reference for evaluating the quality of research designs. In this section we will examine briefly the characteristics of good design from a somewhat less technical point of view.

Appropriateness for research question

The requirement that the research design should be appropriate for the questions being asked seems so obvious that it may be overlooked. Generally a given research problem can be handled adequately with a number of different designs, so that the researcher typically has some flexibility in selecting a design. Yet many designs will be completely unsuitable for dealing with the research problem. For example, if a researcher were interested in comparing the effects of two drugs on sleep promotion, it is unlikely that a repeated measures design would be recommendable, given the interactive nature of many drugs. As another example, a loosely structured research design such as those often used in field studies might be inappropriate to address the question of whether nonnutritive sucking opportunities among premature infants facilitate early oral feedings. On the other hand, a tightly controlled study may unnecessarily restrict the researcher interested in understanding the *processes* by which nurses make diagnoses. This chapter has emphasized techniques of control normally associated with highly structured, scientific research, but there are many research questions of interest to nurses for which such designs may be unsuitable.

Lack of bias

A second characteristic of good research design in traditional scientific studies is that it results in data that are not biased. Bias can operate in a variety of ways, some of which are very subtle. The most pervasive source of bias is in the allocation of subjects to groups. When groups are formed on a nonrandom basis, the risk of selection bias is always present. Note

that we do not mean that the investigator is necessarily responsible for the bias. In ex post facto studies in which subjects "self-select" themselves into groups, the biases might be quite beyond the researcher's control.

In studies in which the data are collected by means of observation, the researcher's preconceptions might unconsciously bias the objective collection of data. In such a case, the researcher should take a number of steps to minimize this risk. Whenever possible, *double-blind* procedures are highly recommended. This technique removes observer biases by virtue of the fact that neither the subject nor the observer (or person collecting the data) knows in which group a given subject is. When this approach is not feasible, it is a good practice to have two or more observers so that at least an estimation of the biases can be made.

Bias can enter the data whenever there is an opportunity for something other than the independent variable of interest to affect the outcomes in a systematic way. The techniques discussed in the first section of this chapter, such as randomization, counterbalancing, and so forth, should be built into the structure of the research to eliminate or reduce problems of bias.

Precision

The first section of this chapter dealt with the notion of control over extraneous variables. What this control is actually all about is *control over variability in the dependent measures*. In an example used repeatedly, we talked about the variability from one elderly individual to another on measures of cardiovascular functioning. The various control mechanisms discussed represented attempts to isolate that portion of the variability in cardiovascular status that could be attributable to participation in a physical training program. Let us express what the researcher is attempting to do in the form of a ratio:

Variability in cardiovascular status
due to training program

Variability in cardiovascular status
due to age, sex, prior occupation,
initial level of cardiovascular status

This ratio, though greatly simplified here, captures the essence of many statistical procedures. The researcher wants to make the variability in the numerator (the upper half) as large as possible relative to the variability in the denominator (the lower half) in order to demonstrate most clearly the relationship between program participation and cardiovascular functioning. The smaller the variability caused by extraneous variables such as age and sex, the easier it will be for the researcher to detect differences in cardiovascular functioning between those who did and those who did not participate in the physical training program. Designs that enable the researcher to reduce the variability caused by the extraneous variables are said to increase the precision of the research. As a purely hypothetical illustration of why this is so, we will attach some numerical values* to the ratio above:

$$\frac{\text{Variability due to training program}}{\text{Variability due to extraneous variables}} = \frac{10}{4}$$

Now, if we can make the bottom number smaller, say from four to two, we will have a purer and more precise estimate of the effect of program participation on physical fitness. How can a research design help to reduce the variability caused by extraneous variables?

A randomized block design is one example of a design that increases the precision of an analysis. Let us say we performed the physical fitness study as a true experiment, using two age groups. The total variability in cardiovascular functioning (that is, the extent to which individuals had different heart rates and maxi-

* The reader should not be concerned at this point with how these numbers can be obtained in a real analysis. The procedure will be explained at length in Chapter 21.

mal oxygen consumption) can be conceptualized as having three components.

Total Variability in cardiovascular status
= Variability due to program + Variability
due to age + Variability due to other extraneous variables

This equation can be taken to mean that part of the reason why some individuals did well and others did less well on measures of cardiovascular functioning is that (1) some participated in the training program and others did not; (2) some people are older and some younger; and (3) other factors such as sex, prior occupation, and so forth had an effect.

The randomized block procedure allows us to segregate the variability that is due to age and remove it from the variability resulting from all other extraneous variables. By doing this, the effect of the training program becomes greater, relative to the extraneous variability. Thus, we can say that the randomized block design has enabled us to get a more precise estimate of the effect of participation in the training program. Research designs differ considerably in the sensitivity with which the treatment effects can be detected with statistical tools.

Power

We use power here to describe the ability of a research design to detect relationships among variables. Precision contributes to the power of a design. Power is also increased when a large sample is used. This aspect of power is discussed in Chapters 12 and 22.

One other aspect of a powerful design concerns the construction (in experimental research) or definition (in nonexperimental research) of the independent variable. For both statistical and theoretical reasons, results are clearer and more conclusive when the differences in the results between two groups are large. The researcher should generally aim to maximize group differences on the dependent variables by maximizing differences on the independent variable. In other words, the results are likely to be more clear-cut if the treatments can be made as different as possible. This advice is clearly more easily followed in experimental than in ex post facto research. Research manipulation allows the investigator to devise treatments that are distinct and as strong as time, money, ethics, and practicality permit. However, even in nonexperimental research there are frequently opportunities to operationalize the independent variables in such a way that power to detect differences is enhanced.

□

The time dimension

Certain research problems are concerned with phenomena that evolve over time: healing, learning, growth, recidivism, physical development, and so on, are all variables that involve a time dimension. There are various designs available to researchers interested in such phenomena. These designs fall into two broad categories: cross-sectional and longitudinal.

Cross-sectional designs

Cross-sectional studies involve the collection of data at one point in time. The phenomena under investigation are captured, as they manifest themselves, during one period of data collection. Suppose, for example, we are interested in studying the changes in nursing students' attitude toward professionalism as they progress through a four-year baccalaureate program. One way to investigate this issue would be to survey students when they are freshmen and resurvey them every year until they graduate. On the other hand, we could use a *cross-sectional design* by surveying members of the four classes at one point in time and then comparing the responses of the four groups. If seniors manifested more positive attitudes toward nursing professionalism than freshmen, it might be inferred that nursing students become increasingly socialized professionally by their educational experiences. In order to make this kind of inference, the researcher must assume that the senior students would have responded as the freshmen responded had they been questioned three years earlier, or, conversely, that freshmen students would demonstrate increased favorability toward professionalism if they were surveyed three years later.

The main advantage of cross-sectional designs is that they are practical. They are relatively easy to manage and economical. There are, however, a number of problems in inferring changes and trends over time using a cross-sectional design. The overwhelming amount of social and technological change that characterizes our society frequently makes it questionable to assume that differences in the behaviors, attitudes, or characteristics of different age groups are the result of the passage through time rather than to cohort or "generational" differences. In the above example, seniors and freshmen may have different attitudes toward the nursing profession, independent of any experiences they had during their four years of education. In cross-sectional studies there are frequently several rival hypotheses for any observed differences. Furthermore, ex post facto studies aimed at shedding light on causal relationships are handicapped when a cross-sectional design is adopted because the doubtful temporal ordering of phenomena mitigates against drawing causal conclusions.

Longitudinal designs

Research projects that are designed to collect data at more than one point in time are referred to as *longitudinal studies.* As the preceding discussion suggested, the main value of longitudinal designs lies in their ability to shed light upon (1) trends or changes over time and (2) the temporal sequencing of phenomena, which is an essential criterion for establishing causality.

Four types of longitudinal designs deserve special mention — trend, cohort, panel, and follow-up studies. *Trend studies* are investigations in which samples from a general population are studied over time with respect to some phenomenon. Different samples are selected at repeated intervals, but the samples are always drawn from the same population. Trend studies permit researchers to examine patterns and rates of change over time and to make predictions about future directions. For example, trend studies have been initiated to analyze the number of students entering nursing programs and to forecast future supplies of nursing personnel.

Cohort studies are a particular kind of trend study in which specific subpopulations are examined over time. Once again, different samples are selected at different points in time, but the samples are drawn from specific subgroups that are often age-related. For example, the cohort of women born during the 1946–1950 period may be studied at regular intervals with respect to health care utilization. As another example, the cohort of nursing students receiving their bachelor's degree in 1960 may be periodically surveyed to determine their employment/unemployment patterns. A sophisticated design known as the *cross-sequential design* combines the features of cohort studies with a cross-sectional approach. In cross-sequential studies two or more different age cohorts are studied longitudinally so that both changes over time and "generational" or cohort differences can be detected.

Panel studies differ from trend and cohort studies in that the *same* subjects are used to supply the data at two or more points in time.

The term "panel," which is used almost exclusively in the context of longitudinal survey projects, refers to the sample of subjects involved in the study. Panel studies typically yield more information than trend studies because the investigator can usually reveal patterns of change and reasons for the changes. Because the same individuals are contacted at two or more points in time, the researcher can identify the subjects who did and did not change and then isolate the characteristics of the subgroups in which changes occurred. As an example, a panel study could be designed to explore over time the nutritional habits of a sample of women during their childbearing years. Panel studies are intuitively appealing as an approach to studying change but are extremely difficult and expensive to manage. The most serious problem is the loss of participants at different points in the study, a difficulty referred to as *attrition* or *subject mortality.* Attrition is problematic for the researcher because those who drop out of the study may differ in important respects from the individuals who continue to participate; hence, the generalizability of the findings may be impaired.

Follow-up studies are quite similar in design to panel studies except that the former term is usually associated with experiments or other types of nonsurvey research. Follow-up investigations are generally undertaken to determine the subsequent development of individuals with a specified condition or who have received a specified intervention. For example, patients who have received a particular nursing intervention or clinical treatment may be followed up to ascertain the long-term effects of the treatment. To take a nonexperimental example, samples of premature babies may be followed up to assess their later perceptual and motor development.

In sum, longitudinal designs are useful for studying the dynamics of a variable or phenomenon over time. The number of data collection periods and the time intervals in between the data collection points depend upon the nature of study. When change or development is rapid, numerous time points at short intervals may be required to document the pattern and make accurate forecasts.

□
Research examples

We conclude with examples of two research studies that highlight some of the points made in this chapter. The first example illustrates a design that carefully controlled extraneous variables. The second example deals with a longitudinal study.

Example of a randomized block, factorial design

Johnson and her colleagues (1985) were interested in learning the effects of interventions that provided different means of patients' exerting personal control over postoperative experiences. Their study was built on the premise that personal control can modify reactions to stressful experiences, such as hospitalization. The factorial experiment they designed involved a $2 \times 3 \times 2$ design. That is, they were interested in three different independent variables: (1) the presence or absence of concrete sensory information about the hospitalization experience; (2) three modes of instruction relating to coping strategies—a cognitive technique, a behavioral technique, or no specific instruction; and (3) experimental and control information about postdischarge experiences. A total of 168 hysterectomy patients participated in the research and were randomly assigned to one of the treatment groups, in this case to one of 12 possible conditions. The dependent variables in this study included patients' ratings of pain; self-reported mood

states such as anxiety and depression; ratings on a physical recovery index; and information from hospital records, such as medications used and length of hospitalization.

The investigators exerted strong control over the research situation through a number of techniques. First and foremost, subjects were randomly assigned to conditions. Through randomization, the researchers were able to maximize the likelihood that subjects in all treatment groups were as similar as possible with regard to all variables that could influence perceptions of the hospitalization experience. Second, the investigators introduced a blocking variable (race) in their design. By using race as a blocking variable (i.e., by randomly assigning black and white patients separately to experimental conditions), the researchers ensured that both racial groups would be proportionately represented in all conditions. Finally, the researchers exerted some control through homogeneity. By restricting the sample to hysterectomy patients, Johnson and her colleagues controlled patient gender and type of operation. The results suggested that different strategies of introducing personal control had positive effects on different patient outcomes. For example, the behavioral coping strategy was associated with a reduction in patients' pain medication, but the cognitive coping strategy was associated with greater physical recovery during hospitalization.

Example of a cross-sequential design

Mercer (1985) conducted a longitudinal study to explore the transition to the maternal role over the first year of a first-born infant's life. We call her design cross-sequential because, in addition to the fact that she gathered information longitudinally, she also followed the transition to the maternal role for three age groups—women who became mothers at age

15 to 19, 20 to 29, and 30 to 42. By using this design, she could examine how both time and maturation affected the process of role attainment.

The sample in Mercer's study consisted of 242 women, all of whom had delivered their first normal infant at a university-affiliated hospital. Interview data were obtained from subjects at 1, 4, 8, and 12 months postpartum. The interviews included a number of standardized measures, including such scales as Feelings About My Baby and Gratification in the Mothering Role. By examining trends in the reporting of the subjects' feelings, the researcher was able to learn about the process of becoming a mother. Among the reported results was the finding that positive feelings about the baby and perceived maternal competency peaked at four months for mothers in all three age groups. Although the three age groups functioned at somewhat different levels, their patterns of functioning over the year were very similar, leading the researcher to conclude that the maternal role presented similar challenges for all women.

☐
Summary

The purpose of research design in scientific studies is to guide the collection and analysis of data in such a way that the results it yields are interpretable and generalizable. We plan and design studies, rather than simply rush out to collect information, because research that is carefully designed increases our confidence in the conclusions. The researcher must design a study that controls *extraneous variables,* that is, the unwanted or irrelevant variables in the research setting, or irrelevant characteristics of the participants, that could influence the results of the study.

One important type of control relates to the constancy of conditions under which a study is performed. A number of aspects of the study, such as the environment, timing, communications, and the implementation of treatment, should be held constant or kept as similar as possible for each participant.

The most problematic and pervasive extraneous variables are intrinsic characteristics of the subjects. Several techniques are available to control such characteristics. First, the ideal method of control is through the random assignment of subjects to groups. Randomization effectively controls for all possible extraneous variables because it tends to produce groups in which individual variation is cancelled out. Second, a homogeneous sample of subjects can be used such that there is no variability relating to characteristics that could affect the outcome of a study. Third, the extraneous variables can be built into the design of a study so that a direct assessment of their impact can be made. One such design that accomplishes this is the *randomized block design,* in which the extraneous variable is referred to as the *blocking variable.* The fourth approach, *matching,* is essentially an after-the-fact attempt to approximate a randomized block design. This procedure matches subjects on the basis of one or more extraneous variables in an attempt to secure comparable groups. A fifth technique is to control extraneous variables by means of a statistical procedure known as an *analysis of covariance.* The last four procedures for controlling extraneous individual characteristics share one disadvantage, and that is that the researcher must know which variables need to be controlled. Finally, in some types of studies subjects can be exposed to more than one level of a treatment and thus serve as their own controls. This design, known as a *repeated measures design,* is efficient because it reduces the number of subjects required but may be unsuitable because of the potential problem of carry-over effects.

The control mechanisms reviewed here help to improve the *internal validity* of studies. Internal validity is concerned with the question of whether or not the results of a project are attributable to the independent variable(s) of interest or to other, extraneous factors. *External validity* refers to the generalizability of the research findings to other individuals and other settings. A research study possesses external validity to the extent that the sample is representative of the broader population, and to the extent that the study setting and experimental arrangements are representative of other environments. A useful distinction can be made between the *accessible population,* the population from which a sample is drawn, and the *target population,* which represents a larger group of individuals in whom the investigator is interested. The researcher should define the target population in terms of those characteristics that are present in the accessible population.

A research design must balance the need for internal and external validity in order to produce useful scientific results. In addition, a good design must be appropriate for the question being asked, free from bias, sufficiently powerful, and capable of enhancing statistical precision. This latter term refers to the sensitivity with which treatment effects, relative to the effects of extraneous variables, can be detected.

Research designers need to consider what time frame is best suited to their problem. *Cross-sectional studies* involve the collection of data at one point in time, whereas *longitudinal studies* collect data at two or more points in time. Research problems that involve trends, changes, or development over time are best addressed through longitudinal designs. *Trend studies* investigate a particular phenomenon over time by repeatedly drawing different samples from the same general population. *Cohort studies* represent a type of trend study in which a particular subpopulation is studied over time with respect to some phenomenon. Longitudinal survey studies in which the *same* sample of subjects is questioned twice (or more often) are known as *panel studies. Follow-up studies* similarly deal with the same subjects studied at two or more points in time, and generally refer to those investigations in which subjects who have received a treatment or who have a particular characteristic of interest are followed-up in order to study their subsequent development. Longitudinal studies are typically expensive, time-consuming, and plagued with such difficulties as *attrition* but are often extremely valuable with respect to the information they produce.

□
Study suggestions

1. How do you suppose the use of identical twins in a research study can enhance control?
2. Suppose you were planning to conduct a nonexperimental study concerning the effects of three types of ambulation devices (cane, walker, and crutch) on feelings of control or security for persons requiring such assistive devices. What types of extraneous variables relating to characteristics of the subjects would be important to consider and, if possible, control?
3. With respect to the preceding question, how would you go about controlling for the extraneous variables you have identified?
4. Read a research report suggested under "Substantive References" in Chapters 8 through 10. Assess the adequacy of the control mechanisms used by the investigator and recommend additional ones if appropriate.
5. Suppose that you are studying the effects of range of motion exercises on radical mas-

tectomy patients. You start your experiment with 50 experimental subjects and 50 control subjects. Your intervention requires the experimental subjects to come for daily sessions over a 2-week period, while control subjects come only once at the end of 2 weeks. Your final group sizes are 40 for the experimental group and 49 for the control group. The results of your study indicate that the experimental group did better in raising arm, affected side, above head level. What effects, if any, do you think the subject attrition would have on the internal validity of your study?

6. A nurse researcher wants to study how nurses' attitudes toward death change as a function of years of nursing experience. Design a cross-sectional study to research this question, specifying the samples that you would want to include. Now design a longitudinal study to research the same problem. Identify the problems and strengths of each approach.

7. For each of the examples below, indicate (a) the types of research approach that could be used to study the problem (experimental, quasi-experimental, etc.); (b) the type of approach you would recommend using; and (c) how you would go about obtaining a sample, collecting data and establishing control procedures.

   a. What effect does the presence of the newborn's father in the delivery room have on the mother's subjective report of pain?

   b. What is the effect of different types of bowel evacuation regimes on quadriplegics?

   c. Does the reinforcement of intensive care unit nonsmoking behavior in smokers affect postintensive care unit behaviors?

   d. Is the degree of change in body image of surgical patients related to their need for touch?

□
Suggested readings

Methodological references

Braucht, G.H., & Glass, G.V. (1968). The external validity of experiments. *American Educational Research Journal, 5,* 437–473.

Campbell, D.T., & Stanley, J.C. (1963). *Experimental and quasi-experimental designs for research.* Chicago: Rand McNally.

Dayton, C.M. (1970). *The design of educational experiments.* New York: McGraw-Hill.

Hinshaw, A.S. (1979). Control by constancy: Will it work in clinical research? *Western Journal of Nursing Research, 1,* 142–145.

Kempthorne, O. (1961). The design and analysis of experiments with some reference to educational research. In R.O. Collier & S.M. Elan (Eds.), *Research design and analysis* (pp. 97–126). Bloomington, IN: Phi Delta Kappa.

Kerlinger, F.N. (1973). *Foundations of behavioral research.* (2nd ed.). New York: Holt, Rinehart and Winston. (Chapters 17–21).

Kirk, R.E. (1968). *Experimental design: Procedures for the behavioral sciences.* Belmont, CA: Wadsworth.

Rosenthal, R. (1976). *Experimenter effects in behavioral research.* New York: Halsted Press.

Substantive References*

Baker, N.C. *et al.* (1984). The effect of type of thermometer and length of time inserted on oral temperature measurements of afebrile subjects. *Nursing Research, 33,* 109–111 (Constancy of conditions).

Greenleaf, N.P. (1983). Labor force participation among registered nurses and women in comparable occupations. *Nursing Research, 32,* 306–311 (Trend study).

Johnson, J.E., Christman, N.J., & Stitt, C. (1985). Personal control interventions: Short- and long-term effects on surgical patients. *Research in*

* These studies illustrate some of the points made in this chapter. A parenthetical comment after each citation designates the design feature of interest.

Nursing and Health, 8, 131–145 (Factorial experiment; randomized block).

Kirchhoff, K.T., Rebenson-Piano, M., & Patel, M.K. (1984). Mean arterial pressure readings: Variations with positions and transducer level. *Nursing Research, 33,* 343–345 (Repeated measures).

Lewis, M.A. *et al.* (1985). The immediate and subsequent outcomes of nursing home care. *American Journal of Public Health, 75,* 758–762 (Follow-up study).

Mercer, R.T. (1985). The process of maternal role attainment over the first year. *Nursing Research, 34,* 198–203 (Cross-sequential design).

O'Brien, M.E. (1980). Hemodialysis regimen compliance and social environment. *Nursing Research, 29,* 250–255 (Panel study).

Rice, V.H. & Johnson, J.E. (1984). Preadmission self-instruction booklets, postadmission exercise performance, and teaching time. *Nursing Research, 33,* 147–151 (Randomized block design).

Schraeder, B.D. (1986). Developmental progress in very low birth weight infants during the first year of life. *Nursing Research, 35,* 237–241 (Follow-up study).

Chapter 12
□
Sampling designs

Sampling is a complex and technical topic, to which entire texts have been devoted. At the same time, it is a topic whose basic features are familiar to us all. In the course of our daily activities we gather knowledge, make decisions, and formulate predictions through sampling procedures. A nursing student may decide on an elective course for a semester by sampling two or three classes on the first day of the semester. Patients may generalize about the quality of nursing care as a result of their exposure to a sample of nurses during a one-week hospital stay. In short, we all come to conclusions about phenomena on the basis of exposure to a limited portion of those phenomena.

The scientist, too, must derive knowledge from samples. For example, in testing the efficacy of a medication for asthma patients, a scientific researcher must come to some conclusion without administering the drug to every asthmatic. However, the scientist cannot afford to draw conclusions based on a sample size of three or four subjects. Therefore, research methodologists have devoted considerable attention to the development of sampling plans that produce accurate and meaningful information. In this chapter we review some of these plans.

□
Basic sampling concepts

Sampling is an indispensable step in the research process, and a step to which too little attention is typically paid. To understand the importance of sampling, the reader must first become familiar with the terms associated with sampling. Much of this terminology has been introduced in earlier chapters but will be explained in more detail here to avoid any possible confusion in subsequent discussions.

Populations

A *population* is the entire aggregation of cases that meet a designated set of criteria. For instance, if a nurse researcher were studying American nurses with doctorates, the population could be defined as all United States citizens who are RNs and who have acquired a Ph.D., D.Sc.N., D.Ed., or other doctoral-level degree. Other possible populations might be all the male patients who had undergone surgery in hospital X during the year 1978; all the women in New York state who gave birth to a live baby during the past decade; all women over 60 years old who are under psychiatric care; or all the children in the United States with cystic fibrosis. As this list illustrates, a population may be broadly defined, involving millions of individuals, or may be narrowly specified to include only several hundred people.

It is important in defining a population to be specific about the criteria for inclusion in the population. Consider a population defined as "American nursing students." Would this population include students in all three types of basic programs? Would part-time students be included? How about RNs returning to school for a bachelor's degree? Or those students who dropped out of school for a semester? Would foreign students enrolled in American nursing programs qualify? Insofar as possible, the researcher must consider the exact criteria by which it could be decided whether an individual person would or would not be classified as a member of the population in question.

The definition of population given above by no means restricts populations to human subjects. A population might consist of all of the hospital records on file in the Belleville Hospital; or all of the blood samples taken from clients of a health maintenance organization; or all of the correspondence of Florence Nightingale. Populations may be defined in terms of actions, words, organizations, groups, and so on. Whatever the basic unit, the population is always composed of a specific aggregate of elements in which the researcher is interested.

In Chapter 11 a distinction between target and accessible populations was made. It is an important distinction for nurse researchers, who seldom have access to the target population about which they would like to draw conclusions. The *accessible population* is the aggregate of cases that conform to the designated criteria *and* that are accessible to the researcher as a pool of subject for a study. The *target population* is the entire specified aggregate of cases about which the researcher would like to make generalizations. A target population might consist of all RNs currently employed in the United States, but the more modest accessible population might be restricted to employed RNs working in San Francisco. The utility of identifying both the target and accessible populations will be discussed in a later section of this chapter.

Samples and sampling

Sampling refers to the process of selecting a portion of the population to represent the entire population. A *sample,* then, consists of a subset of the units that make up the population. In sampling terminology, the units that make up the samples and populations are usually referred to as *elements.* The element is the most basic unit about which information is collected. As we have seen, the most common element in nursing research is individuals, but other entities can form the basis of a sample or population.

Samples and sampling plans vary in their adequacy. The overriding consideration in assessing a sample is its representativeness. A representative sample is one whose key characteristics closely approximate those of the population. If a population in a study of family-planning practices consisted of 50 percent females, 25 percent of whom had used oral contraception, then a representative sample would reflect these attributes in the same proportions.

Unfortunately, there is no method for really being sure that a sample is representative without obtaining the information from the entire population. Certain sampling procedures are less likely to result in biased samples than others, but there is never any guarantee of a representative sample. This may sound somewhat discouraging, but it must be remembered that the scientist always operates under conditions in which error is possible. An important role of the scientist is to minimize or control those errors, or at least to estimate the magnitude of their effects. With certain types of sampling plans it is possible to estimate through statistical procedures the *margin of error* in the data obtained from samples. Advanced texts such as those by Kish (1965) or Cochran (1963) elaborate upon the procedures for making such estimates.

Sampling plans can be grouped into two categories: probability sampling and nonprobability sampling. *Probability sampling* involves some form of random selection in choosing the sampling units. The hallmark of a probability sample is that a researcher is in a position to specify the probability that each element of the population will be included in the sample. Probability sampling is the more respected of the two types of sampling plans because greater confidence can be placed in the representativeness of probability samples. In *nonprobability samples,* elements are selected by nonrandom methods. There is no way of estimating the probability that each element has of being included in a nonprobability sample, and there is no assurance that every element *does* have a chance for inclusion.

Strata

Sometimes it is useful to think of populations as consisting of two or more subpopulations or strata. A *stratum* refers to mutually exclusive segments of a population established by one or more specification. For instance, suppose our population consisted of all RNs currently employed in the United States. This population could be divided into two strata based on the gender of the nurse. Alternatively, we could specify three strata consisting of nurses younger than 30, nurses aged 30 to 45, and nurses 46 or older. Within a sampling context, strata are often identified and used in the sample selection process to enhance the representativeness of the sample.

Sampling rationale

Scientists work with samples rather than with populations because it is more economical and efficient to work with a small group of elements than with an entire set of elements. The typical researcher does not have the time or resources required to study all possible members of a population. The need for data in a specified time period usually makes it imperative for the researcher to sample. Furthermore, it is usually unnecessary to gather information about some phenomenon from an entire population. It is almost always possible to obtain a reasonably accurate understanding of the phenomena under investigation by securing information from a sample. Samples, thus, are practical and efficient means of collecting data.

Still, despite all of the advantages of sampling, the data obtained from samples can lead to erroneous conclusions. Finding 100 willing subjects to participate in a research project seldom poses any difficulty at all to even a novice researcher. It is considerably more problematic to select 100 subjects who adequately represent the population. Biases in sample selection may be conscious or unconscious. Bias in sampling refers to the systematic overrepresentation or underrepresentation of some segment of the population in terms of a characteristic relevant to the research question. Suppose a nurse researcher is investigating patients' responsivity to touch by nurses and decides to use as a sample the first 50 patients meeting certain criteria who are admitted to a specific hospital unit. Our fictitious researcher decides to omit Mr. Z from the sample because of his hostility to nurses. Mrs. X, who has just lost a spouse, is also excluded from the study out of consideration for her psychological discomfort. The researcher has made conscious decisions to exclude certain types of individuals, and the decisions reflect personal biases rather than bona fide criteria for selection. Sampling bias is more likely to occur unconsciously than consciously, however. If a researcher studying student nurses systematically interviews every tenth student who enters the nursing school library, the sample of students will be strongly biased in favor of librarygoers, even though the researcher may exert a conscientious effort to include every tenth entrant irrespective of their appearance, sex, or other characteristics.

The extent to which sampling bias is likely to give cause for concern is a function of the homogeneity of the population with respect to the attributes under investigation. If the elements in a population were all identical with respect to some critical attribute, then any sample would be as good as any other. Indeed, if the population were completely homogeneous, that is, exhibited no variability at all, then a single element would constitute a sufficient sample for drawing conclusions about the population. With regard to many physical or physiological attributes, it may be safe to assume a reasonably high degree of homogeneity and to proceed in selecting a sample on the basis of this assumption. For example, the blood in a person's veins is relatively homogeneous. A single blood sample chosen haphazardly is usually adequate for clinical purposes. As another illustration, the physiology of laboratory rats is sufficiently similar that elaborate sampling procedures are unnecessary when testing physiological processes with a sample of rats. For most human attributes, however, homogeneity is the exception rather than the rule. Variables, after all, derive their name from the fact that traits vary from one individual to the next. Age, income, religion, health condition, stress, attitudes, needs, smoking habits — all of these attributes reflect the heterogeneity of human beings. The researcher must be concerned with the problem of sampling bias to the degree that a population is heterogeneous on key variables. Whenever variation occurs in the population, then the same variation should be reflected in a sample.

Nonprobability sampling

The nonprobability approach to selecting a sample is less likely than probability sampling to produce accurate and representative samples. Despite this fact, the vast majority of samples in most disciplines, including nursing research, are nonprobability samples. There are three primary methods of nonprobability sampling: accidental, quota, and purposive.

Accidental sampling

Accidental sampling entails the use of the most readily available persons or objects for use as subjects in a study. The faculty member who distributes questionnaires to the nursing students in her or his class is using an accidental sample, or a *sample of convenience,* as it is sometimes called. The nurse who conducts an observational study of husbands whose wives are delivering a baby at the local hospital is also relying on an accidental sample. The problem with accidental sampling is that available subjects might be atypical of the population with regard to the critical variables being measured.

Accidental samples are not necessarily composed of individuals known to the researchers. Stopping people at a street corner to ask their opinion on some issue is sampling by convenience. Sometimes a researcher seeking individuals with certain characteristics will place an advertisement in a newspaper or place signs in supermakets, laundromats, or community centers. Both of these approaches are subject to problems of bias, because people self-select themselves as pedestrians on certain streets or as volunteers in response to public notices.

Another type of accidental sampling is known as *snowball sampling* or *network sampling*. This approach is used when the research population consists of individuals with specific traits who are difficult to identify by ordinary means. Suppose a researcher was interested in studying mothers who had stopped breastfeeding their infants within one month of being released from a hospital. There are no lists or directories of persons who meet these specifications. Therefore, the researcher might use a snowballing technique to get in touch with prospective subjects. Let us say that the researcher personally knows ten women who meet the designated criteria. These women are invited to participate and also asked to provide the names of any of their friends or acquaintances who also meet the criteria. The snowballing process continues until the desired sample size has been obtained. Like other types of accidental sampling, snowball sampling offers the researcher convenience at the risk of sample bias.

Accidental sampling is the weakest form of sampling. It is also probably the most commonly used sampling method. In cases in which the phenomena under investigation are fairly homogeneous within the population, the risks of bias may be minimal. In heteroge-

neous populations, there is no other sampling approach in which the risk of bias is greater.

When a researcher believes that there is no alternative to accidental sampling, several steps should be taken to enhance the likelihood of a representative sample. First, identify important extraneous variables. That is, identify the factors that influence the heterogeneity of the population with respect to the dependent variable. For example, in a study of the relationship between stress and health, a person's socioeconomic status is likely to be an important extraneous variable because poor people are likely to be less healthy and more stressed than more affluent ones. Then, make a decision about how to account for this source of variation in the sampling design. One solution is to define the population such that variation resulting from extraneous variables is reduced. In the above example, we might, for instance, restrict the sample to middle-class subjects. Alternatively, we could select the sample from communities known to differ in socioeconomic characteristics, so that our sample would be known to reflect the experiences of both lower- and middle-class subjects. In other words, if the population is known to be heterogeneous, we should take steps to either make it more homogeneous or to capture the full variation in the sample. Finally, we should attempt to gather information about the distribution of the research and extraneous variables in the population, so that general estimates of the direction and magnitude of any biases can be made. For example, if we knew that 40 percent of the target population were of low-income, but only 20 percent of the accidental sample were of low-income, it would be possible to make some inferences about the nature of biases in the results.

These recommended steps reinforce a point made earlier in this text: the function of research design (of which sampling design is a special case) is to control variability. Accidental sampling generally provides limited oppor-

Table 12-1
Numbers and percentages of students in strata of a population, accidental sample, and quota sample

		Freshmen	Sophomores	Juniors	Seniors	Total
Population	Males	25(2.5%)	25(2.5%)	25(2.5%)	25(2.5%)	100(10%)
	Females	225(22.5%)	225(22.5%)	225(22.5%)	225(22.5%)	900(90%)
	TOTAL	250(25%)	250(25%)	250(25%)	250(25%)	1000(100%)
Accidental	Males	2(1%)	4(2%)	3(1.5%)	1(.5%)	10(5%)
Sample	Females	98(49%)	36(18%)	37(18.5%)	19(9.5%)	190(95%)
	TOTAL	100(50%)	40(20%)	40(20%)	20(10%)	200(100%)
Quota	Males	5(2.5%)	5(2.5%)	5(2.5%)	5(2.5%)	20(10%)
Sample	Females	45(22.5%)	45(22.5%)	45(22.5%)	45(22.5%)	180(90%)
	TOTAL	50(25%)	50(25%)	50(25%)	50(25%)	200(100%)

tunity for such control. If accidental samples can be avoided, it is wise to do so. If not, the researcher should attempt some of the steps described above and should be cautious in analyzing and interpreting the resultant data.

Quota sampling

Quota sampling is, like accidental sampling, a form of nonprobability sampling. Quota sampling goes one step beyond the suggestions made above in terms of efforts to use knowledge about the population to build some representativeness into the sampling plan. The quota sample is one in which the researcher identifies strata of the population and determines the proportions of elements needed from the various segments of the population. By using information about the composition of a population, the investigator can ensure that diverse segments are represented in the sample in the proportions in which they occur in the population. Quota sampling gets its name from the procedure of establishing "quotas" for the various strata from which data are to be collected.

Let us use as an example a researcher interested in studying the attitudes of undergraduate nursing students toward the role of the industrial nurse. The accessible population is a single school of nursing that has an undergraduate enrollment of 1000 students. A sample size of 200 students is desired. The easiest procedure would be to use an accidental sample, by distributing questionnaires in classrooms or catching students as they enter or leave the library. The researcher may believe, however, that male and female students will have different attitudes toward the industrial nurse's role, as will members of the four different classes. An accidental sample could easily oversample and undersample these diverse population sectors. Table 12-1 presents some fictitious data showing the proportions of each stratum for the population and for an accidental sample. As this table shows, the accidental sample very seriously overrepresents freshmen and women, while underrepresenting men and members of the sophomore, junior, and senior classes. In anticipation of a problem of this type, the researcher can guide the selection of subjects such that the final

Table 12-2
Students willing to consider industrial nurse role

	Number in Population	Number in Accidental Sample	Number in Quota Sample
Freshmen males	2	0	0
Sophomore males	6	1	1
Junior males	8	1	2
Senior males	12	0	3
Freshman females	6	2	1
Sophomore females	16	2	3
Junior females	30	4	7
Senior females	45	3	9
Number of willing students	125	13	26
Total number of students	1000	200	200
PERCENTAGE	12.5%	6.5%	13.0%

sample will include the correct number of cases from each stratum. The bottom of Table 12-1 shows the number of cases that would be required for each stratum in a quota sample for this example.

If we pursue this same example a bit further, the reader may perhaps better appreciate the dangers of inadequate representation of the various strata. Suppose that one of the key questions in this study was "Do you think you might ever consider taking a position as an industrial nurse?" The percentage of students in the population who would respond "yes" to this inquiry is shown in the first section of Table 12-2. Of course, these values would never be known by the researcher; they are displayed to illustrate a point. Within the population, males and older students are more willing to consider the industrial nurse's role, yet these are the very groups that are underrepresented in the accidental sample. As a result, there is a sizable discrepancy between the population and sample values: nearly twice as many students are favorable toward the role of the industrial nurse (12.5%) than one would suspect based on the results obtained from the accidental sample (6.5%). The quota sample, on the other hand, does a reasonably good job

of mirroring the viewpoint of the population. In actual research situations, the distortions introduced by accidental sampling may be much smaller than in this fictitious example but, conceivably, could be larger as well.

Quota sampling does not require sophisticated skills or an inordinate amount of time or effort. Many researchers who claim that the use of an accidental sample is unavoidable for their projects could probably design a quota sampling plan, and it would be to their advantage to do so. The characteristics chosen to form the strata are necessarily selected according to the researcher's judgment. The basis of stratification should be some variable that, in the estimation of the investigator, would reflect important differences in the dependent variable under investigation. Such variables as age, sex, ethnicity, socioeconomic status, educational attainment, medical diagnosis, and occupational rank are likely to be important stratifying variables in nursing research investigations.

Except for the identification of the strata and the proportional representation for each, quota sampling is procedurally quite similar to accidental sampling. Subjects are not recruited into the study according to any systematized scheme. The subjects in any particular cell constitute, in essence, an accidental sample from that stratum of the population. Referring back to the example in Table 12-1, the accidental sample of 200 students constituted a sample of convenience from the population of 1000. In the quota sample, the 45 female seniors would constitute an accidental sample of the 225 female seniors in the population. Because of this fact, quota sampling shares many of the same weaknesses as accidental sampling. For instance, if a researcher is required by a sampling plan to interview ten males between the ages of 65 and 80, a trip to a nursing home might be the most convenient method of obtaining those subjects. Yet this approach would fail to give any representation to those many senior citizens who are living independently in the community. Despite its problems, quota sampling represents an important improvement over accidental sampling and should be considered by any researcher whose resources prevent the utilization of a probability sampling plan.

Purposive sampling

Purposive or *judgmental sampling* derives from the belief that a researcher's knowledge about the population and its elements can be used to handpick the cases to be included in the sample. The researcher might decide to purposely select the widest possible variety of respondents, or might choose subjects who are judged to be "typical" of the population in question. An underlying assumption in purposive sampling is that any errors of judgment will, in the long run, tend to balance out. Methodological research on this approach suggests, however, that this assumption may be unwarranted. Sampling in this subjective manner provides no external, objective method for assessing the typicalness of the selected subjects.

The purposive sampling method is not a generally recommended approach but can be used to advantage in certain limited instances. Newly developed instruments can be effectively pretested and evaluated with a purposive sample of divergent types of people. As another example, purposive sampling is often used when the researcher wants a sample of experts, as, for example, in conducting a needs assessment using the key informant approach or in doing a Delphi survey (see Chapter 16). Field researchers often use purposive sampling in their collection of data in the field.

The question of whether purposive samples tend to produce more accurate, representative data than accidental samples is open to conjecture. In a purposive sample there is certainly a risk of conscious sample biases, but perhaps the necessity of making individual decisions minimizes the risk of unconscious biases. The same advice given earlier still pertains: (1) purposive samples, like accidental samples, should be avoided if possible, particularly if the population is heterogeneous; and (2) if they are unavoidable, the data should be treated with circumspection.

Evaluation of nonprobability sampling

We have repeatedly stressed the disadvantages of using nonprobability samples in scientific research. The difficulty stems from the fact that not every element in the population has a chance of being included in the sample. Therefore, it is likely that some segment of the population will be systematically underrepresented. If the population is homogeneous on the critical attributes, then systematic biases may be negligible. But only a small fraction of the characteristics in which nursing researchers are interested are sufficiently homogeneous to render sampling bias an irrelevant consideration.

Why then are nonprobability samples used at all? Clearly, the advantage of this group of sampling designs lies in their practicality and economy. Probability sampling, which will be discussed in the next section, requires skill, resources, time, and opportunity. In many situations, especially in studies of a clinical nature, there may be no option but to use a nonprobability approach or to abandon the project altogether. Even hard-nosed research consultants would hesitate to advocate a total abandonment of one's ideas in the absence of a random sample. The researcher using a nonprobability sample out of necessity must be cautious about the inferences and conclusions drawn from the data. With care in the selection of the sample, a conservative interpretation of the results, and replication of the study with new samples, the researcher may find that nonprobability samples work reasonably well.

Probability sampling

The hallmark of probability sampling is the random selection of elements from the population. Random selection should not be confused with random assignment, which was described in connection with experimental research in Chapter 8. Random assignment, it will be recalled, refers to the process of allocating subjects to different experimental conditions on a random basis. Random assignment has no bearing on how the subjects participating in an experiment are selected in the first place. A random selection process is one in which each element in the population has an equal, independent chance of being selected. The four most commonly used probability sampling methods are simple random, stratified random, cluster, and systematic sampling.

Simple random sampling

Simple random sampling is the most basic of the probability sampling designs, although it is not particularly common in the research lit-

erature. Because the more complex probability sampling designs incorporate the features of simple random sampling, the procedures involved will be described here in some detail.

After the population has been identified and defined, it is necessary to establish what is known as a sampling frame. The term *sampling frame* is the technical name for the actual list of the sampling units or elements from which the sample will be chosen. If nursing students attending Wayne State University constituted the accessible population, then a roster of those students would be the sampling frame. If the sampling unit was 400-bed (or larger) general hospitals in the United States, then a list of all such hospitals would be the sampling frame. In actual practice, a population may be defined in terms of an existing sampling frame rather than starting with a population and then developing a list of sampling units. For example, if a researcher wanted to use a telephone directory as a sampling frame, the population would have to be defined as the residents of a certain community who are clients of the telephone company and who have a listed number. All members of a community do not own a telephone and others fail to have their numbers listed, so it would be inappropriate to consider a telephone directory the sampling frame for the entire community population.

Once a listing of the population elements has been developed or located, the elements must all be numbered consecutively. A table of random numbers would then be used to draw a sample of the desired size. An example of a sampling frame with 50 individuals is presented in Table 12-3. Let us assume that a sample of 20 persons is sufficient for our purposes. As in the case of random assignment, we would find a starting place in the table of random numbers by blindly placing our finger at some point on the page. In order to include all numbers between one and 50, two-digit com-

Table 12-3
Sampling frame for simple random sampling example

①. N. Alexander	㉖. F. Bradley
2. J. Behnke	27. M Couty
3. J. Carter	28. G. Dobbs
4. E. Dirk	29. L. Erikson
⑤. J. Enochs	㉚. H. Ferguson
⑥. T. Falbo	㉛. J. Gitelman
7. D. Gurieva	32. G. Hickenlooper
8. P. Hudgins	㉝. B. James
9. T.Insley	㉞. J. Kahn
10. A. Jenkins	35. M. Larson
11. C. Kivlahan	36. S. Mandell
12. F. Lafser	37. N. Nagel
⑬. J. Miller	㊳. J. O'Hara
⑭. P. Nelson	39. B. Pope
15. H. Ouellette	40. J. Quint
16. V. Pelzer	41. J. Riccio
17. R. Reed	42. E. Scruggs
18. J. Storey	㊸. S. Turner
19. W. Trumbower	44. N. Vessell
20. D. Udry	㊺. B. Webster
㉑. N. Volkart	㊻. D. Zumwalt
22. H. Woods	47. D. Abraham
㉓. R. Yoder	48. J. Barth
㉔. L. Zulauf	49. L. Conley
25. R. Asel	㊿. P. Dallmeyer

binations would be read. Suppose, for the sake of the example, that we began the random selection with the very first number in the random number table of Table 8-1 (in Chapter 8), which is 46. The person corresponding to the number, D. Zumwalt is the first subject selected to participate in the study. Number 05, J. Enochs is the second selection, and number 23, R. Yoder is the third. This process would continue until the 20 required subjects were chosen. The selected elements are circled in Table 12-3.

It should be clear that a sample selected randomly in this fashion is not subject to the biases of the researcher. There is no chance for the operation of personal preferences. Despite the fact that systematic biases do not operate in a properly drawn random sample, there is no guarantee that the sample will be representative. Random selection does, how-ever guarantee that differences in the attributes of the sample and the population are purely a function of chance. The probability of selecting a markedly deviant sample is normally quite low, and this probability decreases as the size of the sample increases.

Simple random sampling usually is a laborious process. The development of the sampling frame, enumeration of all the elements, and selection of the sample elements are time-consuming chores, particularly if the population is large. Imagine enumerating all of the telephone subscribers listed in the New York City telephone directory. If the elements can be arranged in computer-readable form, the computer can easily be programmed to automatically select the sample. In actual practice, simple random sampling is seldom used because it is a relatively inefficient procedure. Furthermore, it is often impossible to get a complete listing of every element in the population, so other methods may be required.

Stratified random sampling

Stratified random sampling is a variant of simple random sampling in which the population is first divided into two or more strata or subgroups. As in the case of quota sampling, the aim of stratified sampling is to obtain a greater degree of representativeness. Stratified sampling designs subdivide the population into homogeneous subsets from which an appropriate number of elements can be selected at random

The stratification may be based upon a wide variety of attributes, such as age, gender, occupation, and so forth. The chosen variable should be one that will result in internally homogeneous strata on the attributes about which information is being sought. The difficulty lies in the fact that the variables of interest may not be readily discernible or available. If one is working with a telephone directory, it would be risky to make decisions about a person's gender, and certainly age, ethnicity, or other personal information is not listed. One might be able to use the telephone exchange as an indicator of the area of residence, but perhaps the residential area would not be a relevant stratifying variable. Patient listings, student rosters, or organizational directories might contain the information needed for a meaningful stratification. Quota sampling does not have the same problem because the prospective subject can be asked questions that determine his or her eligibility for a particular stratum. In stratified sampling, however, decisions about a person's status in a stratum must be made before a sample is chosen.

Various procedures for drawing a stratified sample have been used. The most common is to group together those elements that belong to a stratum and to select randomly the desired number of elements. The researcher may take either the same number of elements from each stratum, or may decide to select unequal numbers, for reasons that will be discussed below. To illustrate the procedure used in the simplest case, suppose that the list in Table 12-3 consisted of 25 males (numbers 1 through 25) and 25 females (numbers 26 through 50). Using gender as the stratifying variable, we could guarantee a sample of ten males and ten females by randomly sampling ten numbers from the first half of the list and ten from the second half. As it turns out, our simple random sampling did result in ten elements being chosen from each half of the list but this was purely by chance. It would not have been unusual to draw, say, seven names from one half and thirteen from the other. Stratified sampling can guarantee the appropriate representation of different segments of the population.

In many cases the stratifying variables will divide the population into unequal subpopulations. For example, if the person's race were used to stratify the population of U.S. citizens, the subpopulation of white persons would be larger than that of black and other nonwhite persons. In such a situation, the researcher might decide to select subjects in proportion to the size of the stratum in the population. This procedure is referred to as *proportional stratified sampling.* If an undergraduate population in a school of nursing consisted of 10 percent blacks, 5 percent Hispanics, and 85 percent whites, then a proportional stratified sample of 100 students, with racial/ethnic background as the stratifying variable, would consist of ten, five, and eighty-five students from the respective subpopulations.

When the researcher's prime concern is to understand differences between the strata, proportional sampling may result in an insufficient base for making comparisons. In the previous example, would the researcher be justified in coming to conclusions about the characteristics of Hispanic nursing students based on only five cases? It would be extremely unwise to do so in most types of research. When random selection procedures are used, the probability of obtaining a representative sample increases as the sample size increases. For this reason, researchers often adopt a *disproportional sampling design* whenever interstratum comparisons are sought between strata of greatly unequal membership size. In the example at hand, the sampling proportions might be altered to select twenty blacks, twenty Hispanics, and sixty whites. This design would ensure a more adequate representation of the viewpoints of the two racial/ethnic minorities. When disproportional sampling is used, however, it is necessary to make an adjustment to the data in order to arrive at the best estimate of overall population values. This adjustment process, known as *weighting,* is a simple mathematic computation that is described in detail in most texts on sampling.

Stratified random sampling offers the researcher the opportunity to sharpen the precision and representativeness of the final sample. When it is desirable to obtain reliable information about subpopulations whose membership is relatively small, stratification provides a means of including a sufficient number of cases in the sample by oversampling for that stratum. Stratified sampling may, however, be impossible if information on the critical variables is unavailable. Furthermore, a stratified sample requires even more labor and effort than a simple random sampling, because the sample must be drawn from multiple enumerated listings.

Cluster sampling

For many populations, it is simply not possible to obtain a listing of all of the elements. The population consisting of all full-time nursing students in the country would be quite difficult to list and enumerate for the purpose of drawing a simple or stratified random sample. In addition, it would often be prohibitively expensive to sample nursing students in this way, because the resulting sample would include no more than one or two students per institution. If interviews were involved, the interviewers would have to travel to individuals scattered throughout the country. Because of these considerations, large-scale studies almost never use simple or stratified random sampling. The most common procedure for large-scale surveys is cluster sampling.

In *cluster sampling,* there is a successive random sampling of units. The first unit to be sampled is large groupings, or "clusters." In drawing a sample of nursing students, the researcher might first draw a random sample of nursing schools. Or, if a sample of nursing supervisors was desired, a random sample of hospitals might first be obtained. Usually, the procedure for selecting a general sample of citizens is to successively sample such administrative units as states, cities, districts, blocks, and then households.

The clusters can be selected either by simple or stratified methods. For instance, in selecting clusters of nursing schools it might be advisable to stratify on program type. The final selection from within a cluster may also be performed by simple or stratified random sampling.

Typically, cluster sampling proceeds through a series of different sampling units. One begins with the largest, most inclusive unit (such as a state), moving on to less inclusive units (such as counties, then hospitals), down to the most basic unit or element of the population (such as cardiac patients). Because of the successive stages of sampling, this approach is often referred to as *multi-stage sampling.*

For a specified number of cases, cluster sampling tends to contain more sampling errors than simple or stratified random sampling. Despite these disadvantages, cluster sampling is considerably more economical and practical than other types of probability sampling, particularly when the population is large and widely dispersed.

Systematic sampling

The final type of sampling design to be discussed can be classified as either a probability or nonprobability sampling approach, depending upon the exact procedure used. *Systematic sampling* involves the selection of every *k*th case from some list or group, such as every tenth person on a patient list, or every hundredth person listed in a directory of ANA members. Systematic sampling is sometimes used to sample every *k*th person entering a bookstore, or passing down the street, or leaving a hospital, and so forth. In such situations, unless the population is narrowly defined as consisting of all those people entering, passing by, or leaving, the sampling is nonprobability in nature. If college students were sampled systematically upon entering a bookstore, the resulting sample could not be called a random selection because not every student would have a chance of being selected.

Systematic sampling designs can, however, be applied in such a way that an essentially random sample is drawn. If the researcher has a list, or sampling frame, the following procedure can be adopted. The desired sample size is established at some number (n). The size of the population must be known or estimated (N). By dividing N by n, the sampling interval width (k) is established. The *sampling interval* is the standard distance between the elements chosen for the sample. For instance, if we were seeking a sample of 200 from a population of 40,000, then our sampling interval would be:

$$k = 40,000/200 = 200$$

In other words, every 200th element on the list would be sampled. The first element should be selected randomly, using a table of random numbers. Let us say that we randomly selected number 73 from a table. The persons corresponding to number 73, 273, 473, 673, and so forth would be included in the sample.

In actual practice, systematic sampling conducted in this manner is essentially identical to simple random sampling. Problems may arise if the list is arranged in such a way that a certain type of element is listed at intervals coinciding with the sampling interval. For instance, if every tenth nurse listed in a nursing personnel roster was a head nurse, and the sampling interval was ten, then head nurses would either always or never be included in the sample. Problems of this type are not too common, fortunately. In most cases, systematic sampling is preferable to simple random sampling because the same results are obtained in a more convenient and efficient manner. Systematic sampling procedures can also be applied to lists that have been stratified.

Evaluation of probability sampling

Probability sampling is really the only viable method of obtaining truly representative samples. The superiority of probability sampling lies in its avoidance of conscious or unconscious biases. If all of the elements in the population have an equal probability of being selected, then the likelihood is high that the resulting sample will do a good job of representing the population.

A further advantage is that probability sampling allows the researcher to estimate the magnitude of sampling error. *Sampling error* refers to differences between population values (such as the average age of the population) and sample values (such as the average age of the sample). It is a very rare sample that is perfectly representative of a population and contains no sampling error on any of the attributes under investigation. Probability sampling does, however, permit estimates of the degree of expected error.

Probability sampling is at the heart of most statistical testing. Strictly speaking, it is inappropriate to apply inferential statistics to data obtained from nonprobability samples, although most researchers ignore this issue in their treatment of data. Chein (1976) has discussed this problem at some length, and the concerned reader would profit by reading this discussion.

The great drawback of probability sampling is its expense and inconvenience. Unless the population is very narrowly defined, it is usually beyond the scope of small-scale research projects to sample using a probability design. A researcher adopting a nonprobability sampling design might well be able to argue that the homogeneity of the attribute under consideration makes an elaborate sampling scheme unnecessary. This justification will probably not be acceptable, however, if psychological, social, or economic attributes are being studied.

It might also be pointed out that the *selection* of elements that is representative of the population does not guarantee the participation of all of those elements. Biased samples can result from probability samples if certain segments of the population systematically refuse to cooperate. In sum, probability sampling is the preferred and most respected method of obtaining sample elements, but it may in some cases be impractical or unnecessary.

☐
Sample size

A major concern to beginning researchers is the number of subjects to be selected in a sample. The specification of a sample size is a complex issue that cannot be described in de-tail here. Below we offer some guidelines to beginning researchers. The advanced student should review the discussion of power analysis in Chapter 22 or consult an advanced sampling or statistical text.

Although there is no simple equation that can automatically tell the researcher how large a sample is needed, we can offer a simple piece of advice: you should always use the largest sample possible. The larger the sample, the more representative of the population it is likely to be. Every time a researcher calculates a percentage or an average based on sample data, the purpose is to estimate a population value. Smaller samples will tend to produce less accurate estimates than larger samples. In other words, the larger the sample, the smaller the sampling error.

Let us illustrate this notion with a simple example of, say, annual aspirin consumption in a class of 15 nursing students, as shown in Table 12-4. The population consists of 15 values, the average of which is 16. Two simple random samples with sample sizes of 2, 3, 5, and 10 each have been drawn. Each sample average on the right represents an estimate of the population, which we know is 16. Under ordinary circumstances, the population value would be unknown to us, and we would draw only one sample. With a sample size of 2, our estimate might have been wrong by as many as 8 aspirins in sample 1B—a 50% error. As the sample size increases, the averages not only get closer to the true population value, but the differences in the estimates between samples A and B get smaller as well. As the sample size increases, the probability of getting a markedly deviant sample diminishes. Large samples permit the principle of randomization to do the job for which it is designed: to counterbalance, in the long run, atypical values. The safest procedure is to obtain data from as large a sample as is economically and practically feasible, unless you have reason to believe that the population is relatively homogeneous

Table 12-4
Comparison of population and sample values/averages

Number in Group	Group	Values (annual number of aspirins consumed)	Average
.15	Population	2, 4, 6, 8, 10, 12, 14, 16, 18, 20, 22, 24, 26, 28, 30	16.0
2	Sample 1A	6, 14	10.0
2	Sample 1B	20, 28	24.0
3	Sample 2A	16, 18, 8	14.0
3	Sample 2B	20, 14, 26	20.0
5	Sample 3A	26, 14, 18, 2, 28	17.6
5	Sample 3B	30, 2, 26, 10, 4	14.4
10	Sample 4A	22, 16, 24, 22, 2, 8, 14, 28, 20, 2	15.8
10	Sample 4B	14, 18, 12, 20, 6, 14, 28, 12, 24, 16	16.4

with respect to the variables under investigation.

A consideration that can sometimes help in establishing a sample size is to consider how the resulting data will be analyzed. We have seen in the above example that results based on sample sizes of 5 or smaller tend to be unstable. That is, with small samples, the values fluctuate from one sample to the next. It is generally recommended that a sample size of at least 10, and preferably 20 to 30, be selected for every subdivision of the data, or cell of the design. If we had an experimental and control group and also wanted to consider male and female subjects separately, we would need as a bare minimum forty subjects (4 cells × 10 subjects). Or, if we were interested in comparing the levels of empathy of nurses with three different types of educational background and four clinical specialty areas, a sample size of at least 120 would be recommended (4 × 3 × 10).

Nursing research studies often use samples that are too small to reliably determine important relationships. In a survey of nursing studies published over four decades (the 1950s to the 1980s), Brown and her colleagues (1984) found that the average sample size was under 100 subjects in all four decades. While in some cases a small sample size may be justified by the nature of the problem (e.g., a study of a homogeneous population) or the nature of the inquiry (e.g., an in-depth field study), in many cases a small sample is not appropriate and can lead to misleading results.

We must hasten to add that large samples are no assurance of accuracy. When nonprobability sampling methods are used, even a large sample can harbor extensive bias. The famous example illustrating this point is the 1936 presidential poll conducted by the magazine *Literary Digest,* which predicted that Alfred M. Landon would defeat Franklin D. Roosevelt by a landslide. Approximately 2½ million individuals participated in this poll—a rather substantial sample. Biases resulted from the fact that the sample was drawn from telephone directories and automobile registrations during a depression year when only the well-to-do had a car or telephone.

A large sample cannot correct for a faulty sampling design. The researcher should make decisions about the sample size and designs with the following in mind: the ultimate criterion for assessing a sample is its representativeness, not the quantity of data it produces.

☐
Steps in sampling

The steps to be accomplished in drawing a sample vary somewhat from one sampling design to the next. However, the general outline of procedures involved can be described. The first phase of the sampling process involves the identification of the target population. The target population, it will be recalled, is the entire group of people or objects about whom the researcher would like to draw conclusions or make generalizations. The target population could consist of all RNs currently unemployed in the United States, or all diabetics, or all women who have had a miscarriage.

Unless the researcher has a large amount of resources at his or her disposal, access to the entire target population usually is not possible. Therefore, it is useful to identify a portion of the target population that is accessible to the researcher. In essence, an accessible population is a sample from the larger target population. An accessible population might consist of unemployed RNs in the state of Ohio, or all diabetics under the care of a specific health maintenance organization, or women who had a miscarriage in Centerville Hospital last year, or all mentally retarded children in a state school for the learning disabled.

Once the accessible population has been identified, the researcher must decide how the sample will be chosen and how large it will be. If the researcher can perform a power analysis to determine the desired number of subjects, it is highly recommended that he or she do so. Similarly, if probability sampling is an option, that option should be exercised. The typical nurse researcher is not in a position to do either. In such a situation, we recommend using as large a sample as possible and taking steps to build representativeness into the design (for example, by using quota sampling).

Once the sampling design has been specified, the next step is to recruit the subjects according to the designated plan and ask them for their cooperation. It is generally important to record some information about all individuals approached, including those who refuse to participate. If possible, obtain such information as age, gender, education, and occupation. This information may help you to estimate the extent of biases in your results.

One final point concerns the interpretation of results. Ideally, the sample is representative of the accessible population, and the accessible population is representative of the target population. By using an appropriate sample size and sampling plan, the researcher can have some assurance that the first part of this ideal has been realized. A much greater risk is involved in assuming that the second part of the ideal is also realized. Are the unemployed nurses of Ohio representative of all unemployed nurses in the United States? One can never be sure. The researcher must exercise judgment in assessing their degree of similarity.

There are, of course, no rules that a researcher can use as a guideline in making such judgments. The best advice is to be realistic and somewhat conservative. The researcher should interpret the findings and come to conclusions after asking: Is it reasonable to assume that the accessible population is representative of the target population? In what ways might they be expected to differ? And how would such differences affect the conclusions? If the researcher decides that the differences in the two populations are too great, it would be prudent to identify a more restricted target population to which the findings could be meaningfully generalized.

☐
Research example

Duxbury and her colleagues (1984) studied the effect of head nurse leadership style (as perceived by staff) on staff nurses' "burnout" and job satisfaction. The study focused on nurses working in neonatal intensive care units (NICUs). The aim was to distribute questionnaires to a national sample of nurses working in such units.

The investigators began with a simple random sample of level III NICUs in the United States. From that random sample, a subsample of 20 NICUs was drawn, using judgmental procedures. The sample was selected so as to ensure that both high-turnover and low-turnover junits would be represented in the study sample. Of the 20 NICUs selected, only 14 agreed to participate by distributing the questionnaires to staff nurses.

The final sample consisted of 283 RNs employed in staff nurse positions in the 14 NICUs. The method of distribution of questionnaires was not described in the report, but presumably all nurses meeting the study criteria in the 14 NICUs were asked to complete a questionnaire. Among those nurses to whom a questionnaire was given, 57.3 percent responded.

The investigators clearly took some steps to ensure that the results of their study would not be limited to a single institution or to several institutions in a single geographic area. Furthermore, although the questionnaire response rate was fairly low, the researchers instituted procedures to assess response bias. They compared the background characteristics of those nurses who completed the questionnaire with those of all who did not and found that, for the most part, there were few differences. However, the investigators did not indicate the extent to which the 14 NICUs were representative of all NICUs in this country.

□
Summary

Sampling is the process of selecting a portion of the population to represent the entire popu-

lation. A *population*, in turn, is the entire aggregate of cases that meet a designated set of criteria. In a sampling context, an *element* is the most basic unit about which information is collected.

The overriding consideration in assessing the adequacy of any sample is the degree to which it is representative of the population. Sampling plans vary in their ability to reflect adequately the population from which the sample was drawn. *Sampling bias* refers to the systematic overrepresentation or underrepresentation of some segment of the population. The greater the heterogeneity of the population with respect to the critical attributes, the greater the risk of sampling bias.

Sampling plans may be classified as either nonprobability or probability sampling. In *nonprobability sampling,* elements are selected by nonrandom methods. Accidental, quota, and purposive sampling are the principal nonprobability methods. *Accidental sampling* consists of using the most readily available or most convenient group of subjects for the sample. *Quota sampling* divides the population into homogeneous *strata* or subpopulations in order to ensure representative proportions of the various strata in the sample. Within each stratum, the researcher selects subjects by accidental sampling. In *purposive sampling,* subjects or objects are handpicked to be included in the sample, based upon the researcher's knowledge about the population. Nonprobability sampling designs have the advantage of being convenient and economical. The major disadvantage of nonprobability sampling designs is their potential for serious biases.

Probability sampling designs involve the random selection of elements from the population. A *simple random sample* involves the selection of elements on a random basis from a *sampling frame* that enumerates all the elements. A *stratified random sample* divides the population into homogeneous subgroups from which elements are selected at random. *Cluster sampling* involves the successive selection of random samples from larger to smaller units by either simple random or stratified random methods. *Systematic sampling* is the selection of every *k*th case from some list or group. By dividing the population size by the desired sample size, the researcher is able to establish the *sampling interval,* which is the standard distance between the elements chosen for the systematic sample. Probability sampling designs are preferred to nonprobability methods because the former sampling plans tend to result in more representative samples and because they permit the researcher to estimate the magnitude of sampling error. Probability samples, however, are time-consuming, expensive, inconvenient, and, in some cases, impossible to obtain.

There is no simple equation that can be used to determine how large a sample is needed for a particular research project. One rule of thumb is to use as large a sample as possible and practical. In general, the larger the sample, the more representative of the population it is likely to be. Even a very large sample, however, does not guarantee representativeness.

□
Study suggestions

1. Draw a simple random sample of 25 persons from the sampling frame of Table 12.3 using the table of random numbers that appears in Table 8.1. Begin your selection by blindly placing your finger at some point on the table.
2. Suppose you have decided to use a systematic sampling design for a research project. The known population size is 4400 and the sample size desired is 200. What is the sampling interval? If the first element selected is 23, what would be the second, third, and fourth elements to be selected?

3. Read the article by Yarcheski and Mahon (1985) listed in the substantive references. What were the successive clusters used to draw the sample?
4. Suppose a researcher is interested in studying the attitude of clinical specialists toward autonomy in the work situation. Suggest a possible target and accessible population. What strata might be identified by the researcher if quota sampling were used?
5. What type of sampling design was used to obtain the following samples?
   a. Fifteen persons known by the researcher to have hypertension and 15 persons known not to have hypertension.
   b. The couples attending a particular prenatal class.
   c. One hundred nurses from a list of nurses registered in the state of Pennsylvania, using a table of random numbers.
   d. Twenty head nurses randomly selected from a random selection of ten hospitals located in one state.
   e. Every fifth article published in *Nursing Research* during the 1970s beginning with the first article.

□
Suggested readings

Methodological references

Babbie, E. (1973). *Survey research methods.* (Chapters 5 & 6). Belmont, CA: Wadsworth.

Brown, J.S., Tanner, C.A., & Padrick, K.P. (1984). Nursing's search for scientific knowledge. *Nursing Research, 33,* 26–32.

Brown, R.C., Jr. (1976). Research Q and A on sampling. *Nursing Research, 25,* 62.

Chein, I. (1976). In Selltiz, C., Wrightsman, L.S., & Cook, S.W. *Research methods in social relations* (3rd ed.). New York: Holt, Rinehart & Winston, pp. 512–540.

Cochran, W.G. (1963). *Sampling techniques* (2nd ed.). New York: John Wiley and Sons.

Cohen, J. (1977). *Statistical power analysis for the behavioral sciences* (Rev. ed.). New York: Academic Press.

Kish, L. (1965). *Survey sampling.* New York: John Wiley and Sons.

Levey, P.S. & Lemeshow, S. (1980). *Sampling for health professionals.* New York: Lifetime Learning.

Sudman, S. (1976). *Applied sampling.* New York: Academic Press.

Williams, B. (1978). *A sampler on sampling.* New York: John Wiley and Sons.

Substantive references

Benoliel, J.Q., McCorkle, R., & Young, K. (1980). Development of a social dependency scale. *Research in Nursing and Health, 3,* 3–10 (Accidental sampling).

Beyer, J.A. (1981). Interpersonal communication as perceived by nurse educators in collegial interactions. *Nursing Research, 30,* 111–117 (Simple random sampling)

Duxbury, M.L. *et al.* (1984). Head nurse leadership style with staff nurse burnout and job satisfaction in neonatal intensive care units. *Nursing Research, 33,* 97–101 (Purposive sampling).

Dawson, C. (1985). Hypertension, perceived clinician empathy, and patient self-disclosure. *Research in Nursing and Health, 8,* 191–198 (Accidental sampling).

Fuller, S.S., & Larson, S.B. (1980). Life events, emotional support, and health of older people. *Research in Nursing and Health, 3,* 31–39 (Simple random sampling).

Hanson, S. (1981). Single custodial fathers and the parent–child relationship. *Nursing Research, 30,* 202–204 (Quota sampling).

Holzemer, W.L., Schleutermann, J.A., Farrand, L.L. & Miller, A.G. (1981). A validation study: Simulation as a measure of nurse practitioners' problem-solving skills. *Nursing Research, 30,* 139–144 (Stratified random sampling).

Kelley, B.A. (1979). Nurses' knowledge of glycosuria testing in diabetes mellitus. *Nursing Research, 28,* 316–319 (Quota sampling).

King, I. (1984). Philosophy of nursing education: A national survey. *Western Journal of Nursing Research, 6,* 387–400 (Stratified random sampling).

Thompson, T. (1980). An ordinal evaluation of the consumer participation process in community health programs. *Nursing Research, 30,* 50–54 (Systematic random sampling).

Yarcheski, A., & Mahan, N.E. (1985). The unification model in nursing. *Nursing Research, 34,* 120–125 (Multi-stage sampling).

Part IV

Measurement and data collection

Chapter 13
☐
Interviews and questionnaires

The concepts in which a researcher is interested must ultimately be translated into phenomena that can be observed and recorded. The tasks of defining the research variables and selecting or developing appropriate methods for collecting data are among the most challenging in the research process. Without high-quality data collection methods, researchers must always question the accuracy and robustness of the conclusions. As in the case of research and sampling design, the researcher must often choose from an array of alternatives in deciding how data are to be collected.

Data collection methods vary along several important dimensions:

- *Structure*. Research data are often collected according to a highly structured plan that indicates what information is to be gathered and exactly how to gather it. Sometimes, however, it is appropriate to impose a minimum of structure and to provide subjects with opportunities to reveal relevant information in a naturalistic way, as in the case of field studies.
- *Quantifiability*. Data that will be subjected to statistical analysis must be gathered in such a way that it can be quantified. On the other hand, data that are to be analyzed qualitatively are typically collected in narrative form. Structured data collection approaches generally yield data that are more easily quantified. However, it is often possible and useful to quantify unstructured information as well.
- *Researcher Obtrusiveness*. Data collection methods differ in terms of the degree to which subjects are aware of their subject

status. If subjects are fully aware of their role in a study, their behavior and responses might not be "normal." When data are collected unobtrusively, however, ethical problems may emerge.

• *Objectivity.* Some data collection approaches require more subjective judgment than others. Scientists generally strive for methods that are as objective as possible. However, in some research (especially, phenomenologically based research), the subjective judgment of the investigator is considered a valuable component of data collection.

Sometimes the nature of the research question will dictate where on these four continua the method of data collection will lie. For example, questions that require a field study will normally be low on all dimensions, whereas questions that require a survey will normally be high on all four. Often, however, the researcher has considerable latitude in selecting or designing a suitable data collection plan.

In addition to the above dimensions, nurse researchers must consider the form of data collection to use. Three types of approach have been used most frequently by nurse researchers: self-report, observation, and physiological measures. This chapter describes in detail options with respect to two types of self-report: interviews and questionnaires. Subsequent chapters in this section deal with other forms of self-report (standardized scales), as well as with observational methods, biophysiological measures, and other less frequently used methods.

☐
Introduction
to the self-report approach

In the human sciences, a good deal of information can be gathered by direct questioning of people. If, for example, we are interested in learning about patients' perceptions of hospi-
tal care, patients' level of hunger or preoperative fears, or nursing students' attitudes toward gerontological nursing, we are likely to try to find answers by posing our questions to a group of relevant persons. For some research variables, alternatives to direct questions exist. However, the unique ability of humans to communicate verbally on a sophisticated level makes it unlikely that systematic questioning will ever be eliminated from the repertoire of data collection techniques. A recent analysis of published nursing studies spanning four decades revealed that the majority of nursing investigations involve data collected by means of self-reports (Brown et al., 1984).

The self-report method is strong with respect to its directness and versatility. If we want to know what people think, feel, or believe, the most direct means of gathering the information is to ask them about it. Perhaps the strongest argument that can be made for the self-report method is that it frequently yields information that would be difficult, if not impossible, to gather by any other means. Current behaviors can be directly observed, but only if the subject is willing to manifest them publicly. For example, it may be impossible for a researcher to observe such behaviors as child abuse, contraceptive practices, or drug usage. Furthermore, observers can only observe behaviors occurring at the time of the study; self-report instruments can gather retrospective data about activities and events occurring in the past, or gather projections about behaviors in which subjects plan to engage in the future. Information about feelings, values, opinions, and motives can sometimes be inferred through observation, but behaviors and feelings do not always correspond exactly. People's actions do not always tell us about their state of mind. Here again, self-report instruments are designed to measure psychological characteristics through direct communication with the subject.

Self-reports are also versatile with respect to content coverage. People can be asked to report on facts about their personal background; facts about other persons known to them; facts about events or environmental conditions; beliefs about what the facts are; attitudes, feelings, and opinions; reasons for opinions, attitudes, or behaviors; level of knowledge about conditions, situations, or practices; and intentions for future behaviors.

Despite these advantages, verbal report instruments share a number of weaknesses. The most serious issue is the question of the validity and accuracy of self-reports: How can we really be sure that respondents feel or act the way they say they do? How can we trust the information that respondents provide, particularly if the questions could potentially require them to reveal an unpopular position on a controversial issue? Investigators often have no alternative but to assume that the majority of their respondents have been frank. Yet we all have a tendency to want to present ourselves in the best light, and this may conflict with the truth. Researchers who find it necessary or appropriate to gather self-report data should be cognizant of the limitations of this method and should be prepared to take these shortcomings into consideration when interpreting the results. And consumers of research reports should similarly be alert to potential biases introduced when subjects are asked to describe themselves, particularly with respect to behaviors or feelings that our society judges to be wrong.

As noted in Chapter 10, self-report data can be gathered either orally by interview or in writing by questionnaire. Interviews (and, to a lesser extent, questionnaires) vary considerably with respect to their degree of structure, as discussed below.

□
Unstructured and semistructured self-report techniques

A researcher using a tightly structured approach always operates with a written docu-

ment to guide the collection of data. With a non-oral format, the document is the questionnaire itself. With an oral format, the document is referred to as the *interview schedule. Standardized* or tightly *structured* schedules consist of a set of items in which the wording of both the question and the alternative responses is predetermined. When structured interviews or questionnaires are used, all subjects are asked to respond to exactly the same questions, in exactly the same order, and have the same set of options for their responses. In this section we consider six approaches to collecting self-report data using unstructured or loosely structured methods.

Unstructured interviews

When a researcher proceeds with no preconceived view of the content or flow of information to be gathered, he or she may conduct *unstructured interviews* with respondents (in self-report studies, subjects are generally referred to as *respondents*). Unstructured interviews are typically conversational in nature and are conducted in naturalistic settings. Their aim is to elucidate the respondents' perceptions of the world without imposing any of the researcher's views on them. A researcher using a completely unstructured approach may informally ask a broad question relating to the topic under investigation, such as "Tell me about what happened when you first learned you had AIDS?" Field studies generally rely heavily on unstructured interviews. Leininger (1984), for example, used unstructured interviews (as well as other methods) in her field study of the health-care values, beliefs, and practices of southern rural black and white cultures.

Focused interviews

A researcher often wants to be sure that a given set of topics is covered in interviews with research subjects. In a *focused interview,* the interviewer is given a list of areas or questions to be covered with each respondent; the list is referred to as a *topic guide.* The interviewer's function is to encourage participants to talk freely about all of the topics on the list and to record the responses (often on a tape recorder). For example, Kroska (1985) used a topic guide to study the role of "granny" midwives in rural Alabama.

A variant of the focused interview is the *focus group interview,* a technique that is becoming increasingly popular in the study of some health problems. In a focus group interview, a group of usually ten to 20 individuals is assembled for a group discussion, led by an interviewer who is guided by a written series of questions. The advantage of a group format is that it is efficient — the respondent obtains the viewpoint of many individuals in a short space of time. Its disadvantage is that some people are not comfortable about expressing their views in front of a group. Folch-Lyon and Trost (1981) provide guidelines for using focus group sessions for research purposes.

Life histories

Life histories are narrative self-disclosures about a person's life experiences. Anthropologists frequently use the life history approach to learn about cultural patterns. With this approach, the researcher asks the respondents to provide, in chronological sequence, a narration of their ideas and experiences vis-a-vis some theme, either orally or in writing. Leininger (1985) has noted that comparative life histories are especially valuable for the study of the patterns and meanings of health and health care among the elderly. Her highly regarded essay provides a protocol for obtaining a life health-care history.

Critical incidents

The *critical incidents technique* is a method of gathering information about people's be-

haviors by an examination of specific incidents relating to the behavior under investigation. The data for a critical incidents study are typically collected in a semi-structured interview.

The technique, as the name suggests, focuses on a factual incident, which may be defined as an observable and integral episode of human behavior. The word "critical" means that the incident must have a discernible impact on some outcome; it must make either a positive or negative contribution to the accomplishment of some activity of interest.

An example should clarify the purpose of this technique. Suppose we were interested in understanding why patients do not always follow their medication regime, and we wanted to develop teaching strategies to improve compliance. We might ask a sample of patients the following questions:

> Think of the last time you failed to take your medications as prescribed.
> What led up to the situation?
> Exactly what did you do?
> Why did you feel it would be alright to miss taking the medicine?

The technique differs from other self-report approaches in that it focuses on something specific about which the respondent can be expected to "testify" as an expert witness. The primary concern is to collect one or more descriptions about factual incidents that can enlighten our understanding about why, and under what circumstances, people act the way they do. Clark and Lenburg (1980), for example, used the critical incidents technique to explore knowledge-informed behavior among nurses.

Diaries

Personal diaries have long been used as a source of data in historical research. It is also possible to generate new data for a nonhistorical study by asking subjects to maintain a diary over a specified period of time. The diaries may be completely unstructured; for example, individuals who have undergone an organ transplant could be asked simply to spend ten minutes a day jotting down their thoughts and feelings. Frequently, however, subjects are requested to make entries into a diary regarding some specific aspect of their experience, sometimes in a semi-structured format. For example, studies of the effect of nutrition during pregnancy on fetal outcomes frequently require subjects to maintain a complete diary of everything they ate over a one-to-two week period. Boyle (1985) used a Family Health Calendar over a one-month period to collect information about how families prevent illness, maintain health, experience morbidity, and treat health problems.

Evaluation of unstructured approaches

Unstructured interviews are an extremely flexible approach to gathering data, and in many research situations offer distinct advantages. In many clinical situations, for example, it may be appropriate to let individuals talk freely about their problems, allowing them to take much of the initiative in directing the flow of information. In general, unstructured interviews are of greatest utility, from a researcher's point, when a new area of research is being explored. In such situations an unstructured approach may allow the investigator to ascertain what the basic issues or problems are, how sensitive or controversial the topic is, how easy it is to secure respondents' cooperation in discussing the issues, how individuals conceptualize and talk about the problems, and what range of opinions or behaviors exist that are relevant to the topic. Unstructured methods may also help elucidate the underlying meaning of a pattern or relationship repeatedly observed in survey research.

However, unstructured methods are extremely time consuming and very demanding of the researcher's skill in analyzing and interpreting qualitative materials. Samples tend to be small because of the quantity of information produced, so it is often difficult to know whether findings can be generalized at all. Unstructured methods do not generally lend themselves to the rigorous testing of hypotheses concerning cause-and-effect relationships.

☐
Research example: semistructured self-report

Tripp-Reimer (1982) investigated barriers to health care among an American subcultural group, the Appalachians. An earlier study had found that Appalachians tended to use professional health-care services less than other minority groups. Tripp-Reimer's investigation explored the possible reasons for this finding by examining perceptions of health-care professionals working within this subculture.

Her study involved intensive, semi-structured interviews with 37 health-care professionals, who were interviewed at various health-care agencies that targeted their services toward Appalachian migrants. The interviews averaged two-and-a-half hours in length. Each interview, which was guided by a topic guide, was either tape recorded or recorded by shorthand and then later transcribed verbatim in full.

The interviews probed into the health-care professionals' perceptions of Appalachian lifestyles, customs, characteristics, and beliefs. The perceptions of those of Appalachian origin were contrasted with those of non-Appalachian origin. Although both groups agreed on many objective facts about the lifeways of the Appalachian migrants, they differed considerably in their interpretation of those facts. For example, both groups agreed that the Appalachians have large families, but non-Appalachian health-care professionals viewed this as a symptom of irresponsibility, whereas the Appalachian health-care professionals interpreted this as the importance of children within the Appalachian culture. Tripp-Reimer concluded that the closed-mindedness and ethnocentrism of the non-Appalachian health care workers might be detrimental to health-care delivery to Appalachian clients.

□
Structured self-report instruments

The majority of nurse researchers who collect self-report data use instruments with a moderate to high degree of structure. In developing structured instruments, a great deal of effort is usually devoted to the content, form, and wording of the questions being posed. This section provides some guidelines for the development and use of structured interview schedules and questionnaires.

Question form

Structured instruments vary in their degree of structure through their combination of open-ended and closed-ended questions. *Open-ended* questions (or *items,* as they are sometimes called), allow subjects to respond to the question in their own words. The question "What aspect of your professional relationship with physicians do you feel is most in need of improvement?" is an example of an open-ended question that might be used in a study investigating nurse-physician relations. In questionnaires, the respondent is asked to give a written reply to open-ended items and, therefore, adequate space must be provided to allow the expression of opinions. In interviews, the interviewer is normally expected to quote the response verbatim or as closely as possible.

Closed-ended (or *fixed-alternative*) questions offer respondents a number of alternative replies from which the subjects must choose the one that most closely approximates the "right" answer. The alternatives may range from the simple yes-no variety ("Have you

smoked a cigarette within the past 24 hours?") to rather complex expressions of opinion or behavior.

Both open and closed questions have certain strengths and weaknesses. Closed-ended items are difficult to construct but easy to administer and, especially, to analyze. With closed-ended questions, the researcher needs only to tabulate the number of responses to each alternative in order to gain some understanding about what the sample as a whole thinks about an issue. The analysis of open-ended items, on the other hand, is often difficult and time consuming. The procedure that is normally followed is the development of categories and the assignment of the open-ended responses to those categories. That is, the researcher essentially transforms the open-ended responses to fixed categories in a post hoc fashion so that tabulations can be made. This classification process takes considerable time and skill. Furthermore, because the ultimate classification decision lies in the hands of the researchers rather than the respondents, there is the possibility of inappropriate categorization caused by misinterpretation of the responses or an inadequate classification system.

Closed-ended items are generally more efficient than open-ended questions in the sense that a respondent is normally able to complete more closed- than open-ended questions in a given amount of time. In questionnaires, subjects may be less willing to compose a written response than to simply check off or circle the appropriate alternative. With respondents who are unable to express themselves well verbally, closed-ended items have a distinct advantage. Furthermore, there are some types of questions that may seem less objectionable in closed form than in open form. Take the following example:

1. What was the gross annual income of your family last year?

2. In what range was your family's gross annual income last year?
   ( ) under $5,000
   ( ) $5,000 to $9,999
   ( ) $10,000 to $14,999
   ( ) $15,000 to $19,999
   ( ) $20,000 to $24,999
   ( ) $25,000 or over

The second question is more likely to be answered by respondents because the range of the options allows them a greater measure of privacy than the blunter open-ended question.

These various advantages of the fixed-alternative question are offset by some corresponding shortcomings. The major drawback of closed-ended questions lies in the possibility of the reseacher neglecting or overlooking some potentially important responses. It is often difficult to see an issue from multiple points of view. The omission of possible alternatives can, of course, lead to inadequate understanding of the issues and to outright bias if the respondents choose an alternative that misrepresents their position. When the researcher is unable to pretest the instrument thoroughly or when the area of research is relatively new, open-ended questions may be more suitable than closed-ended items for avoiding bias.

Another objection to closed-ended items is that they are sometimes considered too superficial. Open-ended questions allow for a richer and fuller perspective on the topic of interest, if the respondents are verbally expressive and cooperative. Some of this richness may be lost when the researcher later tabulates answers by developing a system of classification, but excerpts taken directly from the open-ended responses can be extremely valuable in the final report in imparting the "flavor" of the replies.

Finally, some respondents will often object to being forced into choosing from among responses that do not reflect their opinions precisely. Open-ended questions give a lot of freedom to the respondent and, therefore, offer the possibility of spontaneity, which is unattainable when a set of responses is provided.

In conclusion, the decisions to use open and closed questions are based on a number of important considerations such as the sensitivity of the topic, the verbal ability of the respondents, the amount of time available, and so forth. Combinations of both types are highly recommended to offset the strengths and weaknesses of each. Questionnaires typically use fixed-alternative questions predominantly in order to minimize the respondent's writing burden. Interview schedules, on the other hand, are more variable in their mixture of these two question types.

Question wording

Unquestionably the most difficult aspect of constructing a schedule is the actual wording of the questions and, for closed-ended items, the wording of the alternative responses. In this section we confine our discussion to the first problem and review a number of considerations that should be borne in mind as the questions are being designed.

1. *Clarity.* It seems fairly obvious that the designer of a questionnaire or interview schedule should strive for clarity and unambiguity. A question that can be interpreted differently by different people is unlikely to produce meaningful information. Unfortunately clarity is more easily discussed than achieved. Even seemingly simple and straightforward questions may be ambiguous or open to various interpretations to respondents who do not have the same perspective on the issue as the researcher. The question "When do you usually eat your evening meal?" might bring forth such responses as "around 6 p.m.," "when my husband

gets home from work," or "during the evening television news broadcast." The question itself contains no words that are technical or difficult but the question is unclear because the intent of the researcher is not apparent. A few suggestions might help to improve the precision of questions:

a. Clarify in your own mind the information that you are trying to obtain. If you are unclear about exactly what you want to find out, you can hardly expect respondents to guess your intentions.

b. Avoid long sentences or phrases.

c. Avoid "double-barreled" questions that contain two distinct ideas or concepts. The statement "The mentally ill are essentially incapable of caring for themselves and should, therefore, be denied of any responsibilities or rights," might generate expressions of both agreement and disagreement by the same persons.

d. Avoid technical terms if more common terms are equally appropriate.

e. Try to state your questions in the affirmative rather than the negative.

2. *Ability of Respondents to Reply or Give Information.* A second important consideration is whether respondents can reasonably be expected to answer the questions accurately and meaningfully. Research participants are often reluctant to say "I don't know" or "I don't understand." Therefore, the designer of the research instrument must give some thought to the characteristics of the sample in deciding whether or not to include certain questions and how to word them. The respondent may not be competent to answer questions for different reasons, each of which has implications for the wording of the question.

a. *Language:* Try to use words that are simple enough for the *least* educated respondents in your sample. Do not assume that even members of your own profession will have extensive knowledge on all aspects of nursing and medical terminology.

b. *Level of Information:* It should not be assumed that respondents will be aware of, or informed about, issues or questions in which you are interested. Furthermore, you should avoid giving the impression that respondents *ought* to have the information. Questions dealing with complex or specialized issues can be worded in such a way that a respondent will be comfortable admitting ignorance. Here is one illustration: "Many people have not had an opportunity to learn much about the physiological side-effects of oral contraceptives, but some people have picked up information on this subject. Do you happen to know of any such side effects?" Such face-saving devices can be invaluable in making the respondent's lack of knowledge acceptable. Another approach is to preface a question by a short statement of explanation about terminology or issues.

c. *Memory:* You should not take for granted that respondents will be able to remember events, situations, or previous activities and feelings with a high degree of accuracy. To put respondents at ease, you could preface a question requiring memory with a statement such as "For many of us, communications are so varied and rapid that it is difficult to remember very much in detail."

3. *Bias.* Bias is an extremely serious problem in verbal self-report instruments. Respondents, after all, can distort the results very easily by giving misinformation.

Some techniques are useful in minimizing any biases that the researchers might inadvertently introduce themselves.

   a. Avoid leading questions that suggest a particular kind of answer. A question like "Do you agree that nurse-midwives play an indispensable role in the health team?" is not neutral.

   b. Avoid identifying a position or attitude with a prestigious person or group.

   c. State a range of alternatives within the question itself when possible. For instance, the question "Do you normally prefer to get up early in the morning?" is more suggestive of the "right" answer than "Do you normally prefer to get up early in the morning or to sleep late, or does it depend on the circumstances?"

4. *Handling Sensitive or Personal Information.* As researchers we must always keep in mind that respondents are doing us a favor by taking time to reply to our questions. Questionnaires and interviews always represent an intrusion on people's privacy. Schedules are not only time consuming, they are also designed to probe personal areas of the respondents' experience. On the other hand, many people are not only willing, but happy, to have the opportunity to express their views on certain topics. In any event, the researcher must strive to be courteous, considerate, and sensitive to the needs and rights of research participants. The following concepts might be kept in mind.

   a. For questions that deal with socially unacceptable behavior or attitudes (for example, excessive drinking habits, premarital sexual behavior, noncompliance with physician's instructions, and the like), the researcher can usually elicit more frankness if the schedule creates an atmosphere of permissiveness or nonjudgment. The use of response alternatives may once again be useful in this regard because (1) it is easier to merely check off having engaged in socially disapproved actions than to verbalize them in response to an open-ended question and (2) the appearance of the behavior printed on an official-looking schedule is likely to make respondents aware that they are not alone in their behaviors or attitudes, so that admitting to them becomes less difficult.

   b. Impersonal wording of a question is often useful in minimizing embarrassment and encouraging honesty. To illustrate this point, compare these two statements with which respondents would be asked to agree or disagree: (1) "I am personally quite satisfied with the nursing care I received during my hospitalization;" (2) "The quality of nursing care in this hospital is quite good." A respondent might feel more comfortable about admitting dissatisfaction with nursing care in the less personally worded second question.

   c. Politeness and encouragement help to motivate a respondent to cooperate. Include phrases such as "Would you mind . . . ," "We would appreciate . . . ," and "please" often.

Response alternatives

If closed-ended questions are used, the researcher needs to make decisions about the form that the response alternatives will take. Below are some suggestions for preparing alternatives to closed-ended items.

1. *Coverage of Alternatives.* The responses should adequately encompass all of the

significant alternatives. If respondents are forced to choose a response from among options provided by the researcher, they should feel reasonably comfortable with the available options. As a safety measure, the researcher can have as one response option a phrase such as "Other—please specify."

2. *Overlapping Responses.* The alternatives should be mutually exclusive.
3. *Ordering Responses.* There should be some underlying rationale for the order in which the alternatives are presented to the respondent. Very often the options can be placed in order of decreasing or increasing favorability, agreement, or intensity. When the respondent is asked to choose from options that have no "natural" sequence or order, alphabetic ordering of the alternatives is less likely to "lead" the respondent to a particular response.
4. *Response Length.* The response alternatives should not be too lengthy. One sentence or phrase for each alternative should almost always be sufficient to express a concept. In general, the response alternatives should be approximately equal in length.

Examples of closed-ended questions

It is often difficult to design good-quality closed-ended questions because the researcher must pay careful attention not only to the wording of the question but also to the content, wording, and formatting of the fixed alternatives. Nevertheless, the analytic advantages of closed-ended questions make it compelling to include at least some on most structured instruments. In this section we illustrate several different types of closed-ended questions.

The simplest type of closed-ended questions requires the respondent to make a choice between two alternatives. *Dichotomous items,* as such questions are called, are considered most appropriate for gathering factual information, as in the following example:

Have you ever been hospitalized?
( ) Yes
( ) No

Dichotomous items often are considered too restrictive by respondents, who may resent being forced to see an issue as either yes or no. Graded alternatives are preferable for opinion or attitude questions because they give the researcher more information and because they give the respondent the opportunity to be more accurate. A range of alternatives provides more information in that the researcher can measure intensity of feeling as well as direction. Multiple-choice questions most commonly offer three to five alternatives, as in the example below:

How important is it to you to avoid a pregnancy at this time?
( ) Extremely important
( ) Very important
( ) Somewhat important
( ) Not at all important

A special type of multiple choice item is the "cafeteria" question, which asks respondents to select a response that most adequately states their view:

People have different opinions about the use of estrogen replacement therapy for women in menopause. Which of the following statements best represents your point of view?
1. Estrogen replacement is dangerous and should be totally banned.
2. Estrogen replacement may have some undesirable side-effects that suggest the need for caution in its use.
3. I am undecided about my views on estrogen replacement therapy.

Here are some characteristics of birth-control devices that are of varying importance to different people. How important a consideration has each of these been for you in choosing a birth-control method?

	Of Very Great Importance	Of Great Importance	Of Some Importance	Of No Importance
1. Comfort				
2. Cost				
3. Ease of use				
4. Effectiveness				
5. Noninterference with spontaneity				
6. Safety to you				
7. Safety to partner				

Figure 13-1. Example of a checklist.

4. Estrogen replacement has many beneficial effects that merit its promotion.
5. Estrogen replacement is a wonder cure that should be administered routinely to menopausal women.

Rank-order questions ask respondents to rank their responses along a continuum from most favorable to least favorable (or most/least important, beneficial, familiar, etc.). They can be quite useful but need to be carefully handled because they are often misunderstood by respondents. Here is an example:

People value different things about life. Below is a list of principles or ideas that are often cited when people are asked to name the things they value most. Please indicate the order of importance of these values to you by placing a "1" beside the most important, "2" beside the next most important, and so forth.
( ) Achievement and success
( ) Family relationships
( ) Friendships and social interaction
( ) Health
( ) Money
( ) Religion

Checklists are items that encompass several questions on a topic and require the same response format. Checklists are relatively efficient and easy for respondents to understand. Because checklists are difficult for an interviewer to read, they are used more frequently in self-administered questionnaires than in interviews.

A checklist is often a two-dimensional arrangement in which a series of questions is listed along one dimension (usually vertically) and response alternatives are listed along the other. It is this two-dimensional character that is being referred to when the term *matrix question* is used by some writers instead of the term "checklist." Figure 13-1 is an example of a checklist.

Instrument format

The appearance and layout of the schedule may seem a matter of minor administrative importance. However, a poorly designed format can have substantive consequences if respondents (or interviewers) become confused, miss questions, or answer questions that they should have omitted. The format is more important in the case of questionnaires because respondents who are unfamiliar with the researcher's intent will not usually have an opportunity to ask questions. A few suggestions may assist the beginning investigator's efforts to lay out a schedule.

1. Try not to compress too many questions into too small a space. An extra page of questions is better than a schedule that appears cluttered and confusing and that provides inadequate space for open-ended questions.

2. In the formatting of alternative responses, the response options should be set off from the question or stem itself, and are usually aligned vertically. Respondents can be asked either to circle the appropriate answer or to place a check in the appropriate box, illustrated below as Methods A and B:

Are you a member of the American Nurses' Association?

a. yes	[ ] yes
b. no	[ ] no
Method A	Method B
(Circling)	(Checking)

3. Special care should be given to formatting *filter questions,* which are designed to route respondents through different sets of questions depending on their response to earlier questions. Probably the least confusing approach is to set off

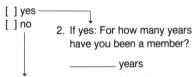

1. Are you a member of the American Nurses' Association?

[ ] yes
[ ] no   2. If yes: For how many years have you been a member?

_____ years

3. Do you subscribe to any nursing journals?

[ ] yes
[ ] no

questions appropriate to only a subset of respondents from the main series of questions, as shown at the bottom of the first column.

There are alternative procedures, but they are more likely to give rise to difficulties. Instructions such as "Skip to question 3" might be misunderstood by some respondents. (However, "Skip to" instructions are commonly used in interview schedules because interviewers are generally thoroughly trained in the use of the instrument.) It is also best to avoid forcing all readers to go through inapplicable questions. That is, question 2 in the example could have been worded "If you are a member of ANA, for how long have you been a member?" The person who is not an ANA member might not be sure how to handle this question and might be annoyed at having to read through material that is not relevant.

Steps in instrument development

A careful, well-developed schedule cannot be prepared in minutes or even in hours. A researcher interested in designing a useful and accurate instrument must devote considerable time to analyzing the research requirements and attending to minute details. If a researcher is sloppy or haphazard in designing an instrument, little confidence can be placed in the obtained data. Imagine how wary you might be in using a piece of technical equipment — say a sphygmomanometer — that had been designed in haste and inadequately tested. The following steps are normally required to develop a sound self-report instrument:

1. *Preliminary Decisions.* Decide whether to collect the data by means of interview or questionnaire. (The advantages and disadvantages of each are described in a

later section.) Then, decide on the form the instrument will take. If the instrument is to be self-administered, the questions probably will be more structured and fewer open-ended questions will be included than if an interview were used.

2. Next, decide on the type of information that needs to be collected. There is a tendency to want to ask too many questions, so try to think ahead about how each question will be used to address your research problem.

3. *Drafting the Schedule*. The actual development of questions should not be done hastily. The content of the question needs to be matched to the most appropriate question type. Because there is a considerable variety of closed-question types, there is ample room here for ingenuity and creativity. The wording of each question needs to be carefully monitored. The researcher should not feel compelled to develop entirely original questions. Existing instruments on the same or a similar topic should be consulted. Particularly in the case of basic background information, it makes little sense for every questionnaire developer to struggle anew with the wording of virtually universal questions.

4. The questions are seldom written in their order of presentation, so the next step should be to decide how to sequence the questions. A questionnaire or interview schedule is not a random set of questions that the researcher pulls out of a hat. Some thought needs to be given to the sequencing of the questions so as to arrive at an order that is psychologically meaningful to respondents and encourages candor and cooperation. For example, the schedule should begin with questions that are interesting and motivating. The instrument also needs to be arranged in such a way that distortions and biases are minimized. The possibility that earlier questions will influence replies to the subsequent questions is an ever-present problem. Whenever both general and specific questions about a topic are to be included, the general question should be placed first to avoid putting ideas into people's heads. Once the questions have been ordered the instrument can be formatted.

5. An introduction should then be written and, for questionnaires, instructions on how to complete the form should be prepared. Every schedule should be prefaced by some introductory comments about the nature and purpose of the study. In face-to-face or telephone interviews the introductory comments would normally be read to the respondents by the interviewer. In questionnaires the introduction usually takes the form of a cover letter accompanying the instrument. The introduction should be given considerable care and attention, because it represents the first point of contact between the researcher and potential respondents. The introduction would normally answer the following questions:

- What is the purpose of the study? Why should the respondent spend time providing the information; that is, what contribution is the respondent making?
- How did the respondent come to be selected? Where did you get his or her name? (People are sometimes puzzled by or suspicious about being selected to participate in a study.)
- What will be done with the information? Will confidentiality or anonymity be maintained?
- What is the deadline for the return of the schedule (in the case of a questionnaire)? How should the respondent go about returning the questionnaire?

• Has the respondent been adequately thanked for participating in the study?

6. *Revising and Pretesting.* When a first draft of the instrument is in reasonably good order, it should be critically discussed with individuals who are knowledgeable about the construction of questionnaires and with persons who are familiar with the substantive content of your schedule. The instrument should also be reviewed by someone who is capable of detecting technical difficulties such as spelling mistakes, grammatical errors, and so forth. When these various persons have provided feedback, a revised version of the instrument can be pretested.

7. A *pretest* of an instrument is a trial run to determine, insofar as possible, its clarity, research adequacy, and freedom from bias. The pretest provides an opportunity for detecting at least gross inadequacies or unforeseen problems before going to the expense of a full-scale study. The pretest should be administered to individuals who are similar to those who will ultimately participate in the study. Ordinarily, ten to twenty pretested schedules should be sufficient, although more may be necessary if the instrument is complex and if the sample is heterogeneous. If extensive revisions are suggested by the reactions and responses to the pretest, a second pretest may be required. If minor revisions are sufficient, the instrument should be given one final editing and can then be reproduced for the final administration.

☐
The administration of self-report instruments

Interview schedules and questionnaires require different skills and different considera-

tions in their administration. The successful collection of the data is clearly as important to the research endeavor as is the design of the instruments. Both the quantity and the quality of the data gathered are influenced by the data collection procedures and the competencies of the research personnel. In this section we will examine some of the problems involved in instrument administration and some ways of handling those difficulties.

Collecting interview data

The quality of interview data depends to a great extent upon the proficiency of the interviewers. Interviewers for large survey organizations receive extensive general training in addition to more specific training for individual studies. In this introductory text we cannot adequately cover all of the principles of good interviewing, but we can identify some of the major issues.

A primary task of the interviewer is to put respondents at ease so that they will feel comfortable in expressing their honest opinions. The respondents' personal reaction to the interviewer can seriously affect their willingness to participate. Interviewers, therefore, should always be neat (but not overdressed), punctual (if an appointment has been made), courteous, and friendly. The interviewer should strive to appear unbiased and to create a permissive atmosphere that encourages candor. The job of the interviewer is to serve as a neutral medium of communication. All opinions of the respondents should be accepted as natural — the interviewer should generally not express surprise, disapproval, or even approval.

Interviewers should follow the wording of the questions in the schedule precisely. Similarly, interviewers should not offer spontaneous explanations of what the questions mean. Repetitions of the questions are usually adequate to dispel any misunderstanding, particularly if the instrument has been properly pretested. The interviewer should not read the questions from the schedule. A naturalistic, conversational tone is essential in building rapport with respondents, and this tone is impossible to achieve if the questions are not thoroughly familiar to the interviewer.

When questions with lengthy or complicated response alternatives are posed, the interviewers should hand the subjects a card that lists all of the options. Individuals cannot be expected to remember detailed unfamiliar material and are sometimes inclined to choose the last alternative if they cannot recall earlier ones. Closed-ended items can be recorded by checking or circling the appropriate alternative, but responses to open-ended questions need to be recorded in full. The interviewer should not paraphrase or summarize the respondent's reply.

The interviewer undoubtedly will find that obtaining complete and relevant responses is not always an easy matter. Respondents often reply to seemingly straightforward questions with irrelevant discussions or partial answers, or they may say "I don't know" to avoid giving their opinions on sensitive topics or to stall while they think over the question. In such cases the job of the interviewer is to *probe*. The purpose of a probe is to elicit more useful information from a respondent than was volunteered during the first reply. A probe can take many forms: sometimes it involves a repetition of the original question and sometimes it is a long pause intended to communicate to respondents that they should continue. Frequently it is necessary to encourage a more complete response by a nondirective supplementary question such as "How is that?" "Anything else?" or "Could you explain a bit further?" The interviewer must be careful to insert only *neutral* probes that do not influence the subject's response. The ability to probe well is perhaps the greatest test of an interviewer's skill. In order to know when to probe and how to select the best probes, the interviewers must comprehend fully the purpose of each question and the type of information being sought.

The guidelines for handling telephone interviews are essentially the same as those for face-to-face interviews, although additional effort usually is required to build rapport over the telephone. In both cases, the interviewer should strive to make the interview a pleasant and satisfying experience in which respondents are made to feel as though the information they are providing is important.

Collecting questionnaire data

Self-administered questionnaires can be distributed in a number of ways. The most convenient procedure is to administer the questionnaire to a group of respondents who complete the instrument together at the same time. This approach has the obvious advantage of maximizing the return rate and allowing the researcher to clarify any possible misunderstandings about the instrument. Group administrations are often possible in educational settings and might also be feasible in some hospital or community situations.

Personal presentation of questionnaires to individual respondents is another alternative. Personal contact with respondents has been found to have a positive effect on the rate of questionnaires returned. Furthermore, the availability of the researcher or an assistant can be an advantage in terms of explaining and clarifying the purposes of the study or particular items. This method may, however, be relatively time consuming and expensive if the questionnaires have to be delivered and picked up at respondents' homes. However, the distribution of questionnaires in a clinical setting is often inexpensive and efficient, and likely to yield a high rate of completed questionnaires.

Questionnaires are often mailed to respondents. A problematic feature of this approach is that the completion rates tend to be very low. When only a small subsample of respondents return their questionnaires, it may be unreasonable to assume that those who did respond were somehow "typical" of the sample as a whole. In other words, the researcher is faced with the possibility that those individuals who did not complete a questionnaire would as a group have answered the questions differently from those who did return the schedule. In such a situation, it may be inappropriate to generalize the results of the study to the target population.

If the response rate is high, the risk of serious response bias may be negligible. A response rate greater than 60 percent is probably sufficient for most purposes, but lower response rates are common. The researcher generally should attempt to discover how representative the respondents are, relative to the target population, in terms of basic demographic characteristics such as age, sex, marital status, and the like. This comparison might lead the researcher to conclude that respondents and nonrespondents are similar enough to assume the absence of serious biases. If demographic differences are found, the investigator will at least be in a position to make some inferences about the direction of the biases.

The response rate can be affected by the manner in which the questionnaires are designed and mailed. The physical appearance of the questionnaire can influence its appeal, so some thought should be given to the layout, quality and color of paper, method of reproduction, and typographic quality of the instrument. The standard procedure for distributing the questionnaire is to include with the schedule a cover letter and a stamped, addressed return envelope. Failure to enclose a return envelope could have a serious effect upon the response rate. Also, you should be sure that both your main envelope and the return envelope carry sufficient postage.

The use of *follow-up reminders* has been found to be effective in achieving higher response rates for mailed questionnaires. This procedure involves the mailing of additional letters urging nonrespondents to complete and return their schedules. Follow-up letters or notices are typically sent two to three weeks after the initial mailing. A number of techniques have been adopted for follow-ups, the simplest being a letter of encouragement to nonrespondents. It is preferable, however, to enclose a second copy of the questionnaire with the reminder letter since most people will have misplaced the original copy. Telephone follow-ups can be quite successful, but they are costly and involve a considerable amount of time.

In the event that the questionnaire is anonymous, the investigator may be unable to distinguish respondents and nonrespondents for the purpose of sending follow-up letters. Although several techniques for dealing with this problem exist, the simplest procedure is to send out a follow-up letter to the entire sample, thanking those individuals who have already answered and asking others to cooperate.

As questionnaires are returned, the investigator should keep a log of the incoming receipts on a daily basis. Each questionnaire should be opened, checked for usability, and assigned an identification number. This record-keeping activity will assist the researcher in assembling the results, monitoring the return rate, and making decisions about the timing of follow-up mailings and cut-off dates.

The problems associated with mailed questionnaires are not ones that can be handled by interpersonal skills. Building rapport in a questionnaire situation in order to enhance the completion rate is a difficult chore and often is dependent upon attention to details. Even though these procedural matters may seem trivial, the success of the project may depend upon their careful execution.

□
Questionnaires versus interviews: an assessment

Self-administered questionnaires offer a number of advantages over personal interviews, but they have some drawbacks as well. First, let us consider some of the strong points of questionnaires.

1. Questionnaires, relative to interviews, are generally much less costly and require less time and energy to administer. Group-administered questionnaires are clearly the least expensive and time consuming of any procedure. With a fixed amount of funds and/or time, a larger and more geographically diverse sample can usually be obtained with mailed questionnaires than with interviews.
2. Questionnaires, unlike interview schedules, offer the possibility of complete anonymity. Sometimes a guarantee of anonymity is crucial in obtaining candid responses, particularly if the questions are of a highly personal or sensitive nature. Anonymous questionnaires often result in a higher proportion of socially unacceptable responses (that is, responses that place the respondent in an unfavorable light) than face-to-face interviews.
3. The absence of an interviewer ensures that there will be no interviewer bias. Ideally, an interviewer is a neutral agent through whom questions and answers are passed. Studies have shown, however, that this ideal is difficult to achieve. Respondents and interviewers interact as

human beings, and this interaction can affect the subject's responses. This problem clearly is not present for questionnaires.

Despite these advantages, the strengths of interviews far outweigh those of mailed questionnaires. It is true that interviews are costly, prevent respondent anonymity, and are subject to interviewer biases. Nevertheless, the numerous advantages outlined below have led many researchers to conclude that interviews are superior to questionnaires for most research purposes.

1. The response rate tends to be quite high in face-to-face interviews. Respondents are apparently more reluctant to refuse to talk to an interviewer who is directly in front of them than to discard or ignore a questionnaire. A well-designed and properly conducted interview study normally achieves a response rate in the vicinity of 80 to 90 percent. Since nonresponse is not a random process, low response rates may introduce serious biases.
2. There are many individuals who simply cannot fill out a questionnaire. Examples include young children, the blind, the very elderly, the illiterate, or the uneducated. Interviews, on the other hand, are normally feasible with most people.
3. Interviews offer a protection against ambiguous or confusing questions. The interviewer can determine whether questions have been misunderstood and clarify matters. In questionnaires, items that are misinterpreted may go undetected by the researchers and the responses may, thus, lead to erroneous conclusions.
4. The information obtained from questionnaires tends to be somewhat more superficial than interview data. This is

due partly to the fact that questionnaires ordinarily contain a preponderance of closed-ended items. Open-ended questions often engender resentment among questionnaire respondents, who dislike having to compose and write out a reply. Much of the richness and complexity of the human experience can be lost if closed-ended items are used exclusively. Furthermore, interviewers can enhance the quality of their data through probing.

5. Respondents are less likely to give "don't know" responses or to leave a question unanswered in an interview situation than on questionnaires.
6. In an interview the researcher has strict control over the order of presentation of the questions. Questionnaire respondents are at liberty to skip around from one section of the instrument to another. It is possible that a different ordering of questions from the one originally intended could bias the responses.
7. Interviews permit greater control over the sample in the sense that the interviewer knows whether or not the person being interviewed is the intended participant. It is not unusual to have individuals who receive questionnaires pass the instrument on to a friend, relative, secretary, and so forth. This kind of activity can change the characteristics of the sample.
8. Finally, face-to-face interviews have an advantage in their ability to produce additional data through observation. The interviewer is in a position to observe or judge the respondents' level of understanding, degree of cooperativeness, social class, lifestyle, and so forth. These kinds of information can be useful in interpreting the responses.

It should be pointed out before concluding that many of the advantages of face-to-face interviews also apply to telephone interviews.

Complicated or detailed schedules clearly are not well suited for telephone interviewing but, for relatively brief instruments, the telephone interview combines the economy and ease of administration of questionnaires with relatively high response rates.

☐
Research example: structured self-report

Robarge and her colleagues (1982) studied whether extremely close birth spacing was an important risk factor in child abuse. They hypothesized that if spacing were a critical variable, then twins ought to be especially at risk of being abused by their parents. To test this hypothesis, the investigators mailed questionnaires to a sample of mothers who had had a recent birth. The questionnaires included 25 questions, designed to elicit information in five areas: (1) the mother's feelings about her pregnancy and delivery; (2) the mother's perceptions of her relationship with the baby or babies and other family members; (3) the mother's perception of difficulty in caring for the infant(s); (4) the mother's evaluation of infant health; and (5) the mother's perception of family and peer support. The questionnaires were mailed to mothers whose infants were delivered in a specific hospital and whose infants were at least six months of age. To be eligible for the study, the mothers had to have given birth to twins whose birth weights exceeded 2000 grams and whose 5-minute Apgar score was at least 6. For each set of twins, two or three single birth infants (matched in terms of race, social class, maternal age, and birth date) were also included in the study. The sample consisted of mothers of 38 sets of twins and 97 comparison group mothers.

The questionnaire was pretested with a sample of similar patients to evaluate clarity, question relevancy, and ease of response. The finalized version of the questionnaire was mailed with a cover letter indicating that signature of the questionnaire was optional. However, the questionnaires were precoded so that the respondent could be identified and later matched to records on child abuse available from the county child protection agency. Eight weeks after the first mailing, a second questionnaire was mailed to those who had not responded to the first request. In a handful of cases, mothers who failed to respond but who attended the hospital clinic were personally requested to complete the questionnaire. The investigators also attempted to locate the addresses of any subjects who had moved after delivery. Thus, these investigators took steps to ensure that their questionnaires were workable with the study population and initiated several activities to increase the rate of response to their mailed questionnaires. The final response rate was 61 percent; the supplementary steps taken by the investigators (such as the second mailing) boosted their response rate by about 50 percent. The researchers were able to document response biases that underscore the difficulty with mailed questionnaires: in the entire original sample, there were nine reported cases of child abuse or neglect, but only one of the nine mothers responded to the questionnaire.

☐
Summary

A wide variety of data collection approaches are available to nurse researchers. Data collection methods vary along four important dimensions: structure, quantifiability, research obtrusiveness, and objectivity. Nurse researchers must consider these dimensions as well as the method of data collection to be used; the three principal data collection approaches are self-report, observation, and biophysiological measures. This chapter focused on self-reported data obtained through interviews or questionnaires.

The majority of nursing research studies involve the collection of self-reported data — that is, data obtained by directly questioning subjects regarding the desired information. The self-report method is strong with respect to its directness and versatility, but the major drawback is the potential for deliberate or unconscious distortions.

Self-reported data are collected by means of an oral interview or written questionnaire. Self reports vary widely in terms of their degree of structure or standardization. Tightly structured methods provide little flexibility for respondents, while unstructured methods provide both respondent and interviewer latitude in the formulation of questions and answers. Several methods of collecting unstructured or loosely structured self-report data were described: (1) *unstructured interviews,* which are conversational discussions on the topic of interest, generally in naturalistic settings; (2) *focused interviews,* in which the interviewer is guided by a broad *topic guide* of questions to be asked; (3) *focused group interviews,* which involve discussions with small groups about topics covered in a topic guide; (4) *life histories,* which encourage respondents to narrate, in chronological sequence, their life experiences vis-à-vis some theme; (5) *critical incidents,* which involves probes about the circumstances surrounding a behavior or incident that is critical to some outcome of interest; and (6) *diaries,* in which respondents are asked to maintain daily records about some aspects of their lives. Unstructured methods tend to yield data of considerable depth and are useful in gaining an understanding about little-researched phenomena. These methods are, however, time-consuming and suffer from the fact that the data are difficult to analyze and are often from small and perhaps unrepresentative samples.

Most self-report data in nursing studies are collected through structured interview schedules or questionnaires. Questions in the instrument also vary in their degree of structure. *Open-ended* questions permit respondents to reply to questions in their own words. *Closed-ended* (or *fixed-alternative*) questions offer a number of alternative responses from which respondents are instructed to make a decision.

One of the most problematic aspects of schedule construction is the wording of questions and response options. Several suggestions for question wording were offered under the general rubrics of clarity, respondents' ability to reply, biases, and the handling of sensitive or personal information. With regard to response alternatives, the major considerations dealt with were the adequate coverage of alternatives, overlapping responses, the ordering of responses, and response length.

Closed-ended questions can take a number of different forms. The simplest type of fixed alternative requires a choice between two options, such as "yes/no"; this type is referred to as *dichotomous* items. *Multiple-choice* questions provide respondents with a range of alternatives. "Cafeteria" questions are a special type of multiple choice item in which respondents are asked to select a statement that best represents their view. Respondents are sometimes requested to *rank order* a list of alternatives along a continuum from (usually) most favorable to least favorable. A *checklist* groups together several questions that require the same response format and that can be answered by placing a check in the appropriate space.

The construction of an interview schedule or questionnaire normally proceeds through a number of systematic steps. First, some preliminary decisions must be made: the researcher needs to decide whether the data will be collected via interviews or questionnaires, how structured the schedule should be, and what type of information should be collected. Next, the questions should be drafted and put into a suitable sequence, and an introduction or cover letter should be prepared. Finally, the draft of the instrument should be subjected to critical review and pretesting so that appropriate revisions can be made.

The collection of interview data depends quite heavily on the interpersonal skills of the interviewer. In order to secure participants' cooperation and trust, the interviewer must take pains to put people at ease. The interviewers should be thoroughly trained and familiar enough with the schedule so that they do not need to read questions from the schedule. When respondents give incomplete or irrelevant replies to a question, the interviewer must use a technique known as *probing* to solicit additional information.

Self-administered questionnaires can be distributed in various ways. Group administration to an intact group is the most convenient and economical procedure. The most common approach is to mail questionnaires to individuals in their home or place of work. The main problem with mailed questionnaires is that many people fail to respond to them, leading to the risk of a biased sample. A number of techniques, such as the use of *follow-up reminders,* are designed to reduce the problem of nonresponse.

Methods of direct questioning are probably indispensable as a means of collecting data on human subjects. These methods are open to a number of criticisms, particularly in regard to their validity and accuracy. On the whole, interviews suffer from fewer weaknesses than questionnaires. Questionnaires are less costly and time consuming than interviews, offer the possibility of anonymity, and run no risk of interviewer bias. However, interviews yield a higher response rate, are suitable for a wider variety of individuals, are less likely to lead to misinterpretations of questions, and provide richer data than questionnaires. The researcher with a limited budget and time constraints will have to consider these important advantages carefully.

☐ Study suggestions

1. Identify which unstructured method(s) of self-report might be appropriate for the following research problems:
   a. What are the coping strategies of parents who have lost a child through the Sudden Infant Death Syndrome?
   b. How do nurses in emergency rooms make decisions about their activities?
   c. What are the health beliefs and practices of Hmong immigrants in the U.S.?
2. Suppose you were interested in studying the experiences of young women suffering perimenstrual distress. Outline what you might do to collect data by means of a highly structured and highly unstructured self-report method.
3. Suggest ways of improving the following questions:
   a. When do you usually administer your injection of insulin?
   b. Would you disagree with the statement that nurses should not unionize?
   c. Do you agree or disagree with the following statement: Alcoholics deserve more pity than scorn and should be encouraged to seek medical rather than spiritual assistance?
   d. What is your opinion about the new health insurance bill recently passed by Congress?
   e. Don't you think that the role of nurses ought to be expanded?
4. For the study suggested in No. 2 above, develop two open-ended and two closed-ended questions.
5. The underutilization of nursing skills because of voluntary nonemployment is sometimes the cause of some concern. Suppose that you were planning to conduct a statewide study concerning the plans and intentions of nonemployed registered nurses in your state. Would you adopt an interview or questionnaire approach? How structured would your schedule be? Why?
6. Suppose that the investigation of nonemployed nurses were to be accomplished by means of a mailed questionnaire. Draft a cover letter to accompany the schedule.

☐ Suggested readings

Methodological references

Bradburn, N.M. & Sudman, S. (1979). *Improving interview method and questionnaire design.* San Francisco: Josey Bass.

Brown, J.S. *et al.* (1984). Nursing's search for Scientific knowledge. *Nursing Research, 33,* 26–32.

Denzin, N.K. (1972). *The research act* (2nd ed.). New York: McGraw-Hill.

Dillman, D. (1978). *Mail and telephone surveys: The total design method.* New York: John Wiley.

Flanagan, J.C. (1954). The critical-incident technique. *Psychological Bulletin, 51,* 327–358.

Folch-Lyon, E. and Trost, J.F. (1981). Conducting focus group sessions. *Studies in Family Planning, 12,* 443–448.

Gordon, R.L. (1980). *Interviewing: Strategy, techniques and tactics* (3rd ed.). Homewood, IL: Dorsey Press.

Institute for Social Research (1976). *Interviewer's manual, Survey Research Center* (Rev. ed.). Ann Arbor: University of Michigan.

Kornhauser, A. & Sheatsley, P.B. (1976). Questionnaire construction and interview procedure. In C. Selltiz, L.S. Wrightsman, & S.W. Cook (Eds.). *Research methods in social relations* (Appendix B). (3rd ed.). New York: Holt, Rinehart & Winston.

Leininger, M.M. (1985). Life-health-care history: Purposes, methods and techniques. In M.M. Leininger (Ed.). *Qualitative Research Methods in Nursing.* New York: Grune & Stratton.

Oppenheim, A.N. (1966). *Questionnaire design and attitude measurement.* New York: Basic Books.

Payne, S. (1951). *The art of asking questions.* Princeton, NJ: Princeton University Press.

Schuman, H. (1981). *Questions and answers in attitude surveys: Experiments in questions form, wording, and context.* New York: Academic Press.

Woods, N.F. (1981). The health diary as an instrument for nursing research. *Western Journal of Nursing Research, 3,* 76–92.

Substantive references

Unstructured methods

Bramwell, L. (1984). Use of the life history in pattern identification and health promotion. *Advances in Nursing Science, 6,* 37–44.

Boyle, J.S. (1985). Use of the family health calendar and interview schedules to study health and illness. In M.M. Leininger (Ed.). *Qualitative Research Methods in Nursing.* New York: Grune & Stratton.

Clark, N.M. & Lenburg, C.B. (1980). Knowledge-informed behavior and the nursing culture: A preliminary study. *Nursing Research, 29,* 244–249.

Kroska, R.A. (1985). Ethnographic research method: A qualitative example to discover the role of "granny" midwives in health services. In M.M. Leininger (Ed.). *Qualitative Research Methods in Nursing.* New York: Grune & Stratton.

Leininger, M.M. (1984). *Care: The essence of nursing and health.* Thorofare, NJ: Charles B. Slack.

Savitz, J. & Friedman, M.I. (1981). Diagnosing boredom and confusion. *Nursing Research, 30,* 16–20.

Tripp-Reimer, T. (1982). Barriers to health care: Variations in interpretation of Appalachian client behavior by Appalachian and non-Appalachian health professionals. *Western Journal of Nursing Research, 4,* 179–191.

Structured methods

Beyer, J.E. (1981). Interpersonal communication as perceived by nurse educators in collegial interactions. *Nursing Research, 30,* 111–117.

Broom, B.L. (1984). Consensus about the marital relationship during transition to parenthood. *Nursing Research, 33,* 223–228.

Craft, M. (1981). Preferences of hospitalized adolescents for information providers. *Nursing Research, 30,* 205–211.

La Rocco, S.A., & Polit, D.F. (1980). Women's knowledge about the menopause. *Nursing Research, 29,* 10–13.

Fuller, S.S. & Larson, S.B. (1980). Life events, emotional support, and health of older people. *Research in Nursing and Health, 3,* 81–89.

Hanson, S. (1981). Single custodial fathers and the parent-child relationship. *Nursing Research, 30,* 202–204.

Robarge, J.P., Reynolds, Z.B., & Groothuis, J.R. (1982). Increased child abuse in families with twins. *Research in Nursing and Health, 5,* 199–203.

Smith, H.L. (1981). Nurses' quality of working life in an HMO. *Nursing Research, 30,* 54–58.

Woods, N.F., Most, A., & Dery, G.K. (1982). Toward a construct of perimenstrual distress. *Research in Nursing and Health, 5,* 123–136.

Chapter 14
□
Scales and standardized self-report measures

Self-report instruments frequently include one or more psychosocial scales. A *scale* is a device designed to assign a numerical score in order to place subjects along a continuum with respect to the attribute being measured. The purpose of psychosocial scales is to quantitatively distinguish among people in terms of the degree to which they can be characterized by some personal trait. Scales have been constructed to discriminate among people with different attitudes, fears, motives, perceptions, personality traits, and needs. Just as a thermometer is a scale that permits a quantitative differentiation between two different temperatures, so a scale that measures attitudes attempts to distinguish between individuals who are more or less favorable toward some concept.

In this chapter we will examine scales that combine more than one measurement in order to form a single composite score. We will discuss a number of different scaling approaches in order to assist researchers interested in devising their own measures. In a later section of this chapter we also describe existing scales and other standardized self-report measures, together with procedures for locating them.

□
Methods of scaling psychosocial traits

Many of the sophisticated techniques developed by social psychologists for quantifying psychological states have focused on the measurement of attitudes. These techniques are versatile and have proved to be quite useful to researchers in nursing and other disciplines. Our discussion, therefore, will focus on attitude scales,* although the procedures described below have been profitably applied to other psychological domains as well.

Likert scales

The most common form of attitude measurement is the Likert scale, named after social psychologist Rensis Likert, who developed its use. A Likert scale consists of several declarative statements expressing a viewpoint on a topic. Respondents are asked to indicate the degree to which they agree or disagree with the opinion expressed in the statement. Table 14-1 presents a ten-item Likert scale for measuring attitudes toward the mentally ill. A number of features of this table will be discussed in the following paragraphs, but let us briefly consider the procedure for constructing a Likert scale.

The first step is to develop a large pool of items or statements that clearly state favorable and unfavorable attitudes toward the issue under consideration. Neutral statements or statements so extreme that virtually everyone would agree or disagree with them should be avoided. The aim is to spread out people with various attitudes along a continuum of favorability. Approximately equal numbers of positively and negatively worded statements should be chosen to avoid biasing the responses. It is also important to select only items that focus on one concept.† Usually ten to 20 items are sufficient for a Likert scale.

There are differences of opinion concerning the appropriate number of response alternatives to use. Likert used five categories of agreement-disagreement, such as are shown in Table 14-1. Some investigators prefer a seven-point scale, adding the alternatives "slightly agree" and "slightly disagree." There is also a diversity of opinion about the advisability of including an explicit category labeled "uncertain." Some researchers argue that the inclusion of this option makes the task less objectionable to people who cannot make up their minds or have no strong feelings about an issue. Others, however, feel that the use of this "undecided" category encourages fence-sitting, or the tendency to not take sides. Investigators who do not give respondents an explicit alternative for indecision or uncertainty proceed in principle as though they were working with a five- or seven-point scale, even though only four or six alternatives are given: nonresponse to a given statement is *scored* as though the neutral response were there and had been chosen.

After the items are administered to respondents, the responses to the Likert scale must be scored. Typically, the responses are scored in such a way that endorsement of positively worded statements, and nonendorsement of negatively worded statements, are assigned a higher score. Table 14-1 illustrates what this procedure involves. The first statement is phrased such that agreement is indicative of a favorable attitude toward the mentally ill. The "+" in the first column of the table signifies that this is a positively worded item. We would, therefore, assign a higher score to a person agreeing with this statement than to someone disagreeing with it. Since the scale has a maximum of five points, we would give a

---

* Among the earliest types of attitude scales were the Thurstone scales, named after the psychologist L.L. Thurstone, who developed them during the 1920s. The Thurstone approach to scaling is elaborate and time-consuming, and has fallen into relative disuse. The interested reader can learn about the Thurstone technique in Selltiz *et al.,* 1976.

† It is possible to present statements relating to two or more concepts together in the same section of a question-

naire. However, it is important that separate *scoring* be performed for the various concepts. This distinction will hopefully become clearer in the subsequent discussion on scoring.

Table 14-1

¬ example of a Likert scale to measure attitudes toward the mentally ill

				Responses†				Score	
on ¬oring*		SA	A	?	D	SD		(✓) Person 1	(X) Person 2
+	1. People who have had a mental illness can become normal, productive citizens after treatment.		✓			X		4	1
−	2. People who have been patients in mental hospitals should not be allowed to have children.		X		✓			5	3
−	3. The best way to handle patients in mental hospitals is to restrict their activity as much as possible.		X		✓			4	2
+	4. Many patients in mental hospitals develop normal, healthy relationships with staff members and other patients.			✓	X			3	2
+	5. There should be an expanded effort to get the mentally ill out of institutional settings and back into their communities.	✓				X		5	1
−	6. Since the mentally ill can't be trusted, they should be kept under constant guard.		X			✓		5	2
−	7. There is really very little that can be done to help a person once they have had a mental disorder.		X			✓		5	2
−	8. Too much money is being spent on research to help the mentally ill.	X				✓		5	1
+	9. Mental illness could happen to anyone.	✓		X				5	2
+	10. The condition of most facilities for the mentally ill is critically in need of improvement.	✓	X					5	3
								$\overline{46}$	$\overline{19}$

Total Score for Person 1 = 46
Total Score for Person 2 = 19

* The researcher would not indicate the direction of scoring on a Likert scale administered to subjects. The scoring direction is indicated in this table for illustrative purposes only.
† SA—Strongly Agree; A—Agree; ?—Uncertain; D—Disagree; SD—Strongly Disagree

"5" to someone strongly agreeing, "4" to someone agreeing, and so forth. The responses of two hypothetical respondents are shown by a check or an "X," and their score for each item is shown in the right-hand columns of the table. Person 1, who agreed with the first statement, is given a score of 4, while Person 2, who strongly disagreed, is given a score of 1.

The second item is negatively worded in that someone who agreed with the statement would tend to have a negative attitude toward the mentally ill. For this question the scoring must be *reversed,* assigning a score of "1" to those who strongly agree, and so forth. This reversal is necessary so that a high score will consistently reflect positive attitudes toward the mentally ill. When each item has been handled in this manner, a person's total score can be determined by adding together individual item scores. The arithmetic derivation of total scores in this manner has led to the term *summated rating scale,* which is sometimes used to refer to Likert scales. The total scores of the two hypothetical respondents to the items in Table 14-1 are shown at the bottom of that table. These scores reflect a considerably more positive attitude toward the mentally ill on the part of Person 1 than Person 2.

Once the scoring is completed, the investigator should make some assessment of which items should be retained in the final scale and which statements should be discarded. There are a number of sophisticated procedures for accomplishing this selection task.* The researcher who lacks statistical skills can use a few basic criteria for eliminating non-useful items. First, the responses to items should reflect some variability. That is, some people should agree while others disagree with each statement. If variability is lacking, the item is not making a contribution toward a scale designed to discriminate among individuals on the basis of their attitudes. The researcher should also check to make sure that the *a priori* decision concerning the directionality of the item is justified. People who agree with positively worded statements should tend to get higher total scores than those who disagree. If the opposite is found to be the case, the item should be reversed entirely and new total scores computed. If some items are endorsed about equally by those with high total

scores and those with low total scores, the item is probably irrelevant to the attitude being measured or ambiguously worded. Such items should be eliminated from the scale.

The fact that item responses are added together should indicate why it is inappropriate to score together responses relating to two or more different concepts. As an exaggerated example, if question 10 in Table 14-1 were replaced with the statement "Abortion should be available to all women seeking to terminate a pregnancy," it would make little sense to score the responses to this statement together with the other nine. It is unfortunately not always easy to tell which items are conceptually related. Complex topics often embrace a number of different dimensions and may need separately scored scales for each dimension. Some statistical procedures such as factor analysis are useful in this regard but cannot be treated here. Beginning researchers who lack statistical expertise should use their logical skills to attempt to build scales that are unidimensional, that is, those having items that are all measuring the same thing.

Likert scales may appear to involve a lot of work and trouble but they are actually quite powerful. The summation feature of these scales makes it possible to make very fine discriminations among individuals with different points of view. A single Likert question allows people to be put into only five (or seven) categories. A ten-item scale such as the one in Table 14-1 permits much finer gradations: from a minimum possible score of ten (10 × 1) to a maximum possible score of 50 (10 × 5).

Cumulative or Guttman scales

A second method for measuring attitudes was developed by Louis Guttman during the 1940s. Like the other scaling procedures examined, Guttman scales are made up of a set of items with which respondents are asked to ei-

---

* The advanced student who is developing a Likert scale for general use should consult a reference on psychometric procedures, such as *Psychometric Theory* by Nunnally (1978).

ther agree or disagree. To construct a cumulative scale, a number of items of increasing intensity with regard to some attitude object are developed. Typically, the number of items is quite small: four or five items are common. The statements should form a homogeneous set relating to one (and only one) variable or concept. The goal is to generate a hierarchy of items such that an individual who endorses an item of a given intensity should endorse *all* less-extreme items. The scoring procedure with cumulative scores is quite simple: a person is given a score equivalent to the number of items with which he or she agrees.

The items below form a hypothetical cumulative scale:

1. A nursing research course at the undergraduate level should be available to students.
2. Students would very likely benefit from taking an undergraduate nursing research course.
3. A nursing research course would be in the best interests of undergraduate students.
4. A course in nursing research should be mandatory for all undergraduate nursing students.

A person who *disapproved* of undergraduate nursing research courses would probably disagree with all four statements and would be assigned a score of 0. On the other hand, persons who felt that such a course is essential in the undergraduate curriculum would probably agree with all four statements and would be assigned a score of four.

Guttman developed a procedure known as *scalogram analysis* for ascertaining whether the attitude under investigation really is unidimensional (that is, measures a single concept). According to this procedure, if the cumulative scale is unidimensional, it should be possible to *reproduce* a person's response pattern based on the assigned score. For instance, in the above illustration a score of "3" should signify that the individual endorsed items one, two, and three but not four. If the score of three were attained in any other way (say, by endorsing items one, three, and four) by a large number of respondents, then the scale is probably faulty. If an investigator can reproduce exactly the specific items with which a subject agreed by knowing the respondent's total score, the scale is said to exhibit a high degree of *reproducibility*. It is rare, in practice, to find a cumulative scale that is perfectly reproducible across all subjects, but approximations are feasible. The function of scalogram analysis is to apply various statistical criteria in making a decision as to whether or not a set of items may be appropriately regarded as approximating a unidimensional scale.

The Guttman technique offers an interesting approach to the measurement of attitudes but, like other techniques, has received its share of criticisms. First of all, the Guttman procedure offers no guidance for the selection or generation of items that are likely to form a cumulative scale. Furthermore, these scales do not permit fine discriminations among individuals to be made: the scores range from a low of zero to a high equal to the number of items, which is typically small. A number of other technical weaknesses have limited the usage of cumulative scales as attitudinal measures.

Semantic differential

The semantic differential (SD) is a technique that is often used to measure attitudes. Osgood, Suci, and Tannenbaum (1957), who developed the semantic differential, describe it more generally as a technique for measuring the psychological meaning of concepts or objects to an individual.

The building blocks of semantic differentials are *graphic rating scales*. With graphic rating scales respondents are asked to give a judgment of something along an ordered dimension. The task is to place a check at the appropriate point along the line that extends from one extreme of the characteristic or dimension in question to the other extreme. Graphic rating scales are *bipolar* in nature because they specify the two opposite ends of a continuum. Here is an example of an item that might be used in a questionnaire with discharged patients:

How would you rate the overall quality of your nursing care?
(Place a check in the appropriate space on the scale.)

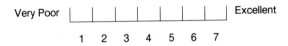

The semantic differential consists of a set of graphic rating scales. The respondent is asked to rate a given concept (for example, primary care nursing, integrated curriculum, four-day work schedule) on a series of bipolar rating scales. The scales consist of bipolar adjectives such as good-bad, important-unimportant, strong-weak, beautiful-ugly, and so forth. An example of the format for a complete semantic differential is shown in Figure 14.1. Seven scale points are most commonly used, as in this example, but five or nine might also be employed.

The semantic differential has the advantage of being highly flexible and easy to construct. The concept being rated can be virtually anything—a person, place, situation, abstract idea, controversial issue, and so forth. Furthermore, the concept can be a single word, a phrase, a sentence, or even a picture or sketch. Typically, several concepts are included on the same schedule so that comparisons can be made (if the same bipolar scales are used) across concepts. For instance, a researcher may be interested in contrasting the reactions of respondents to the concepts male nurse, female nurse, male physician, and female physician.

The researcher also has considerable freedom in constructing bipolar scales. However, two considerations should guide the selection of the adjectives. First, the adjectives should be appropriate for the concepts being used and for the information being sought. The addition of the adjective pair tall-short in Figure 14-1 would add little understanding of how people react to the role of nurse practitioners. When the scales are used to rate two or more concepts, adjective pairs that were considered relevant for one concept may be inappropriate for another and may need to be discarded or replaced.

The second consideration in the selection of adjective pairs is the extent to which the adjectives are measuring the same dimension or aspect of the concept. Osgood and his colleagues, through extensive research with semantic differential scales, have found that adjective pairs tend to cluster along three principal and independent dimensions which they have labeled Evaluation, Potency, and Activity. The most important group of adjectives are those that are Evaluative, such as valuable-worthless, good-bad, fair-unfair, and so forth. Potency adjectives include strong-weak and large-small, and examples of Activity adjectives are active-passive or fast-slow. The reason these three dimensions need to be considered separately is that a person's evaluative rating of a concept (such as a nurse practitioner) is independent of the activity or potency ratings of that concept. Two persons who associate high levels of activity with the concept of nurse practitioner might have divergent views with regard to how valuable they perceive the role to be. The researcher must decide whether to represent all three of these dimensions or whether only one or two are needed. Each dimension or aspect must be scored separately.

NURSE PRACTITIONERS

competent	7*	6	5	4	3	2	1		incompetent
worthless	1	2	3	4	5	6	7		valuable
important									unimportant
pleasant									unpleasant
bad									good
cold									warm
responsible									irresponsible
successful									unsuccessful

*The score values would not be printed on the form administered to actual subjects. The numbers are presented here solely for the purpose of illustrating how semantic differentials are scored.

Figure 14-1. Example of a semantic differential.

The scoring procedure for semantic differential responses is essentially the same as for Likert scales. Scores from one to seven are assigned to each bipolar scale response. Usually, the positively-worded adjective is associated with higher scores, so that a check to the extreme left for the competent-incompetent combination in Figure 14-1 would be scored "7," and a check to the extreme right would be scored a "1." Note that in this figure the direction of the adjective pairs has been randomly reversed to prevent response biases. Thus, for the next set of adjectives, worthless-valuable, checks on the extreme *right* would be scored as "7." After proceeding in this fashion, subgroups of scale responses associated with the same dimension can be summed to yield a total score. Potentially, then, each concept could provide three scores (Evaluation, Potency, and Activity) if adjective pairs representing these three dimensions are included. In this example, only evaluative adjectives are listed, so that all scale responses could be added together.

Semantic differentials produce a large quantity of information with relatively little effort. The data from semantic differentials can be analyzed in a wide variety of ways. Different groups of respondents (for example, males versus females) can be compared in terms of their ratings of a concept. The ratings of two or more different concepts also can be compared. Various sophisticated analytic techniques have also been devised expressly for handling semantic differential data. While the semantic differential is versatile, respondents can become confused or bored with these questions and may manifest their discomfort by placing all of their checks in the middle scale position. Clear instructions are essential and an explicit example may be required.

Other scaling approaches

The techniques described above are by far the most common methods of measuring attitudes currently in use. Other approaches do exist, however. The advanced student may want to refer to the references at the end of this chapter for a more extended discussion of advanced scaling procedures, such as ratio scaling, unfolding technique, multidimensional scaling, and multiple scalogram analysis.

The problem of response sets

Scaling procedures are subject to several common problems, the most troublesome of which is referred to as *response sets*. The scale scores that represent individuals' attitudes toward some phenomenon are seldom totally accurate and pure measures of the critical variable. A number of irrelevant factors are also being "measured" at the same time. Since these response-set factors can sometimes influence or bias resposes to a considerable degree, investigators who construct scales must attempt to eliminate them or reduce their impact.

One influence on responses is a person's tendency to present a favorable image of himself or herself. The *social desirability* response set refers to the tendency of some individuals to misrepresent their attitudes by giving answers that are consistent with prevailing social mores. This problem is a thorny one and often difficult to combat. Subtle, indirect, and delicately worded questioning sometimes can help to alleviate this response bias. The creation of a permissive atmosphere and provisions for respondent anonymity also encourage frankness.

Extreme responses constitute a second type of response set. This biasing factor results from the fact that some individuals consistently express their attitudes in terms of extreme response alternatives (e.g., "strongly agree"), while others characteristically endorse middle-range alternatives. This response style is a distorting influence in that extreme responses may not necessarily signify the most intense attitude toward the phenomenon under investigation. There appears to be little that a researcher can do to counteract this bias, although there are procedures for detecting its existence. There is some evidence that the distortion introduced by the extreme-response set is not powerful.

Some people have been found to agree with statements regardless of the content. In the research literature, these people are sometimes referred to as "yea-sayers"; the bias is known as the *acquiescence response set*. A less common problem is the opposite tendency for other individuals, called "nay-sayers," to disagree with statements independently of the question content. While there apparently are some people for whom such tendencies are stable and enduring personality characteristics, acquiescence and its opposite counterpart can often be avoided or minimized by the simple strategy of *counterbalancing* positively and negatively worded statements.

The effects of response biases should not be exaggerated, but it is important that researchers who are constructing a scale give these issues some thought. If the investigator is developing a scale for general use by other researchers, it is recommended that evidence be gathered demonstrating that the scale is sufficiently free from the influence of response sets to measure the critical variable.

☐
Existing scales and measures

The preceding section described some of the principles underlying the construction of scales for measuring people's attitudes. In an emerging field like nursing research, investigators will often find that no suitable scale exists to measure the concepts in which they are interested or that existing scales are in need of adaptation or improvement. In such a case, the researcher may be forced to develop a new scale or instrument. Nevertheless, it should be pointed out that the design and testing of an accurate and valid measure of personal traits or states is a difficult and time-consuming activity. Beginning researchers, in particular, should be careful to exhaust all other possibilities before developing a new instrument. There are thousands upon thousands of existing scales and standardized instruments already in existence, many of which have documentation concerning their accuracy, validity, response biases, and usages. This section will describe general classes of psychosocial measures and provide some clues concerning where to find them.

Attitude scales

Since we have already treated attitude scales extensively in the preceding section, we only need mention here a few sources for locating existing instruments. For attitudinal variables that are strictly related to nursing, the researcher should consult the various nursing indexes described in Chapter 5 or the books discussed in the concluding section of this chapter.

There are a number of more general concepts in which nurses share an interest with researchers from other disciplines. Examples of this second type of variable include attitudes toward death or attitudes toward alcoholics. Both the nursing and non-nursing indexes and abstracting services should be consulted for references to studies that have developed scales to measure such variables. *Psychological Abstracts* is particularly useful, since it has separate sections entitled ''Attitude Measurement'' and ''Attitude Measures.'' In addition, several useful anthologies of attitude scales have been prepared, including Robinson and Shaver's (1973) *Measures of Social Psychological Attitudes* and Shaw and Wright's (1967) *Scales for the Measurement of Attitudes.* These reference books present the actual items appearing on scales, together with a critique of the scale's technical adequacy. Another useful reference is Beere's (1979) *Women and Women's Issues: A Handbook of Tests and Measures.* Scales measuring the following kinds of attitudes are included in these sources: attitudes toward birth control, socialized medicine, death, old people, blind-

ness, mentally retarded persons, sexuality, abortion, and traditional sex roles.

Personality measures

For the purpose of our present discussion we will define personality as the relatively enduring attributes of individuals that dispose them to respond in a certain way to their environment. A number of nursing research studies have employed an instrument to assess the personality characteristics of such groups as practicing nurses, nursing faculty members, nursing students, and clients. For example, Meleis and Dagenais (1981) compared graduates of diploma, associate degree, and baccalaureate degree programs with regard to their sex-role identity using the Omnibus Personality Inventory.

There are literally hundreds of personality measures in existence. Personality tests differ in their comprehensiveness (e.g., measurement of one versus multiple personality dimensions) and structure. The majority of instruments that nurse researchers have used are of the type known as a personality *inventory.* In an inventory respondents are typically presented with a number of descriptive statements that they rate as either characteristic or uncharacteristic of them. For example, a tense individual would be likely to answer ''yes'' or ''agree'' to a statement such as ''I often worry about what the future holds for me.'' A person's score is usually calculated by summing the number of affirmative responses to statements relating to a trait. Major tests of this type include the *California Psychological Inventory,* the *Sixteen Personality Factor Questionnaire,* and *Edwards Personal Preference Inventory.*

Most of the tests we have discussed so far are intended to measure traits of psychologically healthy, normal individuals, but there are also several clinically oriented instruments to measure different forms of psychopathology, such as paranoia, schizophrenia, and the like. The most commonly used measure of psychopathology is the *Minnesota Multiphasic Personality Inventory.*

Several references on psychological measurements offer a thorough discussion and explicit information on available measures. Among these sources are Anastasi's (1982) fifth edition of *Psychological Testing,* a textbook on various types of available tools; Cattell and Warburton's (1967) *Objective Personality and Motivation Tests;* Chun, Cobb, and French's (1975) *Measures for Psychological Assessment,* which indexes tests in terms of the traits they measure; Buros' (1974) *Tests in Print,* a guide to published commerical tests; and Buros' *Mental Measurement Yearbooks,* which describe and review available psychological tests. Additionally, information on many standardized testing instruments can be retrieved through a computerized literature search of the data base called *Mental Measurement Yearbook,* produced by the Buros Institute of Mental Measurements.

Intelligence, developmental, and achievement tests

Occasionally nurse researchers are interested in assessing the cognitive abilities and attainments of a group of subjects. For example, Alichnie and Bellucci (1981) used several ability measures, such as SAT scores and scores on the Aptitude Test for Nursing, to predict achievement in a baccalaureate nursing program.

Intelligence tests represent attempts to evaluate the general, global ability of individuals to perceive relationships and solve problems. Of the many such tests available, some have been developed for individual administration while others have been designed for group use. There are also a number of developmental tests for measuring the cognitive and motor development in young preschool children, such as the Denver Developmental

Screening Test and Bayley's Scale of Infant Development. Good sources for learning more about ability and developmental tests are the Buros' books and the Anastasi text listed in the reference section at the end of this chapter.

Nurse researchers are sometimes interested in tests of achievement. Achievement tests are designed to measure the subject's present level of proficiency or mastery of various areas of knowledge. Since both practicing nurses and nurse educators are involved, to differing degrees, in teaching, the measurement of instructional effectiveness is an area in which some nurse researchers are interested. Achievement tests are either standardized or specially constructed. Standardized tests are instruments that have been carefully developed and tested, and that normally cover broad achievement objectives. The test constructors of such tests establish *norms,* which make possible the comparison of individuals and groups with a reference group. The NLN Achievement Test is an example of a standardized test. For specific learning objectives, the researcher may be forced to construct a new test. The development of an achievement test that is objective, accurate, and valid is a laborious task. Ebel's (1986) book entitled *Essentials of Educational Measurement* is a useful reference for those readers interested in achievement test construction.

Other types of psychosocial measures

In addition to measures of attitudes, personality, and cognitive functioning, there are numerous tests to measure other aspects of a person's psychosocial and health status. It is beyond the scope of this book to identify all psychosocial attributes that have attracted the interest of nurse researchers, but some attributes have received repeated attention because of their relevance to clinical nursing practice. Table 14-2 lists 15 variables that were used in at least five nursing research studies

Table 14-2
Examples of concepts frequently measured in nursing studies with psychosocial scales

Concept	Research Example Reference	Instrument Used
Anxiety	Levesque, L. *et al.,* 1984	State-Trait Anxiety Inventory
	Rudy & Estok, 1983	Zuckerman's General Anxiety Scale
Body image	Strang & Sullivan, 1985	Attitude Toward Body Image Scale
	Krouse & Krouse, 1982	Body Image Questionnaire
Coping	Chiriboga *et al.,* 1983	Lazarus Ways of Coping Scale
	Ventura, 1982	Family Coping Inventory
Depression	Newman & Gaudiano, 1984	Beck Depression Inventory
	Tilden, 1984	Lubin Depression Adjective Checklist
	Murphy, 1984	Hopkins Symptom Checklist
Health locus of control	Itano *et al.,* 1983	Health Locus of Control Scale
	Thomas & Hooper, 1983	Multidimensional Health Locus of Control Scale
Job satisfaction	Duxbury *et al.,* 1984	Minnesota Satisfaction Questionnaire
	Riesch, 1984	Job Satisfaction Index
Locus of control	Thomas & Hooper, 1983	Rotter I-E Scale
	LaMontagne, 1984	Nowicki-Strickland Locus of Control Scale for Children
Menstrual distress	Jordan & Meckler, 1982	Moos Menstrual Distress Questionnaire
	O'Rourke, 1983	Moos Menstrual Distress Questionnaire
Mood states	Sime & Libera, 1985	Profile of Mood States
	Johnson *et al,* 1985	Profile of Mood States
Morale/life satisfaction	Ryden, 1984	Philadelphia Geriatric Center Morale Scale
	Burckhardt, 1985	Life Satisfaction Index
Pain	Laborde & Powers, 1985	McGill Pain Questionnaire
	Burckhardt, 1985	McGill Pain Questionnaire
Parent-child relations	Hanson, 1981	Parent-Child Interaction Rating Scale
	Ellison, 1983	Family Peer Relationship Questionnaire
Self-esteem	Rudy & Estok, 1983	Rosenberg Self Esteem Scale
	Riffee, 1981	Coopersmith Self Esteem Inventory
Social support	Brandt, 1984	Personal Resource Questionnaire
	Tilden, 1984	Social Support Questionnaire
	Thomas & Hooper, 1983	Interview for Social Interaction
Stress	Owen & Damron, 1984	Holmes-Rahe Life Events Inventory
	VanOs, 1985	Schedule of Recent Experiences
	Tilden, 1984	Sarason's Life Experiences Survey

published in the 1980s. The middle column provides references for some of the nursing studies that used an existing measure of the variable. The methodological references at the end of this chapter should be useful in locating measures of other psychosocial variables not discussed in this chapter.

Instruments about nursing care and patient functioning

Nurse researchers have made tremendous strides over the past decade in developing instruments to evaluate nursing behaviors and competencies, as well as the behaviors, experiences, and affective states of people under their care. An excellent reference for locating such measures is the book by Waltz, Strickland, and Lenz (1984) entitled *Measurement in Nursing Research.* The instruments that have been developed by nurse researchers include highly structured scales that yield a quantified score as well as more loosely structured protocols for diagnosis and decision-making. An important advantage of using or adapting a previously developed measure is

Table 14-3
Self-report instruments for measuring nursing variables

Name of Instrument	Concept Measured	Source
Hospital Stress Rating Scale	Patients' levels of stress	Volicer & Bohannon, 1975
Health Behavior Choice Scale	Patients' practice of health behaviors	Laffrey, 1985
Chronicity Impact and Coping Questionnaire	Parents' coping during child's long-term illness	Hymovich, 1984
Uncertainty in Illness Scale	Adults' uncertainty regarding their illness	Mishel, 1981
Risser Patient Satisfaction Scale	Patients' satisfaction with primary nursing	Risser, 1975
Patient Satisfaction Instrument	Patients' satisfaction with nursing care	Hinshaw & Atwood, 1982
Values in the Choice of Treatment Inventory	Predominant values in medical/surgical conditions	Gortner *et al.,* 1984
Health Self-Determinism Index	Motivation in health behavior	Cox, 1985
Judgments About Nursing Decisions	Nursing actions in ethical dilemmas	Ketefian, 1981
Nurse's Self-Description Form	Self-assessed nursing performance	Dagenais & Meleis, 1982
Bereavement Health Assessment Scale	Changes in health after a major loss	Miles, 1985
Clinical Skills Inventory	Self-assessed nursing skills	Benner & Benner, 1979
Collaborative Practice Scales	Nurse/physician interaction in patient care	Weiss & Davis, 1985
Patient Recovery Index	Patients' self-assessment of recovery from surgery	Wolfer, 1973

(in addition to ease and efficiency) that it facilitates the comparison of findings among studies and creates a greater potential for knowledge accumulation. While we cannot list the many self-report instruments that have been developed specifically by or for nurses, Table 14-3 does provide some examples. This table gives the name of the instrument, the concepts it is designed to measure, and the source for the full description of the instrument.

☐
Research example

Andreoli (1981) was interested in determining whether hypertensive patients who practiced compliance with a prescribed therapy were different than those who did not in terms of their self-concepts and health beliefs. Her aim was to try to identify variables that could be used to predict noncompliance, so that ap-

propriate interventions could be developed. The research sample for this study consisted of 71 male hypertensive patients enrolled in a VA clinic.

Two instruments were administered to the subjects. The first was a standardized measure of self-concept, the Tennessee Self-Concept Scale. This scale consists of 100 self-descriptive statements, which an individual rates on a five-point scale ranging from completely false to completely true.

Andreoli found no acceptable measure of health beliefs to use in her study. Therefore, she developed a 15-item Likert scale that she referred to as the Health Beliefs Questionnaire (HBQ). The HBQ consists of perceptual statements on which the respondent is asked to give a self-rating in three categories of health belief: susceptibility to hypertension, severity of hypertension, and benefits of regimen compliance. Each category consisted of five items, balanced in terms of the positive and negative wording within each category. Andreoli scored the HBQ to yield a subscore for each of the three categories and a total health belief score.

Findings from this research failed to confirm Andreoli's hypotheses. The compliers and noncompliers had similar scores on the self-concept and health belief measures.

□
Summary

Scales are tools for quantitatively measuring the degree to which individuals possess or are characterized by target traits or attributes. Psychosocial scaling procedures have been most fully developed in connection with the measurement of attitudes.

The most common form of attitude measure is the *Likert scale,* or *summated rating scale.* Likert scales present the respondent with a series of items (normally between 10 and 20) that are worded either favorably or unfavorably toward some phenomenon. Respondents are asked to indicate their degree of agreement or disagreement with each statement. Five or seven response alternatives are typically used. The responses can then be combined to form a composite score, the aim of which is to signify the individual's position, relative to that of others, on the attitudinal favorability/unfavorability continuum. A total score is derived by the summation of scores assigned to all items, which in turn are scored according to the direction of favorability expressed.

Cumulative scales or *Guttman scales* are composed, once again, of attitudinal statements with which respondents must agree or disagree. This type of scale employs a relatively small number of positively *or* negatively worded items that are graduated in terms of the intensity expressed. The aim is to select statements such that a person endorsing an item of a given intensity will also agree with all items of a lesser intensity. A person's score is

equal to the total number of items endorsed. *Scalogram analysis* is applied to Guttman scales as a method of ascertaining their adequacy and unidimensionality. The analysis makes use of the concept of *reproducibility,* which is the degree to which knowledge of a person's score allows the investigator to designate which specific statements were approved.

The *semantic differential* is a procedure for measuring the meaning of concepts to individuals and has been used widely in the area of attitude measurement. The technique consists of a series of *graphic rating scales* on which respondents are asked to indicate their reaction toward some phenomenon. Normally five to fifteen bipolar adjectival scales are included for each concept. The adjectives may be measuring an Evaluation (good/bad), Activity (active/passive), or Potency (strong/weak) dimension. Scoring of the semantic differential proceeds in a fashion similar to that of Likert scales.

The researcher interested in constructing new psychological measures must contend with a number of difficulties, some of which are referred to as *response set* biases. This problem concerns the tendency of certain individuals to respond to items in characteristic ways, independently of the item's content. The *social desirability* response set is a bias stemming from a person's desire to appear in a favorable light. The *extreme-response* set results when persons characteristically endorse extreme response alternatives. A third type of response bias is known as *acquiescence,* which designates an individual's tendency to agree with statements regardless of their content. A converse problem arises less frequently when a person disagrees with most statements.

The researcher should give sufficient consideration to existing measures before embarking on a project to construct new scales. The development of good instruments is both arduous and time consuming. Since literally thousands of existing measures are available, some effort should be made to identify potentially useful instruments that tap the variables of interest. Scales and tests that measure attitudes, personality traits, abilities, development, achievement, psychological states, health behaviors, and nursing activities were discussed and sources for their location were identified in this chapter.

□
Study suggestions

1. Below are twenty attitudinal statements that relate to attitudes toward menopause. Respond to these 20 statements, and then score yourself in terms of overall favorability toward the menopause.

   1. Menopause is simply a normal period of biological development.
   2. I look forward to menopause as a relief from the nuisance of menstruation.
   3. I resent the thought of menopause.
   4. Menopause to me means the opportunity for greater freedom of sexual expression.
   5. I am ashamed to talk about the subject of menopause.
   6. I am indifferent to the thought of menopause.
   7. The idea of menopause frightens me a little.
   8. I dread the loss of my ability to reproduce.
   9. Menstruation makes me feel womanly, and I will regret its cessation.
   10. I am annoyed that menopause is a process over which I have no control.
   11. I am frightened by stories I have heard about the menopause.
   12. When I reach the menopause, I will consider myself an old woman.
   13. Menopause is a process about which I know very little.
   14. Menopause will give me a feeling of kinship with women of my age group.
   15. The thought of menopause revolts me.
   16. I am sure that when I reach the menopause I will not feel abnormal or peculiar.
   17. To me, menopause means that I will have reached a new level of maturity.
   18. I will want a lot of sympathy during the menopause.
   19. My life will probably change very little, if at all, because of menopause.
   20. I can talk freely about menopause with my friends or family.

2. From the twenty statements listed above, select four that you feel might constitute a Guttman scale. Ask a friend to agree or disagree with the items. Are you able to perfectly reproduce your friend's score?
3. List ten pairs of bipolar adjectives that would be appropriate for rating *all* of the following concepts for a semantic differential scale: cigarettes, alcohol, marijuana, heroin.
4. Using the references cited at the end of this chapter, find the names of four or five instruments that measure a person's level of marital adjustment.
5. Suppose that you were interested in studying the attitudes of men toward witnessing the birth of their children in a hospital delivery room. Develop five positively worded and five negatively worded statements that could be used in constructing a Likert scale for such a study.

□
Suggested readings

Methodological references

Anastasi, A. (1982). *Psychological testing* (5th ed.). New York: Macmillan.
Batey, M.V. (1979). Acquiescent response set: A

source of measurement error. *Western Journal of Nursing Research, 1,* 247–249.

Beere, C.A. (1979). *Women and women's issues: A handbook of tests and measures.* San Francisco: Josey Bass.

Buros, O.K. (Ed.). (1978). *The eighth mental measurements yearbook.* Hyland Park, N.J.: Gryphon Press.

Buros, O.K. (1974). *Tests in print II.* Highland Park, N.J.: Gryphon Press.

Cattell, J.B., & Warburton, F.W. (1967). *Objective personality and motivation tests.* Chicago: University of Illinois Press.

Chun, K.T., Cobb, S., & French, J.R.P., Jr. (1975). *Measures for psychological assessment.* Ann Arbor: Survey Research Center.

Davison, M.L. (1983). *Multidimensional scaling.* New York: John Wiley & Sons.

Ebel, R. (1986). *Essentials of educational measurements* (4th ed.). Englewood Cliffs, N.J.: Prentice-Hall.

Edwards, A.L. (1982). *Techniques of attitude scale construction.* New York: Irvington.

Karoly, P. (1984). *Measurement strategies in health psychology.* New York: John Wiley & Sons.

Nunnally, J.C. (1978). *Psychometric theory.* New York: McGraw-Hill.

Osgood, C.E., Suci, G.J., & Tannenbaum, P.H. (1957). *The measurement of meaning.* Urbana, Ill.: University of Illinois Press.

Reeder, L.G., *et al.* (1976). *Handbook of scales and indices of health behavior.* Pacific Palisades, CA.: Goodyear.

Robinson, J.P., & Shaver, P.R. (1973). *Measures of social psychological attitudes* (Rev. ed.). Ann Arbor: University of Michigan.

Selltiz, C., Wrightsman, L.S., & Cook, S.W. (1976). *Research methods in social relations* (3rd ed.) New York: Holt, Rinehart & Winston (Chapter 12).

Shaw, M.E., & Wright, J.M. (1967). *Scales for the measurement of attitudes.* New York: McGraw-Hill.

Waltz, C.F., Strickland, O.L. & Lenz, E.R. (1984). *Measurement in nursing research.* Philadelphia: F.A. Davis.

Ward, M.J. & Felter, M.E. (1979). *Instruments for use in nursing education research.* Boulder, CO:

Western Interstate Commission for Higher Education.

Ward, M.J., & Lindeman, C.A. (Eds.). (1978). *Instruments for measuring nursing practice and other health variables.* Washington: Government Printing Office.

Substantive references

Studies with original scales

Andreoli, K.G. (1981). Self-concept and health beliefs in compliant and noncompliant hypertensive patients. *Nursing Research, 30,* 323–328 (Likert scale).

Godschalx, S.M. (1984). Effect of a mental health educational program upon police officers. *Research in Nursing and Health, 7,* 111–117 (Semantic differential).

Hott, J.R. (1980). Best laid plans: Pre- and post-partum comparison of self and spouse in primiparous Lamaze couples who deliver and those who do not. *Nursing Research, 29,* 20–27. (Semantic differential).

Jacobson, S.F. (1984). A semantic differential for external comparison of conceptual nursing models. *Advances in Nursing Science, 6,* 58–70 (Semantic differential).

Mishel, M.H. (1981). The measurement of uncertainty in illness. *Nursing Research, 30,* 258–263 (Likert scale).

Morgan, B.S. (1984). A semantic differential measure of attitudes toward black American patients. *Research in Nursing and Health, 7,* 155–162 (Semantic differential).

Schmidt, A. (1981). Predicting nurses' charting behavior based on Fishbein's model. *Nursing Research, 30,* 118. (Semantic differential).

Williams, R.A. & Wikolaisen, S.M. (1982). Sudden Infant Death Syndrome: Parents' perceptions and responses to the loss of their infant. *Research in Nursing and Health, 5,* 55–61 (Likert scale).

Studies using existing scales

Alichnie, M.C. & Bellucci, J.T. (1981). Prediction of freshman students' success in a Baccalaureate nursing program. *Nursing Research, 30,* 49–53.

Brandt, P.A. (1984). Stress-buffering effects of social support on maternal discipline. *Nursing Research, 33,* 229–234.

Burckhardt, C.S. (1985). The impact of arthritis on quality of life. *Nursing Research, 34,* 11–16.

Chiriboga, D.A., Jenkins, G. & Bailey, J. (1983). Stress and coping hospice nurses: Test of an analytic model. *Nursing Research, 32,* 294–299.

Duxbury, M.L., *et al.* (1984). Head nurse leadership style with staff nurse burnout and job satisfaction in neonatal intensive care units. *Nursing Research, 33,* 97–101.

Ellison, E.S. (1983). Parental support and school-aged children. *Western Journal of Nursing Research, 5,* 145–153.

Hanson, S. (1981). Single custodial fathers and the parent-child relationship. *Nursing Research, 30,* 202–204.

Itano, J. *et al.* (1983). Compliance of cancer patients to therapy. *Western Journal of Nursing Research, 5,* 5–16.

Johnson, J.E., Christman, N.J. & Stitt, C. (1985). Personal control interventions. *Research in Nursing and Health, 8,* 131–145.

Jordan, J. & Meckler, J.R. (1982). The relationship between life change events, social supports, and dysmenorrhea. *Research in Nursing and Health, 5,* 73–79.

Krouse, H.J. & Krouse, J.H. (1982). Cancer as crisis: The critical elements of adjustment. *Nursing Research, 31,* 96–101.

Laborde, J.M. & Powers, M.J. (1985). Life satisfaction, health control orientation, and illness-related factors in persons with osteoarthritis. *Research in Nursing and Health, 8,* 183–190.

LaMontagne, L.L. (1984). Children's locus of control beliefs as predictors of preoperative coping behavior. *Nursing Research, 33,* 76–79.

Levesque, L. *et al.* (1984). Evaluation of a presurgical group program given at two different times. *Research in Nursing and Health, 7,* 227–236.

Meleis, A.I., & Dagenais, F. (1981). Sex-role identity and perception of professional self in graduates of three nursing programs. *Nursing Research, 30,* 162–167.

Murphy, S.A. (1984). Stress levels and health status of victims of a natural disaster. *Research in Nursing and Health, 7,* 205–215.

Newman, M.A. & Gaudiano, T.K. (1984). Depression as an explanation for decreased subjective time in the elderly. *Nursing Research, 33,* 137–139.

O'Rourke, M.W. (1983). Subjective appraisal of psychological well-being and self-reports of menstrual and non-menstrual symptomatology in employed women. *Nursing Research, 32,* 288–292.

Owen, B.D. & Damron, C.F. (1984). Personal characteristics and back injury among hospital nursing personnel. *Research in Nursing and Health, 7,* 305–313.

Riesch, S.K. (1984). Occupational commitment and the quality of maternal-infant interaction. *Research in Nursing and Health, 7,* 295–303.

Riffee, D.M. (1981). Self-esteem changes in hospitalized school-age children. *Nursing Research, 30,* 94–97.

Rudy, E.B. & Estok, P.J. (1983). Intensity of jogging: Its relationship to selected physical and psychosocial variables in women. *Western Journal of Nursing Research, 5,* 325–336.

Ryden, M.B. (1984). Morale and perceived control in institutionalized elderly. *Nursing Research, 33,* 130–136.

Sime, A.M. & Libera, M.B. (1985). Sensation information, self-instruction and responses to dental surgery. *Research in Nursing and Health, 8,* 41–47.

Strang, V.R. & Sullivan, P.L. (1985). Body image attitudes during pregnancy and the postpartum period. *Journal of Obstetric, Gynecologic, and Neonatal Nursing, 14,* 332–337.

Thomas, P.D. & Hooper, E. M. (1983). Healthy elderly: Social bonds and locus of control. *Research in Nursing and Health, 6,* 11–16.

Tilden, V.P. (1984). The relation of selected psychosocial variables to single status of adult women during pregnancy, *Nursing Research, 33,* 102–106.

VanOs, D.K. *et al.* (1985). Life stress and cystic fibrosis. *Western Journal of Nursing Research, 7,* 301–315.

Ventura, J.N. (1982). Parent coping behaviors, parent functioning, and infant temperament characteristics. *Nursing Research, 31,* 269–273.

References for nursing instruments

Benner, P. & Benner, R. (1979). *The new nurse's work entry.* New York: Tiresias Press.

Cox, C.L. (1985). The Health Self-Determinism Index. *Nursing Research, 34,* 177–183.

Dagenais, F. & Meleis, A.I. (1982). Professionalism, work ethic and empathy in nursing. *Western Journal of Nursing Research, 4,* 407–422.

Gortner, S.R., Hudes, M. & Zyzanski, S.J. (1984). Appraisal of values in the choice of treatment. *Nursing Research, 33,* 319–324.

Hinshaw, A.S. & Atwood, J.R. (1982). A Patient Satisfaction Instrument: Precision by replication. *Nursing Research, 31,* 170–175.

Hymovich, D.P. (1984). Development of the Chronicity Impact and Coping Instrument: Parent questionnaire (CICI: PQ). *Nursing Research, 33,* 218–222.

Ketefian, S. (1981). Moral reasoning and moral behavior among selected groups of practicing nurses. *Nursing Research, 30,* 171–176.

Laffrey, S.C. (1985). Health behavior choices as related to self-actualization and health conception. *Western Journal of Nursing Research, 7,* 279–300.

Miles, M.S. (1985). Emotional symptoms and physical health in bereaved parents. *Nursing Research, 34,* 76–81.

Mishel, M. (1981). The measurement of uncertainty in illness. *Nursing Research, 30,* 258–263.

Risser, N. (1975). Development of an instrument to measure patient satisfaction with nurses and nursing care in primary care settings. *Nursing Research, 24,* 45–52.

Volicer, B.J. & Bohannon, M.W. (1975). A hospital stress rating scale. *Nursing Research, 24,* 352–359.

Weiss, S.J. & Davis, H.P. (1985). Validity and reliability of the Collaborative Practice Scales. *Nursing Research, 34,* 299–305.

Wolfer, J.A. (1973). Definition and assessment of surgical patients' welfare and recovery. *Nursing Research, 22,* 394–401.

Chapter 15
☐
Observational methods

Observational methods are the methodological backbone in a number of scientific disciplines, such as in earth sciences, ethnology, anthropology, and zoology. Many kinds of information required by nurse researchers as evidence of nursing effectiveness or as clues to improving nursing practices can be obtained through direct observation. Suppose, for instance, we were interested in studying mental patients' methods of defending their personal territory; or children's reactions to the removal of a leg cast; or a patient's mode of emergence from anesthesia. These data could all be collected by the direct observation of the relevant behaviors.

Scientific observation involves the systematic selection, observation, and recording of behaviors and settings relevant to a problem under investigation. Like self-report methods, observational methods can vary in terms of structure, from highly unstructured to highly structured approaches. Both structured and unstructured methods are discussed in this chapter. First, however, we present an overview of some general issues.

☐
Selection of phenomena for observation

When a nurse researcher observes an event — let us say a nurse administering an injection to a patient — he or she must have a clear idea about what is to be observed. A single incidence or occurrence encompasses a variety of aspects and dimensions. The researcher cannot absorb and record an infinite number of details and must, therefore, have some guidelines specifying the manner in which the observations are to be focused or edited.

The choice of the phenomena to be observed will be guided by the problem being investigated, but even after the problem area is defined there is a need for further specification and selection. Suppose we were interested in understanding how the educational preparation of nurses was related to their empathic behavior in administering injections to patients. We have now focused our attention on a specific dimension of nursing behavior, but how will we define and observe "empathic behavior?" We might select a number of alternatives, such as the frequency, content, or tone of the nurses' statements to the patients, or the nurses' facial expressions as they prepare and administer the injections, or their frequency and manner of touching the patients. Any of these behaviors, as well as several others, could be used as an observational measure of empathy among nurses. In this section we will try to demonstrate the versatility of observational methods by pointing out some considerations for the selection of observable phenomena.

Phenomena amenable to observations

In nursing research, observational records usually are made of either human behaviors or the characteristics of individuals, events, environments, or objects. The following list of observable phenomena is meant to be suggestive rather than exhaustive.

1. *Characteristics and Conditions of Individuals.* A broad variety of information about people's attributes and states can be gathered by direct observation. We refer not only to relatively enduring traits of individuals, such as their physical appearance, but also to more temporary conditions, such as physiological symptoms that are amenable to observation. We include here physiological conditions that can be observed either directly through the senses, or aided by observational apparatus, such as by means of an x-ray. To illustrate this class of observable phenomena, the following could be used as dependent or independent variables in a nursing research investigation: the sleep or wake state of patients, the presence of edema in congestive heart failure, turgor of the skin in dehydration, the manifestation of decubitus ulcers, alopecia during cancer chemotherapy, or symptoms of infusion phlebitis in hospitalized patients.

2. *Verbal Communication Behaviors.* One of the most commonly observed types of human behavior is linguistic behavior. The content and structure of people's conversations are readily observable, easy to record, and, thus, are an obvious source of data. Among the kinds of verbal communications that a nurse researcher might be interested in observing are: information-giving of nurses to patients; nurses' conversations with grieving relatives; exchange of information among nurses at change of shift report; the dialogue of residents in a nursing home; and conversations in a rural public health clinic.

3. *Nonverbal Communication Behaviors.* People communicate their fears, wants, and emotions in many ways other than just with words. For nursing researchers, nonverbal communication represents an extremely fruitful area for research, since nurses are often called upon to be sensitive to nonverbal cues. The kinds of nonverbal behavior amenable to observational methods include facial expressions; touch; posture; gestures and other body movements; and extralinguistic behavior (i.e., the manner in which people speak, aside from the content, such as the

intonation, loudness, and continuity of the speech).

4. *Activities.* There are many actions that are amenable to observation and that constitute valuable data for nursing researchers. Activities that serve as an index of health status or physical and emotional functioning are particularly important. As illustrations, the following constitute the kinds of activities that lend themselves to an observational study: patients' eating habits and trends; bowel movements in postsurgical patients; self-grooming activities of nursing home residents; length and number of visits by friends and relatives to hospitalized patients; and aggressive actions among children in the hospital playroom.

5. *Skill Attainment and Performance.* Nurses and nurse educators are constantly called upon to develop skills among clients and students. The attainment of these skills is often manifested behaviorally, such that an observational assessment is necessary. For example, a nursing researcher might want to observe the following kinds of behaviors: the ability of student nurses to properly insert a urinary catheter; the ability of stroke patients to scan a food tray if homonymous hemianopsia is present; the ability of diabetics to test their urine for sugar and acetone; or the ability of a newborn to exhibit sucking behavior when positioned for breastfeeding.

6. *Environmental Characteristics.* An individual's surroundings may have a profound effect on her or his behavior and, therefore, a number of studies have explored the relationship between certain observable attributes of the environment on the one hand and human beliefs, actions, and needs on the other. Examples of observable environmental attributes include the following: the noise levels in different areas of a hospital; the existence of architectural barriers in the homes of individuals with a disability; the color of walls in a nursing home; the laboratory facilities in a school of nursing; or the cleanliness of the homes in a community.

Units of analysis

In selecting behaviors, attributes, or situations to be observed, the investigator must make a decision concerning what constitutes a unit. There are two basic approaches, which are perhaps best considered as the end-points of a continuum. The *molar approach* entails observing large units of behavior and treating them as a whole. For example, psychiatric nurse researchers might engage in a study of patient mood swings. A whole constellation of verbal and nonverbal behaviors might be construed as signalling aggressive behaviors, while another set might constitute passive behaviors. At the other extreme, the *molecular approach* uses small and highly specific behaviors as the unit of observation. Each movement, action, gesture, or phrase is treated as a separate entity, or perhaps broken down into even smaller units. The choice of approaches depends to a large degree on the nature of the problem and the preferences of the investigator. The molar approach is more susceptible to observer errors and distortions because of the greater ambiguity in the definition of the units. On the other hand, in reducing the observations to more concrete and specific activities, the investigator may lose sight of the activities that are at the heart of the inquiry.

☐
The observer/observed relationship

The observer/researcher can interact with individuals in the observational setting to varying degrees. The issue of the relationship between the observer and those observed is an important one, and one that has stirred much controversy. The two most important aspects of this issue are intervention and concealment. The decisions a researcher makes in establishing a strategy for handling these considerations should be based on an understanding of the ethical and methodological implications.

In observational studies, intervention may involve an experimental intervention of the type described in Chapter 8 on experimental designs. For example, a nurse researcher may observe patients' postoperative behaviors following an intervention designed to improve the patients' ability to cough and breathe after surgery. However, in observational studies, the researcher sometimes intervenes to structure the research setting, without necessarily introducing an experimental treatment, that is, without manipulating the independent variable. This approach is sometimes referred to as the use of "directed settings." For instance, researchers sometimes "stage" a situation in order to provoke specific behavioral patterns. Certain events or activities are rare in naturalistic settings and, therefore, it becomes inexpedient to wait for their manifestation. Investigators in such studies typically make every attempt to maintain the outward appearance of a natural event. For example, a large number of social psychological investigations have studied the behavior of bystanders in crisis or emergency situations. Crises are not very common, and their occurrence is not predictable. Therefore, in order to observe the determinants of helping behavior (or lack of it) among onlookers, investigators have created "emergencies." Such studies are considered high on the intervention dimension.

Studies in which the researcher intervenes to elicit behaviors of interest may be practical when there is little opportunity to observe activities or events as they unfold naturalistically. However, such studies are sometimes criticized on the grounds of artificiality and may

suffer from serious problems of external validity.

The second dimension that concerns the relationship between the observer and the observed is the degree to which subjects are aware of the observation and their subject status. In naturalistic settings, observer/researchers are often concerned that their presence, if known, would alter the behaviors of interest. In some situations, therefore, observers may adopt a completely passive role, attempting insofar as possible to become unobtrusive bystanders. The problem of behavioral distortions owing to the known presence of an observer has been called a reactive measurement effect or, more simple, *reactivity.*

One approach to minimizing the problem of reactivity is to make the observations without the subjects' knowledge, through some type of concealment. For example, a nurse could monitor patients' conversations by means of the call system located at the nurses' station, thereby concealing the fact that the conversations were being overheard. In laboratory environments or in some "directed settings," concealed observations can be accomplished through the use of one-way mirrors.

Concealment offers the researcher a number of distinct advantages, even beyond the reduction of reactivity. Some individuals might deny a researcher the privilege of observing them altogether, so that the alternative to concealed observation might be no observation at all. Total concealment, however, may be difficult to attain except in highly structured or active observational settings. Furthermore, concealed observation, without the knowledge and consent of those observed, is often questionable from an ethical point of view.

A second situation is one in which the subjects are aware of the researcher's presence but may not be aware of the investigator's underlying motives. This approach offers the researcher the opportunity of getting more in-depth information than is usually possible with total concealment. Also, because the researcher is not totally concealed, there may be fewer ethical problems. Nevertheless, the issues of subject deception and failure to obtain informed voluntary consent remain thorny ones. Furthermore, a serious drawback of this second approach is the possibility that the interaction between the observer and the observed will alter the subjects' behavior. Even when the observed individuals are unaware of being participants in a research study, there is always a risk that the researcher's presence will alter their normal activities, mannerisms, or conversations.

The researcher will be confronted with methodological, substantive, or ethical issues at every point along the concealment/intervention dimensions. Some of these problems will be irrelevant in particular projects, but the careful investigator should assess the relative weaknesses of an approach against the possible advantages it might offer.

☐
Observational methods: Unstructured observations

Field research (see Chapter 10) usually involves the collection of unstructured or loosely structured observational data. The aim of field research is typically to understand the behaviors and experiences of people as they actually occur in naturalistic settings. Therefore, the field researcher's aim is to observe and record information about people and their environments with a minimum of structure and researcher-imposed interference.

The gathering of observational data in field settings is often referred to as participant observation. In such research, the investigator participates in the functioning of the social group under investigation, and strives to observe and record information within the contexts, structures, and symbols that are relevant

to the group members. Although it is beyond the scope of this book to describe in detail the methods used in participant observation research, we describe some of the salient issues. Textbooks on field research methods, such as that by Schatzman and Strauss (1982), should be consulted for a more thorough elaboration of methods.

The observer/participant role

The role that an observer plays in the social group under investigation is important because the social position of the observer determines what he or she is likely to see. That is, the behaviors that are likely to be available for observation will depend on the observer's position in a network of relations.

Leininger (1985) has noted that the observer's role typically evolves through a sequence of four phases:

- Primarily observation
- Primarily observation with some participation
- Primarily participation with some observation
- Reflective observation

In the initial phase, the researcher observes and listens to obtain a broad view of the situation. This initial phase allows both observers and subjects to "size up" each other, to become acquainted, and to become more comfortable in interacting. In phase II, observation is enhanced by a modest degree of participation. As the researcher participates more actively in the activities of the social group, the reactions of people to specific researcher behaviors can be more systematically studied. In phase III, the researcher strives to become a more active participant, learning by the actual experience of "doing" rather than just watching and listening. In the final phase, the researcher reflects on the total process of what transpired and how people interacted with and reacted to the researcher.

The observer must overcome at least two major hurdles in assuming a satisfactory role vis-à-vis subject-informants. The first is to gain entrée into the social group under investigation; the second is to establish rapport and develop trust within the social group. Without gaining entrée, the study cannot proceed; but without the trust of the group, the researcher will typically be restricted to what Leininger (1985) refers to as "front stage" knowledge, that is, information that is distorted by the group's protective facades. The goal of the participant observer is to "get back stage," to learn about the true realities of the group's experiences and behaviors.

Clearly, interpersonal skills play an important role in overcoming both these hurdles. Wilson (1985) has noted that successful participant observation research may require researchers to "go through channels, cultivate relationships, contour [their] appearances, withhold evaluative judgments, and be as unobtrusive and charming as possible" (p. 376).

Gathering and recording unstructured observational data

During the initial phase of a field study, it is often useful to gather some written or pictorial descriptive information that provides an overview of the environment. In an institutional setting, for example, it may be helpful to obtain a floor plan, an organizational chart, an annual report, and so on. Then, a preliminary personal tour of the site should be undertaken to gain familiarity with the ambience of the site and to note major activities, social groupings, transactions, and events.

The next step is to identify a meaningful way to sample observations and to select observational locations. Sampling by time and by event are common strategies for observational sampling (these are discussed later in this chapter). It is generally useful to use a combination of positioning approaches in selecting observational locations. *Single positioning* means staying in a single location for a period to observe behaviors and transactions in that location. *Multiple positioning* involves moving around the site to observe behaviors from different locations. *Mobile positioning* involves following a person throughout a given activity or period.

It should be noted that, because participant observers cannot spend a lifetime in one site and because they cannot be in more than one place at a time, observation is almost always supplemented with information obtained in unstructured interviews or conversations. For example, an *informant* may be asked to describe what went on in a meeting that the observer was unable to attend; or informants may be asked to describe an event that occurred before the observer entered the field. In such a case, the informant functions as the observer's observer.

The participant observer typically places few restrictions on the types of data collected, in keeping with the goal of minimizing observer-imposed meanings and structure. Given this aim, the most common forms of record-keeping in participant observation studies are logs and field notes. A *log* is a daily record of events and conversations that took place. *Field notes* may include the daily log but tend to be much broader, more analytic, and more interpretive than a simple listing of occurrences. Field notes represent the participant observer's efforts to record information and also to synthesize and understand the data.

Field notes are sometimes categorized according to the purpose they will serve during the analysis and integration of information. *Observational notes* are objective descriptions of events and conversations; information such as time, place, activity, and dialogue are recorded as completely and objectively as possible. *Theoretical notes* are interpretive attempts to attach meaning to observations. *Methodological notes* are instructions or re-

Table 15-1
Example of field notes: study of an in vitro fertilization facility

• Observational notes	Couple A entered the center for the first time at around 7:00 PM on a Tuesday evening. Mrs. A sat very stiffly on the chair next to the receptionist's desk, and Mr. A sat beside her. Both parties looked uncomfortable and tense. There was little interaction between them until they were called in for the initial consultation. While in the waiting area, Mrs. A picked up several magazines, thumbed through them absently, and then put them down again. Mr. A spent most of the time smoking cigarettes, staring at the ceiling or at the entrance to the office. Couple A spent approximately 15 minutes in the waiting area. When their name was called, Mrs. A jumped as though startled and then moved quickly toward the door. She turned back once to make sure Mr. A was following, and when she saw that he was just rising, motioned for him to follow her.
• Theoretical notes	Tension is a common feature among couples waiting for their initial consultation. However, the tension seems to stem from different sources and manifests itself in different ways. Some couples seem not to be persuaded that *in vitro* fertilization (IVF) is right for them; these couples seem embarrassed and tend not to communicate with one another. Among others, the source of tension seems to stem less from conflict about whether to try IVF but rather from the fear of disappointment. These couples tend to engage in continuous *soto voce* discussions about what they've heard about IVF while waiting for their intake.
• Methodological notes	I decided yesterday to make more systematic observations of couples immediately after they complete their initial interview. This decision was spurred by an incident yesterday in which both partners left the office in tears.
• Personal notes	My progress in understanding what these couples seeking IVF treatment are going through is very uneven. Two days ago, I was confident that patterns were falling into place. But this afternoon a little girl in the waiting room (an adopted daughter of a couple undergoing treatment) made me painfully aware of how much more complex the phenomenon of infertility and its social and psychological meanings really are.

minders about how subsequent observations will be made. *Personal notes* are comments about the researcher's own feelings during the research process. Table 15-1 presents some examples of all four types of field notes from a fictitious study of an *in vitro* fertilization treatment facility.

The success of any participant observation study is highly dependent upon the quality of the logs and field notes. It is clearly essential to record observations while the researcher is still in the process of collecting information, since memory failures are bound to occur if there is too long a delay. On the other hand, the participant observer cannot usually per-

form the recording function by visibly carrying a clipboard, pens and paper, since this procedure would undermine the observer's role as an ordinary participating member of the group. The researcher, therefore, must develop the skill of making detailed mental notes that can later be committed to paper or recorded on tape. Alternatively, the observer can try to jot down unobtrusively a phrase or sentence that will later serve as a reminder of an event, conversation, or impression. At a later point — preferably as soon as possible — the observer can utilize the brief notes and mental recordings to develop the more extensive field notes. The use of portable computers with word processing capabilities can greatly facilitate the recording and organization of notes in the field.

Evaluation of unstructured observation

The methods described in this section have both strong opponents and proponents. Those researchers who support the use of unstructured methods point out that these techniques usually provide a deeper and richer understanding of human behaviors and social situations than is possible with more rigorous procedures. Participant observation is particularly valuable, according to this view, for its ability to "get inside" a particular situation and lead to a more complete understanding of its complexities. Furthermore, unstructured observational approaches are inherently flexible and, therefore, permit the observer greater freedom to reconceptualize the problem after becoming more familiar with the situation. Advocates of qualitative observational research also claim that structured, quantitatively-oriented methods are too mechanistic and superficial to render a meaningful account of the intricate nature of human behavior.

Critics of the unstructured approach point out a number of methodological shortcomings. Observer bias and observer influence are prominent difficulties. Not only is there a concern that the observer may lose objectivity in recording actual observations, there is also the question that the observer will inappropriately sample events and situations to be observed. Once the researcher begins to participate in a group's activities, the possibility of emotional involvement becomes a salient issue. The researcher in the new "member" role may fail to attend to many scientifically relevant aspects of the situation or may develop a myopic view on issues of importance to the group. Participant observation techniques, thus, may be an unsuitable approach to study problems when one suspects that the risks of identification are

strong. Memory distortions represent another possible source of inaccuracy. Finally, unstructured observational methods are more highly dependent on the observational and interpersonal skills of the observer than are highly structured techniques. A highly skilled and sensitive observer can develop extremely valuable knowledge about human experiences in much the same way that a talented novelist does. But talent of this kind is not common.

There is obviously no "right" or "wrong" answer to the question of which approach should be adopted. The researcher should choose an approach that, given the research problem and the researcher's own skills and interests, is most likely to yield meaningful and useful data. The above arguments may be useful in making this decision. On the whole, it would appear that unstructured observational methods are extremely profitable for exploratory research in which the investigator wishes to establish an adequate conceptualization of the important variables in a social setting or wants to develop a set of hypotheses. The more rigorous observational methods, discussed in the following section, are probably better suited in most cases to the testing of research hypotheses.

☐
Observational methods: structured observations

Structured observational methods differ from the unstructured techniques in the specificity of behaviors or events selected for observation, in the advanced preparation of record-keeping forms, and in the kinds of activities in which the observer engages. The observer utilizing a structured observational procedure may still have ample room for making inferences and exercising judgment but is restrained with regard to the kinds of phenomena that will be watched and recorded. The creativity of structured observation lies not in the observation itself but, rather, in the formulation of a system for accurately categorizing, recording, and encoding the observations and sampling the phenomena of interest. Since structured techniques are highly dependent upon plans developed prior to observations, they are not considered appropriate when the investigator has limited or no knowledge about the phenomena under investigation.

Categories and checklists

The most common approach to making structured observations of ongoing events and behaviors consists of the construction of a category system to which the observed phenomena can be assigned. A category system represents an attempt to designate in a systematic or quantitative fashion the qualitative behaviors and events transpiring within the observational setting.

Considerations in using category systems

One of the most important requirements of a category system is the careful and explicit definition of the behaviors and characteristics to be observed. Each category should be explained in detail with an operational definition so that observers will have relatively clear-cut criteria for assessing the occurrence of the phenomenon in question. For example, Borgatta (1962) presented a category system for the observation of verbal communication and social interaction involving two or more individuals. The Interaction Process Score system involves a total of 18 categories of interactive behavior. Category four, which designates the observed subject's "acknowledgment, understanding or recognition" within a social interaction, is defined as follows:

This category includes all passive indicators of having understood or recognized the

communication directed toward the recipient. The most common score for this category is a nod or saying "Uhuh," "Yes," "O.K.," "Mum," "Right," "Check," "I see," "That may be, but . . ." In general, items are scored into this category if they indicate the acceptance of an item of communication, but this does not require agreement with the communication, the presence of which would place the response in Category 5 (Borgatta, 1962, p. 273).

In developing or selecting a categorization scheme, the researcher must make a number of important decisions. One decision concerns the exhaustiveness of the phenomena to be observed and the number of categories to be included. Some category systems, such as Borgatta's interaction procedure, are constructed such that *all* observed behaviors can be classified into one (and only one) of eighteen categories. Another example of an exhaustive system is the Downs and Fitzpatrick (1976) observation tool for analyzing body position and motor activity in mobile subjects. Their instrument was developed with the objective that all postural and motor behavior could be classified into one or another of their categories. A contrasting technique is to develop a system in which only particular types of behavior are categorized. For example, Gill, White, and Anderson (1984) used a more restrictive category system for the observation of crying behaviors in newborn infants. Their system categorized 25 different crying behaviors, but noncrying behaviors are not included. As another example, if we were observing the aggressive behavior of autistic children, we might develop such categories as "strikes another child," "kicks or hits walls/floors," "calls other children names," "throws objects around the room," and so forth. In this more restricted category system, many behaviors (all those that are nonaggressive) would not be classified. It might be pointed out that while nonexhaustive systems may be adequate for many research purposes, they run the risk of providing data that are difficult to interpret. When a large number of observed behaviors are unclassified, the investigator may have difficulty in placing the categoried behaviors into a proper perspective.

Virtually all category systems require that some inferences be made on the part of the observer, but there is considerable variability on this dimension. The Downs and Fitzpatrick (1976) observational instrument for body position and motor activity consists of a category system that requires only a modest amount of inference. For example, total body position is classified in one of six relatively straightforward categories: upright, lying down, leaning, sitting, leaning over, and kneeling. On the other hand, a category system such as the Abnormal Involuntary Movement Scale (AIMS) requires considerably more inference. The AIMS system, which was developed by the National Institue for Mental Health and used in a study by Whall and associates (1983) for detecting tardive dyskinesia associated with the prolonged use of neuroleptic drugs, contains such categories as "global judgments" and "trunk movements." Even when such categories are accompanied by detailed definitions and descriptions, there is clearly a heavy inferential burden placed upon the observer. The decision concerning how much observer inference is appropriate will depend on a number of factors, including the research purposes and the skills of the observers. Beginning researchers are advised to construct or use category systems that require only a moderate degree of inference. In general, category systems that use molecular units of behavior tend to require less inference than those that use molar units.

Once a category system has been developed or selected, the researcher can proceed to construct a checklist, which is the instrument used by the observer to record observed phenom-ena. Whether one constructs a new category system or uses a well-developed method, the system should be subjected to pilot runs to assess its suitability for the intended study.

Checklists for exhaustive systems

When an observer uses an exhaustive system (that is, when all behaviors are observed and recorded), the researcher must be especially careful to define the categories in such a way that the observers know when one behavior ends and a new one begins. Another essential feature of exhaustive systems is that the referent behaviors should be mutually exclusive. If overlapping categories are not eliminated, the observer may have difficulty in deciding how to classify a particular observation. The underlying assumption in the use of such a category system is that behaviors, events, or attributes that are allocated to a particular category are equivalent to every other behavior, event, or attribute in that same category.

The checklist is generally formatted with the list of behaviors or events from the category system on the left, and space for tallying the frequency and/or duration of occurrence of behaviors on the right. In complex social situations with multiple actors, the right-hand portion may be divided into panels according to characteristics of the actors (e.g., nurse/physician; male patients/female patients) or by individual subjects' names or assigned identification numbers.

The task of the observer using this approach is to place all behaviors in only one category for each element. By element, we refer here to either a unit of behavior, such as a sentence in a conversation, or to a time interval. To illustrate suppose that we were interested in studying the problem-solving behavior of a group of public health workers developing a maternal-child health program in a rural area. We might construct a category system such as the following: (1) information seeking; (2) information giving; (3) problem describing; (4) sugges-

Table 15-2
Examples of categories for a sign analysis

Activity	Frequency
Eating Behaviors	
Eats with hand	
Eats with spoon or fork	
Cuts soft food	
Cuts meat	
Drinks from a straw	
Drinks from a cup or glass	
Hygiene	
Washes hands or extremities	
Brushes teeth	
Cleans fingernails	
Brushes or combs hair	
Shaves	
Dressing Skills	
Fastens or unfastens buttons	
Fastens or unfastens snaps	
Pulls zipper up or down	
Ties or unties shoelace	
Puts on or takes off eyeglasses	
Fastens or unfastens buckle	
Puts in or takes out dentures	

tion proposing; (5) suggestion opposing; (6) suggestion supporting; (7) summarizing; and (8) miscellaneous. The observer would be required to classify every group member's contribution to the problem-solving process in terms of one of these eight categories. By employing such a system, it would be possible to analyze, for example, the relationship between a group member's role, status, or characteristics on the one hand and the types of problem-solving behaviors engaged in on the other.

The second manner in which this approach can be used is to categorize the relevant behaviors at regular time intervals. The observational system for analyzing motor activity developed by Downs and Fitzpatrick (1976) uses 15-second time intervals as the basic recording unit. That is, the observer is expected to record all body positions and movements occurring within a 15-second period. Checklists based on exhaustive category systems are demanding of the observer, since the recording task is continuous.

Checklists for nonexhaustive systems

The second approach, which is sometimes referred to as a *sign system,* begins with a listing of categories of behaviors that may or may not be manifested by the subjects. The observer's task is to watch for instances of the behaviors on the list. When a behavior occurs, the observer either places a checkmark beside the appropriate behavior to designte its occurrence, or makes a cumulative tally of the number of times the behavior was witnessed. The product of this type of endeavor is a kind of demography of events transpiring within the observational period. With this type of checklist, the observer does not classify *all* the behaviors or characteristics of the individuals being observed but rather identifies the occurrence and frequency of particular behaviors. A hypothetical example of a checklist using the sign system for describing patients' ability to perform selected activities of daily living is presented in Table 15-2.

Rating scales

Structured observations can be recorded in a number of ways other than through the use of category systems and checklists. The major alternative is to employ rating scales. A *rating scale* is a tool that requires the observer to rate some phenomenon in terms of points along a descriptive continuum. The ratings usually are quantified during the subsequent analysis of the observational data.

Rating scales normally are used in one of two ways. The observer may be required to make ratings of behavior or events at frequent intervals throughout the observational period in much the same way that a checklist would be used. Alternatively, the observer may use the rating scales to summarize an entire event or transaction after the observation is completed. Post-observation ratings require the observer to integrate a number of activities and to make a judgment as to which point on a scale most closely resembles the interpretation given to the overall situation. For example, suppose that we were interested in comparing the behaviors of nurses working in intensive care units with those of nurses in other units. After 15-minute observation sessions, the observer might be asked to rate the perceived anxiety level of the nursing staff in each unit as a whole, or that of individual members. The rating scale item might take the following form:

According to your perceptions, how tense were the nurses in the observed unit?
(1) extremely relaxed
(2) rather relaxed
(3) somewhat relaxed
(4) neither relaxed nor tense
(5) somewhat tense
(6) rather tense
(7) extremely tense

The same information could be solicited using a graphic rating scale format:

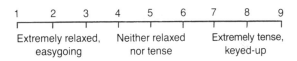

Rating scales can also be used as an extension of checklists wherein the observer records not only the occurrence of some behavior but also some qualitative aspect of it such as its magnitude or intensity. The Downs and Fitzpatrick (1976) instrument for motor activity once again provides a good example. Their category scheme is composed of eight body movement categories: head active, right arm active, left arm active, both arms active, right leg active, left leg active, both legs active, and both arms and legs active. Observers must both classify the subjects' activity in terms of these categories *and* rate the intensity of the movement on a three-point scale: minimally active, moderately active, and very active. When rating scales are coupled with a category scheme in this fashion, considerably more information about the phenomena under investigation can be obtained. The disadvantage of this approach is that it places an immense burden on the observer, particularly if there is an extensive amount of activity.

Constructing versus borrowing structured observational instruments

The development, testing, refining, and retesting of a new category scheme or rating scale may require weeks or even months of effort, particularly if the system is intended to be used in a variety of settings and with a variety of subjects. In some cases, a researcher may have no alternative but to design new observational instruments. For example, the researcher may be investigating a relatively new area or may be expanding an area of inquiry with a new population of subjects for whom existing tools may not be appropriate. However, as in the case of self-report instruments, we encourage researchers to fully explore the literature for potentially usable observational instruments.

Many observational systems have been constructed with the intent of being applied to a variety of research situations. Generalized systems, such as those of Downs and Fitzpatrick and Borgatta described earlier, should be scrutinized before proceeding to design a new system. The use of an existing system not only saves a considerable amount of work but also facilitates comparisons among investigations.

There are a few source books that describe

Table 15-3
Examples of observational category systems used by nurse researchers

Name of Instrument	Concept(s) Measured	Source
Recovery Room Activity Schedule	Behaviors observed in recovery room	Elms, 1972
Index of Activities of Daily Living (ADL)	Level of independence of the chronically ill or aged	Katz and Akpom, 1976
Sleep Status Observation Form	Sleep/wake behaviors	McFadden & Giblen, 1971
Quality of Patient Care Scale (Qual Pacs)	Quality of nursing care	Wandelt and Ager, 1974
Home Observation for Measurement of the Environment (HOME)	Child-rearing environment	Elardo *et al.,* 1977
Nurse Practitioner Rating Form	Performance in the nurse practitioner role	Prescott *et al.,* 1981
Parent-Child Communication Schedule	Parent–child interaction	O'Brien, 1980
The Nonverbal Behavior Worksheet	Nonverbal behavior of patients	McCorkle, 1974

available observational checklists for certain research applications. For example, the reference book by Ward and Lindemann (1979), which describes instruments for measuring variables of relevance to nursing, includes some observational instruments. Perhaps the best source for such tools, however, is the current research literature on the topic of interest. For example, if you wanted to conduct an observational study of maternal bonding behavior, a good place to begin is by reviewing recently completed research on this or similar topics to get clues about how "maternal bonding" was operationalized. Table 15-3 provides examples of some concepts of interest to nurse researchers for which observational instruments have been developed and lists the appropriate references for locating them.

Observational sampling

Structured observational methods rarely involve the recording of all behaviors or activities that take place in a given situation. The investigator must often make some decisions concerning how and when the system will be applied. Observational sampling methods represent a mechanism for obtaining representative examples of the behavior being observed without having to observe an entire event.

The most frequently used system is the *time-sampling method.* This procedure involves the selection of time periods during which the observations will take place. The time frames may be systematically selected (for example, every 30 seconds at 2-minute intervals) or may be selected at random. As a hypothetical example, suppose we were studying the interaction patterns of mothers and their handicapped children. Some of the mothers have received specific preparation from a community health nurse for dealing with their conflict over the child's dependence-independence needs, while a control group of mothers has not received this preparation. In order to examine the effects of this intervention, the behavior of the mothers and children are observed in a playground setting. During a 1-hour observation period, we decide to sample behaviors rather than to observe the entire session. For the sake of simplicity, let us say that 3-minute observations will be made. If we use a systematic sampling approach, we would observe for 3-minutes, then cease observing for a prespecified period, say 3 minutes. Using this scheme, a total of ten 3-minute observations would be made. A second approach is to randomly sample 3-minute periods from the total of twenty such periods in an hour. The decision with regard to the length and number of periods comprising a suitable sample must be influenced by the aims of the research. In establishing time units, one of the most important considerations is determining what a psychologically meaningful time frame would be. A good deal of pretesting and experimentation with different sampling plans is essential in developing or adapting observational strategies.

Event sampling is a second system for obtaining a set of observations. This approach selects integral behaviors or events of a prespecified type for observation. Event sampling requires that the investigator either have some knowledge concerning the occurrence of events or be in a position to wait for their occurrence. Examples of "integral events" that may be suitable for event sampling include shift changes of nurses in a hospital, cast removals of pediatric patients, epileptic seizures, and cardiac arrests in the emergency room. This sampling approach is preferable to time sampling when the events of principal interest are infrequent throughout the day and are at risk of being missed if specific time-sampling frames are established. In addition, event sampling has the advantage that the observation treats whole situations in their entirety rather than fragmenting them into discontinuous segments. Still, when behaviors and events are relatively frequent, time sampling does have the virtue of enhancing the representativeness of the observed behaviors. Time sampling and event sampling can sometimes be profitably combined.

Training observers

Observational methods are more vulnerable to human perceptual errors than virtually any other data collection procedure. If persons are to become good "instruments" for measuring observational data, then they must be trained to observe in such a way that accuracy is maximized and biases are minimized. The training of observers is a crucial phase in the preparation of a study and should not be neglected. Even when the investigator who designed the study does most or all of the observations, training and "dry runs" are essential.

The observers must be familiarized thoroughly with the aims of the project, the nature of the behaviors or events to be observed, the sampling strategy, and the formal instrument. For large projects that involve more than one or two observers, it is wise to produce an "observer's manual" with detailed instructions and examples. When category systems are used, the observers should memorize the scheme, since they are typically called upon to record observations virtually simultaneous with the occurrence of the observed behaviors. Training sessions are useful for clarifying any ambiguities, for explaining how to deal with marginal cases, and for alerting the observers to the need to perceive familiar behaviors within the constraints imposed by the observation schedule.

After this initial training, the observers are ready for a trial use of the instrument. The setting during this trial period should resemble as closely as possible the settings that will be the focus of the final observations. Sometimes it may be possible to use role-playing techniques to simulate events and behaviors. This approach has the advantage that the trainees can interrupt the interaction to ask questions if difficulties arise. Thorough discussions of the trial experience are recommended in order to address any problems and to allow the observers an opportunity to make suggestions for improving the instruments' efficiency or quality. During a practice session, the comparability of the observers' recordings should be assessed. That is, two or more observers should watch a trial event or situation, and the notations on the checklist or rating scales should be compared. This procedure is referred to as an evaluation of *interrater reliability* and will be described more fully in Chapter 17.

Structured observations by nonresearch personnel

The research we have discussed thus far involves situations in which the researchers (or an observer assistant) observes ongoing events or behaviors of relevance to the research problem and then codes information relating to what has been seen in some specified time period. There are other forms of observational data-gathering methods that provide more global information about the characteristics and behaviors of individuals. Often such methods involve asking nonresearch personnel to summarize on structured scales their knowledge of a person or group, based on their own observations. This method has much in common (in terms of format and scoring procedures) with the self-report scales described in the preceding chapter; the primary difference is that the person completing the scale describes the attributes and behaviors of persons other than themselves. For example, a mother might be asked to describe the temperament of her infant, or staff nurses might be asked to evaluate the functional capacity of nursing home residents, or a nursing supervisor might be asked to assess the nursing competency of nurses on the unit. As with self-report instruments, a researcher might decide to construct his or her own behavior rating scale for a specific research purpose, or might choose to use or adapt an existing scale. Some of the references cited in Chapter 14 and at the end of this chapter identify observa-

tional instruments. Table 15-4 lists several such global rating scales that have been used in nursing studies.

The use of nonresearch personnel to provide observational data has a number of practical advantages. It is an economical method compared to using trained observers. For example, an observer might have to watch children for hours or days to fully describe the nature and intensity of certain behavior problems while a parent or teacher could readily do this. In some situations the behaviors of interest might never be capable of observation by an outsider, because of reactivity problems, because they involve private situations, or because they constitute rare events (e.g., sleep walking). Also, there are some populations for whom self-report data cannot be obtained, such as infants, the mentally retarded, or the very old. On the other hand, such methods may have all of the same problems as self-report scales (such as response set biases) *plus* the additional problem of observer bias. Nonresearch observers are typically not "trained" and interobserver reliability cannot usually be determined. Thus, this approach has a number of problems but will inevitably continue to find many research applications because in many cases there are no alternatives.

☐ Mechanical aids in observations

Our discussion has focused thus far on those types of observations in which the observers and coders are the same person, in which the coding and observing occur simultaneously, and which are made by observers directly through the use of their sensory organs. There are observational studies that do not meet all three of these conditions. In this section we will look at mechanical devices or other equipment that can be used either as an extension of the human senses or as a means of

Table 15-4
Examples of behavioral rating scales that can be completed by nonresearch personnel

Name of Instrument	Concept(s) Measured	Source
Nursing Rating Scale (nurses)*	Psychopathological disturbance in hospitalized psychiatric patients	Hargreaves, 1968
Child Health Questionnaire (teachers)	Psychological health of grade school children	Butler, 1975
Infant Characteristics Questionnaire (parents)	Infant temperament	Pates *et al.,* 1979
Eyberg Child Behavior Inventory (parents)	Children's conduct problems	Eyberg & Ross, 1978
Blank Infant Tenderness Scale (mothers)	Infants' need for tenderness	Blank, 1983
Parents' Perception of Uncertainty Scale (parents)	Children's uncertainty in illness	Mishel, 1983
Ibe Behavioral Checklist (nurses)	Patients' level of dependence	Clough & Derdiarian, 1980
Six-Dimension Scale of Nursing Performance (supervisors)	Nursing performance	Schwirian, 1978

* Parentheses indicate person normally asked to complete the instrument.

securing permanent records of observational data.

The health-care field has a rich store of devices and equipment designed to make available to observers conditions or attributes that are ordinarily imperceptible. Nasal speculums, stethoscopes, bronchoscopes, radiographic equipment, and a myriad of other medical instruments make it possible for health care personnel to gather observational information concerning the health status and bodily functioning of patients.

In addition to equipment for enhancing physiological observations, several mechanical devices are available for recording behaviors and events. These techniques make possible categorization at a later point in time. When the behavior of interest is primarily auditory, tape recordings can be obtained and used as a permanent observational record. Transcripts from such recordings can then be prepared to facilitate the classification process. Other technological instruments to aid auditory observation have been developed, such as laser devices that are capable of recording sounds by being directed on a window to a room, and voice tremor detectors that are sensitive to stress.

When a visual record is desired, motion picture films or videotapes are suitable media. Both of these techniques—and particularly videotapes—have gained increased acceptability as their advantages have become apparent. Films and videotapes, in addition to being permanent, offer the possibility of capturing complex behaviors that would elude categorization by an on-the-spot observer. Visual records are also capable of capturing finer units of behavior than the naked eye, such as micromomentary facial expressions. Videotapes and films offer the possibility of checking the accuracy of the coders and, thus, are quite useful as an aid to training. Finally, it is often easier to conceal a camera than a human observer, and in some situations this feature would constitute a major advantage. Film records also have a number of drawbacks, some of which are fairly technical, such as lighting requirements, lens limitations, and so forth. Other serious problems result from the fact that the camera angle adopted could present a lopsided view of an event or situation. The ability of films and videotapes to capture complex or fleeting behaviors is at once an advantage and a disadvantage. The analysis of motion picture records, frame by frame, can become a complicated and time-consuming process. Still, for many applications permanent visual records offer unparalleled opportunities to expand the range and scope of observational studies.

It might also be mentioned that there is a growing technology for assisting with the encoding and recording of observations made directly by on-the-spot observers. For example, there is equipment that permits the observer to enter observational data directly into a computer as the observation is taking place, and in some cases the equipment can be used to record physiological data concurrently. The research example at the end of this chapter describes how such a system was used in one nursing study.

☐
Evaluation of observational methods

The field of nursing is well-suited to observational research: observation has always been an integral part of the nursing process. Observational methods have both weaknesses and strengths, however, as is the case for so many approaches to obtaining data on human beings. The investigator about to embark on a research project should carefully weigh both the negative and positive aspects of this approach before data are collected.

Advantages of observational methods

One of the main reasons for using observational methods is that it may be impossible to obtain the desired information in any other way. Self-report measures such as questionnaires and interviews are often inadequate for dealing with activities and behaviors of which individuals may themselves be unaware or unable to verbalize. For certain research questions there simply may be no acceptable substitute for observation.

Observational methods have an intrinsic appeal with respect to their ability to capture directly a record of behaviors and events. Furthermore, there is virtually no other data collection method that can provide the depth and variety of information as observation. With this approach, human beings — the observers — are used as "measuring instruments," and provide a uniquely sensitive and intelligent (if fallible) tool.

Although we have used examples in this chapter that may suggest that observational methods are most suitable for descriptive naturalistic studies, the techniques described here are quite flexible and may be appropriately used for both experimental and nonexperimental research. Both laboratory and field studies have put observational methods to creative and skillful use. Within the area of nursing research, observational methods have broad applicability for clinical inquiries, as well as for educational and administrative studies.

Disadvantages of observational methods

Some of the problems with which an observational researcher must contend were described in our discussion of the observer/observed relationship. These include possible ethical difficulties, reactivity of the observed when the observer is conspicuous, and lack of consent to being observed. Observational data are very clearly vulnerable to many distortions and biases. Human perceptual errors and inadequacies are a continuous threat to the quality of obtained information. Observation and interpretation are very demanding tasks, requiring attention, sensation, perception, and conception. To accomplish these activities in a completely objective fashion is probably impossible, though structured category systems and sampling procedures help to reduce observer subjectivity. A number of factors interfere with objective observations: (1) emotions, prejudices, attitudes, and values may result in faulty inference; (2) personal interest and commitment may color what is seen in the direction of what the observer wants to see; (3) anticipation of what is to be observed may affect what is observed; and (4) hasty decisions before adequate information is collected may result in erroneous classifications or conclusions.

Several types of observational biases are especially common. One bias is referred to as the *enhancement of contrast effect*. The observer may tend to distort the observation in the direction of dividing the content into clear-cut entities. The converse effect—a bias toward *central tendency*—occurs when extreme events are distorted toward a middle ground. A series of biases are in a category described as *assimilatory*. The observer may tend to distort observations in the direction of identity with previous inputs. This bias would have the effect of miscategorizing information in the direction of regularity and orderliness. Assimilation to other "objects" also occurs: expectations and attitudes of the observer are the most common.

Rating scales are susceptible to several distinct types of error. The *halo effect* refers to the tendency of the rater to be influenced by one characteristic in rating other nonrelated characteristics. For example, if we formed a very positive general impression of a person, we would probably be likely to rate that person as "intelligent," "loyal" and "dependable" simply because these traits are positively valued. Rating scales may reflect the personality traits of the observer. The *error of leniency* is the

tendency for the observer to rate everything positively and the *error of severity* is the contrasting tendency to rate too harshly.

Needless to say, these biases are much more likely to operate when a high degree of observer inference is required by the observational tasks. The careful construction and pretesting of checklists and rating scales, the development of an adequate sampling plan, the proper training of observers, and interrater comparisons are techniques that can play an important role in minimizing or estimating these problematic biases. While the degree of observer bias is not necessarily a function of the degree of structure imposed on the observation, the difficulty with unstructured methods is that it is generally more difficult to assess the extent of bias.

□
Research examples

Unstructured observation

Cohen (1982) studied the birthing beliefs and practices of the Black Caribs of Central America as a participant observer. During seven months of fieldwork, she talked with villagers and observed their behaviors with regard to pregnancy, delivery, postpartum care, and immediate infant care. Some mechanical equipment (camera and tape recorder) was used occasionally, but the primary means of recording observations was through written field notes that were analyzed and catalogued every evening. During the course of the fieldwork, Cohen increased her participation in the birthing activities of the village. She assisted in the delivery of three infants, at the invitation of the village midwife, and eventually helped one woman single-handedly in the delivery of her baby.

Cohen's report summarized the process of prenatal care, labor, delivery, and postpartum care of Black Carib village women. Cohen noted the numerous differences that exist between birthing practices in this village as compared with standard North American practices. For example, the Carib mother is encouraged by the midwife to walk during the entire course of labor. Women deliver in a squatting position and delivery takes place in the home, attended by friends and relatives. Forceps are not used and no medications are given to ease the pain of labor. Based on her research, Cohen encouraged self-examination of some of our practices, such as birth positioning.

Structured observation

White and her colleagues (1983) tested whether a tape-recorded bedtime story read by a parent would help to ease separation anxiety and facilitate falling asleep among hospitalized children whose parents were not rooming-in. A sample of 18 children aged 3 to 8 (seven of whom had a tape-recorded story read by a parent; the control children had no special treatment) were observed for three nights during the falling asleep period (event sampling) for 15 minutes. The investigators used an exhaustive structured instrument called the Falling Asleep Inventory that encompassed 54 behaviors in which the child could engage during the observation session. Examples include "Eye rubbing," "Verbally seeking assistance," and "Getting out of bed." The inventory was designed for use with the Senders Signals and Receivers System (SSR), an observational and data management system that permitted automatic entry into a computer of observational codes relating to the children's falling asleep behaviors. Rather than using manual recording forms, observers entered codes for observed behaviors into an SSR keyboard. Duration and sequence of entries were automatically incorporated into the encoding system. The observer entered when a given behavior began, who exhibited the behavior, what the action was, and what the ob-

ject of the behavior was (e.g., the nurse). For example, the following code entered onto the keyboard would mean that the child began to stroke a toy:

$$+ \qquad 05 \qquad ST \qquad 06$$

Findings from this research indicated that children who had stories read to them fell asleep sooner, exhibited more sleepy behaviors, and displayed fewer active behaviors than the control group children. The investigators concluded that hospitalized children who hear a recorded bedtime story use self-soothing behaviors to cope with the separation experience.

☐
Summary

Observational methods are techniques for acquiring information for research purposes through the direct observation and interpretation of phenomena in the environment. A wide variety of human activity and experience can be researched using observational methods.

In any observational setting—whether it be in a natural field situation or laboratory setup—the observer cannot possibly attend to every behavior or event. Therefore, the investigator usually specifies in advance the nature of the phenomena to be observed. The researcher must also select an appropriate *unit of analysis*. The *molar approach* entails the observation of large segments of behaviors and events as integral units. The *molecular approach,* on the other hand, treats small, specific actions as separate entities.

The investigator must make decisions concerning the relationship between the observer and the subjects. The decisions relate primarily to the dimensions of *concealment* and *intervention*. Concealment refers to the degree to which the observed persons are aware that they are being observed and/or that they are the subjects of a research study. The problem of behavioral distortions stemming from the presence of an observer (known as *reactivity*) is a major reason for making concealed observations. Intervention refers to the degree to which the investigator structures the observational setting in line with research demands as opposed to being a passive observer.

Like self-reports, observational data vary on a structured/unstructured dimension. Field studies generally collect observational data that are unstructured, using a procedure known as participant observation. *Participant observation* is a method that has been used extensively by anthropologists and sociologists as a means of understanding cultures, institutions, and social groups. The participant observer endeavors to obtain information about the dynamics of the social group within the subject's own frame of reference, without imposing a preconceived structure based on the researcher's world view.

In participant observation studies, the researcher must pay careful attention to his or her role in the social group under study, because the behaviors available for observation will generally be contingent on the role. The researcher must first gain entrée into the group and then develop the trust of group members in order to get at the "back stage" realities of the group's experiences.

In the initial phase of a participant observation study, the researcher is primarily an observer and gathers a preliminary understanding of the site. As time passes, the researcher typically becomes a more active participant, and also develops a plan for sampling events and selecting observational positions. The observer usually combines *single positioning, multiple positioning,* and *mobile positioning.* The final phase of the research involves reflective observation about the activities that transpired.

Participant observation places few restrictions on the type or amount of data collected.

Logs of daily events and *field notes* are the major methods of recording data. Field notes have multiple purposes and may be categorized as *observational notes, theoretical notes, methodological notes* and *personal notes.*

Proponents of the participant observation approach claim it represents both a source of data *and* a basis for understanding what the data mean. Although unstructured methods can yield extremely rich and useful information, particularly when used by insightful observers, they are nevertheless subject to a number of methodological difficulties. The most prominent difficulties are observer bias in sampling, recording, and interpreting phenomena; observer influence (reactivity); and observer identification with the observed group.

Structured observational methods impose a number of constraints upon the observer for the purpose of maximizing observer accuracy and objectivity and for obtaining an adequate representation of the phenomena of interest. Two types of record-keeping forms are used most commonly by observers in structured situations. *Checklists* are tools for recording the appearance and/or frequency of prespecified behaviors, events, or characteristics. Checklists are based upon the development of *category systems* for encoding the observed phenomena. The researcher constructing a category system must make a number of decisions concerning its exhaustiveness, generality, inference requirements, and training demands. One type of checklist is based on the *sign system* and is used as a demographic record of the types of behavior that occurred during the observational session. A second format is used to exhaustively analyze ongoing events and activities.

Rating scales are the second most common record-keeping tool for structured observations. The observer using a rating scale is required to rate some phenomenon according to points along a dimension that is typically bipolar (for example, passive/aggressive or excellent health/poor health). Ratings are generally made either during the observational setting at specific intervals (e.g., every 5 minutes) or after the observation is completed.

Most structured observations make use of some form of *sampling plan* for selecting the behaviors, events, and conditions to be observed. The most frequently used approach is *time sampling,* which involves the specification of the duration and frequency of both the observational periods and the intersession intervals. *Event sampling* selects integral behaviors or events of a special type for observation.

It is crucial that observers be properly trained. The training should include thorough familiarization with the research aims and sensitization to perceiving common occurrences in an unusual way. The category scheme (if one is used for recording information) should be memorized and trial runs made with the instrument before the observers proceed to make the observations.

Technological advances have greatly augmented the researcher's capacity to collect, record, and preserve observational data. Such devices as tape recorders, movie cameras, videotape cameras, laser devices, and so forth permit behaviors and events to be categorized after their occurrence.

Perhaps the greatest strength of observation is that it allows for the collection of data that would be impossible to obtain in any other way. Important descriptive information about behavioral patterns and the human condition can be made available to scientific researchers through direct observation. The methods outlined in this chapter are flexible and can be applied to a wide variety of research problems and designs.

On the other hand, the researcher using observational techniques must be aware of their limitations. In addition to problems of an ethical nature, observation is subject to a variety of biasing effects. The greater the degree of observer inference and judgment, the more likely it is that perceptual errors and distortions will occur.

□
Study suggestions

1. Suppose you were interested in observing the behavior of fathers in the delivery room during the birth of their first child. Identify the observer/observed relationship along the concealment/intervention dimensions that you would recommend adopting for such a study and defend your recommendation. What are the possible drawbacks of your approach and how might you deal with them?

2. Would a psychiatric nurse researcher be well suited to conduct a participant observation study of the behavior of psychiatric nurses and their interactions with clients? Why or why not?

3. A nurse researcher is planning to study temper tantrums displayed by hospitalized children. Would you recommend using a time-sampling approach? Why?

4. Suppose you were interested in studying pain-related behaviors using observational methods. Develop some categories of behavior that could be used for classifying the observations.

5. Below are a list of problem statements. Indicate which of these problems could be studied by using some form of observational method. For each problem that is amenable to observation, specify whether you think a structured or unstructured approach would be preferable.

   a. Does team nursing versus primary nursing affect the type of communication patterns between nurses and patients?

   b. Is there a relationship between prenatal instruction and delivery room behaviors of primiparas?

   c. Is the number of hours of direct clinical

practice for student nurses related to their performance on the licensure examination?

d. Do the attitudes of nurses toward abortion affect the quality of care given to abortion patients?

e. Do industrial alcohol programs have a positive impact on on-the-job accident rates?

f. Is the touching behavior of nurses related to their ethnic or cultural background?

□
Suggested readings

Methodological references

General references

Bickman, L. (1976). Observational methods. In C. Selltiz, L.S. Wrightsman & S.W. Cook (Eds.), *Research methods in social relations*. New York: Holt, Rinehart & Winston (Chapter 8).

Byerly, E.L. (1976). The nurse researcher as participant-observer in a nursing setting. In P.J. Brink (ed.), *Transcultural nursing: A book of readings*. Englewood Cliffs, NJ: Prentice-Hall.

Dowrick, P. & Biggs, S.J. (Eds.) (1983). *Using video: psychological and social applications*. New York: John Wiley & Sons.

Gold, R.L. (1971). Roles in sociological observations. In B.J. Franklin & H.W. Osborne (Eds.), *Research methods: Issues and insights* pp. 255–267). Belmont, CA: Wadsworth.

Godsmith, J.W. (1981). Methodological considerations in using videotape to establish rater reliability. *Nursing Research, 30,* 124–127.

Jackson, B.S. (1973). Participant observation in nursing research. *Supervisor Nurse, 4,* 30–40.

Kerlinger, F. (1973). *Foundations of behavioral research* (2nd ed.). New York: Holt, Rinehart & Winston (Chapter 31).

Leininger, M. (1985). Ethnography and ethnonursing: Models and modes of qualitative data analysis. In M. Leininger (Ed.) *Qualitative Research Methods in Nursing*. New York: Grune & Stratton.

Lofland, J. (1971). *Analyzing social settings: A guide to qualitative observation and analysis*. Belmont, CA: Wadsworth.

McCall, G.J. & Simmons H.L. (Eds.). (1969). *Issues in participant observation: A text and reader*. Reading, MA: Addison-Wesley.

Pearsall, M. (1965). Participant observation as role and method in behavioral research. *Nursing Research, 14,* 37–42.

Schatzman, L. & Strauss, A. (1982). *Field research: Strategies for a natural sociology,* (2nd ed.). Englewood Cliffs, NJ: Prentice-Hall.

Ward, M.J. & Lindemann, C. (eds.) (1979). *Instruments for measuring nursing practice and other health care variables*. Hyattsville, MD:DHEW.

Wilson, H.S. (1985). *Research in nursing*. Menlo Park, CA: Addison-Wesley (Chapter 13).

References to observational instruments

Bates, J.E., Freeland, C.A., Lounsbury, M.L. (1979). Measurement of infant difficultness. *Child Development, 50,* 794–803.

Blank, D.M. (1985). Development of the Infant Tenderness Scale. *Nursing Research, 34,* 211–216.

Borgatta, E.F. (1962). A systematic study of interaction process scores, peer and self-assessments, personality and other variables. *Genetic Psychology Monographs, 65,* 219–291.

Butler, A.C. (1975). The Child Health Questionnaire. *Psychology in the Schools, 12,* 153–160.

Clough, D.H. & Derdiarian, A. (1980). A behavioral checklist to measure dependence and independence. *Nursing Research, 29,* 55–58.

Downs, F. & Fitzpatrick, J.J. (1976). Preliminary investigation of the reliability and validity of a tool for the assessment of body position and motor activity. *Nursing Research, 25,* 404–408.

Elardo, R., Bradley, R. & Caldwell, B. (1977). A longitudinal study of the relationship of infants' home environment to language development at age three. *Child Development, 48,* 595–603.

Elms, R.R. (1972). Recovery room behavior and postoperative convalescence. *Nursing Research, 21,* 390–397.

Eyberg, S.M. & Ross, A.W. (1978). Assessment of child behavior problems: The validation of a new inventory. *Journal of Clinical Child Psychology, 7,* 113–116.

Gill, N.E., White, M.A. & Anderson, G.C. (1984). Transitional newborn infants in a hospital nursery: From first oral cue to first sustained cry. *Nursing Research, 33,* 213–217.

Hargreaves, W.A. (1968). Systematic nursing observation of psychopathology. *Achives of General Psychiatry, 18,* 518–531.

Katz, S. & Akpom, A. (1976). A measure of primary socio-biologic functions. *International Journal of Health Services, 6,* 493–508.

McCorkle, R. (1974). The effects of touch on seriously ill patients. *Nursing Research, 23,* 125–132.

McFadden, E.H. & Giblin, E. (1971). Sleep deprivation in patients having open-heart surgery. *Nursing Research, 20,* 249–254.

Mishel, M.H. (1983). Parents' perception of uncertainty concerning their hospitalized child. *Nursing Research, 32,* 324–330.

O'Brien, R.A. (1980). Relationship of parent–child and self-differentiation. *Nursing Research, 29,* 150–156.

Prescott, P.A. *et al.* (1981). The Nurse Practitioner Rating Form. *Nursing Research, 30,* 223–228.

Schwirian, P.M. (1978). Evaluating the performance of nurses. *Nursing Research, 27,* 347–351.

Wandelt, M.A. & Ager, J.W. (1974). *Quality Patient Care Scale.* New York: Appleton-Century-Crofts.

Whall, A.L. *et al.* (1983). Development of a screening program for Tardive Dyskinesia: Feasibility issues. *Nursing Research, 32,* 151–156.

Substantive references

Bowen, S.M. & Miller, B.C. (1980). Paternal attachment behavior as related to presence at delivery and parenthood classes. *Nursing Research, 29,* 307–311 (Structured observation).

Cohen, F.S. (1982). Childbirth belief and practice in a Garifuna (Black Carib) village on the north coast of Honduras. *Western Journal of Nursing Research, 4,* 193–208 (Unstructured observation).

Hardin, S.B. (1980). Comparative analysis of nonverbal interpersonal communication of schizophrenics and normals. *Research in Nursing and Health, 3,* 57–68 (Structured observation).

Jordan-Marsh, M. (1983). Factors in the delivery of comprehensive services through child care programs. *Western Journal of Nursing Research,* 337–354 (Unstructured observation).

Kerr, J.A.C. (1985). Space use, privacy, and territoriality. *Western Journal of Nursing Research, 7,* 199–219 (Structured and unstructured observation).

Niemeier, D.F. (1983). A behavioral analysis of staff–patient interactions in a psychiatric setting. *Western Journal of Nursing Research, 5,* 269–277 (Unstructured observation).

Rice, V.H. & Johnson, J.E. (1984). Preadmission self-instruction booklets, postadmission exercise performance, and teaching time. *Nursing Research, 33,* 147–151 (Structured observation)

Salyer, J. & Stuart, B.J. (1985). Nurse–patient interaction in the intensive care unit. *Heart & Lung, 14,* 20–24 (Structured observation).

Tulman, L.J. (1985). Mothers' and unrelated persons' initial handling of newborn infants. *Nursing Research, 34,* 205–209 (Structured observation).

White, M.A., Wear, E. & Stephenson, G. (1983). A computer-compatible method for observing falling asleep behavior of hospitalized children. *Research in Nursing and Health, 6,* 191–198 (Structured observation).

Chapter 16
□
*Biophysiological
and other
data collection
methods*

The vast majority of nursing research studies involve the collection of data by means of methods discussed in the preceding chapters — interviews, questionnaires, psychosocial scales, and observational methods. However, there are other methods of measuring research variables of interest to nurse researchers, and several of these are reviewed in this chapter. The most important alternative method is the use of biophysiological instrumentation and apparatus.

□
Biophysiological measures

The trend in nursing research has been toward increased clinical, patient-centered investigations, and this trend is likely to continue in years to come. One result of this trend is expanded use of methods to assess the physiological status of subjects. In this section we discuss a particular class of measures, namely those physiological and physical variables that require specialized technical instruments and equipment for their measurement and, generally, specialized training for the interpretation of results.

Settings in which nurses operate are typically filled with a wide variety of technical instruments for measuring physiological functions. It is beyond the scope of this book to describe in any detail the many kinds of biophysiological measures available to nurse researchers. Our objective is to present an overview of potential criterion measures for clinical nursing studies, to illustrate their usage in a research context, and to direct the interested reader to more comprehensive sources for further information.

Even these objectives are not easily achieved. We have unavoidably omitted many tests and measures that would be of great interest to clinical researchers in nursing. A unique difficulty we faced in preparing this section (as opposed to the previous three chapters) is that here we are concerned with instrument identification as opposed to instrument development. Nurse researchers *do* design their own observational instruments and interview schedules, and it is possible to present general guidelines for developing such measuring tools. It is unlikely that many nurse researchers will develop technical apparatus and electronic instruments. Thus, just as it was impossible to catalogue all available psychosocial instruments, it is likewise impractical to adequately cover all physiological measures. Still, we believe that a consideration of physiological tools is extremely important, and so we have had to accept incompleteness and the inevitability of being outdated by rapid technological advances.

We should also note that a good many clinical variables do not require specialized equipment for their measurement. Data on physiological functioning can often be gathered either by self-report or through direct observation, methods described in previous chapters. For instance, the presence/absence or intensity of physiological activity or dysfunction is often amenable to observational methods. Examples include such phenomena as vomiting, cyanosis, postcardiotomy delirium, edema, and wound status. Other biophysiological data can be gathered by asking people directly. Examples of possible self-report measures include time of first postoperative voiding, assessment of pain, ratings of fatigue, and reports of nausea, to name a few. This section focuses on phenomena that require the use of specialized technical apparatus.

Purposes of using biophysiological measures

Clinical nursing studies often involve specialized equipment and instruments both for creating independent variables (e.g., an intervention using biofeedback equipment) and for measuring dependent variables. For the most part, our discussion focuses on the use of biophysiological measures as dependent variables.

The majority of nursing studies in which biophysiological measures have been used fall into one of four classes. The first involves the study of basic physiological processes that have relevance for nursing care. Such studies often involve subjects who are healthy and normal or some subhuman animal species. For example, Geden (1982) studied the effect of alternative lifting techniques (mechanical lift, rocking axillary, self-lift, shoulder assist, and straight pull) on the energy expenditure of normal subjects. Heitkemper and Marotta (1985) studied the effect of a choline-deficient diet on the enzymes that synthesize and degrade neurotransmitters in the gastrointestinal tract.

A second class of studies includes explorations of the ways in which nursing actions affect the health outcomes of patients. For example, Osborne (1984) investigated whether there were differences in the cardiovascular responses of patients ambulated 32 versus 56 hours after coronary artery bypass surgery. Castle and Osterhout (1974) studied the incidence of urinary tract infection following catheterization.

The third class of studies concerns an evaluation of a specific nursing procedure or intervention. These studies differ from the studies in the preceding class in that they generally involve a hypothesis stating that a new nursing procedure will result in improved biophysiological outcomes among patients. For example, one group of researchers (Clemente *et al.,* 1979) studied the relation between prone immersion physical exercise and respiratory volume in children with cystic fibrosis. Levesque and coworkers (1984) evaluated the recovery outcomes of cholecystectomy patients who participated in a preadmission teaching program.

Finally, a fourth class of studies in which biophysiological measures have been used focuses on the improvement in measuring and recording physiological information that is normally gathered by nurses. For example, Baker and her colleagues (1984) studied the difference in temperature readings taken using mercury-in-glass and electronic thermometers. Tachovsky (1985) compared indirect auscultatory blood pressure measurement at the forearm with measures obtained at the traditional upper arm site.

The physiological phenomena that interest nurse researchers run the full gamut of available measures. Some of these measures are discussed below.

Types of biophysiological measures

Physiological measurements can be classified in one of two major categories. *In vivo* measurements are those that are performed directly within or on living organisms themselves. One example of an *in vivo* measure is blood flow determination through radiography. An *in vitro* measurement, by contrast, is performed outside of the organism's body, as in the case of measuring serum potassium concentration in the blood drawn from a patient.

In vivo measures

In vivo measurements often involve the use of highly complex instrumentation systems. An *instrumentation system* may be defined as the apparatus and equipment used to measure one or more attributes of a subject and the presentation of that measurement data in a manner that humans can interpret. Organism-instrument systems involve up to six major components: subject; stimulus; sensing equipment; signal-conditioning equipment; display equipment; and recording, data processing, and transmission equipment. These components and their interrelationships are presented in Figure 16-1. The role of each component is briefly described below.

1. The Subject: The bodies of humans (and other organisms) consist of chemical, electrical, mechanical, thermal, hydraulic, pneumatic, and other systems interacting with each other and with the outside world. Communication of the human organism with the external environment consists of various inputs (e.g., sensory inputs, inspired air, liquid and food intake) and outputs (e.g., speech, body movements, expired air, wastes). The majority of these inputs and outputs are easily amenable to measurements. The major bodily systems—circulatory, respiratory, and so forth—also communicate with each other internally, as do smaller subsystems, such as organs and cells. Biomedical instrumentation constitute the tools for measuring the information communicated by these diverse elements.

2. The Stimulus: Many physiological measurements require some type of external stimulus. The stimulation may be engendered by another human being, as in the case of requests for deep and rapid breathing by the patient when recording electrical activity from the brain. The stimulus may also be produced by electrical or mechanical equipment, such as an external pacemaker and cardiac defibrillator.

| Stimulus | Subject | Sensing Equipment | Signal Conditioning Equipment | Display Equipment | Recording & Data Processing Equipment |

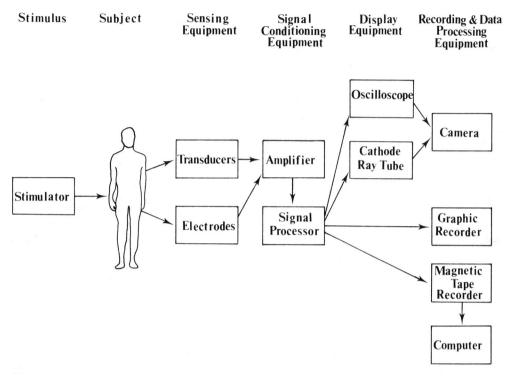

Figure 16-1. Schema of the Organism-Instrument System.

3. The Sensing Equipment: Sensing equipment normally consists of one or more transducers. Generally defined, a *transducer* is a device that converts one form of energy into another. Transducers are used in organism-instrument systems to measure physical phenomena by producing an electrical signal proportional to these phenomena. Electrical signals permit presentations of the desired physiological information in a highly useful form. With an electrical analog of the critical physiological event, the scientist can store the event on magnetic tape for later inspection and analysis.

A few examples of methods used to convert a physiological characteristic into electrical output should suffice to illustrate the underlying principles. A *displacement transducer* converts volume displacement of some element into an electrical signal. A fluid column blood pressure transducer operates on a displacement principle by converting fluid pressure into force, which is then converted to linear displacement. *Temperature transducers* are exemplified by the thermistor, which is an element whose resistance varies proportionately with temperature. To measure *bioelectric potentials* produced by the heart, brain, or other organs, a transducer consisting of two electrodes is used. *Electrodes* are devices for converting bioelectric (ionic) potentials into electronic potentials. In sum, the transducer plays a key role in instrumentation systems designed to make biophysical measurements.

4. Signal-Conditioning Equipment: Signal-conditioning or signal-processing equipment is used to amplify or modify the transducer's electrical signal. Both the input to and the output from signal conditioning equipment are electrical signals. However, the output signal usually is modified in some respect in order to prepare the signals for operating display and recording equipment. Physiological signals acquired by transducers are typically below 10 millivolts in amplitude and must, therefore, be amplified in order to be compatible with display units and recorders. In virtually all physiological measurements, two signals are produced by the subject: the key physiological signal, such as the electrocardiographic signal, and an interference signal. An important function of signal conditioning equipment is to reject the interference signal and to amplify the desired physiological signal.

5. Display Equipment: Display devices convert the modified electrical signals into visual or auditory output. The most common display device is the oscilloscope. An *oscilloscope* is a device that allows for the visual observation of the wave form of a signal. It is used to display and measure the time, phase, voltage, or frequency of a physiological signal. The information is presented on a *cathode-ray tube* (CRT). The face of the display is typically calibrated in centimeters with voltage (amplitude) on the ordinate (the vertical plane) and time on the abscissa (horizontal plane). With sophisticated equipment, a television screen that shows interpretation of the various physiological functions being monitored is often available.

6. Recording, Data Processing, and Transmission Equipment: For research purposes, it is usually necessary to obtain a permanent record of the physiological measurements for subsequent scrutiny and analysis. The recording equipment can either be a unit separate from the display device or integrated with it. A *strip recorder* is an example of a device that both displays electrical potentials and provides a permanent record of them. Other devices supplement oscilloscopes or other display units. For example, a signal may often be stored on magnetic tape. The use of a magnetic tape recorder or other computer-linked equipment has the advantage of permitting information to be transmitted and replayed for convenient and detailed analysis.

Not all instrumentation systems involve all six components. Some systems, such as an electronic thermometer, are quite simple; other systems are extremely complex. For example, there are some electronic monitors that, though they are miniaturized and can be put in place during ambulation, yield simultaneous measures of such physiological variables as cardiac responsivity, respiratory rate and rhythm, core temperature, and muscular activity.

In vivo instruments have been developed to measure all bodily functions, and technological improvements continue to advance our ability to measure biophysiological phenomena more accurately, more conveniently, and more rapidly than ever before. It is not possible to catalogue all such instruments, but Table 16-1 presents a list of some commonly used instruments and the variables they measure, according to six physiological systems.

The uses to which such instruments have been put by nurse researchers is richly diverse and impressive. Table 16-2 presents examples of research questions that have been posed by nurse researchers relating to the six physiological systems, together with a list of the physiological variables measured. Of course, most

Table 16-1
Examples of instruments for in vivo *measurements*

Bodily Function	Variable	Example(s) of Instrumentation
Circulatory	Blood pressure	Sphygmomanometer/stethoscope
	Blood volume	Plethysmograph
	Blood flow velocity	Laser Doppler velocimeter
	Cardiac potential	Electrocardiograph (ECG or EDG); cardiotachometer; cardiac ultrasound Holter monitor
Respiratory	Respiratory volume	Spirometer
	Respiratory air flow	Spirometer; pneumotachometer
	Oxygen consumption	Max Planck respirometer; Douglas bag technique
Neurological	Systemic body temperature	Thermometer; thermo-couple; thermistor
	Skin surface temperature	Infrared thermometer
	Bioelectric brain potential	Electroencephalograph (EEG)
	Tumors	Nuclear magnetic resonance (tomography)
Musculoskeletal	Muscular contractions	Myograph
	Electrical muscular potential	Electromyograph (EMG)
	Muscle tremors	Accelerometer; tromometer
	Muscle strength	Dynamometer
	Motor response	Steadiness tester; pursuit rotor
	Range of motion	Goniometer; actometer
	Reaction time	Chronoscope
Gastrointestinal	Gastric motility	Pressure transducer/Dynograph recorder
	Electrical potential of stomach muscles	Electrogastrograph (EGG)
	Gastrointestinal activity	Endoradiosones
Genitourinary	Renal function	Renoscan
	Renal obstruction	Renal arteriograph

nurse researchers who have gathered physiological data have used data from two or more physiological systems. For example, it is common for nurses to use data on vital signs (temperature, heart rate, blood pressure) in their investigations. It is also common for nurses to combine information from *in vivo* measures with that from *in vitro* measures.

In vitro measures

With *in vitro* measures, data are gathered from subjects by extracting some physiological material from subjects and subjecting it to laboratory analysis. Nurse researchers may or may not be involved in the extraction of the material; however, the analysis is normally done by highly specialized laboratory technicians. Generally, each laboratory establishes normal values for each measurement, and this information is critical for interpreting the results of laboratory tests.

Several classes of laboratory analysis have been used in studies by nurse researchers. These include:

* *Chemical measurements,* such as the measure of hormone levels, sugar levels, or potassium levels;
* *Microbiological measures,* such as bacterial counts and identification; and
* *Cytological or histological measures,* such as tissue biopsies.

Table 16-2
Examples of nursing research studies using in vivo *measures*

Research Problem	Measurements	Reference
What are the effects of position changes on the cerebrovascular status of patients with severe closed head injuries?	Circulatory Function: heart rate; arterial blood pressure; intracranial pressure; cerebral perfusion rate	Parsons & Wilson, 1984
What is the effect of biofeedback training on the respiratory patterns of patients with chronic obstructive pulmonary disease?	Respiratory Function: respiratory rate; tidal volume; alveolar ventilation; end-tidal CO_2; thoracic displacement	Sitzman, Kamiya & Johnston, 1983
What are the physiological effects of physical versus therapeutic touch following exposure to a stressful stimulus?	Neurological Function: peripheral skin temperature; skin conductance levels	Randolph, 1984
Will a hand-positioning device placed in the palm of a patient with nonprogressive brain damage decrease wrist and finger hypertonicity?	Musculoskeletal Function: range of joint mobility; composite extension of hand; grip strength	Jamison & Dayhoff, 1980
What is the effect of nasogastric tube feedings administered at three different temperatures on gastric motility and total gastrointestinal transit time?	Gastrointestinal Function: gastric motility; intragastric pressure	Kagawa-Busby, *et al.,* 1980
What variables are related to the employment potential of patients receiving hemodialysis?	Genitourinary Function: mean arterial pressure	Ferrans & Powers, 1985

Because nurse researchers as a rule are not responsible for the analysis of *in vitro* extractions, it is not necessary to explain relevant instrumentation or procedures; nor is it possible to catalogue the thousands of laboratory tests available. However, to give students a flavor of how *in vitro* measures have been used by nurse researchers, we present some examples in Table 16-3. Laboratory analyses of blood and urine samples are the most frequently used *in vitro* measures in nursing investigations.

Selecting a biophysiological measure

For nurses unfamiliar with the hundreds of biophysiological measures available in institutional settings, the selection of one or more appropriate measures of important research variables may pose a real challenge. There are, unfortunately, no comprehensive handbooks to guide interested researchers to the measures, instruments, and interpretations that might be required in collecting physiological data. Among the best sources of information

Table 16-3
Examples of nursing research studies using in vitro *measures*

Type of Test	Research Problem	Measurement	Reference
Blood tests	· What is the magnitude of changes in hemodynamic and respiratory variables that occur during and after endotracheal suctioning?	Blood gas analysis; acid-base blood	Baun, 1984
	· Does the timing of drawing a blood sample after inserting an intracath affect the accuracy of blood values?	Levels of plasma glucose, plasma insulin, free fatty acid levels	Tallman, 1982
Urine tests	· What is the physiological response of pacemaker implantation?	Levels of urinary cortisol, epinephrine, and norepinephrine	Lanuza & Marotta, 1983
	· Is there a relationship between the degree of circadian alteration in acute-care surgical patients and their reentrainment to typical circadian profiles?	Levels of urinary catecholamine metabolites, adrenal cortical hormones, sodium, potassium, and creatinine	Farr *et al.,* 1984
Sputum culture	· Does the type of tracheotomy care affect postoperative pulmonary infection?	Growth of specific organism changes under normal colonization	Harris & Hyman, 1984
Umbilical cord culture	· Does sibling contact affect the bacterial colonization rates of neonates?	Bacterial colonization rates (*Staphylococcus aureus* and Group B Streptococcus)	Kowba & Schwirian, 1985
Cell histology	· What is the effect of the epidermal growth factor on wound healing in a pig model?	Histologic measurement of the migration of keratinocytes over the wound; rate of differentiation of keratinocytes; mitotic index	Gill & Atwood, 1981

on measures that might be useful are original research articles on a problem similar to your own, a review article on the central phenomenon under investigation, manufacturers' catalogues, and exhibits of manufacturers at professional conferences.

Obviously, the most basic issue to address in selecting a physiological measure is whether the measure will yield good information about the research variable under investigation. In some cases, the researcher will need to consider whether the variable should be measured by observation or self-report instead of (or in addition to) using biophysiological equipment or apparatus. For example, stress could be measured by asking people questions (e.g., using the State–Trait Anxiety Inventory); by observing their behavior during exposure to stressful stimuli; or by measuring heart rate, blood pressure, or levels of ACTH in urine samples.

Several other considerations should be kept in mind in selecting a biophysiological measure, several of which have been noted by Lindsey and Stotts (1985). These include the following:

- Is the equipment and/or laboratory analysis you will need readily available to you? If not, can it be borrowed, rented, or purchased?
- If equipment must be purchased, is it affordable? Can funding be acquired to cover the purchase (or rental) price?
- Can you operate the required equipment and interpret its results, or will you need training? Are there resources available to help you with operation and interpretation?
- Will you encounter any difficulties in obtaining permission to use the necessary equipment from an Institutional Review Board or other institutional authority?
- Does the measure need to be direct (e.g., a direct measure of blood pressure via an arterial line) or is an indirect measure (e.g., blood pressure measurement via a sphygmomanometer) sufficient?
- Will continuous monitoring be necessary (for example, ECG readings) or is a point-in-time measure adequate?
- Will your activities during data collection permit you to be recording data simultaneously or will you need an instrument system with recording equipment (or a research assistant)?

- Will a mechanical stimulus be needed in order to get appropriate or meaningful measurements? Does available equipment include the required stimulus?
- Will a single measure of your dependent variable be sufficient or is it preferable to operationalize your research variable using multiple measures? If multiple measures are better, what burden does this place on you as a researcher and on patients as research subjects?
- Are your measures likely to be influenced by reactivity (i.e., the subjects' awareness of their subject status)? If so, can alternative or supplementary nonreactive measures be identified, or can the extent of reactivity bias be assessed?
- Can your research variable be measured using a noninvasive procedure or is an invasive procedure required?
- Is the measure you plan to use sufficiently accurate and sensitive to variation?
- Are you thoroughly familiar with rules and safety precautions, such as grounding procedures, especially when using electrical equipment?

The difficulty in choosing biophysiological measures for nursing research investigations lies not in their shortage, or in their questionable utility, or in their inferiority to other methods. Indeed they are plentiful, often highly reliable and valid, and extremely useful in clinical nursing studies. However, great care must be exercised in selecting appropriate instruments or laboratory analyses with regard to practical, ethical, medical, and technical considerations.

Evaluation of physiological measures

A major strength of physiological measures is their objectivity. Objectivity refers to the degree of agreement between the final "scores" assigned by two independent observers. Nurse A and Nurse B, reading from the same spirometer output, are likely to record the same or highly similar tidal volume measurements for a patient. Furthermore, barring the possibility of equipment malfunctioning, two different spirometers are likely to produce identical tidal volume readouts.

Another advantage of physiological measurements is the relative precision and sensitivity that they normally offer. By "relative," we are implicitly comparing physiological instruments with devices for obtaining various psychological measurements, such as self-report measures of anxiety, pain, attitudes, and so forth. Patients are unlikely to be able to deliberately distort measurements of physiological functioning. Furthermore, researchers are generally quite confident that physiological instrumentation provides measures of those variables in which they are interested: thermometers can be depended upon to measure temperature and not blood volume, and so forth. This characteristic may seem so obvious as to render its mention unnecessary. However, for nonphysiological measurements, the question of whether a measuring tool is really measuring the target concept is a continuously perplexing problem.

In comparison with other types of data collection tools, the equipment for obtaining physiological measurements is rather costly. However, because such equipment is generally available in hospital settings, the costs to nurse researchers may be quite small or nonexistent.

Physiological measures also have some disadvantages. For example, the highly technical nature of the equipment may constitute a difficulty, because the failure of nonengineers to understand the limitations of the instruments may result in greater faith in their accuracy than is warranted.

A problem that physiological measures share with other data collection approaches is the effect that the measuring tool itself has on the variables it is attempting to measure. The presence of a sensing device such as a transducer can change the variable of interest. For instance, a flow transducer located in a blood vessel partially blocks that vessel and, hence, alters the pressure-flow characteristics being measured. Some researchers have erroneously assumed that physiological measures are unobtrusive, based upon the argument that the patients are unaware of the research purposes to which the measurements will be applied. From the body's point of view, however, physiological measures are rarely unobtrusive.

Another difficulty is that there are normally interferences that create artifacts in physiological measurements. For example, "noise" generated within a measuring instrument interferes with the signal being produced. The subject may also create artifactual signals, particularly when the subject's movements result in movements of the sensing devices. Many transducers are highly sensitive to motion and may produce signal variations that confound or obscure variations from the critical variable.

Despite the presentation in Tables 16-1 and 16-2 in terms of bodily functions, there is clearly a high degree of interaction among the major physiological systems. These interrelationships can result in problems if the stimulation of one system leads to responses in other systems. Sometimes such responses are unpredictable and poorly understood, resulting in a confounding of effects that are difficult to unravel. Measuring devices themselves can produce interactions in other systems.

Energy must often be applied to the organism when making the physiological measurements. The energy requirements mean that extreme caution must continually be exercised to avoid the risk of damaging cells by high energy concentrations. Any researcher utilizing electrical equipment should be thoroughly familiar with safety rules and considerations such as grounding specifications.

Research example

Baun and her colleagues (1984) explored whether a human/pet bond can have positive physiological effects on people. They noted that there has been much speculation but little empirical evidence that human/pet bonding can have therapeutic effects that would be especially helpful with certain types of populations, such as nursing home residents, children undergoing psychiatric care, and residents in extended-care facilities. To investigate this issue, they designed an experiment, using a repeated measures design, in which 24 healthy subjects were exposed, in a randomized sequence, to three 9-minute conditions. The three conditions were: (1) quiet reading of a magazine; (2) petting an unknown dog; and (3) petting their own dog. Three physiological measures were used to evaluate the subjects' well-being during the experimental procedures. Blood pressures were measured at 3-minute intervals by use of an electronic blood pressure instrument. Heart rates were measured by three electrodes placed posteriorly over the upper back and recorded continuously. Respiratory rate was measured by a respiration transducer placed in the subject's nostril and recorded continuously. It was found that the protocol in which subjects petted their own dogs exhibited the greatest blood pressure decreases over time.

□
Records and available data

Thus far we have examined a number of data collection strategies for which it was assumed that the researcher would be responsible for actually collecting the data and, in some cases, developing the data collection instruments. However, it is not always necessary for a researcher to collect fresh data. A wealth of data is gathered for nonresearch purposes and can be fruitfully exploited to answer research questions. Nurse researchers are particularly fortunate in the amount and quality of existing data available to them for exploration. Hospital records, patient charts, physicians' order sheets, care plan statements, nursing students' grades, NLN examination scores, and so forth, all constitute rich data sources to which nurse researchers may have access.

Data sources

The places where a nurse researcher is likely to find useful records are too numerous to list here, but a few suggestions might be helpful. Within a hospital or other health care setting, excellent records are kept routinely and systematically. In addition to medical records, hospitals maintain financial records, personnel records, nutritional records, and so forth. Educational institutions maintain records of varying quality. Most schools of nursing have permanent files on their students. Public school systems also keep records, but the smaller school systems are less likely to keep extensive and accurate records than the larger ones. Industries and businesses normally maintain a variety of records that might interest industrial nurse researchers, such as information on employees' absenteeism, health status, on-the-job accidents, job performance ratings, alcoholism or drug problems, and so forth. The state and federal governments also maintain records that have been used frequently by researchers. In addition to institutional records, personal documents such as diaries and letters should be considered as possible data sources.

Advantages and disadvantages of using records

The use of information from records is advantageous to the researcher for several reasons. The most salient advantage of existing records is that they are an economical source of information. The collection of data is often the most time-consuming and costly step in the research process. The use of preexisting records also permits an examination of trends over time, if the information is of the type that is collected repeatedly. Problems of reactivity and response biases may be completely absent when the researcher obtains information from records. Furthermore, the investigator does not have to be concerned with obtaining cooperation from participants.

On the other hand, because the researcher has not been responsible for the collection and recording of information, he or she may be unaware of the limitations, biases, or incompleteness of the records. Two of the major sources of biases in records are *selective deposit* and *selective survival.* If the records available for use do not constitute the entire set of all *possible* such records, the investigator must somehow deal with the question of how representative the existing records are. Many record keepers intend to maintain an entire universe or set of records rather than a sample but may fail to adhere to this ideal. The lapses from the ideal may be the result of some systematic biases, and the careful researcher should attempt to learn just what those biases might be.

An additional problem with which researchers must contend is the increasing reluctance of institutions to make their records available for scientific studies. The Privacy Act, a federal regulation enacted to protect individuals against possible misuses of records, has made hospitals, agencies, schools, and industrial organizations sensitive to the possibility of legal action from individuals who feel that their right to privacy has been violated. The major issue here is the divulgence of an individual's identity. If records are maintained with an identifying number rather than a name, permission to use the records may be readily granted. However, most institutions *do* maintain records by their clients' names. In such a situation the researcher may need the assistance of personnel at the institution in order to maintain client anonymity, and some organizations may be unwilling to use their personnel for such purposes.

A number of other difficulties in the use of records for research purposes may be relevant. Sometimes the records have to be verified in terms of their authenticity, authorship, or accuracy, a task that may be difficult to execute if the records are old. The researcher using records must be prepared to deal with forms and file systems that he or she does not understand. Codes and symbols that had meaning to the record keeper may have to be "translated" in order to be usable. In using records to study trends, the researcher should always be alert to the possibility of changes in record-keeping procedures. For example, does a dramatic increase or decrease in the incidence of sudden infant death syndrome reflect changes in the causes or cures of this problem, or does it reflect a change in diagnosis or record keeping?

These considerations suggest that, while existing records may be plentiful, inexpensive, and accessible, they should not be used without paying attention to potential problems and weaknesses.

Research example

Harris and Hyman (1984) used records from ten hospitals to study whether clean tracheotomy care is more effective than sterile tracheotomy care in terms of levels of postoperative pulmonary infection. Ten hospitals with Head and Neck/ENT services in four states

Table 16-4
Example of a distribution of Q sort cards

	Approve of Least								Approve of Most
Category	1	2	3	4	5	6	7	8	9
Number of cards	2		4	7	10	14	10	7	4	2

were selected as the data collection sites. From each hospital, a minimum of 15 patient charts were selected and formed the study sample. The investigators abstracted information from the patients' charts and entered pertinent data into a recording instrument, the Weighted Level of Pulmonary Infection Tool. The instrument consisted of laboratory and clinical parameters that have been used to define pulmonary infection. The instrument could be scored to create level of pulmonary clinical, laboratory, and total infection scores. The variables in the instrument were weighted to give heavier weights to more objective criteria. Among the ten hospitals, three categories of aseptic type emerged: clean, sterile, and mixed. The results indicated no differences among the three aseptic types with regard to clinical data. However, the laboratory data from the records indicated that practicing clean procedures was associated with the lowest level of postoperative infection.

□
Q methodology

Q methodology is the term used by William Stephenson to refer to a constellation of substantive, statistical, and psychometric concepts relating to research on individuals. Q methodology utilizes a procedure known as the *Q sort,* which involves the sorting of a deck of cards according to specified criteria.

Q sort procedures

In a Q sort, the subject is presented with a set of cards on which words, phrases, statements, or other messages are written. The subject is then asked to sort the cards according to a particular dimension, such as approval/disapproval, most like me/least like me, or highest priority/lowest priority. The number of cards to be sorted is typically between 60 and 100. Usually, the subject sorts the cards into 9 or 11 piles, with the number of cards placed in each pile determined by the researcher. A common practice is to have the subjects distribute the cards such that fewer cards are placed at either of the two extremes and more cards are placed toward the middle. Table 16-4 shows a hypothetical distribution of 60 cards, with the specification of the number of cards to be placed in each of the nine piles.

The sorting instructions as well as the objects to be sorted in a Q sort investigation vary according to the requirements of the research. Attitudes can be studied by asking subjects to sort statements in terms of agreement and disagreement or approval and disapproval. The researcher can study personality by developing cards on which personality characteristics are described. The subject can then be requested to sort items on a "very-much-like-me/not-at-all-like-me" continuum. Self-concept can be explored by comparing responses to this "like me" dimension to responses elicited when the instructions are to sort cards according to what subjects consider ideal personality traits. Q sorts can be used to great advantage in studying individuals in depth. For example, subjects could be asked to sort traits as they apply to themselves in different roles such as employee, parent, spouse, friend, and so forth. The technique can also be used to gain information concerning how individuals see themselves, as they perceive others see them, as they believe others would like them to be, and so forth. Other applications include asking patients to rate nursing behaviors on a continuum of most helpful/ least helpful; asking nursing students to rate aspects of their educational preparation along a most useful/least useful continuum; and asking primiparas to rate various aspects of their labor and delivery experience in terms of a most problematic/least problematic dimension.

The number of cards in a Q sort varies according to the research problem. However, it is unwise to use fewer than 50 or 60 items, because it is difficult to achieve stable and reliable results with a smaller number. On the other hand, 100 to 200 cards are normally considered the upper limit, inasmuch as the task becomes tedious and difficult with larger numbers.

The analysis of data obtained through Q sorts is a somewhat controversial matter. The options range from the most elementary, descriptive statistical procedures such as rank orderings, averages, and percentages to highly complex procedures such as factor analysis. Factor analysis, a procedure designed to reveal the underlying dimensions or common elements in a set of items, is described in Chapter 22. Some researchers insist that factor analysis is essential in the analysis of Q sort data.

Evaluation of Q methodology

Q methodology can be a powerful methodological tool but, like other data collection techniques, has a number of drawbacks as well. On the plus side, we have seen that Q sorts are extremely versatile and can be applied to a wide variety of problems. Unlike many other clinical approaches, we find in Q methodology an objective and (usually) reliable procedure for the intensive study of an individual. Q sorts have been used effectively to study the progress of people during different phases of therapy, particularly psychotherapy. The requirement that individuals place a predetermined number of cards in each pile virtually eliminates response set biases that often characterize responses to written scale items. Furthermore, the task of sorting cards is often more agreeable to subjects than completing a paper-and-pencil instrument.

On the other hand, it is difficult and time-consuming to administer Q sorts to a large sample of individuals. Without a sizeable sample, it becomes problematic to generalize the results of the study. The sampling problem is further compounded by the fact that Q sorts cannot normally be administered by the mail, thereby causing difficulties in obtaining a geographically diverse sample of subjects. Some critics have argued that the forced procedure of distributing cards according to the researcher's specifications is artificial and actually excludes information concerning how the subjects would ordinarily distribute their opinions.

Another criticism of Q sort data relates to permissible statistical operations. Most statistical tests and procedures assume that responses to items are independent of one another. Likert-type scales exemplify items that are totally independent: a person's response of agree/disagree to one item does not in any way restrict responses to other items. Techniques of this type are known as *normative measures*. Normative measures can be interpreted by comparing individual scores to the average score for a group. The Q sort technique is a forced-choice procedure, wherein a person's response to one item depends upon, and is restricted by, responses to other items. Referring to Table 16-4, a respondent who has already placed two cards in Category 1 ("approve of least") is not free to place another item in this same category.* Such forced-choice approaches produce what is known as *ipsative measures.* With ipsative measures, the average of a group is not a relevant point of comparison, since the average is identical for all individuals. With a nine-category Q sort such as shown in Table 16-4, the average "value" of the sorted cards will always be five. (The average value of a *particular item* can be meaningfully computed and compared among individuals or groups, however.) Strictly speaking, ordinary statistical tests of significance are not appropriate for use with nonindependent ipsative measures. In practice, many researchers feel that the violation of assumptions in applying standard statistical procedures to Q sort data is not a serious transgression, particularly if the number of items is large.

Research example

Freihofer and Felton (1976) used the Q sort to ascertain the nursing behaviors most and least desired by family members or significant others of dying patients. From a total of 125 statements concerning nursing behaviors obtained through a search of the literature, 37 were eliminated following a pretest because of redundancy or ambiguity. The sample consisted of 25 relatives or close friends of persons dying in a particular hospital. The investigators gave each respondent 88 typed cards, each of which contained a nursing behavior. Respondents were also given a set of written instructions and a video cassette demonstra-

tion tape on the use of the Q sort. The study participants were asked to sort the 88 statements into nine piles according to desirableness of nursing behavior in each statement. The subjects sorted the cards so that pile five (the middle pile) contained the most statements with subsequent decrease in the number of statements placed in piles as he or she progressed to pile one and pile nine. Following completion of the card sort, each statement was scored according to its pile placement. For instance, if statement six was placed in pile three, it was given a score of 3. Each subject's sort of each statement was recorded, and the average for each statement was computed for the total group of subjects.

The findings revealed that the most desired nursing behaviors included keeping the patient free from pain, physically comfortable, and well-groomed and allowing the patient to do as much for herself/himself as possible. The least desired nursing behaviors included encouraging the family member to cry, holding the family member's hand, crying with the family member, and telling the loved one that the suffering would soon be over.

☐ Delphi technique

The method known as the Delphi technique was developed by a research and development organization (the Rand Corporation) as a tool for short-term forecasting. This technique uses self-report questionnaires, but the procedures for data collection and analysis differ from normal survey procedures.

Delphi procedures

The Delphi technique requires the cooperation of a panel of experts who are asked to complete a series of questionnaires. The information solicited in the instruments typically relates to the expert's opinions, predic-

---

* Subjects are usually told, however, that they can move cards around from one pile to another until the desired distribution is obtained.

tions, or judgment concerning a specific topic of interest. The Delphi technique differs from other surveys in several respects. First, the Delphi technique consists of several rounds of questionnaires. Each of the cooperating experts is asked to complete four or more instruments. This multiple iteration approach is employed as a means of effecting group consensus of opinion — without the necessity of face-to-face committee work. A second feature is the use of feedback to members of the panel. Responses to each round of questionnaires are analyzed, summarized, and returned to the experts with a new questionnaire. The experts can then reformulate their opinions with the knowledge of the group's viewpoint in mind. The process of response-analysis-feedback-response usually is repeated three times until a general consensus is obtained.

Evaluation of the Delphi technique

The Delphi technique is a relatively efficient and effective method of combining the expertise of a large group of individuals in order to obtain information for planning and prediction purposes. The experts are spared the necessity of being brought together for a formal confrontation, thus saving considerable time and expense for the panel members. Another advantage is that any one persuasive or prestigious expert cannot have an undue influence on the opinions of others. Each panel member is on an equal footing with all others. Anonymity probably encourages a greater frankness of opinion than might be expressed in a formal meeting. The feedback-response loops allow for multichanneled communication without any risk of the members being sidetracked from their mission.

At the same time, it must be conceded that the Delphi technique is both costly and time-consuming for the researcher. Experts must be solicited, questionnaires prepared and mailed, responses analyzed, results summarized, new questionnaires prepared, and so forth. The cooperation of the panel members may wane in later rounds of the questionnaire mailings. The problem of sample bias through nonresponse is a constant threat, though probably less severe than through ordinary questionnaire procedures. On the whole, the Delphi technique represents a significant methodological tool for solving problems, planning, and forecasting.

Research example

Lindeman (1975) conducted a study using the Delphi technique to ascertain priorities in nursing research. Four rounds of questionnaires were mailed to 433 panel members, a group identified by professional nursing organizations and funding agencies as being knowledgeable about nursing practice and research. Of the original 433 panel members, 341 members responded to all four rounds of questionnaires. The first questionnaire asked members to identify five areas in which nursing research was urgently needed. The respondents identified over 2000 items from which the research team chose the 150 items most frequently mentioned. These 150 items comprised the base of the second questionnaire in which respondents were asked to indicate whether nursing should take leadership for research in the area, the value of the item for the nursing profession, and the impact the item has on patient welfare. An example of an item was "Ascertain effective methods to prevent diaper rash." The second questionnaire was analyzed by the research team for summary statistics, such as average response and range of responses.

The third questionnaire that was sent to the panel members contained the summary statistics as well as each individual panel member's response to the items. During the administration of the third questionnaire, panel members were asked to write comments about their choice if their choices were substantially different from the summary statistics. Round four of the questionnaire contained summarization of round three questionnaires as well as the written comments (considered a minority report) obtained in round three.

Analysis of the results revealed that the following areas received the highest priority in terms of value for the profession: research concerning the nursing process, the research process, and the development of instruments to measure quality nursing care. Patient education, the alleviation of pain, and the development of indicators measuring quality nursing care received high priority in relation to the impact of patient care question.

☐
Projective techniques

Questionnaires, interview schedules, and psychological tests and scales normally depend on the respondents' capacity for self-insight or willingness to share personal information with the researcher. *Projective techniques* include a variety of methods for obtaining psychological measures with only a minimum of cooperation required of the person. Projective methods give free play to the subjects' imagination and fantasies by providing them with a task that permits an almost unlimited number and variety of responses. The rationale underlying the use of projective techniques is that the manner in which a person organizes and reacts to unstructured stimuli is a reflection of the person's needs, motives, attitudes, values, or personality characteristics. A stimulus of low structure is sufficiently ambiguous that respondents can "read in" their own interpretations and in this way provide the researcher with information about their perception of the world. In other words, people project part of

themselves into their interaction with phenomena, and projective techniques represent a means of taking advantage of this fact.

Types of projective techniques

Projective techniques are highly flexible, since virtually any unstructured stimuli or situation can be used to induce projective behaviors. One class of projective methods utilizes pictorial materials. One particularly useful *pictorial device* is the Thematic Apperception Test (TAT). The TAT materials consist of 20 cards that contain pictures. The subject is requested to make up a story for each picture, inventing an explanation of what led up to the event shown, what is happening at the moment, what the characters are feeling and thinking, and what kind of outcome will result. The responses are then scored according to some scheme for the variables of interest to the researchers. The TAT and other similar instruments have been used in a variety of contexts. Variables that have been measured by TAT-type pictures are achievement motivation, need for affiliation, parent-child relations, attitude toward minority groups, creativity, religious commitment, attitude toward authority, and fear of success.

Verbal projective techniques present subjects with an ambiguous verbal stimulus rather than a pictorial one. Verbal methods can be categorized into two classes, according to the type of response elicited—association techniques and completion techniques. *Word-association methods* present subjects with a series of words, to which subjects respond with the first thing that comes to mind. The word list often combines both neutral and emotionally tinged words, which are included for the purpose of detecting impaired thought processes or internal conflicts. The word-association technique has also been used to study creativity, interests, and attitudes.

The most common completion technique is *sentence completion.* The person is supplied with a set of incomplete sentences and is asked to complete them in any desired manner. This approach is frequently used as a method of measuring attitudes or some aspect of personality. Some examples of incomplete sentences include the following:

When I think of a nurse practitioner I think . . .
The thing I most admire about nurses is . . .
A good nurse should always . . .

The sentence stems are designed to elicit responses toward some attitudinal object or event in which the investigator is interested. Responses are typically categorized or rated according to a prespecified plan.

A third class of projective measures falls into a category known as *expressive methods.* These techniques encourage self-expression, in most cases through the construction of some product out of raw materials. The major expressive methods are play techniques, drawing and painting, and role-playing. The assumption is that people express their feelings, needs, motives, and emotions by working with or manipulating various materials.

Evaluation of projective measures

Projective measures are among the most controversial in the behavioral sciences. Critics point out that projective techniques are, by and large, incapable of being scored objectively. A high degree of inference is required in gleaning information from projective tests, and the quality of the data is heavily dependent upon the sensitivity and interpretive skill of the investigator or analyst. It has been pointed out that the interpretation of the responses by the researcher is almost as pro-

jective as the subjects' reactions to original stimuli.

Another problem with projective techniques is that there have been difficulties in demonstrating that they are, in fact, measuring the variables that they purport to measure. If a pictorial device is used to score aggressive expressions, can the researcher be confident that individual differences in aggressive responses really reflect underlying differences in aggressiveness?

Projective techniques have supporters as well as critics in the research community. People have advocated using projective devices, arguing that they probe the unconscious mind, encompass the whole personality, and provide data of a breadth and depth unattainable by more traditional methods. One useful feature of projective instruments is that they are less susceptible to faking than self-report measures. Another strength is that it is often easier to build rapport and gain the subject's interest with a projective measure than with a questionnaire or scale. Finally, some projective techniques are particularly useful with special groups, such as children or persons with speech and hearing defects. Nevertheless, the use of projective techniques for research applications appears to be associated with more disadvantages than advantages.

Research example

Wood (1983) used an expressive projective technique to ascertain what children perceived as the causes of illness. Sixty-five healthy children were shown a series of seven pictures relating to illness. Each picture had an introductory statement that concluded with a question to the children. One picture, for example, showed a girl holding her stomach as she approached her mother. The introductory statement was "Mary has a stomach ache. She is coming to her mother and her mother asks her: 'What do you suppose made it hurt?' What does Mary tell her?" (p. 102).

The children's responses were recorded verbatim and later analyzed and coded according to five categories of causation: outside force, self, traumatic injury, physiologic causes, and uncrystallized ideas. The researcher and another pediatric nurse independently coded each answer and found a 95 percent level of agreement in their coding. Findings from the study revealed that the most frequently perceived cause of illness by the children was self followed by physiologic, outside forces, trauma, and uncrystallized reasons.

□

Vignettes

The final data collection alternative we will examine are called vignettes.

The uses of vignettes

Vignettes are brief (usually no more than one page) descriptions of an event or situation to which respondents are asked to react. The descriptions can either be fictitious or based on fact, but are always structured to elicit information about respondents' perceptions, opinions, or knowledge about some phenomenon under study. The questions posed to respondents following the vignettes may either be open-ended (e.g., How would you recommend handling this situation?) or closed-ended (e.g., On the nine-point scale below, rate how well you believe that nurse in this story handled the situation.). Normally, the number of vignettes included in a study ranges from four to ten.

The purpose of the study in which vignettes are used is sometimes not revealed to subjects.

This technique has sometimes been used as an indirect measure of attitudes, prejudices, and stereotypes through the use of embedded or hidden descriptors. For example, a researcher interested in exploring attitudes toward, or stereotypes of, male nurses could present subjects with a series of vignettes describing fictitious individuals in terms of, say, their education, family, interests, and so forth. The key vignette would describe a nurse. Half of the subjects would be told the nurse was male and the other half would be told the character was female. The subjects could then be asked to describe the fictitious nurse in terms of likableness, friendliness, cheerfulness, effectiveness, and so forth. Any differences in the subjects' descriptions presumably result from attitudes toward appropriate sex-role behavior.

Evaluation of vignettes

Vignettes are often an economical means of eliciting information about how people might behave in situations that would be difficult to observe in daily life. For example, we might want to assess how patients would react to or feel about nurses with different types of personalities and personal styles of interaction. In clinical settings, it would be difficult to expose patients to many different nurses, all of whom have been evaluated as having different personalities. Another advantage of vignettes is that it is possible to experimentally manipulate the stimuli (the vignettes) by randomly assigning vignettes to groups, as in the above example about male nurses. Furthermore, vignettes often represent an interesting task for subjects. Finally, vignettes can be incorporated into mailed questionnaires and are therefore an inexpensive data collection strategy.

Vignettes are handicapped by some of the same problems as other self-report techniques. The principal problem is that of response biases. If a respondent describes how he or she would react in a situation portrayed in the vignette, how accurate is that description of the respondent's actual behavior? Thus, although the use of vignettes can be profitable, researchers should consider how to minimize or at least assess potential response biases.

Research example

Flaskerud (1984) used vignettes to explore cultural and role differences in perceptions of problematic behavior. She incorporated ten vignettes into an interview schedule that was administered to members of six different minority groups (Chinese-Americans, Mexican-Americans, Filipino-Americans, Native-Americans, Black Americans, and Appalachians) and to mental health professionals in three states. The ten vignettes each told in lay language a short fictitious story of a person experiencing problems. Following each vignette, respondents were asked three questions: 1) What do you think of this person's behavior? 2) Do you think anything should be done about it? and 3) If so, what? None of the vignettes or questions specifically suggested a mental illness or a psychiatric treatment response. The analyses of responses indicated substantial differences between minority and mental health professionals, both in the labels attached to the problematic behaviors and in the recommended strategy for managing the behaviors. The mental health professionals tended to perceive the behaviors as symptoms of mental illness and advised psychiatric treatment. The minority groups "viewed the behavior from a broader perspective that encompassed spiritual, moral, somatic, psychological, and metaphysical components" (p. 196). The investigator concluded that health professionals need to be sensitive to culturally relevant explanations of behavior and should design culture-compatible interventions.

☐ Summary

This chapter reviewed several data collection strategies that are used less frequently than those described in the preceding three chapters. Although these techniques are not especially common, they may be the best choice for certain research problems. This is especially true for the first group of methods examined, biophysiological measures.

The trend in nursing research is toward increasing numbers of clinical, patient-centered investigations in which biophysiological indicators of patients' health status are used as dependent variables. Although it is beyond the scope of this book to describe physiological equipment in detail, many examples of instruments and laboratory tests used in nursing studies were described. Particular attention was paid to the *instrumentation systems* used for *in vivo measurements* (those performed within or on living organisms). The components of an organism-instrument system are the subject, stimulus, sensing equipment, signal conditioning equipment, display equipment, and recording equipment. Examples of instrumentation used to assess the functioning of six bodily systems were presented. Blood tests and urine tests are the most frequently used *in vitro measurements* (those performed outside the organism's body), but examples of other chemical, microbiological, and histological analyses were described. Despite the clear-cut utility of biophysiological measures for nursing science, great care must be taken in selecting such measures with regard to practical, technical, and ethical considerations.

One of the greatest advantages of using physiological measures is their objectivity and validity. Independent researchers are apt to obtain the same results using the same measure. Disadvantages associated with the use of physiological instrumentation are malfunctioning of the equipment and artifacts that interfere with the system. The nurse researcher must exercise extreme caution when electrical equipment is used to collect physiological measurements and must be assured that appropriate safety rules and grounding specifications are followed.

Existing *records* are often used by researchers in the conduct of scientific investigations. Such records provide an economical source of information. In using records, the researcher should try to determine how representative and accurate they are.

Q methodology involves having the subject sort a set of statements into piles according to specified criteria. Attitudes, personality, and self-concept are some of the traits that may be measured by Q methodology. The procedure may be used to study an individual in depth or to rate groups of individuals. One limitation in using Q sorts is that it produces *ipsative measures* wherein the average across cards is not a relevant basis of comparison, inasmuch as the forced-choice approach produces the same average for all subjects. This differs from other techniques that produce *normative measures* because each choice is independent of other choices.

The *Delphi technique* is a method in which several rounds of questionnaires are mailed to a panel of experts. Feedback from previous questionnaires is provided with each new questionnaire. This technique is used for problem solving, planning, and forecasting.

Projective techniques encompass a variety of data collection methods that rely upon the subject's projection of psychological traits or states in response to vaguely structured stimuli. *Pictorial methods* present a picture or cartoon and ask the subject to describe what is happening, what led up to the event, or what kind of action is needed. *Verbal methods* present the subject with an ambiguous verbal stimulus rather than a picture. The two categories of verbal methods are *word association* and *sentence completion. Expressive methods* take the form of *play, drawing,* or *role playing.*

Vignettes are brief descriptions of some event, person, or situation to which respondents are asked to react. Vignettes are often incorporated into questionnaires or interview schedules. They may be used to assess respondents' hypothetical behaviors, opinions, and perceptions.

□
Study suggestions

1. Formulate a research problem in which each of the following could be used as the measurements for the dependent variable:
   a. Blood pressure
   b. Electromyograms
   c. Thermograms
   d. Blood sugar levels
2. Identify some of the *in vivo* or *in vitro* measures you might use to address the following research questions:
   a. Does clapping the lungs prior to suctioning result in better patient outcomes than suctioning without clapping?
   b. What is the effect of various bed positions on the development of respiratory acidosis or alkalosis?
   c. What are the cardiovascular effects of administering liquid potassium chloride in three different solutions (orange juice, fruit punch, cranberry juice)?
   d. What is the rate of respiratory increase for designated decreases in the *p*H level of cerebrospinal fluid?
3. Suppose that you were interested in studying the following variables: professionalism in nurses, fear of death in patients, achievement motivation in nursing stu-

dents, job satisfaction among industrial nurses, fathers' reactions to their newborn infants, and patients' needs for affiliation. Describe at least two ways of collecting data relating to these concepts, using the following approaches:

a. Vignettes
b. Verbal projective techniques
c. Pictorial projective techniques
d. Records
e. Q sorts

☐
Suggested readings

Methodological references

Biophysiological references

Abbey, J. (Guest Ed.). (1978). Symposium on bioinstrumentation for nurses. *Nursing Clinics of North America, 13,* 561–640.

Bauer, J.D., Ackermann, P.G. and Toro, G. (1982). *Clinical laboratory methods* (9th ed.). St. Louis: C.V. Mosby.

Cromwell, L., Weibell, F.J. & Pfeiffer, E.A. (1980). *Biomedical instrumentation and measurements* (2nd ed.). Englewood Cliffs, NJ: Prentice-Hall.

Ferris, C.D. (1980). *Guide to medical laboratory instruments.* Boston: Little, Brown & Company.

Lindsey, A.M. & Stotts, N.A. (1985). Collecting data on biophysiologic variables. In H.S. Wilson, *Research in Nursing.* Menlo Park, CA: Addison-Wesley.

Lindsey, A.M. (1984). Research for clinical practice: Physiological phenomena. *Heart & Lung, 13,* 496–507.

Weiss, M.D. (1973). *Biomedical instrumentation.* Philadelphia: Chilton Book Company.

Widmann, F.K. (1983). *Clinical interpretation of laboratory tests* (9th ed.). Philadelphia: F.A. Davis.

Other data collection methods

Anastasi, A. (1982). *Psychological testing* (5th ed.). New York: Macmillan (Chapter 19).

Angell, R.C. & Freedman, R. (1953). The use of documents, records, census materials, and indices. In L. Festinger & D. Katz (Eds.), *Research methods in the behavioral sciences.* New York: Holt, Rinehart & Winston (pp. 300–326).

Block, J. (1961). *The Q-Sort method in personality assessment and psychiatric research.* Springfield, IL: Charles C. Thomas.

Couper, M.R. (1984). The Delphi technique: Characteristics and sequence model. *Advances in Nursing Science, 7,* 72–77.

Flaskerud, J.H. (1979). Use of vignettes to elicit responses toward broad concepts. *Nursing Research, 28,* 210–212.

Kerlinger, F.N. (1973). *Foundations of behavioral research* (2nd. ed.). New York: Holt, Rinehart & Winston (Chapters 30 & 34).

Linstone, H. & Turoff, M. (1975). *The Delphi technique and applications.* Reading, MA: Addison-Wesley.

Semeomoff, B. (1976). *Projective techniques.* New York: John Wiley & Sons.

Stephenson, W. (1975). *The study of behavior: Q technique and its methodology.* Chicago: University of Chicago Press.

Waltz, C.F., Strickland, O.L. & Lenz, E.R. (1984). *Measurement in nursing research.* Philadelphia: F.A. Davis (Chapter 9).

Wittenborn, J. (1961). Contributions and current status of Q methodology. *Psychological Bulletin, 58,* 132–142.

Substantive references

Biophysiological studies

Baker, N.C. *et al.* (1984). The effect of type of thermometer and length of time inserted on oral temperature measurements of afebrile subjects. *Nursing Research, 33,* 109–111.

Baun, M.M. (1984). Physiological determinants of a clinically successful method of endotracheal suctioning. *Western Journal of Nursing Research, 6,* 213–225.

Baun, M.M. *et al.* (1984). Physiological effects of human/companion animal bonding. *Nursing Research, 33,* 126–129.

Castle, M. & Osterhout, S. (1974). Urinary tract catheterization and associated infection. *Nursing Research, 23,* 170–174.

Clemente, M., Jankowski, L.W. & Beaudry, P.H. (1979). Prone immersion physical exercise in three children with cystic fibrosis: A pilot study. *Nursing Research, 28,* 325–329.

Farr, L. *et al.* (1984). Alterations in circadian excretion of urinary variables and physiological indicators of stress following surgery. *Nursing Research, 33,* 140–146.

Ferrans, C. & Powers, M. (1985). The employment potential of hemodialysis patients. *Nursing Research, 34,* 273–277.

Geden, E.A. (1982). Effects of lifting techniques on energy expenditure. *Nursing Research, 31,* 214–218.

Gill, B.P. & Atwood, J.R. (1981). Reciprocy and helicy used to relate mEGF and wound healing. *Nursing Research, 30,* 68–72.

Harris, R.B. & Hyman, R.B. (1984). Clean vs. sterile tracheotomy care and level of pulmonary infection. *Nursing Research, 33,* 80–85.

Heitkemper, M.M. & Marotta, S.F. (1985). Role of diets in modifying gastrointestinal neurotransmitter enzyme activity. *Nursing Research, 34,* 19–23.

Jamison, S.L. & Dayhoff, N.E. (1980). A hard hand-positioning device to decrease wrist and finger hypertonicity. *Nursing Research, 29,* 285–289.

Kagawa-Busby, K.S. *et al.* (1980). Effects of diet temperature on tolerance of enteral feedings *Nursing Research, 29,* 276–280.

Kowba, M.D. & Schwirian, P.M. (1985). Direct sibling contact and bacterial colonization in newborns. *Journal of Obstetric Gynecologic, & Neonatal Nursing, 14,* 418–423.

Lanuza, D.M. & Marotta, S.F. (1983). Psychoendocrine response to pacemaker implantation. *Proceedings of the 1983 Conference of Western Society for Research in Nursing,* p. 76.

Levesque, L. *et al.* (1984). Evaluation of a presurgical group program given at two different times. *Research in Nursing and Health, 7,* 227–236.

Osborne, D. (1984). Cardiovascular responses of patients ambulated 32 and 56 hours after coronary artery bypass surgery. *Western Journal of Nursing Research, 6,* 321–324.

Parsons, L.C. & Wilson, M.M. (1984). Cerebrovascular status of severe closed head injured patients following passive position changes. *Nursing Research, 33,* 68–75.

Randolph, G. (1984). Therapeutic and physical touch: Physiological response to stressful stimuli. *Nursing Research, 33,* 33–36.

Sitzman, J., Kamiya, J. & Johnston, J. (1983). Biofeedback training for reduced respiratory rate in chronic obstructive pulmonary disease. *Nursing Research, 32,* 218–223.

Tachovsky, B.J. (1985). Indirect auscultatory blood pressure measurement at two sites in the arm. *Research in Nursing and Health, 8,* 125–129.

Tallman, V. (1982). Effect of venipuncture on glucose, insulin, and free fatty acid levels. *Western Journal of Nursing Research, 4,* 21–30.

Studies using other data collection methods

Barkauskas, V.H. (1985). Health problems encountered by nurse practitioners and physicians in family practice clinics. *Western Journal of Nursing Research, 7,* 101–115 (Records).

Burokas, L. (1985). Factors affecting nurses' decisions to medicate pediatric patients after surgery. *Heart & Lung, 14,* 373–379 (Vignettes).

Davidson, R.A. & Lauver, D. (1984). Nurse practitioner and physician roles. *Research in Nursing and Health, 7,* 3–9 (Vignettes).

Flaskerud, J.H. (1984). A comparison of perceptions of problematic behavior by six minority groups and mental health professionals. *Nursing Research, 33,* 190–197 (Vignettes).

Freihofer, P. & Felton, G. (1976). Nursing behaviors in bereavement. *Nursing Research, 25,* 332–337 (Q-sort).

George, T.B. (1982). Development of the self-concept of nurse in nursing students. *Research in Nursing and Health, 5,* 191–197 (Projective technique).

Harris, R.B. & Hyman, R.B. (1984). Clean vs. sterile tracheotomy care and level of pulmonary infection. *Nursing Research, 33,* 80–85 (Records).

Jacobson, S. (1978). Stressful situations for neonatal intensive care unit nurses. *American Journal of Maternal–Child Nursing, 3,* 144–150 (Q-sort).

Jacobson, S.F. (1983). Stresses and coping strategies of neonatal intensive care unit nurses. *Research in Nursing and Health, 6,* 33–40 (Q-sort).

Lindeman, C. (1975). Delphi survey of priorities in

clinical nursing research. *Nursing Research, 24,* 434–444 (Delphi technique).

Oberst, M. (1978). Priorities in cancer nursing research. *Cancer Nursing, 1,* 181–190 (Delphi technique).

O'Connor, A.M. (1983). Factors related to the early phase of rehabilitation following aortocoronary bypass surgery. *Research in Nursing and Health, 6,* 107–116 (Records).

Taylor, A.G., Skelton, J.A. & Butcher, J. (1984). Du-
ration of pain condition and physical pathology as determinants of nurses' assessments of patients in pain. *Nursing Research, 33,* 4–8 (Vignettes).

Ventura, M. & Walegora-Serafin, B. (1981). Setting priorities for nursing research. *Journal of Nursing Administration,* 30–34 (Delphi technique).

Wood, S.P. (1983). School-aged children's perceptions of the causes of illness. *Pediatric Nursing, 9,* 101–104 (Projective technique).

Chapter 17
□
Reliability, validity, and other criteria for assessing measuring tools

An ideal measuring instrument is one that results in measures that are relevant, accurate, unbiased, sensitive, unidimensional, and efficient. These requirements are rather stringent. For most of the concepts of interest to nurse researchers, there are few if any data collection procedures that match this ideal. Measures that are physical or physiological in nature have a much higher chance of success in attaining these goals than measures that are psychological or behavioral, but no measurement tools are perfect.

Inasmuch as measurement plays such a central role in the research process, scientists have developed a number of techniques for evaluating the quality of their instruments. The careful researcher usually is hesitant to accept a measuring tool without a critical evaluation of it. This chapter reviews the criteria and procedures for assessing measurement tools. We turn first to some basic concepts from the theory of measurement error.

□
Errors of measurement

The measurement of attributes does not occur in a vacuum. Both the procedures involved in applying the measurement and the object being measured are susceptible to innumerable influences that could alter the resulting information. Some of the factors that impinge upon the measurement process can be controlled to a certain degree, but it must be recognized that scores obtained from most measuring tools are fallible.

Components of scores

If an instrument is not perfectly accurate, then the measures it yields can be said to contain a certain degree of error. Conceptually, an observed or obtained score can be decomposed into two parts—an error component and a true component. This can be written symbolically as follows:

$$\text{Observed score} = \text{True score} \pm \text{Error}$$
$$\text{or}$$
$$X_0 = X_T \pm X_E$$

The first term in this equation represents the actual, observed score for some measurement. For example, it could represent a patient's systolic blood pressure, a nursing student's attitude toward death, a woman's fear of the labor and delivery experience, and so forth. The "X_T" stands for the true value that would be obtained if it were possible to arrive at an infallible measure. The *true score* is a hypothetical entity—it can never be known because measures are *not* infallible, though its value can be estimated. The final term in the equation is the *error of measurement*. The difference between true and obtained scores is the result of factors that affect the measurement and, therefore, result in distortions.

Decomposing obtained scores in this fashion brings to light an important point. When a researcher measures an attribute of interest, he or she is also *measuring* attributes that are not of interest. The true score component is what one hopes to isolate; the error component is a composite of other factors that are also being measured, contrary to the desires of the researcher. This concept can be illustrated with an exaggerated example. Suppose a researcher were measuring the weight of ten people on a spring scale. As each subject stepped on the scale, our fictitious researcher places a hand on the subject's shoulder and applies some pressure. The resulting measures (the X_0s), will all be biased in an upward direction because the scores reflect the influence of both the subject's actual weight (X_T) and the researcher's pressure (X_E). Other errors of measurement probably affected the observed scores as well.

Errors of measurement are problematic because they represent an unknown quantity and also because they are variable. In our fictitious example of the careless weight measurer, the amount of pressure applied would undoubtedly vary from one subject to the next. In other words, the proportion of true score component in an obtained score varies from one person to the next.

If the above example appears too contrived, consider the evaluation of nursing knowledge as measured by the national licensure examination. Perhaps some individuals did not sleep enough the night before the examination; other individuals may misunderstand the directions for responding; yet others may arrive at the test site late. Therefore, the obtained scores reflect not only nursing knowledge, but also represent "measures" of alertness, comprehension of directions, punctuality, and dozens of other attributes. Some of the major influences on measurements are described in the next section.

Sources of measurement error

Many factors contribute to errors of measurement. Among the most common are the following:

1. *Situational Contaminants.* Scores can be affected by the conditions under which they are produced. The subject's awareness of an observer's presence (the reactivity problem) is one source of bias. The anonymity of the response situation, the friendliness of the researchers, or the location of the data gathering can all affect a subject's responses. Other environmental factors such as the temperature,

humidity, lighting, time of day, and so forth can represent sources of measurement error.

2. *Response Set Biases.* A number of relatively enduring characteristics of the respondents can interfere with accurate measures of the target attribute. Response sets such as social desirability, extreme responses, and acquiescence are potential problems in self-report measures, particularly psychological scales (see Chapter 14).

3. *Transitory Personal Factors.* The scores of an individual may be influenced by a variety of nonenduring personal states, such as fatigue, hunger, anxiety, mood, and so forth. In some cases these factors can affect a measurement directly, as in the case of anxiety affecting a measurement of pulse rate. In other cases temporary personal factors can alter individuals' scores by influencing their motivation to cooperate, act "naturally," or do their best.

4. *Administration Variations.* Alterations in the methods of collecting data from one subject to the next could result in variations in obtained scores that have little to do with variations in the target attribute. If observers alter their coding categories or definitions; if interviewers improvise the wording of a question; if test administrators change the test instructions; or if some physiological measures are taken before a feeding and others are taken post-prandially, then measurement errors can potentially occur.

5. *Instrument Clarity.* If the directions for obtaining measures are vague or poorly understood, then scores may reflect this ambiguity and misunderstanding. For example, questions in a self-report instrument may sometimes be interpreted dif-

ferently by different respondents, leading to a distorted measure of the critical variable. Observers may miscategorize observations if the classification scheme is not clear. The training of observers, interviewers, and other research personnel can reduce this source of error but may not eliminate it completely.

6. *Response Sampling.* Sometimes errors are introduced as a result of the sampling of items used to measure an attribute. For example, a nursing student's score on a 100-item test of general nursing knowledge will be influenced to a certain extent by *which* 100 questions are included on the examination. A person might get 95 questions correct on one test but only get 90 right on a similar test.

7. *Instrument Format.* Several technical characteristics of an instrument can influence the obtained measurements. Open-ended questions may yield information different from closed-ended questions. Oral responses to a specific question may be at odds with responses to a written form of the same question. The ordering of questions within an instrument may also influence responses.

This list represents a sampling of the sources of measurement error with which a researcher must deal. Other common problems will come to light in other sections of this chapter.

☐
Reliability

The *reliability** of a measuring instrument is a major criterion for assessing its quality and ad-

* The discussion of reliability presented here is based entirely upon classical measurement theory. Readers concerned with assessing the reliability of instructional measures that can be classified as mastery-type or criterion-referenced should consult Thorndike and Hagen (1977).

equacy. Essentially, the reliability of an instrument is the degree of consistency with which it measures the attribute it is supposed to be measuring. If a scale gave a reading of 120 pounds for a person's weight one minute, and a reading of 150 pounds in the next minute (barring any tampering with the instrument or subject), we would naturally be wary of using that scale because the information would be unreliable. The less variation an instrument produces in repeated measurements of an attribute, the higher its reliability. Thus reliability can be equated with the stability, consistency, or dependability of a measuring tool.

Another way of defining reliability is in terms of accuracy. An instrument can be said to be reliable if its measures accurately reflect the "true scores" of the attribute under investigation. This definition links reliability to the issues raised in our discussion of measurement error. We can make this relationship clearer by stating that an instrument is reliable to the extent that errors of measurement are absent from obtained scores. In other words, a reliable measure is one that maximizes the true score component and minimizes the error component. The greater the error, the greater the unreliability.

These two ways of approaching the concept of reliability (consistency and accuracy) are not so different as they might at first appear. The errors of measurement that impinge upon an instrument's accuracy also affect its consistency. The example of the scale that produced variable weight readings should clarify this point. Let us suppose that the true weight of a subject is 125 pounds, but that two independent measurements yielded 120 and 150 pounds. In terms of the equation presented in the previous section, we could express the measurements as follows:

$$120 = 125 - 5$$
$$150 = 125 + 25$$

The values of the errors of measurement for the two trials are -5 and $+25$, respectively. These errors produced scores that are both inconsistent and inaccurate. We must conclude that our fictitious spring scale is highly unreliable.

Scientists can place little confidence in their findings if the instruments they use are of questionable reliability. Therefore, it has become a customary procedure for developers of new instruments to estimate the reliability of their tools before making them available for general use. Instruments that are psychological or behavioral in nature are in particular need of pretesting and trial runs. It should be pointed out, however, that an instrument's reliability is not a fixed entity. *The reliability of an instrument is not a property of the instrument, but rather of the instrument when administered to a certain sample under certain conditions.* A scale developed to measure dependence in hospitalized adults in the United States may be unreliable for use with hospitalized adults in Mexico, or for hospitalized adolescents, or for the elderly in nursing homes, and so forth.

What are the implications of this fact for researchers? First, in selecting a measuring tool one should always learn about the characteristics of the group with whom or for whom the instrument was developed. If the original group was similar to the researcher's target group, then the reliability estimate provided by the scale developer is probably a reasonably good index of the instrument's accuracy and consistency for the new study. Other things being equal, one should always choose a measure with demonstrated high reliability. However, the prudent scientist is not satisfied with an instrument that will "probably" be reliable in his or her study. The recommended procedure is to compute estimates of reliability whenever data are collected for a scientific investigation. For physiological measures that are relatively impervious to random fluctuations stemming from personal or situational factors, this procedure may be unnecessary. However, observational tools, self-report measures, tests of knowledge or ability, and projective tests — all of which are highly susceptible to errors of measurement — should be subjected to a reliability check as a routine step in the research process. The interpretation of a study's findings can be greatly affected by the knowledge that the instruments were or were not reliable.

The reliability of a measuring tool can be assessed in several different ways. The method chosen depends to a certain extent on the nature of the instrument but also on the aspect of the reliability concept that is of greatest interest. Three aspects that have received major quantitative attention are stability, internal consistency, and equivalence.

Stability

The stability of a measure refers to the extent to which the same results are obtained on repeated administrations of the instrument. The estimation of reliability here focuses on the instrument's susceptibility to extraneous factors from one application to the next.

Assessments of the stability of a measuring tool are derived through procedures referred to as *test-retest reliability*. The researcher administers the same test to a sample of individuals on two occasions and then compares the scores obtained. The comparison procedure is performed objectively by computing a *reliability coefficient*, which is a numerical index of how reliable the test is.

We must pause at this point to briefly explain the concepts underlying the statistic known as the coefficient.* We have pointed

* Computational procedures and additional information concerning correlation coefficients (Pearson *r*) are presented in Chapter 20.

out repeatedly in this text that a scientist often strives to detect and explain the relationships among phenomena: Is there a relationship between patients' gastric acidity levels and incidents of emotional upset? Is there a relationship between body temperature and perceptions of the passage of time? The correlation coefficient is an important tool for quantitatively describing the magnitude and direction of a relationship. The computation of this index does not concern us here. It is more important to understand how to "read" a correlation coefficient.

Two variables that are obviously related to one another are the height and weight of individuals. Tall people tend, on the average, to be heavier than short people. Light persons tend, on the whole, to be shorter than heavy persons. We would say that the relationship was perfect if the tallest person in the world was the heaviest, the second tallest person was the second heaviest, and so forth. The correlation coefficient summarizes how "perfect" a relationship is. The possible values for a correlation coefficient range from a -1.00 through 0.0 to $+1.00$. If height and weight were perfectly correlated, the correlation coefficient expressing this relationship would be 1.00. Since the relationship does exist but is not perfect, the correlation coefficient is probably in the vicinity of $.50$ or $.60$.

When two variables are totally unrelated, the correlation coefficient is equal to zero. One might anticipate that a woman's dress size is unrelated to her intelligence. Large women are as likely to perform well on tests of ability as small women. The correlation coefficient summarizing such a relationship would presumably be in the vicinity of 0.0.

Correlation coefficients running from 0.0 to -1.00 express what is known as *inverse* or *negative relationships*. When two variables are inversely related, increments in one variable are associated with decrements in the sec-

Table 17-1
Fictitious data for test-retest
of a leadership potential scale

Subject Number	Time 1	Time 2	
1	55	57	
2	49	46	
3	78	74	
4	37	35	
5	44	46	
6	50	56	
7	58	55	
8	62	66	
9	48	50	
10	67	63	r = .95

ond variable. Let us suppose that there is an inverse relationship between a nurse's age and attitude toward abortion. This means that, on the average, the *older* the nurse, the *less* favorable the attitude. If the relationship were perfect (that is, if the oldest nurse had the least favorable attitude and so on), then the correlation coefficient would be equal to -1.00. In actuality, the relationship between age and abortion attitudes is probably quite modest —in the vicinity of $-.20$ or $-.30$. A correlation coefficient of this magnitude describes a weak relationship wherein older nurses tend to be unfavorable and younger persons tend to be favorable toward abortion, but a "crossing of lines" is not unusual. That is, many younger nurses oppose abortion while many older nurses defend it.

Now we are prepared to discuss the use of correlation coefficients to compute reliability estimates. In the case of test-retest reliability, a sample of subjects is exposed to the administration of the instrument on two occasions. Let us say we are interested in the stability of a scale to measure leadership potential in nurses. Since leadership potential might be presumed to be a fairly enduring attribute in individuals, we would expect a measure of it to yield consistent scores on two separate test-

ings. As a check on the instrument's stability, the scale is administered to a sample of ten people three weeks apart. Some fictitious data for this example are presented in Table 17-1. It can be seen that, by and large, the differences in the scores on the two testings are not large. The reliability coefficient for test-retest estimates is the correlation coefficient between the two sets of scores. In this example, the computed reliability coefficient is .95, which is quite high.

The value of the reliability coefficient theoretically can range between -1.00 and $+1.00$, just as in the case of other correlation coefficients. A negative coefficient would have been obtained in the above example if persons who had the highest scores in leadership potential at Time 1 had the lowest scores at Time 2. In practice, reliability coefficients normally range between 0.0 and 1.00. The higher the coefficient, the more stable the measure. For most purposes, reliability coefficients above .70 are considered satisfactory. In some situations, a higher coefficient may be required, or a lower one may be considered acceptable.

The test-retest method is a relatively easy and straightforward approach to estimating reliability. It is a method that can be used with self-report, observational, and physiological measures. However, the test-retest approach has certain disadvantages. One problem is that many traits of interest do change over time, independently of the stability of the measure. Attitudes, behaviors, moods, knowledge, physical condition, and so forth can be modified by intervening experiences between the two testings. The procedures used to estimate stability confound changes resulting from random fluctuations and those resulting from true modifications in the attribute being measured. Still, there are many attributes that are relatively enduring characteristics for which a test-retest approach is suitable. The example of leadership potential is one such attribute.

Stability estimates suffer from other problems, however. One possibility is that the subjects' responses or observer's coding on the second administration will be influenced by the memory of their responses/coding on the first administration, regardless of the actual values on the second day. This memory interference will result in a spuriously high reliability coefficient. Another difficulty is that subjects may actually change as a result of the first administration. Finally, people may not be as careful using the same instrument a second time. If they find the procedure boring on the second occasion, the responses could be haphazard, resulting in a spuriously low estimate of stability.

In summary, the test-retest approach is a procedure for estimating the stability of a measure over time. On the whole, reliability coefficients tend to be higher for short-term retests than for long-term retests (i.e., those greater than one or two months) because of actual changes in the attribute being measured. Stability indexes are most appropriate for relatively enduring characteristics such as personality, abilities, or certain physical attributes such as height.

Internal consistency

Psychosocial scales are often evaluated in terms of their internal consistency. Ideally, scales designed to measure an attribute are composed of a set of items, all of which are measuring the critical attribute and nothing else. On a scale to measure the decision-making abilities of nurses, it would be inappropriate to include an item that is a better measure of empathy than skill in decision-making. An instrument may be said to be *internally consistent* or *homogeneous* to the extent that all of its subparts are measuring the same characteristic.

The internal consistency approach to esti-

mating an instrument's reliability is probably the most widely used method among researchers today. The reason for the popularity of the procedures described below is not only that they are economical (they require only one test administration) but also that they are the best means of assessing one of the most important sources of measurement error in psychosocial instruments, the sampling of items.

One of the oldest methods for assessing internal consistency is the *split-half* technique. In this approach, the items comprising a test are split into two groups, scored independently, and the scores on the two half-tests are used to compute a correlation coefficient. To illustrate this procedure, the fictitious scores from the first administration of the leadership potential scale are reproduced in the first column of Table 17-2. For the sake of simplicity, we will say that the total instrument consists of twenty questions. In order to compute a split-half reliability coefficient, the items must be divided into two groups of ten. While a large number of possible "splits" is possible, the most widely accepted procedure is to use odd items versus even items. One half-test, therefore, consists of items 1, 3, 5, 7, 9, 11, 13, 15, 17, and 19, while the even-numbered items comprise the second half-test. The scores on the two halves for our example are shown in the second and third columns of Table 17-2. The correlation coefficient describing the relationship between the two half-tests is an estimate of the internal consistency of the leadership potential scale. If the odd items are measuring the same attribute as the even items, then the reliability coefficient should be high. The correlation coefficient computed on the fictitious data is .67.

The correlation coefficient computed on split-halves of a measure tends to systematically underestimate the reliability of the entire scale. Other things being equal, longer scales

Table 17-2
Fictitious data for split-half reliability of a leadership potential scale

Subject Number	Total Score	Odd-Numbers Score	Even-Numbers Score
1	55	28	27
2	49	26	23
3	78	36	42
4	37	18	19
5	44	23	21
6	50	30	20
7	58	30	28
8	62	33	29
9	48	23	25
10	67	28	39　　$r = .67$

are more reliable than shorter ones. The correlation coefficient computed on the data in Table 17-2 is an estimate of reliability for a ten-item instrument, not a twenty-item instrument. To overcome this difficulty, a formula has been developed for adjusting the correlation coefficient to give an estimate of reliability for the entire test. The correction equation, which is known as the *Spearman-Brown prophecy formula,* is as follows:

$$r^1 = \frac{2r}{1 + r}$$

where r = the correlation coefficient computed on the split-halves
r^1 = the estimated reliability of the entire test.

Using the formula, the reliability for our hypothetical 20-item measure of leadership potential would be:

$$r_1 = \frac{(2)(.67)}{1 + .67} = .80$$

The split-half technique is easy to use and eliminates most of the problems associated with the test-retest approach. However, the split-half technique is handicapped by the fact that different reliability estimates can be ob-

tained by using different "splits"; that is, it makes a difference whether one uses an odd-even split, a first half-second half split, or some other method of dividing the items into two groups. For this reason the split-half approach is increasingly being replaced by formulas that compensate for this deficiency. The two most widely used methods are *coefficient alpha* (or *Cronbach's alpha*) and the *Kuder-Richardson formula 20* (abbreviated KR-20). It is beyond the scope of this text to explain in detail the application of these formulae. However, since coefficient alpha is perhaps the single most useful index of reliability available, the reader is urged to consult Cronbach (1984) or Nunnally (1978).*

---

* The coefficient alpha equation, for the advanced student, is as follows:

$$r = \frac{k}{k - 1}\left[1 - \frac{\Sigma \sigma_i^2}{\sigma y^2}\right]$$
where: r = the estimated reliability
k = the total number of items in the test
σ_i^2 = the variance of each individual item
σy^2 = the variance of the total test scores
Σ = the sum of

Both the coefficient alpha and KR-20 produce a reliability coefficient that can be interpreted in the same fashion as other reliability coefficients described here. That is, the normal range of values is between 0.0 and +1.00, and higher values reflect a higher degree of internal consistency. Coefficient alpha (and KR-20, which is actually a special case of the more general coefficient alpha used with dichotomous items) is preferable to the split-half procedure because it gives an estimate of the split-half correlation for *all possible* ways of dividing the measure into two halves.

In summary, indices of homogeneity or internal consistency estimate the extent to which different subparts of an instrument are equivalent in terms of measuring the critical attribute. The split-half technique frequently has been used to estimate homogeneity, but the coefficient alpha is a preferable method. None of these approaches take into consideration fluctuations over time as a source of unreliability.

Equivalence

A researcher may be interested in estimating the reliability of a measure via the *equivalence* approach under one of two circumstances: (1) when different observers or researchers are using an instrument to measure the same phenomena at the same time or (2) when two presumably parallel instruments are administered to individuals at about the same time. In both situations, the aim is to determine the consistency or equivalence of the instrument(s) in yielding measurements of the same traits in the same subjects.

In the chapter on observational methods it was pointed out that a potential weakness of this data collection approach is the fallibility of the observer. The greater the interpretive burden upon the observer, the higher is the risk of observer error or bias. The accuracy of observer ratings and classifications can be enhanced by careful training, the development of clearly defined and nonoverlapping categories, the use of a small number of categories, and the use of behaviors that tend to be molecular rather than molar. Even when great care is taken to design an observational system that minimizes the possibility of error, the researcher should assess the reliability of the instrument. In this case the instrument includes both the category system developed by the researcher and the observer making the measurements.

Interrater (or *interobserver*) *reliability* is estimated by having two or more trained observers watching some event simultaneously and independently recording the relevant variables according to a predetermined plan or coding system. The resulting records can then be used to compute an index of equivalence or agreement. Several procedures for arriving at such an index are possible. For certain types of observational data, correlation techniques may be suitable. That is, a correlation coefficient may be computed to demonstrate the strength of the relationship between one observer's ratings and another's.

Another procedure is to compute reliability as a function of agreements, using the following equation:

$$\frac{\text{number of agreements}}{\text{number of agreements} + \text{disagreements}}$$

This simple formula unfortunately tends to overestimate observer agreements. If the behavior under investigation is one that observers code for absence or presence every, say, 10 seconds, then by chance alone the observers will agree 50 percent of the time. Other approaches for estimating interrater reliability may be of interest to advanced students. Guilford (1964) has described the use of such techniques as analysis of variance, intraclass correlations, and rank-order correlations to assess the reliability of observational measures.

The second situation in which the equivalence of measures is evaluated is when two alternative, parallel forms of a single instrument are available. This type of research problem is not likely to present itself frequently in nursing research, except perhaps in an educational context. For example, the development of alternate forms of a test of nursing knowledge might sometimes be needed. In such a case, the two forms should be administered to a sample of individuals in immediate succession, randomly alternating the order of presentation of the forms. The correlation coefficient between the two sets of scores would be an index of reliability of equivalence. This procedure is adopted to determine whether the two instruments are, in fact, measuring the same attribute. The researcher uses this technique to assess the errors of measurement resulting from errors in item sampling.

Interpretation of reliability coefficients

The reliability coefficients computed according to the procedures just described can be used as an important indicator of the quality of an instrument. A measure that is unreliable interferes with an adequate testing of a researcher's hypotheses. If data fail to confirm a research prediction, one possibility is that the measuring tools were unreliable — not necessarily that the expected relationships do not exist. There is no standard for what a reliability coefficient should be. If a researcher is only interested in making group-level comparisons, then coefficients in the vicinity of .70 or even .60 would probably be sufficient. By group-level comparisons, we mean that the investigator is interested in comparing the scores of such groups as male versus female, nurse versus physician, heavy smoker versus light smoker versus nonsmoker, and so forth.

However, if measures were to be used as a basis for making decisions about individuals, then the reliability coefficient should be .90 or better. For instance, if a score on a test were to be employed as a criterion for admission to a graduate nursing program, then the accuracy of the test is of critical importance to both individual applicants and the school of nursing.

The reliability coefficient has a special interpretation that should be briefly explained without elaborating upon technical details. This interpretation relates to the earlier discussion of decomposing an observed score into an error and true component. Suppose that we have just administered to 50 nurses a scale that measures empathy. It would be expected that the scores would vary from one nurse to another, since some nurses are more empathic than others. Some of that variability is "true" variability, reflecting real individual differences in the attribute being measured; some of the variability, however, is error. Thus

$$V_O = V_T + V_E,$$

where V_O = observed total variability in scores

V_T = true variability

V_E = variability owing to random errors

A reliability coefficient is directly associated with this equation. *Reliability is the proportion of true variability to the total obtained variability,* or

$$r = \frac{V_T}{V_O}$$

If, for example, the reliability coefficient were .85, then 85 percent of the variability in obtained scores could be said to represent "true" individual differences, while 15 percent of the variability would reflect random, extraneous fluctuations. Looked at in this way, it should be a bit clearer why instruments with reliabilities of .60 or lower are risky to use.

Knowledge of the reliability of an instrument is useful to researchers not only because it helps them to interpret results, but also because it suggests whether modifications to the instrument are necessary. Instrument developers should be aware of the following issues in improving their measures:

1. The reliability of psychosocial scales is partly a function of their length or number of items. To improve the reliability, more items tapping the same concept should be added.
2. In observational scales, reliability can often be improved by greater precision in the definitions associated with a category system or through increased observer training.
3. The reliability of an instrument is related in part to the heterogeneity of the sample with which it is used. The more homogeneous the sample (that is, the more similar their scores), the lower the reliability coefficient will be. This is because instruments are designed to measure differences among the objects being measured. If the sample is homogeneous, it is more difficult for the instrument to reliably discriminate among those who possess varying degrees of the attribute being measured.
4. Reliability estimates vary according to the procedure used to obtain it. The researcher should determine the aspect of reliability (stability, internal consistency, or equivalence) that is most relevant to the attribute and instrument under consideration.

□
Validity

The second important criterion by which an instrument's quality is evaluated is its validity. *Validity* refers to the degree to which an instrument measures what it is supposed to be measuring. When an instrument to measure the attitudes of nurses toward the mentally retarded has been developed, how can its designer really know that the resulting scores validly reflect these attitudes? Problems of validity relate to the question: are we really measuring the attribute we think we are measuring?

Like reliability, validity has a number of different aspects and assessment approaches. Unlike reliability, however, the validity of an instrument is extremely difficult to establish. Solid evidence supporting the validity of most psychologically oriented measures is rarely available. There are no formulas or equations that can easily be applied to the scores of the hypothetical attitude-toward-the-mentally-retarded scale to estimate how good a job the scale is doing in measuring the critical variable.

The reliability and validity of an instrument are not totally independent qualities of an instrument. *A measuring device that is not reliable cannot possibly be valid.* An instrument cannot validly be measuring the attribute of interest if it is erratic, inconsistent, and inaccurate. An unreliable tool would be "measuring" too many other factors associated with random error to be considered a valid indicator of the target variable. However, an instrument can be reliable without being valid. Suppose we had the idea to measure anxiety in patients by measuring the circumference of their wrists. We could obtain highly accurate, consistent, and precise measurements of their wrists' circumference, but such measures would not be valid indicators of anxiety. Thus, the high reliability of an instrument provides no evidence of its validity for an intended purpose; the low reliability of a measure *is* evidence of low validity.

The methodological literature abounds with terms relating to different facets of the validity question. The classification system adopted here focuses on three types of validity: content, criterion-related, and construct validity.

Content validity

Content validity is concerned with the sampling adequacy of the content area being measured. Content validity is of most relevance to individuals designing a test to measure knowledge in a specific content area. In such a context the validity question being asked is: how representative are the questions on this test of the universe of all questions that might be asked on this topic? Suppose we were interested in testing the knowledge of a group of lay people concerning the seven danger signals of cancer identified by the American Cancer Society. To be representative, or content valid, the questions on the test would have to include items from each of the seven danger signals or "CAUTION":

*C*hange in bowel or bladder habits
A sore that does not heal
*U*nusual bleeding or discharge
*T*hickening or lump in breast or elsewhere
*I*ndigestion or difficulty in swallowing
*O*bvious change in wart or mole
*N*agging cough or hoarseness

The issue of content validity sometimes arises in conjunction with measures of attributes other than knowledge, such as in attitudinal measures, but the developers of attitude scales are usually more concerned with other aspects of validity.

The content validity of an instrument is necessarily based on judgment. There are no objective methods of assuring the adequate content coverage of an instrument. Experts in the content area may be called upon to analyze the items to see if they represent adequately the hypothetical content universe in the correct proportions. Content validity also rests upon the careful consideration and specification of the behavior or attribute that the researcher is interested in and an evaluation of the ways in which the trait might be measured. The test maker, in writing or selecting items for inclusion in an instrument, should aim to build in content validity by careful planning and the careful execution of a prespecified plan.

Criterion-related validity

The *criterion-related* approach to validity assessment is a pragmatic one. The researcher attempting to establish the criterion-related validity of an instrument is not seeking to ascertain how well the tool is measuring a particular theoretical trait. The emphasis is on establishing the relationship between the instrument and some other criterion. The instrument, whatever abstract attribute it is measuring, is said to be valid if its scores correlate highly with some criterion. For example, if a measure of attitudes toward sexuality and birth control among teenage girls correlates highly with subsequent premarital pregnancies, then the attitude measure could be described as having good validity. In terms of the criterion-related validation approach, the key issue is whether the instrument is a useful predictor of subsequent behaviors and health problems.

The essential component of the criterion-related approach to validation is the availability of a reasonably reliable and valid criterion with which the measures on the target instrument can be compared. This is, unfortunately, seldom easy. If we were developing an instrument to predict the nursing effectiveness of nursing students, we might use subsequent supervisory ratings as our criterion. However, how can we be sure that these ratings are themselves valid and reliable? In fact, there is probably a good chance that the ratings are not dependable. The supervisory ratings might

Table 17-3
Fictitious data for criterion-related validity example

Subject	Score on Professionalism Scale	Number of Publications	
1	25	2	
2	30	4	
3	17	0	
4	20	1	
5	22	0	
6	27	2	
7	29	5	
8	19	1	
9	28	3	
10	15	1	r = .83

themselves be in need of validation. Usually the researcher must be content with less than perfect criteria.

Once the criterion is established, the validity can be assessed easily and straightforwardly. The scores on the "predictor" instrument are correlated with scores on the criterion variable. The magnitude of the correlation coefficient is a direct indicator of how valid the instrument is. To illustrate, suppose a team of nurse researchers developed a scale to measure professionalism among nurses. They administer the instrument to a sample of nurses and at the same time ask the nurses to indicate how many articles they have published. The latter variable was chosen as one of many potential objective criteria of professionalism. Fictitious data are presented in Table 17-3. The correlation coefficient of .83 indicates that the "professionalism scale" is a reasonably good predictor of the number of published articles a nurse has authored. Whether the scale is really measuring professionalism is a somewhat different issue — an issue that is the concern of construct validation, discussed below.

Sometimes a distinction is made between two types of criterion-related validity. The dis-

tinction is not a very important one, but the terms are used frequently enough to warrant their mention. *Predictive validity* refers to the adequacy of an instrument in differentiating between the performance or behaviors of individuals on some future criterion. When a school of nursing correlates the incoming SAT scores of students with subsequent grade point averages, the predictive validity of the SATs for nursing school performance is being evaluated. *Concurrent validity* refers to the ability of an instrument to distinguish individuals who differ in their present status on some criterion. For example, a psychological test to differentiate between those patients in a mental institution who can and cannot be released could be correlated with current behavioral ratings of health-care personnel. The difference between predictive and concurrent validity, then, is the difference in the timing of obtaining measurements on a criterion.

Validation by means of the criterion-related approach is most often used in applied or practically oriented research. Criterion-related validity is helpful in assisting decision-makers by giving them some assurance that their decisions will be effective, fair, and, in short, valid.

Construct validity

Validating an instrument in terms of *construct validity* is one of the most difficult and challenging tasks that a researcher faces. The instrument designer adopting this approach is concerned with the questions: What is this measuring device really measuring? Is the abstract concept under investigation being adequately measured with this instrument? Unlike criterion-related validity, construct validity is more concerned with the underlying attribute than with the scores that the instrument produces. The scores are of interest only insofar as they constitute a valid basis for inferring the degree to which a subject possesses some characteristic. Unfortunately, the more abstract the concept, the more difficult it is to establish the construct validity of the measure; at the same time, the more abstract the concept, the less suitable it is to validate a measure by the criterion-related approach. Actually, it is really not so much a question of suitability as it is of feasibility. What objective criterion is there for such concepts as empathy, grief, role conflict, or separation anxiety?

Despite the obstacles and difficulties encountered in assessing the construct validity of instruments, this activity is a vital component of scientific progress. The constructs in which scientists are interested must be measured, and they must be reliably and validly measured. The significance of construct validity is in its linkage with theory and theoretical conceptualization. In validating a measure of death anxiety, we would probably be less concerned with the adequate sampling of items or in relating the resultant scores to a criterion than with the extent to which the measure corresponds to a theory of death anxiety that is acceptable to us.

Construct validation can be approached in several ways, but there is always an emphasis on logical analysis and the testing of relationships predicted on the basis of theoretical considerations. Constructs are usually explicated in terms of other concepts; therefore, the researcher should be in a position to make predictions about the manner in which the construct will function in relation to other constructs. One common approach to construct validation is the *known-groups technique*. In this procedure, groups that are expected to differ on the critical attribute because of some known characteristic are administered the instrument. For instance, in validating a measure of fear of the labor experience, one might contrast the scores of primiparas and multiparas. Because one would expect that women who had never given birth would experience more fears and anxiety than pregnant women who had already had children, one might question the validity of the instrument if such differences did not emerge. There is not necessarily an expectation that the differences would be very great. It would be expected that some primiparas would feel no anxiety at all, while some multiparas would express some fears. On the whole, however, it would be anticipated that some group differences would be reflected in the scores. As another example of the known-groups technique, consider the example of validating a measure concerning limitations in functional ability. One might choose emphysemic and nonemphysemic persons to validate the instrument. The validity of the instrument might be questioned if differences in scores between the two groups did not occur, because one would expect that emphysemic persons would have experienced limitations in functional ability.

A significant advance in the area of construct validation is the procedure developed by Campbell and Fiske (1959) known as the *multitrait-multimethod matrix method*. This procedure makes use of the concepts of convergence and discriminability. *Convergence* refers to evidence that different methods of

Table 17-4
Multitrait-multimethod matrix

	Traits	Method 1		Method 2		Method 3	
		A_1	B_1	A_2	B_2	A_3	B_3
Method 1	A_1	(.88)					
	B_1	−.38	(.86)				
Method 2	A_2	.60	−.19	(.79)			
	B_2	−.21	.58	−.39	(.80)		
Method 3	A_3	.51	−.13	.55	−.12	(.74)	
	B_3	−.14	.49	−.17	.54	−.32	(.72)

A = need for autonomy trait; B = need for affiliation trait; 1 = self-report summated scale; 2 = observational rating; 3 = projective test

measuring a construct yield similar results. Different approaches to measurement should converge on the construct. *Discriminability* refers to the ability to differentiate the construct being measured from other similar constructs. Campbell and Fiske have argued that evidence of both convergence and discriminability should be brought to bear in the construct validity question.

To help explain the multitrait-multimethod approach, fictitious data from a study to validate a "need for autonomy" measure are presented in Table 17-4. In using this approach, the researcher must measure the critical concept by two or more methods. Suppose we measured "need for autonomy" in a sample of graduate nursing students by (1) having the students respond to a self-report summated rating scale (the measure we are attempting to validate), (2) having nursing faculty rate each student after observing them in a task designed to elicit different degrees of autonomy, and (3) having the students write out stories in response to a pictorial (projective) stimulus depicting an autonomy-relevant situation. A second requirement of the multitrait-multimethod approach is that we must also measure constructs from which we wish to differentiate the key construct, employing the same measuring methods. In the present example, it was decided that it would be meaningful to differ-

entiate "need for autonomy" from "need for affiliation." The two concepts are related: one would expect, on the average, that persons who exhibited a high degree of "need for autonomy" would be relatively low in terms of "need for affiliation." The point of including both concepts in a single validation study is to gather evidence that the two concepts are, in fact, distinct rather than two different labels for the same underlying attribute.

The figures in Table 17-4 represent the correlation coefficients between the scores on the six different measures (two traits × three methods). For instance, the coefficient of −.38 at the intersection of A1-B1 expresses the relationship between the self-report scores on the need for autonomy and need for affiliation measures. It will be recalled that a minus sign before the correlation coefficient signifies an inverse relationship. In this case, the −.38 tells us that there was a slight tendency for people scoring high on the need for autonomy scale to score low on the need for affiliation scale. The numbers in parentheses along the diagonal of this matrix are the reliability coefficients.

Various aspects of the multitrait-multimethod matrix have a bearing on the construct validity question. The most direct evidence (convergence) comes from the correlations between two different methods for measuring the same trait. In the case of A1-A2, the coefficient is .60, which is reasonably substantial. Convergent validity should be sufficiently large to encourage further scrutiny of the matrix. Second, the convergent validity entries should be higher (in terms of absolute magnitude*) than those correlations between measures that have neither method nor trait in common. That is, A1-A2 should be greater than A2-B1 or A1-B2. Inspection of the table reveals that, indeed, .60 surpasses the "heterotrait-heteromethod" values of −.21 and −.19. This requirement is a minimum one which, if failed, should cause the researcher to have serious doubts about the validity of the measures. Third, the convergent validity coefficients should be greater than the coefficients between measures of different traits by a single method. Once again, the matrix in Table 17-4 fulfills this criterion: A1-A2 (.60) and A2-A3 (.55) are higher than A1-B1 (−.38), A2-B2 (−.39) and A3-B3 (−.32). The last two requirements provide some evidence for discriminant validity.

The multitrait-multimethod approach can be extended to include more traits and more methods. The difficulty is in administering a large number of measures to a sample of subjects. Also, the evidence is seldom as clear-cut as in this contrived example and, therefore, additional measures may create undesirable confusion. The full matrix as exemplified in Table 17-4 represents a valuable and perhaps unparalleled tool for exploring the validity of instruments. The researcher should not abandon attempts to utilize the concepts underlying the procedure even when the full model is not feasible. Perhaps in some cases only an A1-B1 type of combination is possible, whereas in others A1-A2-A3 would be manage-

able. Without any doubt, the execution of any portion of the model is better than no effort to estimate construct validity, and is even preferable to a content validity approach for the great majority of concepts of interest to nursing researchers.

In addition to the known-groups technique and the multitrait-multimethod procedure there are other approaches to construct validation. A method that does not have a special name to identify it consists of an examination of relationships based on theoretical predictions. A researcher might reason as follows: According to theory, construct X is positively related to construct Y; instrument A is a measure of construct X and instrument B is a measure of construct Y; scores on A and B are correlated positively, as predicted by the theory; therefore, it is inferred that A and B are valid measures of X and Y. This logical analysis is fallible and does not constitute proof of construct validity but is important as a type of evidence, nevertheless.

Another approach to construct validation employs a statistical procedure known as factor analysis. Although factor analysis, which will be discussed in Chapter 22, is computationally complex, it is conceptually rather simple. Factor analysis is essentially a method for identifying clusters of related variables. Each cluster, called a factor, represents a relatively unitary attribute. The procedure, in other words, is used to identify and group together different measures of some underlying attribute. In effect, factor analysis constitutes another means of looking at the convergent and discriminant validity of a large set of measures.

In summary, construct validation employs both logical and empirical procedures. Like content validity, construct validity requires a judgment pertaining to what the instrument is measuring. Unlike content validity, however, the logical operations required by construct validation are typically linked to a theory or conceptual framework. Construct and crite-

---

* The absolute magnitude refers to the value without a plus or minus sign. A value of −.50 is of a higher absolute magnitude than +.40.

rion-related validity share an empirical component, but in the latter case there is usually a pragmatic, objective criterion with which to compare a measure, rather than a second measure of an abstract theoretical construct.

Interpretation of validity

Like reliability, validity is not an all-or-nothing characteristic of an instrument. An instrument cannot really be said to possess or lack validity: it is a question of degree. Furthermore, while we have referred to the process of testing the validity of an instrument as "validation," it is inappropriate to speak of the process as yielding proof of validity. Like all tests of hypotheses, the testing of an instrument's validity is not "proved," "established," or "verified," but rather supported to a greater or lesser degree by evidence.

Strictly speaking, a researcher does not validate the instrument per se but rather some application of the instrument. A measure of anxiety may be valid for presurgical patients on the day before an operation but not be valid for nursing students on the morning of a final examination. Of course, some instruments may be valid for a wide range of uses with different types of samples, but each use requires new supporting evidence. In a sense, validation is a neverending process. The more evidence that can be gathered that an instrument is measuring what it is supposed to be measuring, the more confidence researchers will have in its validity.

□
Other criteria for assessing measures

Reliability and validity are the two most important aspects to consider in evaluating a measuring instrument. If a measure can be shown to be reasonably reliable and valid for a specific purpose, then the researcher can have some assurance that the results of a study will be meaningful. High reliability and validity are a necessary, though not sufficient, condition for good scientific research.

Sometimes a researcher needs to consider other qualities of an instrument in addition to its validity and reliability. These additional criteria are by no means a substitute for reliability and validity but may in some cases be equally important. Indeed, several of these qualities are directly related to the issues raised in the preceding two sections. In many research situations, however, the criteria discussed below may be irrelevant or unimportant.

Efficiency

Instruments of comparable reliability and validity may still differ in their efficiency. An instrument that requires 10 minutes of a subject's time to measure his or her coping capacity is efficient in comparison with an instrument to measure the same attribute that requires 30 minutes to complete. One aspect of efficiency is the number of items incorporated in an instrument. It was mentioned earlier that long instruments tend to be more reliable than shorter ones. There is, however, a point of diminishing returns. As an example, consider a 40-item scale to measure feelings of guilt among parents of handicapped children. Let us say that we find a reliability of .94 for the scale, using coefficient alpha as our index of internal consistency. Using the Spearman-Brown formula discussed earlier, we can estimate how reliable the scale would be with only 30 items:

$$r^1 = \frac{kr}{1 + [(k-1)r]} = \frac{.75(.94)}{1 - [.25(.94)]} = .92$$

(Where k is the factor by which the instrument is being incremented or decreased; in this case k = 30/40 = .75.)

As this calculation shows, a 25 percent reduction in the length of the instrument resulted in this case in a negligible decrease in reliability, from .94 to .92. Most researchers probably would be willing to sacrifice a modest amount of reliability in exchange for the opportunity to substantially reduce the subjects' response burden.

Efficiency is more characteristic of certain types of data collection procedures than others. In a questionnaire or interview, closed-ended questions are more efficient than open-ended items. Self-report scales tend to be less time-consuming than projective instruments for a comparable amount of information. Of course, one may have no choice but to use a procedure that is low on efficiency. Or a researcher may decide that other advantages (such as depth of information) offset the problem of efficiency. Other things being equal, however, it is desirable to select as efficient an instrument as possible.

Sensitivity

The sensitivity of an instrument affects how small a variation in an attribute can be reliably detected and measured. A yardstick marked off with only three divisions for feet would result in a highly insensitive measure of a person's height. The yardstick could be made more sensitive to variations in height by subdividing each foot into twelve equal sections for inches, and the process could be continued until a sufficiently sensitive measuring tool was obtained for the purposes needed. Unfortunately, it is not quite this easy to increase the sensitivity of most instruments.

The sensitivity of an instrument determines how discriminating its measurements will be between individuals with differing amounts of an attribute. Using the yardstick marked off in feet only, it would not be possible to discriminate between a person who is 5 feet 8 inches tall and one who is 6 feet 3 inches tall: both would be measured as 6 feet, measuring to the nearest foot. There are statistical procedures that permit a researcher to enhance the sensitivity of paper-and-pencil measures by assessing the degree to which each item is contributing to the instrument's power to make discriminations. These *item analysis techniques* are described in detail in texts on measurement and psychometric theory. Several references are noted at the end of this chapter.

The sensitivity of an instrument is most likely to become an issue in certain kinds of situations. When changes in the level of an attribute are being closely monitored, as in the case of many physiological measurements, then it is important to use a sensitive device. If important decisions are to be based upon the measures resulting from an instrument, then the sensitivity of the instrument could have serious consequences. Experimenters must also be concerned with the sensitivity of measuring tools whenever the treatments they are introducing are not markedly different from their control conditions. In the nursing research literature there are many examples of studies in which differences between conditions were not detected. Part of the difficulty in many nursing intervention studies is that new interventions are compared with older interventions, rather than with no intervention at all. When experimental and control conditions are not maximally different—as must often be the case in nursing research—then highly sensitive instruments may be required to detect differences in the effects of the treatments.

Other criteria

There is no need to elaborate in detail upon the few remaining qualities that should be considered in developing or selecting a measuring tool. Most of the following criteria are actually aspects of the reliability/validity issues:

1. *Objectivity.* There should be as little room as possible for disagreements between two or more independent researchers applying the instrument to measure the same phenomenon.
2. *Comprehensibility.* The subject and/or the researcher should be able to comprehend the behaviors required to secure accurate and valid measures.
3. *Balance.* The instrument designer should strive for a balanced measure to minimize response set biases and to facilitate content validity.
4. *Speededness.* For most types of instruments, the researcher should be sure that adequate time is allowed to obtain complete measurements without rushing the measuring process.
5. *Unidimensionality.* A measuring tool should be designed to produce separate scores for unitary, isolatable concepts.
6. *Range.* The instrument should be capable of achieving a meaningful measure from the smallest expected value of the variable to the largest.
7. *Linearity.* A researcher normally strives to construct measures that are equally accurate and sensitive over the entire range of values.
8. *Signal-to-Noise Ratio.* In physiological measures it is important to use instruments and procedures that maximize the signal reading and minimize the interference noise.
9. *Frequency Response.* In instrumentation systems, the equipment should be capable of responding quickly enough to reproduce with equivalent sensitivity all frequency components of a waveform.
10. *Reactivity.* The instrument should, insofar as possible, avoid affecting the attribute that is being measured.
11. *Simplicity.* Other things being equal, a simple instrument is more desirable than a complex instrument inasmuch as

complicated measures run a greater risk of having errors.

In conclusion, it is probably fair to say that the development of adequate measuring tools is the single most pressing problem in the field of nursing research—as it is in such fields as education, psychology, sociology, and other disciplines concerned with human behavior. One of the greatest challenges facing this generation of nurse researchers is the construction and utilization of reliable, valid, and sensitive criterion measures of nursing outcomes. Given the improbability of ever finding *the* perfect criterion measure, researchers should strive to employ *multiple criterion measures,* each of whose measurement strengths complement one another.

☐
Assessment of qualitative data collection methods

The methods of assessment described in this chapter apply primarily to structured data collection instruments that yield quantitative scores. For the most part, these procedures cannot be meaningfully applied to such qualitative materials as unstructured interview responses or narrative descriptions from a participant observer's field notes. However, this does not imply that qualitative researchers are unconcerned with the concepts of reliability and validity. The central question underlying the two concepts is this: Do the data collected by the researcher reflect the "truth"? Certainly, qualitative researchers are as eager as quantitative researchers to have their findings reflect the true state of human experience. (Indeed, some qualitative researchers argue that their techniques are superior to others in their ability to really shed light on human behavior and experience.)

Although qualitative methodologists have been less concerned with the issues of reliability and validity than quantitative methodologists, there is a growing interest in addressing these issues. Among the various strategies recommended, perhaps the most important rest upon a principle known as *triangulation.* Triangulation refers to the use of multiple referents to draw conclusions about what constitutes the "truth."

Denzin (1978) has identified four basic types of triangulation:

• *Data triangulation*—use of multiple data sources in a study (e.g., interviewing multiple key informants about the same topic);

• *Investigator triangulation*—the use of multiple individuals to collect and analyze a single set of data;

• *Theory triangulation*—the use of multiple perspectives to interpret a single set of data; and

• *Methodological triangulation*—the use of multiple methods to address a research problem (e.g., observation, interviews, inspection of documents)

The purpose of using triangulation is to provide a basis for convergence on truth. In other words, by using multiple methods and perspectives, it is hoped that "true" information can be sorted out from "error" information. In the final analysis, this is not conceptually different from the process of estimating reliability and validity by quantitative researchers. The reader interested in a further discussion of reliability and validity in qualitative research would be well-advised to consult LeCompte and Goetz (1982) or Kirk and Miller (1985).

☐ Research example

Cox (1985) was interested in developing a scale to measure motivation in health behavior. The author developed a Likert-type questionnaire with five response categories. The content areas of motivation in health behavior were: self-determined health judgments, self-determined health behavior, perceived competency in matters pertaining to health, and responsiveness to internal-external cues. The researcher developed specific items for the four content areas from the existing work of other researchers. Cox chose equal numbers of positive and negative items in an attempt to avoid response-set bias, a source of measurement error.

The 20 items were submitted to graduate students and faculty in nursing and psychology for assessment of the scale's content validity. Cox also conducted a pretest of the scale in an effort to detect problems of clarity in the wording of items and to ensure that responses to each item varied along the continuum of possible responses. Based upon the pretesting of the scale, several items were deleted and new ones developed. The new items were submitted to persons knowledgeable in questionnaire construction and then pretested.

The final instrument, modified on the basis of the pretest, consisted of 20 items. Cronbach's Alpha was used to obtain reliability (internal consistency) coefficients for the total scale. Four of the items were eliminated because they demonstrated low item total score correlations. The Cronbach's Alpha for the total instrument was .84.

In an effort to determine how many dimensions of motivation existed in the scale, irrespective of the researcher's belief, the entire scale was examined by a statistical test to determine the number of dimensions and which items correlated with each other. The same four dimensions emerged and a Cronbach's Alpha was obtained for each dimension. Inter-subscale correlation coefficients were obtained to test for discriminant validation—that is, whether each subscale was measuring a different dimension of motivation in health behavior. The correlation coefficients obtained were lower than any of the subscale reliability coefficients.

In this study, reliability coefficients provided indices of the instrument's internal consistency but not of the instrument's stability over time. Neither test-retest nor equivalence reliability coefficients were calculated. The author used a panel of psychology and nursing graduate students and faculty to help establish content validity. Discriminant validation of the subscales occurred through submission of the items to statistical testing.

□
Summary

Few, if any, measuring instruments used by researchers are pure or infallible. Rather, the "scores" obtained by the measuring tools may be decomposed into two parts—a true score and an error component. The true score is a hypothetical entity that represents the value that would be obtained if it were possible to arrive at a "perfect" measure. The error component, or error of measurement, represents the inaccuracies present in the measurement process. Sources of measurement error include situational contaminants, response set biases, transitory personal factors, and several others.

One important characteristic of a measuring tool is its *reliability,* which refers to the degree of consistency or accuracy with which an instrument measures an attribute. The higher the reliability of an instrument, the lower the amount of error present in the obtained scores. There are several empirical methods for assessing various aspects of an instrument's reliability. The *stability* aspect, which concerns the extent to which the instrument yields the same results on repeated administrations, is evaluated by *test-retest* procedures. The *internal consistency* or *homogeneity* aspect of reliability refers to the extent to which all of the instrument's subparts or items are measuring the same attribute. Internal consistency may be evaluated using either the

split-half reliability technique or *Cronbach's alpha* method. When the focus of a reliability assessment is on establishing equivalence between observers in rating behaviors, estimates of *interrater reliability* may be obtained. The reliability of an instrument is partly a function of its length, the adequacy of the sampling of items, the heterogeneity of the groups to which the instrument was administered, and the procedure used for obtaining the reliability estimate. Most of the methods of estimating reliability rely on the calculation of a *reliability coefficient,* an index that reflects the proportion of true variability in a set of scores to the total obtained variability. Reliability coefficients generally range in value from a low of .00 to 1.00, with higher values reflecting increased reliability.

Validity refers to the degree to which an instrument measures what it is supposed to be measuring. *Content validity* is concerned with the sampling adequacy of the content being measured. *Criterion-related validity* focuses on the relationship or correlation between the instrument and some outside criterion. *Construct validity* refers to the adequacy of an instrument in measuring the abstract construct of interest. One approach to assessing the construct validity of a measuring tool is the *known groups technique,* which contrasts the scores of groups that are presumed to differ on the attribute. Another construct validity approach is the *multitrait-multimethod matrix* technique, which is based upon the concepts of convergence and discriminability. *Convergence* refers to evidence that different methods of measuring the same attribute yield similar results. *Discriminability* refers to the ability to differentiate the construct being measured from other similar concepts.

While high reliability and validity are essential criteria for assessing the quality of an instrument, other characteristics of the tool may also be important. Other criteria for evaluating a measuring tool include its efficiency, sensitivity, objectivity, comprehensibility, balance, speededness, unidimensionality, range, linearity, signal-to-noise ratio, frequency response, reactivity, and simplicity.

Triangulation is the process most frequently used to establish the worth of qualitative data collection approaches. Four types of triangulation have been identified: data triangulation, investigator triangulation, theoretical triangulation, and methodological triangulation. Given the fallibility of data collection methods, the use of *multiple criterion measures* (a form of methodological triangulation) is being increasingly advocated. Such triangulation might profitably involve the use of both qualitative and quantitative methods in a single study.

☐
Study suggestions

1. Explain in your own words the meaning of the following correlation coefficients:
   a. The relationship between intelligence and grade point average was found to be .72.
   b. The correlation coefficient between age and gregariousness was −.20.
   c. It was revealed that patients' compliance with nursing instructions was related to their length of stay in the hospital (r = −.50).
2. Suppose the split-half reliability of an instrument to measure attitudes toward contraception was .70. Calculate the reliability of the full scale by using the Spearman-Brown formula.
3. If a researcher had a 20-item scale whose reliability was .60, approximately how many items would have to be added to achieve a reliability of .80?
4. An instructor has developed an instrument to measure knowledge of research terminology. Would you say that more reliable measurements would be yielded before or after a year of instruction on research methodology, using the exact same test, or would there be no difference? Why?
5. What aspects of the multitrait-multimethod matrix that follows identify weaknesses in the measures?

Traits	Method 1		Method 2	
	A_1	B_1	A_1	B_2
Method 1 A_1	(.40)			
B_1	.38	(.65)		
Method 2 A_2	.36	.50	(.80)	
B_2	.19	.48	.25	(.75)

6. What types of groups do you feel might be useful to employ for a known-groups approach to validating a measure of: (a) emotional maturity; (b) attitudes toward alcoholics; (c) territorial aggressiveness; (d) job motivation; and (e) subjective pain?

☐
Suggested readings

Methodological references

Armstrong, G.D. (1981). The intraclass correlation as a measure of interrater reliability of subjective judgments. *Nursing Research, 30,* 314–315.

Brinberg, D. & McGrath, J.E. (1985). *Validity and the research process.* Beverly Hills, CA: Sage Publications.

Campbell, D.T. & Fiske, D.W. (1959). Convergent and discriminant validation by the multitrait–multimethod matrix. *Psychological Bulletin, 56,* 81–105.

Cronbach, L.J. (1984). *Essentials of psychological testing* (4th ed.). New York: Harper & Row.

Denzin, N.K. (1978). *The research act* (2nd ed.). New York: McGraw-Hill.

Ebel, R.L. (1979). *Essentials of educational measurement* (3rd ed.). Englewood Cliffs, NJ: Prentice-Hall.

Guilford, J.P. (1964). *Psychometric methods* (2nd ed.) New York: McGraw-Hill.

Holm, K. & Kavanagh, J. (1985). An approach to

modifying self-report instruments. *Research in Nursing and Health, 8,* 13–18.

Horn, B.J. (1980). Establishing valid and reliable criteria: A researcher's perspective. *Nursing Research, 29,* 88–90.

Kerlinger, F.N. (1973). *Foundations of behavioral research* (2nd ed.). New York: Holt, Rinehart & Winston (Chapters 26 & 27).

Kirk, J. & Miller, M.L. (1985). *Reliability and validity in qualitative research.* Beverly Hills, CA: Sage Publications.

Le Compte, M.D. & Goetz, J.P. (1982). Problems of reliability and validity in ethnographic research. *Review of Educational Research, 52,* 31–60.

Murdaugh, C. (1981). Measurement error and attenuation. *Western Journal of Nursing Research, 3,* 252–256.

National League for Nursing Measurement and Evaluation Services (1971). Let's examine: Reliability. *Nursing Outlook, 19,* 120–121.

Nunnally, J. (1978). *Psychometric theory.* New York: McGraw-Hill (Chapters 3, 6 & 7).

Thorndike, R.L. & Hagen, E. (1977). *Measurement and evaluation in psychology and education* (4th ed.). New York: John Wiley & Sons.

Waltz, C.F., Strickland, O.L. & Lenz, E.R. (1984). *Measurement in nursing research.* Philadelphia: F.A. Davis (Chapter 5).

Substantive references

Brandt, P.A. & Weinert, C. (1981). The PRQ—a social support measure. *Nursing Research, 30,* 277–280 (Internal consistency reliability—coefficient alpha; content validity; predictive validity; construct validity).

Cox, C.L. (1985). The Health Self-Determinism Index. *Nursing Research, 34,* 177–183 (Cronbach's alpha, content validity, discriminant validity).

Ferrans, C.E. & Powers, M.J. (1985). Quality of life index: Development and psychometric properties. *Advances in Nursing Science, 8,* 15–24 (Test–retest reliability; internal consistency: Cronbach's alpha; content validity; criterion-related validity).

Fox, R.N. & Ventura, M.R. (1984). Internal psychometric characteristics of the Quality Patient Care Scale. *Nursing Research, 34,* 112–117 (Interrater reliability; internal consistency: Cronbach's alpha; construct validity).

Hester, N.O. (1984). Child's health self-concept scale: Its development and psychometric properties. *Advances in Nursing Science, 7,* 45–55 (Test–retest reliability; internal consistency: Cronbach's alpha; content validity; construct validity).

Jalowiec, A., Murphy, S.P. & Powers, M.J. (1984). Psychometric assessment of the Jalowiec Coping Scale. *Nursing Research, 33,* 157–161 (Test–retest reliability; internal consistency: Cronbach's alpha; content validity; construct validity).

Ketefian, S. (1981). Moral reasoning and moral behavior among selected groups of practicing nurses. *Nursing Research, 30,* 171–176 (Internal consistency reliability—coefficient alpha, test–retest reliability; content validity; criterion-related validity; known-groups technique).

Lasky, P. *et al.* (1985). Developing an instrument for the assessment of family dynamics. *Western Journal of Nursing Research, 7,* 40–57 (Internal consistency reliability: Cronbach's alpha; content validity; construct validity).

Mynatt, S. (1985). Empathy in faculty and students in different types of nursing preparation programs. *Western Journal of Nursing Research, 7,* 333–348 (Interrater reliability).

Chapter 18
□
Quantitative measurement

Not all nursing research studies involve the collection of quantitative data, but the majority do. Even studies that use narrative sources of information, such as unstructured interviews or historical documents, often convert some or all of the information to quantified expression. This chapter discusses some of the basic principles of measurement and quantification, in preparation for a discussion on statistical analysis.

The measurement process and the problems it entails are central concerns of the researcher using the scientific approach. Hypotheses are tested through the collection of data, and data are gathered by measuring those variables designated in the hypotheses. This sounds straightforward, and sometimes it is. The measurement of someone's height is easy enough, but how about the measurement of pain, or loneliness, or empathy? The rules for measuring such attributes are neither unanimously agreed upon nor intuitively obvious. The rules for measuring a person's height are not unanimously agreed upon either, but most people accept either the "inches-feet-yards" or metric conventions. Analogous conventions for measuring social and psychological variables do not exist, nor are they likely to be developed. Most social scientists agree that measurement constitutes the most perplexing and enduring problem in the research process. Since much of nursing research is social scientific in nature, the measurement problem in nursing research is a very major concern.

Measurement may be defined as follows: "Measurement consists of rules for assigning numbers to objects to represent quantities of attributes" (Nunnally, 1978, p. 2). In our private lives, we develop our own "rules" for measuring things, but as researchers we must either adopt well-specified rules (as in the case of measuring body temperature in Fahrenheit degrees) or explicitly formulate new ones. Let us consider various aspects of the definition of measurement and the measurement process.

□
Aspects of quantitative measurement

Abstraction and measurement

When we measure something, it is not the object itself that is measured. Rather, we measure abstract attributes or characteristics of the object. The researcher uses the term "concepts" in referring to abstractions of interest. The measurement procedures constitute, in short, the operational definitions of the concepts.

Before measuring the abstractions in which we are interested, it is useful to consider thoroughly the nature of the critical attribute. We should ask ourselves, first, if the attribute really exists. As in the case of all abstractions, we are dealing with human conceptualizations. That is, the abstractions represent a structure that humans impose on objects, and these abstractions may or may not be appropriate or relevant dimensions to consider. The ways in which we normally describe people may not be matched in reality by attributes that can be measured. Is there really such a phenomenon as "women's intuition" or "superego strength?"

A second aspect of the problem is that our abstraction may not be "pure"; that is, it may be a conglomerate of several interrelated concepts rather than a unitary attribute. This problem is an important one for measurement purposes. A good measurement tool should be one that results in a quantitative score for one unitary, isolated attribute. If the concept is complex, then several measures may be required to produce data relating to its various facets. Let us consider for a moment the concept of creativity. Creativity is a term with which we are all familiar and which we use in normal speech, but scientists have had difficulties in dealing with this construct, partly because it is elusive and partly because it manifests itself in vastly different ways in different kinds of people. Is creativity in a nurse researcher similar in any way to creativity in an architect? The researcher seeking a measuring tool should consider if a more modest abstraction might not, in fact, be easier to define and defend. Perhaps instead of dealing with "creativity" the researcher could propose to study "fluidity of verbal expression."

Quantification and measurement

Quantification is intimately associated with measurement. There is an often-quoted statement by an early American psychologist, L.L. Thurstone, which advances a position assumed by many researchers: "Whatever exists, exists in some amount and can be measured." The notion underlying this statement is that attributes of objects are not constant: they vary from day to day, from situation to situation, or from one object to another. This variability is capable of a numerical expression that signifies *how much* of an attribute is present in the object. Quantification is used to communicate that amount.

The purpose of assigning numbers, then, is to differentiate between persons or objects that possess varying degrees of the critical attribute. If Nurse X is a more effective nurse than Nurse Y, then the first nurse should have a higher "score" for effectiveness than the second. The crucial problem is determining *how much* higher the score should be in order to accurately reflect the differences that exist.

Rules and measurement

Numbers must be assigned to objects according to specified rules rather than haphazardly.

Quantification in the absence of rules would be meaningless. The rules for measuring temperature, weight, pressure, and other physical attributes are familiar to us all. Rules for measuring many variables for nursing research studies, however, have to be invented. Whether the data are collected via observation, self-report questionnaire, or some other method, the researcher must specify under what conditions and according to what criteria the numerical values are to be assigned to the characteristic of interest.

As an example, suppose we were studying attitudes toward traditional sex roles and asked nurses to express their extent of agreement with the following statement:

Basically, women are too emotional and dependent to be placed in positions of authority.
[ ] Strongly agree
[ ] Agree
[ ] Slightly agree
[ ] Undecided
[ ] Slightly disagree
[ ] Disagree
[ ] Strongly disagree

The responses to this question can be quantified by developing a system for assigning numbers to them. It should be stressed that *any* rule would satisfy the definition of measurement. We could assign the value of 30 to "strongly agree," 27 to "agree," 20 to "slightly agree," but there is no apparent justification for doing so. Therefore, in measuring attributes we must strive not only to develop rules, but also to develop good, meaningful rules. A simplified scheme of assigning a 1 to "strongly agree" and a 7 to "strongly disagree" is probably the most defensible procedure for the question at hand. This "rule" would quantitatively differentiate, in increments of one point, between people who have seven different reactions to the statement.

In developing a new set of rules for measur-

ing attributes, the researcher seldom knows in advance if his or her rules really are the best possible. In essence, a new set of measurement rules constitutes a researcher's hypothesis concerning how an attribute functions and varies. The adequacy of the hypothesis — that is, the worth of the measuring tool — needs to be assessed, as described in the preceding chapter.

Measurement and reality

The concepts we employ and the rules we develop to quantify those concepts must be linked to the real world. To state this requirement somewhat more technically, the measurement procedures must be isomorphic to reality. The term *isomorphic* signifies equivalence of or similarity between two phenomena. A measurement tool cannot be of scientific utility unless the measures resulting from it have some rational correspondence with reality.

Perhaps the isomorphism criterion strikes the reader as self-evident. Yet researchers continuously face the risk that their instruments are not accurately and validly reflecting real-world phenomena. Failures to meet the requirement for isomorphism generally stem from (1) inadequate conceptualization or definition of attributes, (2) inappropriate rules for assigning numbers to objects, or (3) both of these deficiencies.

To illustrate this point, suppose the Scholastic Aptitude Test (SAT) is administered to ten people, who obtain the following scores: 345, 395, 430, 435, 490, 505, 550, 570, 620, 640. These values are shown at the top of Figure 18-1. Let us further suppose that "in reality" the true scores of these same ten persons in terms of a hypothetical perfect test of scholastic aptitude would be as follows: 360, 375, 430, 465, 470, 500, 550, 610, 590, 670. These values are shown at the bottom of Figure 18-1. This figure shows that, while not perfect, the actual

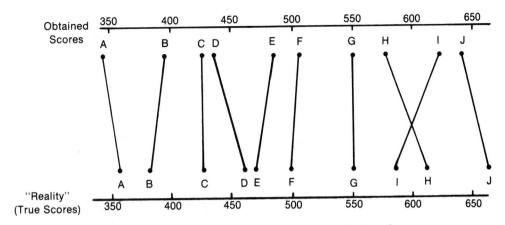

Figure 18-1. *Relationship between obtained and true scores for a hypothetical set of test scores.*

examination came fairly close to representing the "true" scores of the ten subjects. Two obtained scores matched exactly the hypothetical true scores, and no score was off by more than 40 points. Only two individuals (H and I) were improperly ordered as a result of the actual test. This example illustrates a measure whose isomorphism with reality can be considered high, but improvable.

The researcher almost always works with fallible measures. Measuring instruments that measure psychological concepts are less likely to correspond to "reality" than physical measures, but few instruments are immune from error. A person's "true score" on an attribute can never be known, of course, but reliability procedures can be used for estimating the instrument's success in satisfying the isomorphism criterion.

□ Advantages of measurement

What exactly does measurement accomplish that nonmeasurement does not? In this section we examine some answers to the question of what the function of measurement is in science. Before noting the major advantages of measurement, consider what researchers would work with in its absence. What would happen, for example, if there were no measures of body temperature, blood pressure, or respiratory volume? All that would be left is intuition, guesses, personal judgment, and subjective evaluations. With this thought in mind, many of the advantages described below should be apparent.

Objectivity

One of the principal strengths of measurement is that it removes much of the guesswork in gathering scientific data. An objective measure is one that can be independently verified by other researchers. For example, two persons measuring the weight of a subject using the same scale would be likely to get identical or highly similar results. Not all scientific measures are completely objective, but most are likely to incorporate rules for minimizing subjectivity.

In addition to the objectivity that is often built into the measure itself, quantification enhances objectivity in another respect. The numerical results of measurement are amenable to analytic procedures in which subjectivity is all but nonexistent. With purely qualitative information, the organization and analysis are likely to be judgmental. Of course, one of the strengths of qualitative research is that the human mind is capable of making remarkably astute judgments. Nevertheless, even in qualitative research investigators normally take steps to avoid subjective biases and distortions.

Precision

Quantitative measures make it possible to obtain reasonably precise information. Instead of describing John as "rather tall," we can depict him as a man who is 6 feet 1½ inches tall. If we chose, or if the research requirements demanded it, we could obtain even more precise height measurements. Because of the possibility for precision, the researcher's task of differentiating among objects that possess different degrees of an attribute becomes considerably easier.

Communication

Measurement constitutes a language of communication. Science is not a private enterprise, engaged in solely to amuse or satisfy the curiosity of isolated researchers. Communication among scientists is essential if a knowledge base is to be developed. Inasmuch as numbers are less vague than words, quantitative measurement does a reasonably good job of communicating information to a broad audience of people. If a researcher reported that the average oral temperature of a sample of postoperative patients was "somewhat high," different readers might develop different conceptions about the physiological state of the sample. However, if the researcher reported an average temperature of 99.5°F, there is no possibility of ambiguity and subjective interpretations.

☐ Levels of measurement

Scientists have developed a system for categorizing different types of measures. This classification system is important because the analytic operations that can be performed on data depend on the measurement level employed. Four major classes, or levels, of measurement have been identified.

Nominal measurement

The lowest level of measurement is referred to as *nominal measurement*. This level involves the assignment of numbers to simply classify characteristics into categories. For many qualitative attributes, we can do no more than to perform this sorting function. Examples of variables amenable to nominal measurement include gender, race, religion, eye color, blood type, nationality, and medical diagnosis.

The numbers assigned in nominal measurement are not intended to convey any quantitative implications. If we establish a rule to classify males as 1 and females as 2, the numbers in and of themselves have no meaning. The number 2 here clearly does not mean "more than" or "better than" 1. It would be perfectly acceptable to reverse the code and use 1 for females and 2 for males. The numbers are merely symbols that represent two different values of the gender attribute. Indeed, instead of numerical symbols we could as easily have chosen alphabetical symbols such as M and F. We recommend, however, thinking in terms of numerical categories because the subsequent analysis of data will be simplified if such a procedure is adopted when a computer is employed.

Nominal measurement provides no information about an attribute except that of equivalence and nonequivalence. If we were to "measure" the gender of Tom, Mary, Susan, and Jim, we would—according to the rule stated above—assign them the codes, 1, 2, 2, and 1, respectively. Tom and Jim are considered equivalent, at least with respect to the target attribute, but are not equivalent to the other two subjects.

The basic requirements for measuring attributes on the nominal scale are that the classifications must be mutually exclusive and collectively exhaustive. For example, if we were measuring ethnicity, we might establish the following scheme: 1 = whites, 2 = blacks, 3 = Hispanics. Each subject must be classifiable into one and only one of these categories. The requirement for collective exhaustiveness would not be met if, for example, there were several respondents of Chinese descent in the sample.

The numbers used in nominal measurement cannot be treated mathematically. While it might make perfectly good sense to determine the average weight of a sample of subjects, it is meaningless to calculate the average gender of a sample. However, the elements assigned to each category can be enumerated, and statements can be made concerning the frequency of occurrence in each class. In a sample of 50 patients, we might find 30 males and 20 females. We could also say that 60 percent of the sample were male and 40 percent were female. However, no further mathematical operations would be permissible with data from nominal measures.

It might strike some readers as odd to think of the categorization procedure we have been describing as measurement. If our definition of measurement is recalled, however, it can be seen that nominal measurement does, in fact, involve the assignment of numbers to attributes according to rules. The rules are not sophisticated, to be sure, but they are rules nonetheless.

Ordinal measurement

The next level in the measurement hierarchy is *ordinal measurement.* Ordinal measurement permits the sorting of objects on the basis of their standing relative to each other on a specified attribute. This level of measurement goes beyond a mere categorization: the attributes are ordered according to some criterion. If a researcher were to order subjects from the heaviest to the lightest, or the tallest to the shortest, or the most efficient to the least efficient, then we would say that an ordinal level of measurement had been used.

The fundamental difference between nominal and ordinal measurement is that in the latter case information concerning not only equivalence but also concerning relative standing or ordering among objects is implied. When we assign numbers to a person's religious affiliation, the numbers have no inherent meaning or significance. We could develop a scheme whereby Catholics were assigned to category 1, Jews to 2, Protestants to 3, and all others to 4. This nominal measuring scheme is absolutely arbitrary. Now, consider this scheme for measuring a client's ability to perform activities of daily living: (1) completely dependent, (2) needs another person's assistance, (3) needs mechanical assistance, (4) completely independent. In this case the measurement is ordinal. The numbers are not arbitrary—they signify incremental ability to perform the activities of daily living. The individuals assigned a value of four are equivalent to each other with regard to their ability to function *and,* relative to those in all the other categories, have more of that attribute.

Ordinal measurement does not, however, tell us anything about how much greater one level of an attribute is than another level. We do not know if being completely independent is "twice as good" as needing mechanical assistance; neither do we know if the difference between needing another person's assistance and needing mechanical assistance is the same as that between needing mechanical assistance and being completely independent. Ordinal measurement only tells us the relative ranking of the levels of an attribute.

As in the case of nominal scales, the types of mathematical operations permissible with ordinal-level data are rather restricted. Averages are generally meaningless with rank-order measures. Frequency counts, percentages, and several other statistical procedures to be discussed in Chapter 21 are appropriate for analyzing ordinal-level data.

Interval measurement

Interval-level measurement occurs when the researcher can specify both the rank ordering of objects on an attribute and the distance between those objects. Interval scales have numerical values the distances between which represent equal distances in the attribute being measured. Most psychological and educational tests are based on interval scales. The Scholastic Aptitude Test (SAT) is an example of this level of measurement. A score of 550 on the SAT is higher than a score of 500, which in turn is higher than 450. In addition to providing this rank-order information, a difference between 550 and 500 on the test is presumably equivalent to the difference between 500 and 450.

Interval measures, then, are more informative than ordinal measures. One piece of information that interval measures fail to provide is the absolute magnitude of the attribute for any particular object. The Fahrenheit scale for measuring temperature illustrates this point. A temperature of 60° is ten degrees warmer than 50°. A ten degree difference similarly separates 40° and 30°, and the two differences in temperature are equivalent. However, it cannot be said that 60° is twice as hot as

30°, or three times as hot as 20°. The Fahrenheit scale, then, is not a measure of temperature in absolute units. The assignment of numbers to temperature on the Fahrenheit scale involves an arbitrary zero point. Zero on the thermometer does not signify a total absence of heat. In interval scales, there is no real or rational zero point.

The use of interval scales greatly expands the researcher's analytic possibilities. The intervals between numbers can be meaningfully added and subtracted: the interval between 10°F and 5° is 5 degrees, or $10 - 5 = 5$. This same operation could not be performed with ordinal measures. Because of this capability, interval-level data can be averaged. It is perfectly reasonable, for example, to compute an average daily temperature for hospitalized patients from whom temperature readings are taken four times a day. Most sophisticated statistical procedures require that measurements be made on an interval scale.

Ratio measurement

The highest level of measurement is the *ratio scale*. Ratio scales are distinguished from interval scales by virtue of having a rational, meaningful zero. Measures on a ratio scale provide information concerning: (1) the rank ordering of objects on the critical attribute, (2) the intervals between objects, and (3) the absolute magnitude of the attribute for the object. Many physical measures provide ratio-level data. A person's weight, for example, is measured on a ratio scale, because zero weight is an actual possibility. It is perfectly acceptable to say that someone who weighs 200 pounds is twice as heavy as someone who weighs 100 pounds.

Since ratio scales have an absolute zero, all arithmetic operations are permissible. One can meaningfully add, subtract, multiply, and divide numbers on a ratio scale. Consequently, all of the statistical procedures suit-

Table 18-1
Fictitious data for four levels of measurement

	Ratio-Level	Interval-Level	Ordinal	Nominal
Nathan	180	70	10	2
Melissa	110	0	1	1
Dameon	165	55	8	2
Jennifer	130	20	5	1
Jerry	175	65	9	2
Laura	115	5	2	1
Elizabeth	125	15	4	1
Christopher	150	40	7	1
Mark	145	35	6	1
Katy	120	10	3	1

able for interval-level data are also appropriate for ratio-level data. Ratio measurement constitutes the measurement ideal for scientists but is probably an unattainable ideal for the vast majority of attributes of a psychological nature.

Comparison of the levels

The four levels of measurement presented in this section constitute a hierarchy, with ratio scales at the pinnacle and nominal measurement at the base. The basic characteristics of each level have been discussed, but several additional points should be mentioned.

The researcher generally should strive to construct measuring instruments on as high a level of measurement as possible. This guideline is based upon two considerations: higher levels of measurement yield more information and are amenable to more powerful and sensitive analytic procedures than lower levels. When one moves from a higher to a lower level of measurement, there is always an information loss. Let us look at an example relating to data on the weight of a sample of individuals. Table 18-1 presents fictitious data for ten subjects. The first column shows the ratio-level data, that is, the actual weight in pounds. The ratio measure gives us complete information concerning the absolute weight of each subject and the differences in weights between all pairs of subjects.

In the second column the original data have been converted to interval measures by assigning a score of zero to the lightest individual (Melissa), the score of 5 to the person five pounds heavier than the lightest person (Laura), and so forth. Note that the resulting scores are still amenable to addition and subtraction; the differences in pounds are equally far apart, even though they are at different parts of the scale. The data no longer tell us, however, anything about the absolute weights of the persons in this sample. Melissa, the lightest individual, might be a 10-pound infant or a 200-pound Weight Watcher.

In the third column of Table 18-1, ordinal measurements were developed by rank-ordering the sample from the lightest, who was assigned the score of 1, to the heaviest, who was assigned the score of 10. Now even more information is missing. The data provide no indication of how much heavier Nathan is than Melissa. The difference separating them might be as little as five pounds or as much as 150 pounds.

Finally, the last column presents nominal measurements in which all subjects were classified as either "heavy" or "light." The criterion applied in categorizing individuals was arbitrarily set as a weight either greater than

150 pounds (2), or less than/equal to 150 pounds (1). The available information is very limited. Within any one category, there are no clues as to who is heavier than whom. With this level of measurement Nathan, Dameon and Jerry are considered equivalent. They are equivalent with regard to the attribute heavy/light as defined by the classification criterion.

This example illustrates that at every successive level in the measurement hierarchy there is a loss of valuable information. It also illustrates another point: when one has information at one level, one can always manipulate the data to arrive at a lower level, but the converse is not true. If we were only given the nominal measurements, it would be impossible to reconstruct the actual weights. Researchers seldom collapse information to arrive at lower-level data, but it is important to recognize the greater flexibility possible with ratio and interval measures than with ordinal and nominal measures.

One final point should be mentioned. It is not always a straightforward task to identify the level of measurement for a particular instrument. Usually, nominal measures and ratio scales are discernible with little difficulty, but the distinction between ordinal and interval measures is more problematic. Some methodologists argue that most psychological measures that are treated as interval measures are really only ordinal measures. The majority of writers seem to believe that, while such instruments as Likert scales produce data that are, strictly speaking, ordinal level, the distortion introduced by treating them as interval measures is too small to warrant an abandonment of powerful statistical analyses.

☐
Research example

A group of nurse researchers tested the hypothesis that children who experienced a discrepancy between expected and actual physical sensations during orthopedic cast removal would be more distressed than children not experiencing such a discrepancy (Johnson, Kirchoff, & Endress, 1975). They designed a study to test this hypothesis, using a number of measures to evaluate and characterize various attributes of their sample.

Biographical information was measured largely on the nominal scale. The reported characteristics included sex (male/female), age (6–8 years/9–11 years), race (black/white), birth order (firstborn/lastborn), type of cast (arm/leg/spica), and previous cast removed (yes/no). The manipulated variable — the information group to which a subject was assigned — may also be considered nominal, since it was used to classify children into one of three groups (control group/description of procedure group/description of sensation group).

Distress was measured by observational procedures. Separate scores were assigned for signs of minor distress and major distress, as defined by criteria established by the researchers. These two scores were combined to form a single distress score with a range of zero for no distress to 2 for signs of major distress. Since it would be difficult to argue that the difference between no distress (0) and minor distress (1) was equivalent to the difference between minor distress (1) and major distress (2), their distress measure is best described as yielding ordinal-level rather than interval-level data.

The children's degree of fear was measured by showing stick figures of four children on an "equal interval continuum." The researcher explained that the stick figures varied in their degree of fear, ranging from "not at all afraid" to "very, very much afraid." The subjects pointed to the figure which was most like them. This fear measure is strictly speaking an ordinal scale, though it is unlikely that major distortions would result from treating it as an interval scale.

Finally, these researchers used the pulse rate of their sample as a major dependent variable. Pulse rate is a ratio-level measurement, since a score of zero is neither arbitrary nor unfeasible.

□
Summary

Measurement involves a set of rules according to which numerical values are assigned to objects to represent varying degrees of some attribute. Strictly speaking, we do not measure "things," but rather some abstract characteristic of things, such as height, weight, pain, and so on. The quantification aspect of measurement usually focuses on developing a numerical system to indicate how much of the critical attribute the object possesses. This quantification process is not performed haphazardly, but rather according to well-formulated rules. The researcher must strive to locate or develop measures that are *isomorphic* with reality; that is, there must be some correspondence between or equivalence of the actual attributes and the measurements of them.

Measurement offers the research scientist a number of benefits. Objectivity is enhanced through measurement, inasmuch as it permits observations to be independently verified by other researchers. Greater precision can be attained through measurement than through casual observation, making it easier for the researcher to differentiate among the varying degrees of an attribute possessed by objects. Measurement also constitutes an important channel of communication among scientists.

The kinds of rules that can be applied to the measurement of an attribute usually depend on the nature of the attribute. The four major levels of measurement are nominal, ordinal, interval, and ratio. *Nominal measurement* classifies characteristics of attributes into mutually exclusive and collectively exhaustive categories. Nominal measurements, which represent the lowest level of measurement, cannot be manipulated mathematically. *Ordinal measurement* involves the sorting of objects on the basis of their relative standing to each other on a specified attribute. Ordinal-level data yield rank orderings among objects. *Interval measurements* indicate not only the rank-ordering of objects on an attribute but also the amount of distance between each object. Distances between numerical values on the interval scale represent equivalent distances in the attribute being measured. *Ratio-level measurements,* which constitute the highest form of measurement, are distinguished from interval measurements by virtue of having a rational zero point. Since ratio scales have an absolute zero, all arithmetic operations are permissible. In general, researchers should strive to measure key variables on as high a measurement scale as possible.

□
Study suggestions

1. What types of data collection procedure (i.e., observation, self-report, physiological index) might a researcher use to measure the following concepts: fear of death, loneliness, body image, self-esteem, sensitivity to pain, motor coordination, ease of fluid intake, adherence to a nutritional regime, and nursing effectiveness?
2. For one or more of the concepts above, develop rules for quantitatively measuring the variable.
3. Read a research report in a recent issue of *Nursing Research*. Were the levels of measurement used by the author the highest possible? If not, explain how the researcher could have attained higher levels of measurement than were used.
4. For each of the following variables, specify the highest level of measurement that you feel would ordinarily be attainable: number

of siblings, rank in class, color of urine specimen, time to first voiding for postoperative patients, faculty status (i.e., professor, instructor), attitude toward abortion, exposure to genetic counseling, length of stay in hospital, diastolic blood pressure, hospital nursing positions, sleeping state, anxiety level.

5. Below are presented fictitious data for the length in centimeters of ten newborns. Convert this information to interval, ordinal, and nominal measurements.

a) 45 cm. b) 52 cm. c) 61 cm. d) 49 cm.
e) 60 cm. f) 58 cm. g) 63 cm. h) 58 cm.
i) 53 cm. j) 57 cm.

☐
Suggested readings

Allen, M.J. & Yen, W.M. (1979). *Introduction to measurement theory.* Monterey, CA: Brooks-Cole.

Blalock, H.M., Jr. (1982). *Conceptualization and measurement in the social sciences.* Beverly Hills, CA: Sage.

Churchman, C.W. & Ratoosh, P. (Eds.). (1963). *Measurement: Definitions and theories.* New York: John Wiley & Sons.

Johnson, J.E., Kirchhoff, K.T. & Endress, M.P. (1975). Altering children's distress behavior during orthopedic cast removal. *Nursing Research, 24,* 404–410.

Kaplan, A. (1971). Measurement in behavioral sciences. In B.J. Franklin & H.W. Osborne (Eds.)., *Research methods: Issues and insights* (pp. 121–128). Belmont, CA: Wadsworth.

Kerlinger, F.N. (1973). *Foundations of behavioral research* (2nd ed.). New York: Rinehart & Winston (Chapter 25).

Lazarsfeld, P.F. & Barton, A. (1971). Qualitative measurement in the social sciences. In B.J. Franklin & H.W. Osborne (Eds.), *Research methods: Issues and insights* (pp. 140–160). Belmont, CA: Wadsworth.

Nunnally, J.C. (1978). *Psychometric theory.* New York: McGraw-Hill.

Stevens, S.S. (1946). On the theory of scales of measurement. *Science, 103,* 677–680.

Thorndike, R.L. (Ed.). (1971). *Educational measurement* (2nd ed.). Washington: American Council on Education.

Thorndike, R.L. & Hagen, E. (1986). *Measurement and evaluation in psychology and education* (5th ed.). New York: John Wiley & Sons.

Waltz, C.F., Strickland, O.L. & Lenz, E.R. (1984). *Measurement in nursing research.* Philadelphia: J.A. Davis.

Part V

The analysis of research data

Chapter 19
□
Analysis
of qualitative
data

As we saw in the chapters on data collection methods, data for nursing studies vary in their degree of structure. Some research questions and data collection strategies yield loosely structured, narrative materials, such as verbatim dialogue between an interviewer and a respondent, the field notes of a participant observer, or diaries used by historical researchers. At the other extreme are inherently quantified pieces of information, such as those typically provided by biophysiological instrumentation, such as blood pressure readings. This chapter addresses the question: How are qualitative materials analyzed? Remaining chapters in this section of the book describe statistical procedures used to analyze quantitative data. Before proceeding, we briefly discuss the arguments often made in favor of qualitative analysis.

□
The aims of qualitative research

According to Benoliel (1984), qualitative research can be described as "modes of systematic inquiry concerned with understanding human beings and the nature of their transactions with themselves and with their surroundings" (p. 3). Qualitative research is often described as holistic, that is, concerned with humans and their environment in all of their complexities. Qualitative research is often based on the premise that knowledge about humans is not possible without describing human experience as it is lived and as it is defined by the actors themselves.

Qualitative research is often, though not always, allied with a phenomenological perspective. Phenomenological inquiries, because of an emphasis on the subjects' realities, require a minimum of researcher-imposed structure and a maximum of researcher involvement, as the researcher tries to comprehend those people whose experience is under study. Imposing structure on the research situation (for example, by deciding in advance exactly what questions to ask and how to ask them) necessarily restricts the portion of the subjects' experiences that will be revealed.

A debate has emerged in recent years over whether qualitative or quantitative studies are better suited for advancing nursing science (e.g., Webster, Jacox, and Baldwin, 1981; Munhall, 1982), but there is a growing recognition that both approaches are needed (Downs, 1983; Bargagliotti, 1983; Goodwin and Goodwin, 1984; Gorenberg, 1983). The most balanced perspective seems to be that the degree of structure a researcher imposes should be based on the nature of the research question. For example, if the question under investigation is "What are the processes by which infertile couples resolve their infertility?" the investigator is really seeking to understand how men and women make sense of an experience that is complex, interpersonal, and dynamic. It would be possible to investigate this problem with structured instruments, but it is likely that the investigator would never really come to understand the *process* that is the focus of the inquiry.

On the other hand, if the research question is "What is the effect of alternative topical gels applied during wound debridement on the patient's level of pain and extent of debridement accomplished?" it seems appropriate to seek specific, concrete data in a structured format. Both of these hypothetical questions have a place in nursing research, because both can contribute to the improvement of nursing practice. Benoliel (1984) has identified four broad areas in which unstructured, qualitative approaches appear most promising:

- Environmental influences on care-giving systems;
- Decision-making processes;
- People's adaptation to critical life experiences, such as chronic illness or developmental changes; and
- The nature of nurse-client social transactions in relation to stability and change.

☐

Applications of qualitative analysis

Qualitative methods, as suggested above, are more appropriately applied to certain types of research problems than others. There is a fair amount of agreement that qualitative methods are less suitable than quantitative approaches for establishing cause-and-effect relationships, for rigorously testing research hypotheses, or for determining opinions, attitudes, and practices of a large population. The unsuitability of qualitative methods for these purposes is based in part on the difficulties of analyzing qualitative data, as we will discuss below. Another problem, however, is that qualitative research tends to yield vast amounts of data—consequently, it is impractical for the researcher to use large, representative samples for obtaining the data. The extent to which the results can be generalized is therefore often questionable.

We must stress that these shortcomings of qualitative research are offset by some important advantages. Survey-type methods can never yield the rich and potentially insightful material that is generated using an unstructured approach. There are five major purposes for qualitative techniques:

1. *Description.* When little is known about a group of people, an institution, or some

social phenomenon, in-depth interviewing or participant observation are good ways to learn about them. For example, suppose we wanted to learn about the experiences of deinstitutionalized mental patients. How do these people live? What factors facilitate or impede improved mental health? How do they cope with the transition to a new environment? For this type of study, a survey approach might be unfeasible or unprofitable.

2. *Hypothesis Generation.* A researcher using qualitative techniques often has no explicit *a priori* hypotheses. The collection of in-depth information about some phenomenon might, however, lead to the formulation of hypotheses that could be tested more formally in subsequent research. For example, a researcher may be investigating through in-depth interviews the reasons for discontinued use of oral contraceptives among teenage girls. Open-ended discussion with a sample of girls might lead the researcher to hypothesize that girls whose boyfriends have complained about the pill's side effects on the girls (e.g., weight gain, moodiness, headaches) are more likely to stop using the pill than girls whose boyfriends have not made such complaints.

3. *Illustrating the Meaning of Descriptions or Relationships.* Qualitative materials can be useful as illustrations in a quantitatively focused study. Suppose a researcher were studying stress and coping behavior among recently divorced women. The researcher, in analyzing the quantitative materials, might conclude that 80 percent of the sample had experienced considerable distress in the post-separation period, and 30 percent had sought professional assistance for that

stress. These facts are interesting, but the following (real) excerpt illustrating a report of stress would add a perspective that the numbers alone could not provide:

> I've had a lot of emotional problems since my husband left. I can't foresee the future, and I don't want to because I don't think I could keep my sanity if I knew what was ahead. Sometimes when I wake up in the morning I just lie there staring at the ceiling, thinking about everything I've been through; and I'll think, "What am I here for? What's the use of going on? Will anything in my life ever go right for me?"

4. *Understanding Relationships and Causal Processes.* Quantitative methods often demonstrate that variables are systematically related to one another, but they often fail to provide insights about *why* the variables are related. For example, suppose we found that special care unit nurses had higher self-esteem than other nurses. Qualitative methods might yield some understanding about the mechanisms underlying this relationship.

5. *Theory Development.* Qualitative researchers often analyze their data with an eye toward developing an integrated explanatory scheme. The term *grounded theory* is frequently used in connection with a certain approach to analyzing qualitative data, as developed by two sociologists, Glaser and Strauss (1967). This approach involves the generation of theory on the basis of comparative analysis between or among groups within a substantive area, using methods of field research for data collection. The term "grounded theory" refers to the fact that a theoriza-

tion does not spring from the investigator's preconceived hypotheses about a social situation, but rather is "discovered" by being *grounded* in the data.

□
Qualitative data: to quantify or not

One of the decisions a qualitative researcher must make is whether the narrative materials that make up the data will be quantified to some extent. After all, most quantitative measurement methods involve ascribing numbers to *qualities* of persons or objects—for example, their self-esteem, their degree of compliance, or their level of physical fitness. In quantitative research, decisions about how to translate qualities of phenomena into numerical expression are generally made prior to data collection. But researchers who collect qualitative materials often develop schemes for quantifying their narrative materials after the data have been gathered.

There are varying degrees to which qualitative materials can be handled. At one extreme, the researcher can convert all of the narrative information to a numerical system and subject the data to quantitative analysis through statistical procedures. The technique known as *content analysis,* described in a later section of this chapter, often involves the complete quantification of personal communications. At the other extreme, of course, all of the narrative materials can be left intact and can be analyzed through procedures that will be described below. In between are methods for introducing some checks and balances into qualitative analysis. For example, a procedure referred to as *quasi-statistics* resembles an accounting system more than a method of statistical analysis.

Qualitative materials can be quantified in a variety of ways. For example, suppose we asked patients to discuss, in their own words,

the quality of nursing care they received during a long-term hospitalization. Suppose each patient's response was tape-recorded and then transcribed, yielding descriptions ranging from five to ten typewritten pages. How could the material be quantified? We could *count* the number of specific complaints mentioned; we could *count* the number of lines devoted to negative versus positive comments; we could *code* for the presence or absence of specific patient concerns, such as complaints about the time required for the nurse to respond to a call; or we could *rate* the description in terms of overall favorableness toward the care received. The researcher who wants to quantify qualitative material can be extremely creative and ingenious in developing a meaningful approach. The trick is to develop a system that is consistent with the aims of the research and faithful to the message conveyed in the qualitative materials.

Whether or not qualitative data *should* be quantified is a different issue. Some investigators argue that everything can be measured (quantified) and that quantitative analysis is the best way to determine objectively whether relationships between variables exist. This argument aside, it is often useful to quantify qualitative materials purely as a way of coping with the volume of data that is typically produced in qualitative research. Other researchers argue against any quantification, asserting that qualitative materials are richer than numbers and offer more potential for understanding relationships and meanings. They also argue that because data collection and coding procedures are not immune to subjectivity, the use of numbers merely disguises potential bias and gives the illusion of objectivity. We are inclined to disagree with either extreme. We believe that an understanding of human behaviors, problems, and characteristics is best advanced by the judicious use of both qualitative and quantitative data. Sometimes that combination is appropriate in a single study.

□
Qualitative analysis procedures

The purpose of data analysis, regardless of the type of data one has, is to impose some order on a large body of information so that some general conclusions can be reached and communicated in a research report. This task is almost always a formidable one, but is particularly challenging for the qualitative researcher. There are three major reasons for this. First, there are no systematic rules for analyzing and presenting qualitative data. It is at least partly because of this fact that qualitative methods have been described as "soft." The absence of systematic analytic procedures makes it difficult for the researcher engaged in qualitative analysis to present conclusions in such a way that their validity is patently clear. And, the absence of well-defined and universally accepted procedures makes replication difficult.

The second aspect of qualitative analysis that makes it challenging is the sheer amount of work that is required. The qualitative analyst must organize and make sense of pages and pages of narrative materials. In a qualitative study directed by one of the authors (Polit), the data consisted of transcribed, unstructured interviews with over 100 women who had recently divorced. The transcriptions ranged from 40 to 80 pages in length, resulting in over 6000 pages that had to be read, organized, integrated, and synthesized. It is this labor-intensive aspect of qualitative research, combined with the fact that samples must necessarily be rather small, that makes it so difficult to obtain funding for qualitative studies; they are expensive but often of limited generalizability.

The final challenge comes in reducing the data for reporting purposes. The major results of quantitative research can often be summarized in two or three tables. However, if one compresses qualitative data too much, the very point of maintaining the integrity of narrative materials during the analysis phase becomes lost. If one merely summarizes the conclusions reached without including numerous supporting excerpts directly from the narrative materials, the richness of the original data disappears. As a consequence, it is extremely difficult to present the results of qualitative research in a format that is compatible with space limitations in professional journals. Most qualitative researchers find that the best medium for disseminating their results is books rather than journal articles.

Despite the fact that there are no universally accepted rules for the analysis of qualitative materials, numerous systems have evolved. It is beyond the scope of this book to describe all of the major systems in detail, but we present here some guidelines that should provide a basic understanding of the general process. We also describe the major features of two different strategies, analytic induction and grounded theory. However, we strongly encourage interested readers to consult several of the references listed at the end of this chapter.

Data organization

Whether one is working with field notes from a participant observation study, transcriptions from unstructured interviews, historical documents, or some other qualitative material, a critical task is to carefully prepare for the analysis of data by imposing some structure on the mass of information. Some practical tips might prove helpful at this point.

First, as in quantitative studies, it is usually important to check that the data are all there,

Table 19-1
Example of a coding scheme for study of adjustment to divorce

1. Divorce-related issues
   a. Adjustment to divorce
   b. Divorce-induced problems
   c. Advantages of divorce
2. General psychological state
   a. Before divorce
   b. During divorce
   c. Current
3. Physical health state
   a. Before divorce
   b. During divorce
   c. Current
4. Relationship with children
   a. General quality
   b. Communication
   c. Shared activities
   d. Structure of relationship
5. Parenting
   a. Discipline and child-rearing
   b. Feelings about parenthood
   c. Feelings about single parenthood
6. Friendships/social participation
   a. Dating and remarriage
   b. Friendships
   c. Social groups, leisure
   d. Social support
7. Employment/Education
   a. Employment experiences
   b. Educational experiences
   c. Job and career goals
   d. Educational goals
8. Work load
   a. Coping with work load
   b. Schedule
   c. Child care arrangements
9. Finances

are of reasonably good quality, and are in a format that facilitates organization. Make sure that the verbatim transcripts really *are* verbatim (some well-meaning typists are often tempted to "edit" or "clean up" dialogue). You should also make sure that all your field notes have been written up and that there are no glaring holes in the data. It is best to have all of the data typed or printed, double-spaced, and with wide margins so that notes and codes can be inserted into them. You should have at least one backup copy of all the data, but, depending on what system you use to index and analyze your data, you may need a total of three or four copies of the data.

The main task in organizing qualitative data is developing a method to index the materials. That is, the researcher must design a mechanism for gaining access to parts of the data, without having to read and re-read the set of data in its entirety. A standard method is to develop different types of files. One set of files, for example, would contain the master copy of the material and is ordinarily arranged in some administratively relevant manner, such as by chronological date or by subject identification number. The administrative files would ordinarily contain other types of cross-referenced materials, such as listings that link subject identification numbers with other types of information, such as dates and locations of data collection.

A second set of files usually is constructed on a conceptual/analytic basis. To develop such a file, the researcher must develop a coding scheme that relates to the major topics under investigation. An example of the topical coding scheme used in Polit's study of divorced women is presented in Table 19-1. Then, all of the data are reviewed for content and coded according to the topic that is being addressed. A file is subsequently developed for each of the various topics, and all of the materials relating to that topic are inserted into the file. In other words, the researcher "cuts up" one copy of the material by topic area so

Subject 025
June 25, 1980
Page 32

Int: How did you feel right after the separation? Will you tell
       me a little more about that?

025:    Well, you know, when I look back...I mean I think anybody
       would have felt hopeless and helpless...because of, you
       know, emotionally...I think maybe it's a little easier if   *2b*
       you've got more security...more money. I was really stuck.   *9*
       I caught myself thinking..."Oh, if it wasn't for the
       kids..." I love them both dearly, but...I mean there have
       been times when I've said to myself--I think a lot of women   *5c*
       go through this too--I really had thought of giving them
       up. In the beginning I used to think, too, they'd be so
       much better off with somebody that could, you know...When I   *1b.*
       was really struggling--I was on welfare----I used to think,
       "My God, how am I going to educate them? What are they
       going to have? I can't make ends meet now." It's kinda
       projecting the unknown...fear of the unknown. I think you
       can get mixed up.

Figure 19-1. Coded excerpt from an unstructured interview.

that all of the content on a particular topic can be retrieved automatically.

This process of developing conceptual files is often more cumbersome and difficult than the above paragraph suggests, for several reasons. First, the researcher may discover in going through the data that the initial coding system was incomplete or otherwise inadequate. In some cases, this means going back and starting from scratch. For this reason, it is often necessary to review a very large portion of the data before an adequate coding scheme can be developed. It is not unusual for some topics to emerge that were not initially conceptualized. When this happens, it is sometimes risky to assume that the topic failed to appear in materials that have already been coded. That is, a topic might not be identified as important until it has emerged three or four times in the data. In such a case it would be necessary to reread all previously coded material in order to have a truly complete file on that topic.

Another problem stems from the fact that narrative materials are generally not linear. For example, paragraphs from transcribed interviews may contain elements relating to three or four different topics, in which case you would need as many copies of that paragraph as there are topics covered in order to place a copy in each of the topic files. (An example of a multitopic segment of an interview from the study of divorced women, with codes in the margin, is shown in Figure 19-1.) Also, in order to understand the meaning of some statements about a topic, it may be necessary to include a lot of peripherally related material to provide a context, such as material preceding or following the directly relevant materials.

In setting up files based on a conceptual coding scheme, it is important to include pertinent administrative information on each item filed. For example, if your data consisted of transcribed interviews, each informant would ordinarily be assigned an identification number. Each master copy should bear the identification number, and each excerpt from the interview filed in the conceptual file should also include the appropriate identifica-

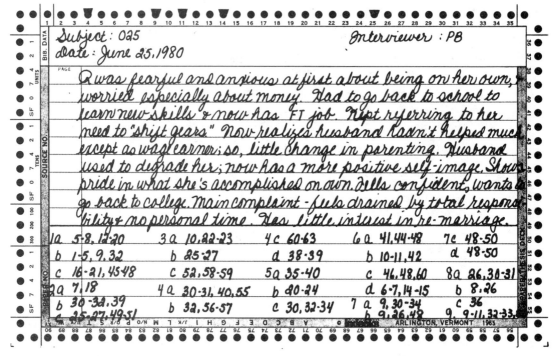

Figure 19-2. Example of interview abstract with code/page summary.

tion number so that you can, if necessary, obtain additional information from the master copy.

In some cases, you would need to develop other types of files in addition to administrative and conceptual files. For example, if your data consisted of field notes from a participant observation study, you would ordinarily need to develop a method for indexing and retrieving methodological and/or personal notes.

While many qualitative researchers find that the development of a complex, multidimensional filing system is an indispensable preliminary task in preparation for the actual analysis, alternative methods have been used. For example, some people prefer to write abstracts of each interview or observation report on index cards, together with a listing of the coded categories and the relevant page numbers. An example, which used a special type of

index card, is shown in Figure 19-2. These index cards have holes on all sides that can be used for easy retrieval of information on a given topic, or on analytic themes. That is, the researcher places notches in the holes corresponding to coded topical categories or concepts. Then, when information relating to a particular topic or theme is needed, all of the cards notched for that topic can easily be pulled from the deck of index cards. (In the example shown in Figure 19-2, the notched holes correspond not to coded categories of content, but to themes developed in the analysis phase. Thematic analysis is described below.) This method has at least three advantages over the use of multiple files. First, files with multiple copies of the data quickly become very bulky and cumbersome. Second, the abstract on the cards provides an immediate and useful overview of the entire observation or interview—an overview that is not available when one works directly from conceptual files. Third, the index cards can also be coded (with appropriate notches, if desired) for different characteristics of the subjects or observational settings. For example, basic demographic information about the respondents such as age, social class, marital status and so on could be recorded for easy reference right on the card. On the other hand, when a researcher is at the point of analysis, it is easier to go directly to the topical files than to start searching through the data with the index cards as a guide. In some cases, it might be worthwhile—if time-consuming—to combine these two approaches.

It is likely that both these approaches will soon be outmoded, given the increasing availability of personal computers that can be used to perform the "filing" and indexing. Suggestions for how qualitative information can be computerized have begun to appear in the literature. For example, one system involves numbering all paragraphs of the researcher's field notes or interviews, coding each paragraph for topical codes, and then entering the information into computer files. This is essentially an automated version of the manual indexing/retrieval systems described above. However, increasingly sophisticated computer programs (LISPQUAL, for example), are being developed that permit the entire data file to be entered onto the computer, each portion of an interview or observation record coded and categorized, and then portions of the text corresponding to specified codes retrieved and printed (or shown on a screen) for analysis.

Analytic procedures

While different approaches to qualitative data analysis have been advocated, there are some elements that are generally common to most approaches. We provide some general guide-

lines below, together with a description of one researcher's steps in performing a qualitative study.

The analysis of qualitative materials generally begins with a search for themes or recurring regularities. In some cases, the thematic analysis takes place in the field as the data are being collected. In other situations, the thematic analysis occurs after the data have been collected, during a reading (or re-reading) of the data set. Themes often develop within categories of data (that is, within categories of the coding scheme used for indexing materials), but sometimes cut across them. For example, a theme that emerged repeatedly in Polit's study of divorced women was that, initially, the women's emotional well-being was so adversely affected by the divorce that they were unable to make plans for more than one day at a time. However, with the passage of time, many of these women became considerably more goal-oriented than they had ever been in their lives, developing long-range plans for their educational, occupational, and financial futures. This theme was one that cut across the coding categories (shown in Figure 19-1) of "Adjustment to divorce" (1.a), "Current psychological state" (2.c), and "Educational and employment goals" (7.c and d).

The search for themes involves not only the discovery of commonalities across subjects, but also a search for natural variation in the data. Themes that emerge from unstructured observations and interviews are never universal. The researcher must attend not only to what themes arise but also to how they are patterned. Does the theme apply only to certain subgroups? In certain types of communities or organizations? In certain contexts? At certain time periods? What are conditions that precede the observed phenomenon, and what are the apparent consequences of it? In other words, the qualitative analyst must be sensitive to *relationships* within the data.

The analyst's search for themes, regularities,

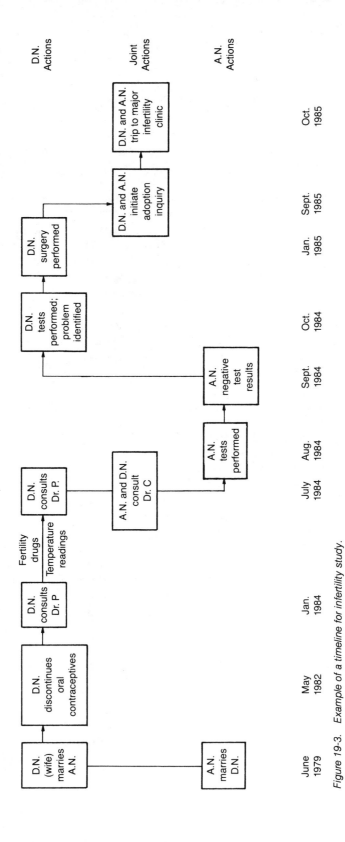

Figure 19-3. Example of a timeline for infertility study.

and patterns in the data can sometimes be facilitated by charting devises that enable the researcher to summarize the evolution of behaviors, events, and processes. For example, for qualitative studies that focus on dynamic experiences — such as decision-making — it is often useful to develop flow charts or time-lines that highlight time sequences, major decision points and events, and factors affecting the decisions. An example of such a flow chart from a study of decision-making among infertile couples is presented in Figure 19-3. The construction of such flow charts for all subjects would help to highlight certain regularities in the subjects' evolving behaviors.

A further step frequently taken involves the validation of the understandings that the thematic exploration has provided. In this phase, the concern is whether the themes inferred are an accurate representation of the perspectives of the people interviewed or observed. Several procedures can be used in this validation step. If there is more than one researcher working on the study, debriefing sessions in which the themes are reviewed and specific cases discussed can be highly productive. Multiple perspectives — what we referred to in Chapter 17 as investigator triangulation — cannot ensure the validity of the themes, but it can minimize any idiosyncratic biases. Using an iterative approach is almost always necessary. That is, the researcher derives themes from the narrative materials, goes back to the materials with the themes in mind to see if the materials really do fit, and then refines the themes as necessary. In some cases, it might also be appropriate to present the preliminary thematic analysis to some of the subjects/informants, who can be encouraged to offer suggestions that might support or contradict this analysis.

It is at this point that some researchers introduce what is referred to as "quasi-statistics." Quasi-statistics involve a tabulation of the frequency with which certain themes, relations, or insights are supported by the data. The frequencies cannot be interpreted in the same way as frequencies generated in survey studies, because of imprecision in the sampling of cases and enumeration of the themes. Nevertheless, as Becker (1970) pointed out,

> quasi-statistics may allow the investigator to dispose of certain troublesome null hypotheses. A simple frequency count of the number of times a given phenomenon appears may make untenable the null hypothesis that the phenomenon is infrequent. A comparison of the number of such instances with the number of negative cases — instances in which some alternative phenomenon that would not be predicted by his theory appears — may make possible a stronger conclusion, especially if the theory was developed early enough in the observational period to allow a systematic search for negative cases. Similarly, an inspection of the range of situations covered by the investigator's data may allow him to negate the hypothesis that his conclusion is restricted to only a few situations, time periods, or types of people in the organization or community (p. 81).

In the final stage of analysis, the researcher strives to weave the thematic pieces together into an integrated whole. The various themes need to be interrelated in a manner that provides an overall structure (theory or model) to the entire body of data. The integration task is an extremely difficult one, because it demands creativity and intellectual rigor if it is to be successful. A strategy that sometimes helps in this task is to cross-tabulate dimensions that have emerged in the thematic analysis. For example, in the study of the emotional well-being of divorced women noted above, one theme that emerged was the the strong goal-orientation of many of the women. Another theme related to the women's interest is the

	Moderate to Strong Goal Orientation	Weak Goal Orientation
Actively seeks remarriage	Strong sense of self-efficacy and belief in own ability to control the future and build on past experiences; ability to cope tied in part to strong social support network; active in work and leisure pursuits.	Strong dependency needs; copes through "fantasies" of an ideal mate and home life; tends to use social supports as crutch; spends a lot of time worrying.
Open to remarriage	Has made explicit efforts to forge a new life which sustains her self-esteem; would consider remarriage to mate willing to share in her personal growth; analytic, problem-solving approach to future decisions.	Focusses most of her energies on her children and derives major sense of self in mother role; would remarry primarily to benefit children; shows a sense of resignation.
Wary about/opposed to remarriage	Fiercely independent and determined not to revert to subservient wifely role; shown an almost martyr-like insistence on self-reliance and personal control.	Intensely bitter about divorce; uses denial and sustained self-righteousness as coping mechanisms; but has not yet adjusted to being divorced; engages in various compulsions (e.g. drinking); has isolationist tendencies.

Figure 19-4. Example of a cross-tabulation of dimensions in a thematic analysis.

possibility of remarriage. When these two dimensions were cross-tabulated, as shown in Figure 19-4, they revealed different mechanisms of women's coping with divorce. A further analysis revealed that the differnt coping mechanisms were linked with different psychological outcomes and differential needs for intervention.

Qualitative researchers seldom discuss in any detail the ways in which they analyze their data. However, one researcher, who studied unmarried, pregnant women, has described the stages of her analytic work (Macintyre, 1977). In this study, Macintyre used a computerized system for indexing (but not for actually analyzing) her massive narrative data. Her analysis involved seven different stages, which actually began prior to entering the field:

- *Stage 1.* A list of research problems and concepts was prepared prior to entering the field. This stage continued as field

work began. After the collection of some preliminary data, she developed the list of categories that could be used to index the data.

- *Stage 2.* Coding took place throughout the data collection period. Categories were constructed from statements and events such that comparisons could be made between the categories. New categories were added on the basis of new concepts emerging from the data.

- *Stage 3.* After data collection and final coding of data, all of the data were re-read. Different types of materials (interview transcripts, fieldnotes, documentary records, etc.) were brought together and linked in terms of conceptual themes and topics. From the various sources, the investigator prepared an account about each of her subjects.

- *Stage 4.* The next phase involved organizing for analysis. The investigator considered four organizational strategies: (1) use of detailed case studies; (2) use of time periods to compare what happened to the women at different points in time; (3) comparison of the accounts of the women themselves versus the professionals with whom they interacted; and (4) use of key concepts or themes that had emerged, such as "bargaining in encounters" and "moral character." (The compromise she reached was to organize by concept, but within a chronological order).

- *Stage 5.* The indexing system she developed was used to locate data that were relevant for the major themes around which the analysis was organized.
- *Stage 6.* The preliminary patterns and interrelationships were checked using quasi-statistical procedures. This approach was used to give credibility to major thematic categories, such as "moral career."
- *Stage 7.* The relationships among the major topics were examined and incorporated into an overall model.

Analytic induction

The general procedures and steps outlined above provide a general outline of how qualitative researchers make sense of their data and distill from them their understandings of processes and behaviors operating in naturalistic settings. However, there are some variations in the goals and underlying philosophies of qualitative researchers that also lead to variations in how the analytic task is handled. One of the major strategies for analyzing qualitative data is referred to as *analytic induction,* an approach that was developed in the 1930s.

The analytic induction approach requires a careful scrutiny of all of the researcher's data, usually according to the following six steps:

1. Definition of the phenomenon to be studied and explained

2. Based on a review of the data, the formulation of a hypothetical explanation of the phenomenon, that is, the development of an inductively derived hypothesis

3. Intensive analysis of individual cases, to see whether the hypothesis fits particular cases

4. A search for negative cases that, if found, lead to a reformulation of the hypothesis *or* a redefinition of the phenomenon in order to exclude the particular case.

5. Continuation of the examination of cases, redefinition of the phenomenon, and the reformulation of hypotheses until a universal pattern of relationships is established.

6. Creation of a higher level of abstraction/ conceptualization through comparison with other settings or groups.

In practice, the use of analytic induction results in a procedure that alternates back and forth between tentative explanation and tentative definition, each refining the other so that a sense of closure can be achieved when an integral relation between the two is established.

Grounded theory

A second major strategy is Glaser and Strauss's (1967) method of generating theories from data, using a procedure that they describe as the discovery of grounded theory. This approach is more than just a method of data analysis; it is an entire philosophy about how to conduct field research. For example, a study that truly follows Glaser and Strauss's precepts does not begin with a highly focused research problem; the problem itself emerges from the data.

One of the fundamental features of the grounded theory approach is that data collection and data analysis occur simultaneously. A procedure referred to as *constant comparison* is used to develop and refine theoretically relevant categories. The categories elicited from the data are constantly compared to data obtained earlier in the data collection so that commonalities and variations can be determined. As data collection proceeds, the inquiry becomes increasingly focused on emerging theoretical concerns.

In contrast to analytic induction, this approach requires "data saturation" rather than the consideration of all data. Glaser and Strauss have identified four stages in the constant comparative method.

1. Establish categories based on similarity of content in incidents and dissimilarity of content with other categories, with the aim of elucidating the theoretical properties of each category.
2. Compare each incident within each category with the dimensions of the category for integration into a unified whole that reflects the relationships of the dimensions or properties of the category.
3. Examine categories and their properties for underlying uniformities that may reduce the number of categories. Look for theoretical saturation of content and add only new incidents to categories when they explicate a new dimension.
4. Produce analytic memos to summarize the theoretical explanations; the memos provide the basis for the writing of publications and reports.

There are some obvious similarities between the grounded theory and analytic induction approach, but there are also some important differences. Of particular importance is their overall aims. Analytic induction is concerned with the testing of inductively derived hypotheses; it is purported to be a method for coming to terms with the problem of causal inference while remaining faithful to qualitative, naturalistic data. The grounded theory method is concerned with the generation of

categories, properties, and hypotheses rather than testing them.

Content analysis

We are devoting a separate section of this chapter to content analysis because, although it is a method of handling narrative, qualitative material, it is a procedure that typically involves quantification. Although some researchers who do not quantify their data sometimes refer to their analytic work as a content analysis, the term in its classic sense refers to "a research technique for the objective, systematic, and quantitative description of the manifest content of communication" (Berelson, 1971, p. 18).

Content analysis is applied to people's written and oral communications. It can be used with such materials as diaries, letters, speeches, dialogues, reports, books, articles, and other linguistic expressions. The technique utilizes a number of controls designed to yield objective and systematic information. The researcher enhances objectivity by conducting the content analysis on the basis of explicitly formulated rules. The rules serve as guidelines to enable two or more persons analyzing the same materials to obtain the same results. The analysis is rendered systematic by the inclusion or exclusion of materials according to consistently applied selection criteria.

Elements of content analysis

Holsti (1968) has pointed out that communications are comprised of six basic elements: a *source*—the sender; an *encoding process* resulting in the *message;* a transmitting *channel;* a *detector*—the recipient of the message; and a *decoding process.* The object of the analysis is the message, but content analysis can be used to answer questions concerning the remaining five elements. The questions one an-

Table 19-2
Content analysis questions, problems, and purposes

Questions	Research Problems	Purposes
What?	To describe trends in communication content To relate attributes of the senders to the messages they produce To relate the message to the characteristics of the recipients To relate the message to the characteristics of situations	To describe characteristics of communication
How?	To analyze techniques of persuasion To analyze style	
To whom?	To relate the message to the characteristics of the recipients To describe patterns of communication	
Why?	To analyze psychological traits of individuals To infer aspects of culture and cultural change	To make inferences as to the antecedents of communication (the encoding process)
Who?	To answer questions of disputed authorship To relate the message to the attributes of the sender	
With what effect?	To analyze the flow of information To assess responses to communication	To make inferences as to the effects of communication (the decoding process)

Adapted from Table 1. O.R. Holsti: "Content analysis." In G. Lindzey and E. Aronson (eds): *The handbook of social psychology,* ed. 2, Vol. 2. Reading, MA: Addison-Wesley, 1968, p. 604.

swers through content analysis are: Who said what? to whom? how? why? and to what effect? Table 19-2, adapted from Holsti (1968), links these questions to research problems and purposes.

The most common applications of content analysis have been directed toward the "what" question, that is, describing the characteristics of the message's content. Several approaches can be used to analyze the attributes of a communication. These approaches share the feature of drawing some type of comparison. Usually a description is meaningless unless it is put into perspective through data compari-

sons. For instance, the fact that ten patients' accounts of their dreams during hospitalization involved death and dying is in itself difficult to interpret. Holsti (1968) has noted that the following types of comparisons are applicable to the "what" question: a comparison of messages from a single source over time, a comparison of messages from a single source in varying situations, a comparison of messages from a single source across audiences, a comparison of two or more concepts within a single message, and the comparison of messages from two or more different sources or types of sources.

Content analysis procedures

The methods used to analyze documents and communications overlap extensively with the procedures described earlier in this chapter, as well as with those used in observational studies. This is not too surprising in light of the fact that observational studies frequently deal with verbal behavior. Like the observational researcher, the investigator performing a content analysis must select the variables or concepts to be recorded, and the *unit* of content that will be employed. There are a variety of units for analyzing verbal expressions, not all of which will be of interest to nurse researchers. The smallest units, such as *letters* and *phonemes,* are unlikely to be useful to researchers in fields other than linguistics. Individual *words,* however, constitute an easy unit to work with and may be serviceable in a number of research applications. A *theme* is a more molar unit of analysis. A theme might be a phrase, sentence, or paragraph embodying ideas or making an assertion about some topic. Some examples of themes that might emerge in patients' accounts of a long-term illness experience include coping with pain, fear of death, loneliness, and loss of motivation for recovery. These are illustrations of themes organized around the content of a message, but it is possible to detect stylistic themes such as different tones (proselytizing, admonishing, informing), different grammatical structures, and so forth.

Another possible unit of analysis is the *item.* This unit refers to an entire message, document, or other production: a letter, editorial, diary entry, conference presentation, issue of a journal, and the like. The whole item can then be categorized in terms of one or more characteristics. For example, articles appearing in the journal *Nursing Research* can be classified according to whether or not the research problem was clinical in nature. Finally, the unit may be a *space-and-time* measure. This last type of unit consists of some physical measurement of content, such as the number of pages, number of words, number of speakers, amount of time spent in a discussion, and so forth. The units referred to here as "item" and "theme" are probably most useful for nurse researchers.

The next step in performing a content analysis is the development of a category system for classifying units of content. It is true that a category system is not always used by content analysts and may in some cases be unnecessary, but the employment of such a system usually enhances the scientific validity of a content analysis study by making the operation more objective and systematic. A coding system enables the researcher to classify messages along relevant dimensions of content. For example, a nurse researcher may classify the descriptions of nursing programs issued in school catalogues in terms of the following variables: NLN accreditation, length of program, size of student body, student/teacher ratio, and state or private institution.

A large variety of coding schemes are possible, even for a specific type of communication. The researcher may develop an original category system based on the idiosyncratic needs of the problem or theoretical framework. However, a criticism that has been levelled at content analyses is the absence of a generally useful and agreed-upon classification system for categorizing and comparing diverse materials. Since a number of systems have already been developed, the investigator might well use an existing scheme rather than generating a new one. Holsti's book (1969, pp. 104–116) provides many examples of category schemes and is a useful starting point for finding a system of classification. The careful training of coders assigned to do the job of categorization is essential to the success of content analysis studies.

Content analyses often apply a sampling plan in selecting materials to be analyzed. The sampling plan adopted will depend upon a number of considerations, the most salient being the extensiveness of the universe of content and the unit of analysis being used. If the unit of analysis is a word or theme, the researcher might use a systematic or random sampling procedure where the *sampling unit* (not to be confused with the unit of analysis) might be pages or paragraphs in a document. That is, the investigator would select only some pages or paragraphs for examination, either on a systematic basis (e.g., every tenth page) or randomly with a table of random numbers.

The quantification of communication materials is normally linked with the category system. The most common form of quantifying materials is the enumeration of recorded occurrences in each category. A second approach is to simply create a binary index (yes/no) of whether the concepts covered in the coding scheme were present or absent in the materials. The ranking of materials according to prespecified criteria is a third possibility. Finally, rating scales can be used to assess various aspects of the communications.

Uses of content analysis

Content analysis can either be used alone or in conjunction with other data collection methods for a variety of applications in nursing research. Historical research, for example, deals almost exclusively with written documents and, therefore, is particularly amenable to content analysis. In psychiatric nursing, or for nurses working with the handicapped, linguistic productions could serve as a criterion for evaluating nursing interventions. Content analysis can be applied to preexisting communications materials such as minutes of meetings, journal articles, and so forth or to messages produced specifically for a research project. For example, the nurses' notes in the records of patients with Alzheimer's disease could be examined for the dimensions of nursing care. The variable types that can be measured through content analysis include a broad range of social and psychological concepts, such as attitudes, emotional stability, motives, needs, expectations, stress, perceptions, values, creativity, and personality traits. This is not to say that content analysis is the *best* approach to measuring such variables. Content analysis suffers from several disadvantages such as the risk of subjectivity and the amount of tedious work involved. However, this technique may be expedient and efficient in its use of available materials, and there may be several research problems for which there are no data collection alternatives.

□
Research examples

Example using grounded theory

Forsythe, Delaney, and Gresham (1984) investigated the perceptions of hospitalized chronically ill patients concerning the effect of the illness on lifestyle, needs during hospitalization, and attitudes toward health care using the grounded theory approach. Data for the study were collected by interviewing patients and observing their interactions with nurses. The researchers audiorecorded both the interviews and observations and maintained a log of field notes. The audiorecords were transcribed for analysis. The initial interviews posed broad questions to the patients, such as "Can you tell me what this hospitalization has been like for you?" As conceptual categories of responses emerged from the interviews, additional questions were asked to help clarify the relationships among the properties of a category and among the categories themselves. For example, the researchers asked additional questions to clarify relationships between type of hospital setting and control of disease management.

Findings that emerged from the data indicated that the hospitalized, chronically ill patients developed strategies to cope with the illness and its unpredictability. The strategies permitted the patients to feel that they were "winning" in terms of controlling the progression of the disease. The specific strategies varied according to person and type of illness. When exacerbations of illness occurred, patients redesigned their strategies according to the lessened functional ability in order to maintain a positive self-image for their lifestyle. Hospitalizations were viewed as a time for restabilization of their conditions in an effort to maintain a "winning position" over their illnesses. In terms of health-care professionals, the patients viewed physicians as a source of hope in symptom control. They viewed nurses as persons who offered subtle support rather than as care-givers.

The researchers concurrently collected and analyzed the data from the interviews, observations, and field notes. They used the constant comparative method to determine the similarity of content in incidents before placing them into a category. The nature of the interviews changed as the study progressed in an effort to clarify relationships among dimensions of a category. Theoretical sampling was used to collect additional data. It is unclear from the article how or if the researchers decided that theoretical saturation had occurred.

Example of content analysis

Swider, McElmurry, and Yarling (1985) used content analysis to categorize the nursing actions that nursing students would take in resolving ethical dilemmas. The sample of 755 senior nursing students from 16 schools was divided into 146 groups. Each group was asked to list the nursing actions it would recommend taking in relation to a hypothetical ethical dilemma that could occur in nursing practice. The groups were instructed to assume that each nursing action they listed was not successful in solving the problem and asked to continue listing actions until all reasonable decisions had been exhausted.

The researchers developed a coding scheme for the content of nursing actions based upon a literature review. The three categories that evolved from the literature were patient-centered, physician-centered, and bureaucratic-centered decisions.

Findings from the study indicated that 12 percent of the responses could not be classified into any of the three categories and were placed into a fourth category labeled "other." The groups made a total of 1163 nursing decisions. The number of decisions for each category were: patient-centered—9 percent; physician-centered—19 percent; and bureaucratic-centered—60 percent. The majority of first nursing actions were bureaucratically oriented. The last nursing decisions suggested by the nursing students spanned all four categories.

In the above research study, the categories evolved from the literature and the researchers were able to classify successfully all but 12 percent of the responses. In addition to sorting the responses according to content, the researchers numerically quantified the number of responses for each category. The article failed to indicate whether more than one person independently sorted the responses into categories according to content.

□
Summary

Qualitative research typically involves the collection and analysis of loosely structured information regarding people in naturalistic settings. Qualitative nursing research has become an increasingly attractive method of inquiry, complementing more quantitative approaches in advancing nursing science.

Qualitative approaches are generally more hoslitic than quantitative approaches, and try to capture the totality of some aspect of human experience. Qualitative research is especially well suited to the following research purposes: description; hypothesis generation; illustrations of outcomes of quantitative studies; understanding causal processes; and theory development. However, qualitative approaches are less suitable for establishing cause-and-effect relationships, for rigorously testing research hypotheses, and for determining the opinions, practices, and attitudes of a large population. Qualitative methods tend to yield in-depth insights into some phenomenon because data collection tends to be intensive. However, qualitative methods have been criticized because of the difficulty of analyzing in an objective and replicable fashion masses of narrative materials. Additional shortcomings of qualitative research are that it is extremely time-consuming, usually restricted to relatively small samples, and difficult to adequately summarize in professional journals.

Although qualitative materials *can* be quantified and subsequently analyzed with statistical procedures, most qualitative researchers prefer to analyze their data through qualitative analysis. The first major step in analyzing qualitative data is to organize the materials according to some plan. One method of organization involves the development of an elaborate file system. In using this system, researchers generally develop a conceptual coding scheme and code all of the narrative materials (e.g., observational notes or transcripts of interviews); then a file is created for each of the topics covered in the coding scheme, so that the researcher can retrieve all of the information on one topic by going to a single file. Other organizational procedures are also possible, including the use of computer files.

The actual analysis of data begins with a search for *themes*. The search for themes involves not only the discovery of commonalities across subjects, but also of natural variation in the data. The next step generally involves a validation of the thematic analysis. Some researchers use a procedure known as *quasi-statistics,* which involves a tabulation of the frequency with which certain themes or relations are supported by the data. In a final step, the analyst tries to weave the thematic strands together into an integrated picture of the phenomenon under investigation.

While this overview summarizes some of the major steps, there are a number of different philosophies underlying qualitative analysis. *Analytic induction* refers to an approach in which the researcher alternates back and forth between tentative definition of emerging hypotheses and tentative explanation, with each iteration making refinements. *Grounded theory* is a term used to describe field investigations, the purpose of which is to discover theoretical precepts grounded in the data. This approach makes use of a technique called *constant comparison:* Categories elicited from the data are constantly compared with data obtained earlier so that commonalities and variations can be determined. Both of these approaches have their intellectual roots in sociological inquiry.

Content analysis is a method for quantifying the content of communications in a systematic and objective fashion. Communications include newspaper articles, diaries, speeches, and verbal expressions. It is systematic in that data are methodically included or excluded according to predetermined criteria. Content analysis is most commonly used to describe the content of the message, although it may be used to answer questions concerning other elements of communication. A variety of units of analysis exist for verbal expressions. The most useful unit for nurse researchers are *themes,* which embody ideas or concepts, and *items,* which refer to the entire message. Once the researcher has chosen the unit of analysis, a classification system to permit the categorization of messages according to content is developed.

□
Study suggestions

1. Suggest five research problems amenable to qualitative research. Explain why you think the problem is better suited to a qualitative than to a quantitative approach.
2. Read a qualitative nursing study (several are suggested in the Substantive References section below). Do you think that if a different investigator had gone into the field to study the same problem, the conclusions would have been the same? How generalizable are the researcher's findings? What did the researcher learn that he or she would probably not have learned with a more structured and quantified approach?
3. As a class assignment, have each student ask two persons to describe their conception of preventive health care and what it means in their daily lives. Pool all of the narrative descriptions and develop a coding scheme to organize the reasons. What are the major themes that emerge?
4. What units of analysis would be appropriate for performing a content analysis of the following materials: letters from nurses stationed in Europe during World War II; the diary of an adolescent dying from leukemia; the minutes of meetings from a state nurses' association; and the articles appearing in the *American Journal of Nursing?*

□
Suggested readings

Methodological references

Bargagliotti, L.A. (1983). The scientific method and phenomenology: Toward their peaceful coexistence in nursing. *Western Journal of Nursing Research, 5,* 409–411.

Becker, H.S. (1970). *Sociological work.* Chicago: Aldine.

Benoliel, J.Q. (1984). Advancing nursing science: Qualitative approaches. *Western Journal of Nursing Research, 6,* 1–8.

Berelson, B. (1971). *Content analysis in communication research.* New York: Free Press.

Downs, F.S. (1983). One dark and stormy night. *Nursing Research, 32,* 259.

Evaneshko, V. & Kay, M.A. (1982). The ethnoscience research technique. *Western Jouranl of Nursing Research, 4,* 51–64.

Fielding, N.G. & Fielding, J.L. (1985). *Linking data.* Beverly Hills, CA: Sage Publications.

Glaser, B.G. & Strauss, A.L. (1967). *The discovery of grounded theory: Strategies for qualitative research.* Chicago: Aldine.

Goodwin, L.D. & Goodwin, W.L. (1984). Qualitative vs. quantitative research or qualitative *and* quantitative research. *Nursing Research, 33,* 378–380.

Gorenberg, B. (1983). The research tradition of nursing: An emerging issue. *Nursing Research, 32,* 347–349.

Holsti, O.R. (1968). Content analysis. In G. Lindzey & E. Aronson (Eds.), *The handbook of social psychology* (2nd ed.). Reading, MA: Addison-Wesley, Vol. II, pp. 596–692.

Holsti, O.R. (1969). *Content analysis for the social sciences and humanities.* Reading, MA: Addison-Wesley (Content analysis).

Klenow, D.J. (1981). Qualitative methodology: A neglected resource in nursing research. *Research in Nursing and Health, 4,* 281–292.

Krippendorff, K. (1980). *Content analysis: An introduction to its methodology.* Beverly Hills: Sage Publications.

Leininger, M.M. (Ed.). (1985). *Qualitative research methods in nursing.* New York: Grune & Stratton.

Miles, M.B. and Huberman, A.M. (1984). *Qualitative data analysis.* Beverly Hills, CA: Sage.

Munhall, P.L. (1982). Nursing philosophy and nursing research: In apposition or opposition? *Nursing Research, 31,* 176–177.

Oiler, C. (1982). The phenomenological approach in nursing research. *Nursing Research, 31,* 178–181.

Simms, L.M. (1981). The grounded theory approach in nursing research. *Nursing Research, 30,* 356–359.

Stern, P.M. (1985). Using grounded theory method in nursing research. In M.M. Leininger (Ed.), *Qualitative research methods in nursing.* New York: Grune & Stratton.

Webster, G., Jacox, A., & Baldwin, B. (1981). Nursing theory and the ghost of the received view. In H. Grace & B. McCloskey (eds.), *Contemporary issues in nursing.* Boston: Blackwell Scientific Publications.

Substantive references

DeVellis, B.M., Adams, J.L., & DeVellis, R.F. (1984). Effects of information on patient stereotyping. *Research in Nursing and Health, 7,* 237–244 (content analysis).

Forsyth, G.L., Delaney, K.D. & Gresham, M.L. (1984). Vying for a winning position: Management style of the chronically ill. *Research in Nursing and Health, 7,* 181–188.

Kalisch, B.J., Kalisch, P.A. & McHugh, M.L. (1982). The nurse as a sex object in motion pictures, 1930 to 1980. *Reserch in Nursing and Health, 5,* 147–154 (content analysis).

Knafl, K.A. (1985). How families manage a pediatric hospitalization. *Western Journal of Nursing Research, 7,* 151–176.

Kus, R.J. (1985). Stages of coming out: An ethnographic approach. *Western Journal of Nursing Research, 7,* 177–198.

Macintyre, S. (1977). *Single and pregnant.* London: Croom Helm.

May, K.A. (1982). Three phases of father involvement in pregnancy. *Nursing Research, 31,* 337–342.

Patterson, E.T. & Hale, E.S. (1985). Making sure: Integrating menstrual care practices into activities of daily living. *Advances in Nursing Science, 7,* 18–31.

Phillips, L.R. & Rempusheski, V.F. (1985). A decision-making model for diagnosing and intervening in elder abuse and neglect. *Nursing Research, 34,* 134–139.

Powers, M.J., Murphy, S.P. & Wooldridge, P.J. (1983). Validation of two experimental nursing approaches using content analyses. *Research in Nursing and Health, 6,* 3–9 (content analysis).

Ritchie, J.A., Caty, S. & Ellerton, M.L. (1984). Concerns of acutely ill, chronically ill, and healthy preschool children. *Research in Nursing and Health, 7,* 265–274 (content analysis).

Schuster, E.A., Kruger, S.F. & Hebenstreit, J.J. (1985). A theory of protection: Parents as sex educators. *Advances in Nursing Science, 7,* 70–77.

Stern, P.N. (1982). Affiliating in stepfather families. *Western Journal of Nursing Research, 4,* 75–89.

Swider, S.M., McElmurry, B.J. & Yarling, R.R. (1985). Ethical decision making in a bureaucratic context by senior nursing students. *Nursing Research, 34,* 108–112 (content analysis).

Weiss, S. & Remen, N. (1983). Self-limiting patterns of nursing behavior within a tripartite context involving consumers and physicians. *Western Journal of Nursing Research, 5,* 77–89.

Chapter 20 □ Descriptive statistics

Statistical methods are techniques for rendering quantitative information meaningful and intelligible. Without the aid of statistics, the quantitative data collected in a research project would be little more than a chaotic mass of numbers. Statistical procedures enable the researcher to reduce, summarize, organize, evaluate, interpret, and communicate numerical information.

A knowledge of basic statistical methods is indispensable for those who want to keep abreast of research developments in their field. Many individuals are intimidated by statistics because they feel they are "no good at math." It is not necessary to have strong mathematical talent to profit from the advantages of statistical analysis. In order to apply and interpret statistics, one needs only basic arithmetic skills and logical thinking ability. In the remainder of this chapter and in the two that follow, there will be no emphasis on the theoretical rationale or mathematical derivation of statistical operations. In fact, even computation will be underplayed because this is not a statistics text and also because statistics are seldom calculated by hand in this era of computers and calculators. The emphasis will be on how to use statistics appropriately in different research situations and how to understand what they mean once they have been applied.

Statistics usually are classified as either descriptive or inferential. *Descriptive statistics* are used to describe and synthesize data obtained from empirical observations and measurements. Averages and percentages are examples of descriptive statistics. Actually, when such indices are calculated on data from a population, they are referred to as *parameters*. A descriptive index from a sample is called a *statistic.* Most scientific questions are about parameters, but researchers usually must be content to calculate statistics to estimate those parameters. When researchers use statistics to make inferences or draw conclusions about a population, then *inferential statistics* are required. This chapter focuses on descriptive statistical procedures.

□
Frequency distributions

Raw data that are neither analyzed nor organized are overwhelming. It is not even possible to discern general trends until some order or structure is imposed on the data. Consider the 60 numbers presented in Table 20-1. Let us assume that these numbers represent the scores of 60 industrial nurses on a 30-item test to measure knowledge about industrial alcoholism and drug abuse. Visual inspection of the numbers in this table is not too helpful in understanding how the nurses performed. The data are too numerous to make much sense of them in this form.

A set of data can be completely summarized in terms of three characteristics: the shape of the distribution of scores, central tendency, and variability. The latter two characteristics are dealt with in subsequent sections.

Constructing frequency distributions

Frequency distributions represent a method of imposing some order on a mass of numerical data with little or no loss of information. A *frequency distribution* is a systematic arrangement of numerical values from the lowest to the highest, together with a count of the number of times each value was obtained. The fictitious test scores of the industrial nurses are presented as a frequency distribution in Table 20-2. It should be apparent that this organized arrangement makes it convenient to see at a

Table 20-1
Test scores for industrial nurses

22	27	25	19	24	25	23	29	24	20
26	16	20	26	17	22	24	18	26	28
15	24	23	22	21	24	20	25	18	27
24	23	16	25	30	29	27	21	23	24
26	18	30	21	17	25	22	24	29	28
20	25	26	24	23	19	27	28	25	26

glance how the nurses performed. We can see what the highest and lowest scores were, where the bulk of scores tended to cluster, and what the most common score was. None of this was easily discernible before the data were organized.

The construction of a frequency distribution is very simple. It consists basically of two parts: the classes of observations or measurements (the Xs) and the frequency or count of the observations falling in each class (the *f*s). The observations are listed in numerical order in one column and the corresponding frequencies are listed in another. Table 20-2 shows the intermediary step in which the observations were actually tallied by the familiar method of four vertical bars and then a slash for the fifth observation. The only requirement for a frequency distribution is that the classes of observation must be mutually exclusive and exhaustive. The sum of the numbers appearing in the frequency column must be equal to the size of the sample. In less verbal terms, $\Sigma f = n$, which translates as the sum of (signified by the Greek letter sigma, Σ) the frequencies (f) equals the sample size (n).

It is often useful to display not only the frequency counts for different values but also the percentages of the total, as shown in the fourth column of Table 20-2. The percents are calculated by the simple formula: $\% = f/n \times 100$. Just as the sum of all frequencies should equal n, the sum of all percentages should equal 100.

Rather than listing frequencies in tabular form, many researchers prefer to display their data graphically. Graphs have the advantage of

Table 20-2
Frequency distribution of test scores

Score (X)	Tallies	Frequency (f)	Percent (%)
15	|	1	1.7
16	||	2	3.3
17	||	2	3.3
18	|||	3	5.0
19	||	2	3.3
20	||||	4	6.7
21	|||	3	5.0
22	||||	4	6.7
23	⊬⊬	5	8.3
24	⊬⊬ ||||	9	15.0
25	⊬⊬ ||	7	11.7
26	⊬⊬ |	6	10.0
27	||||	4	6.7
28	|||	3	5.0
29	|||	3	5.0
30	||	2	3.3
		$n = 60 = \Sigma f$	$100\% = \Sigma\%$

being able to communicate a lot of information almost instantaneously. The most widely used types of graphs are *histograms* and *frequency polygons*. These two types are actually similar forms of presenting the same data.

Both histograms and frequency polygons are constructed in much the same fashion. First, score classes are placed on a horizontal dimension, with the lowest value on the left, ascending to the highest value on the right. Next, the vertical dimension is used to designate the frequency count or, alternatively, percentages. The numbering of the vertical axis usually begins with zero. Using these dimensions as a base, a histogram is constructed by drawing bars above the score classes to the height corresponding to the frequency for that score class. An example is presented in Figure 20-1, using the same fictitious data on test scores for industrial nurses.

Instead of vertical bars, the frequency polygon employs dots connected by straight lines to show frequencies for score classes. A dot corresponding to the frequency is placed above each score, as shown in Figure 20-2. It is

conventional to connect the figure to the base (zero line) at the score below the minimum value obtained and above the maximum value obtained. In this particular example, however, the graph is terminated at 30 and brought down to the base at that point with a dotted line because a score of 31 was not possible.

Shapes of distributions

A distribution of numerical values can assume an almost infinite number of shapes or forms. However, there are general aspects of the shape that can be described verbally. A distribution is said to be *symmetrical* in shape if, when folded over, the two halves of the distribution would be superimposed on one another. In other words, symmetrical distributions consist of two havles that are mirror images of one another. All of the distributions shown in Figure 20-3 are symmetrical. With real data sets, the distributions are rarely as perfectly symmetrical as shown in this figure. However, minor discrepancies are often ig-

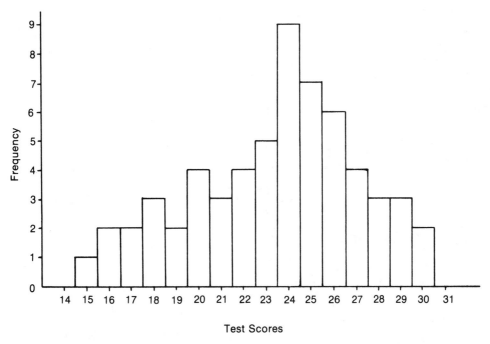

Figure 20-1. Histogram of test scores.

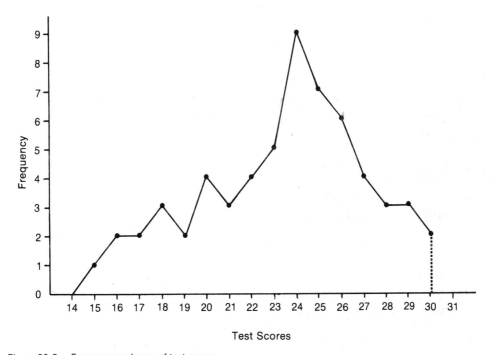

Figure 20-2. Frequency polygon of test scores.

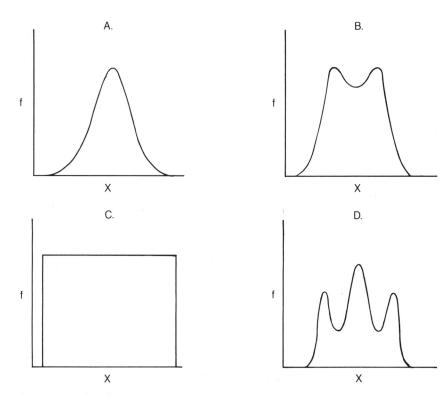

Figure 20-3. *Examples of symmetrical distributions.*

nored in trying to briefly characterize the shape of a distribution.

Nonsymmetrical distributions usually are described as being *skewed*. In skewed distributions, the peak is "off center" and one tail is longer than the other. Distributions that are skewed are usually described in terms of the direction of the skew. When the longer tail is pointing toward the right, the distribution is said to be *positively skewed*. Graph A of Figure 20-4 depicts a positively skewed distribution. If, on the other hand, the tail points to the left, the skew is described as negative. A *negatively skewed* distribution is illustrated in graph B, in Figure 20-4. An example of an actual attribute that is positively skewed is personal income. The bulk of people have low to moderate incomes, with relatively few people in very high income brackets at the tail of the distribution. An example of a negatively skewed attribute is age at death. Here, the bulk of people are at the upper end of the distribution, with relatively few people dying at an early age.

A second aspect of a distribution's shape is its modality. A *unimodal* distribution is one that has only one peak or high point (that is, a value with high frequency), whereas a *multimodal* distribution has two or more peaks (two or more values of high frequency). The most common type of multimodal distribution is one with two peaks, which is called *bimodal*. Graph A in Figure 20-3 is unimodal, as are both graphs in Figure 20-4. Multimodal distributions are illustrated in graphs B and D of Figure 20-3. It should be noted that symmetry and modality are completely independent

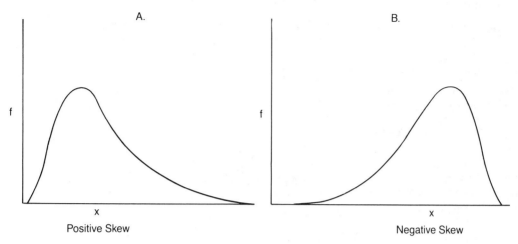

Figure 20-4. *Examples of skewed distributions.*

aspects of a distribution. Knowledge of skewness does not tell you anything about how many peaks the distribution has.

Some distributions are encountered so frequently that special labels are used to designate them. Of particular interest in statistical analysis is the distribution known as the *normal curve.* In terms of the descriptions introduced above, a normal curve is one that is symmetrical, unimodal, and not too peaked, as illustrated by the distribution in graph A of Figure 20-3. Many physical and psychological attributes of human beings have been found to approximate a normal distribution. Examples include height, intelligence, birth weight, and grip strength. As we will see in the next chapter, the normal curve plays a central role in inferential statistics.

□
Central tendency

Frequency distributions are an important means of imposing order on a set of raw data and of clarifying group patterns. For many purposes, however, a group pattern is of less interest to a researcher than an overall summary of a group's characteristics. The researcher usually asks such questions as: What is the average oxygen consumption of myocardial infarction patients during bathing? What is the average blood pressure reading of hypertensive patients during relaxation therapy? or How much information does the average pregnant teenager have about nutrition? Such questions seek a single number that best represents a whole distribution of measures. Because an index of "typicalness" is more likely to be representative if it comes from the center of a distribution than if it comes from either extreme, such indices are referred to as measures of *central tendency.* To lay persons the term *average* is normally used to designate central tendency. Researchers seldom use this term because it is too ambiguous, inasmuch as there are three commonly used kinds of averages, or indices of central tendency: the mode, the median, and the mean. Each can be used as an index to represent a whole set of measurements.

The mode

The mode is that numerical value in a distribution that occurs most frequently. The mode is the simplest to determine of the three measures of central tendency. Actually, the mode is not computed, but rather arrived at through inspection of a frequency distribution. In the following distribution of numbers, one can readily determine that the mode is 53:

50 51 51 52 53 53 53 53 54 55 56

The score of 53 was obtained four times, a higher frequency than for any other number. In the example used earlier in this chapter, the mode of the test scores of industrial nurses is 24 (Table 20-2). The mode, in other words, identifies the most "popular" score (In multimodal distributions, of course, there is more than one score value that has high frequencies). The mode is seldom used in research reports as the only index of central tendency. Modes are a quick and easy method of determining an "average" at a glance but are unsuitable for further computation and are also rather unstable. By unstable we mean that modes tend to fluctuate widely from one sample drawn from a population to another sample drawn from the same population. The mode is infrequently used, except for describing "typical" values on nominal-level measures. For instance, researchers often characterize their samples by providing modal information on nominal-level demographic variables, as in the following example: "The typical subject was a white female, unmarried, living in an urban area, and of a Protestant background."

The median

The median is that point on a numerical scale above which and below which 50 percent of the cases fall. As an example, consider the following set of values:

2 2 3 3 4 5 6 7 8 9

The value that divides the cases exactly in half

is 4.5, which is the median for this set of numbers. The point that has 50 percent of the cases above and below it is halfway between 4 and 5. An important characteristic of the median is that it does not take into account the quantitative values of individual scores. The median is an index of average *position* in a distribution of numbers. The median is insensitive to extreme values. Let us take the previous example to illustrate this point, making only one small change:

2 2 3 3 4 5 6 7 8 99

Despite the fact that the last value has been increased from 9 to 99, the median remains unchanged at 4.5. Because of this property, the median is often the preferred index of central tendency when the distribution is skewed and when one is interested in finding a "typical" value in measures on an ordinal scale or higher.

The mean

The mean is the point on the score scale that is equal to the sum of the scores divided by the number of scores. The mean is the index of central tendency that is usually referred to as an average. The computational formula for a mean — which everyone knows, but whose symbols need to be learned — is:

$$\overline{X} = \frac{\Sigma X}{n}$$

where $\overline{X}$ = the mean
Σ = the sum of
X = each individual raw score
n = the number of cases

The researcher should become familiar with these symbols because they are commonly used to report results in the research literature.

Let us apply the above formula to calculate the mean weight of eight subjects whose individual weights are as follows:

85 109 120 135 158 177 181 195

$$\overline{X} = \frac{85 + 109 + 120 + 135 + 158 + 177 + 181 + 195}{8}$$

$$= 145$$

Unlike the median, the mean is affected by the value of each and every score. If we were to exchange the 195-pound subject in the above example for a subject weighing 275, the mean would increase from 145 to 155. A substitution of this kind would leave the median unchanged.

The mean is unquestionably the most widely used measure of central tendency. Most of the important tests of statistical significance, which will be dealt with in the next chapter, are based upon the mean. When researchers work with interval-level or ratio-level measurements, the mean rather than the median or mode is almost always the statistic reported.

Comparison of the mode, median, and mean

Of the three indices of central tendency, the mean is the most stable. This means that if repeated samples were drawn from a given population, the means would vary or fluctuate less than the modes or medians. Because of its stability, the mean is the most reliable estimate of the central tendency of the population.

The arithmetic mean is the most appropriate index in situations in which the concern is for totals or combined performance of a group. If a school of nursing were comparing two graduating classes in terms of scores on the national licensure examination, then the calculation of two means would be in order. Sometimes, however, the primary concern is learning what a "typical" value is, in which case a median might be preferred. In efforts to understand the economic well-being of United States citizens, for example, we would get a distorted impression of the financial status of the typical individual by considering the mean. The mean in this case would be inflated by the wealth of a small minority. The median, on the other hand, would reflect more realistically how the "average" person fared financially.

When a distribution of scores is symmetrical and unimodal, the three indices of central tendency coincide. In skewed distributions, the values of the mode, median, and mean differ. The mean is always pulled in the direction of the long tail, as shown in Figure 20-5. It is only in skewed distributions, therefore, that one must consider which index to use. When the distribution is nonsymmetrical, it might be preferable to simply report all three values than to select a single index, since all three indices contain some information.

☐ Variability

Although measures of central tendency are of immense importance in descriptions of data, averages do not give a total picture of a distribution. Two sets of data with identical means could be different from one another in several respects. For one thing, two distributions with the same mean could be very different in shape: they could be skewed in opposite directions, for example. The characteristic of concern in this section is how spread out or dispersed the data are. The variability of two distributions could be quite different, whereas the mean values could be identical.

The concept of variability is concerned with the degree to which the subjects in a sample are similar to one another with respect to the critical attribute. Consider the two distributions in Figure 20-6 which represent the hypothetical scores of freshmen students from two schools of nursing on the Scholastic Aptitude

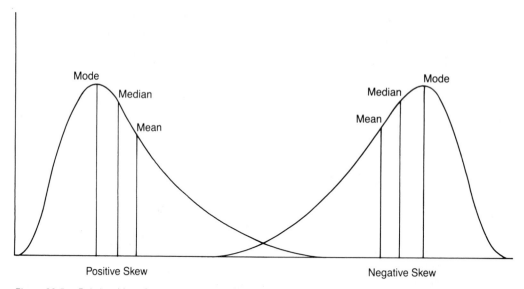

Figure 20-5. *Relationships of central tendency indices in skewed distributions.*

Test. Both distributions have an average of 500, but the outcomes are clearly different. In School A, there is a wide range of obtained scores: from scores below 300 to some above 700. This school has many students who performed among the best, but also has many students who were well below average. In School B, on the other hand, there are few students at either extreme. School A is said to be more *heterogeneous* than School B, but School B may be described as more *homogeneous* than School A.

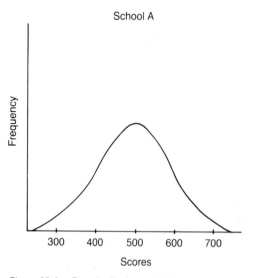

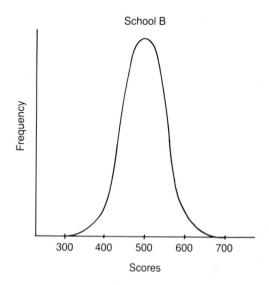

Figure 20-6. *Two distributions of different variability.*

In order to describe a distribution adequately, there is clearly a need for a measure of variability that expresses the extent to which scores deviate from one another. Several such indices have been developed, the most common of which are the range, semiquartile range, and standard deviation.

The range

The range is simply the highest score minus the lowest score in a given distribution. In the examples shown in Figure 20-6 the range for School A is approximately 500 (750−250), while the range for School B is approximately 300 (650−350). The range indicates the distance on the score scale between the lowest and highest values.

The chief virtue of the range is the ease with which it can be computed. As an index of variability, the shortcomings of the range outweigh this modest advantage. The range, being based on only two scores, is a highly unstable index. From sample to sample drawn from the same population, the range tends to fluctuate considerably. Another difficulty with the range is that it ignores completely variations in scores between the two extremes. In School B of Figure 20-6, suppose that one "deviant" student obtained a score of 250, and another obtained a score of 750. The range of both schools would then be 500, despite obvious differences in the heterogeneity of scores. For these reasons, the range is used largely as a gross descriptive index and is typically reported in conjunction with, not instead of, other measures of variability.

Semiquartile range*

In the previous section, the median was described as the point below which 50 percent of

the cases fall. It is computationally possible to determine the point below which any percent of the scores fall. For example, an admissions committee for a school of nursing might establish a minimum standard at the 80th percentile on the Scholastic Aptitude Test for its entrants. The *semiquartile range* is calculated on the basis of quartiles within a distribution. The upper quartile (Q_3) is the point below which 75 percent of the cases fall, and the lower quartile (Q_1) is the point below which 25 percent of the scores lie.* The semiquartile range is half the distance between Q_1 and Q_3, or

$$SQR = \frac{Q_3 - Q_1}{2}$$

The semiquartile range indicates half the range of scores within which the middle 50 percent of scores lie. Because this index is a measure based on middle cases rather than extreme scores, it is considerably more stable than the range. In the case of the two nursing schools in Figure 20-6, School A would have an SQR in the vicinity of 125, while that of School B would be approximately 75. The addition of one deviant case at either extreme for School B would leave the semiquartile range virtually untouched.

Standard deviation

The most widely used measure of variability is the *standard deviation (SD)*. Like the mean, the standard deviation takes into consideration every score in a distribution.

What is needed in a variability index is some way of capturing the degree to which scores deviate from one another. This concept of deviation is represented in both the range and the semiquartile range by the presence of a minus sign, which produces an index of devia-

---

* Some statistical texts use the term semiquartile range, while others refer to this statistic as the semi-interquartile range or the quartile deviation.

* The computational formulas for percentiles are not presented here. Most standard statistics texts contain this information.

Table 20-3
Computation of a standard deviation

X	$x = X - \overline{X}$	$x^2 = (X - \overline{X})^2$
4	−3	9
5	−2	4
6	−1	1
7	0	0
7	0	0
7	0	0
8	1	1
9	2	4
10	3	9

$$X = 63$$
$$\Sigma X/n = \overline{X}$$
$$= 63/9 = 7$$

$$\Sigma x = 0 \qquad \Sigma x^2 = 28$$

$$SD = \sqrt{\frac{28}{9}} = \sqrt{3.11} = 1.76$$

tion, or difference, between two score points. The standard deviation is similarly based upon score differences. In fact, the first step in calculating a standard deviation is to compute *deviation scores* for each subject. A deviation score (usually symbolized with a small x) is the difference between an individual score and the mean. If a person weighed 150 pounds and the sample mean was 140, the person's deviation score would be +10. Symbolically, the formula for a deviation score is: $x = X - \overline{X}$.

Because what one is essentially looking for in an index of variability is a kind of "average" deviation, one might think that a good variability index could be arrived at by summing the deviation scores and then dividing by the number of cases. This gets us close to a good solution, but the difficulty is that the sum of a set of deviation scores is always zero. Table 20-3 presents an example of deviation scores computed for nine numbers. As shown in the second column, the sum of the xs is equal to zero. The deviations above the mean always balance exactly those deviations below the mean.

The standard deviation overcomes this problem by squaring each deviation score before summing. After dividing by the number of

cases, one takes the square root to bring the index back to the original units. The formula for the standard deviation* is:

$$SD = \sqrt{\frac{\Sigma x^2}{n}}$$

The standard deviation has been completely worked out in the example in Table 20-3. First, a deviation score is calculated for each of the nine raw scores by subtracting the mean ($\overline{X} = 7$) from them. The third column shows that each deviation score is squared, thereby converting all values to positive numbers. The squared deviation scores are summed ($\Sigma x^2 = 28$), divided by 9(n), and a square root taken to yield a standard deviation of 1.76.

Most researchers routinely report the standard deviation of a data set along with the mean. Sometimes, however, one will find a reference to an index of variability known as the variance. The *variance*† is simply the value of the standard deviation before a square root has been taken. In other words:

$$Var = \frac{\Sigma x^2}{n} = SD^2$$

In the above example, the variance is $(1.76)^2$, or 3.11. The variance is less widely reported because it is an index that is not the same unit of measurement as the original data. The variance, however, is an important component in many inferential statistical tests and will be encountered later. In any event, once a var-

---

* Some statistical texts indicate that the formula for an unbiased estimate of the population SD is

$$SD = \sqrt{\frac{\Sigma x^2}{n - 1}}$$

Knapp (1970) clarifies when n or $n - 1$ should be used in the denominator. He indicates that n is appropriate when the researcher is interested in *describing* variation in sample data.

† Various symbols are used for the variance and standard deviation. The most common are σ^2 (σ) or s^2 (s), respectively.

iance is obtained, it is a simple step to get a standard deviation, and vice versa.

A standard deviation is typically more difficult for students to interpret than other statistics such as the mean or range. In the example above we calculated an *SD* of 1.76. One might well ask, 1.76 *what?* What does the number mean? We will try to answer these questions from several vantage points. First, as we already know, the standard deviation is an index of how variable the scores in a data set are. If two distributions had a mean of 25.0, but one had a standard deviation of 7.0 while the other had a standard deviation of 3.0, we would immediately know that the second sample was more homogeneous.

A convenient way to conceptualize the standard deviation is to think of it as an average of the deviations from the mean. The mean tells us the single best point for summarizing an entire distribution, whereas a standard deviation tells us how much, on the average, the scores deviate from that mean. A standard deviation might thus be interpreted as an indication of our degree of error when we use a mean to describe an entire data set.

The standard deviation can also be used in interpreting individual scores from within a distribution. Let us suppose we had a set of weight measures from a sample whose mean weight was 125 and whose standard deviation was ten. We can think of the standard deviation as actually providing a "standard" of variability. Weights greater than 1 standard deviation away from the mean (i.e., greater than 135 or less than 115) are greater than the average variability for that distribution. Weights less than one standard deviation from the mean, by consequence, are less than the average variability for that sample.

When the distribution of scores is normal, it is possible to say even more about the standard deviation. A normal curve, it will be recalled, is a symmetric, unimodal curve. There are approximately three standard deviations above

and below the mean with normally distributed data. To illustrate some further characteristics, suppose that we had a normal distribution of scores whose mean was 50 and whose standard deviation was 10. Such a distribution is shown in Figure 20-7. In a normal distribution such as this, a fixed percentage of cases fall within certain distances from the mean. Sixty-eight percent of all cases fall within one standard deviation of the mean. In this example, nearly seven out of every ten scores fall between 40 and 60. Ninety-five percent of the scores in a normal distribution fall within 2 standard deviations from the mean. Only a handful of cases — about 2 percent at each extreme — lie more than 2 SDs from the mean. Using this figure we can see that a person who obtained a score of 70 got a higher score than about 98 percent of the sample.

In sum, the standard deviation is a useful index of variability that can be used to describe an important characteristic of a distribution and that also can be used to interpret the score or performance of an individual vis-à-vis others in the sample. Like the mean, the standard deviation is a stable estimate of a population parameter and also is used extensively in more advanced statistical procedures. The standard deviation is the preferred measure of a distribution's variability.

□
Levels of measurement and descriptive statistics

The kinds of statistics discussed thus far cannot be indiscriminantly applied to a set of data without considering the measurement characteristics of the scores. In an earlier chapter it was pointed out that there are four levels of measurement: nominal, ordinal, interval, and ratio. The level of measurement plays a role in determining the appropriate descriptive statistic for a variable.

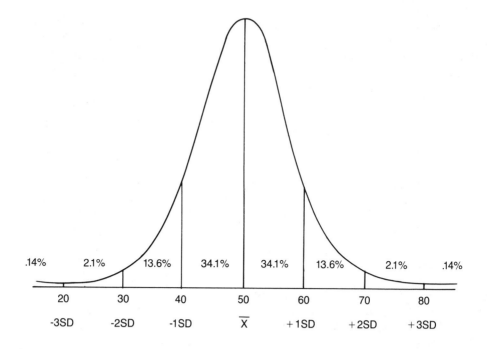

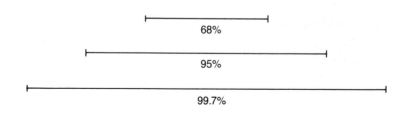

Figure 20-7. *Standard deviations in a normal distribution.*

In general, the higher the level of measurement, the greater the flexibility one has in choosing a descriptive statistic. Variables measured on an interval or ratio scale can use any of the three indices of central tendency, although it usually will be preferable to use the mean. However, for nominal-level data, it would make little sense to compute a mean. If we coded marital status as "1" for single, "2" for married, and "3" for other, a mean marital status of 1.73 would be nonsensical. It would,

however, be reasonable to determine the modal response for nominal data.

Table 20-4 presents a rough guide of the statistics appropriate with different levels of measurement. It should be remembered that it is always possible to choose a statistic from a lower level, but not from a higher one. One could use the range as an index of variability for data on a person's pulse rate (ratio level), but it would not be meaningful to calculate a standard deviation for a measure of ethnicity

Table 20-4
Guide to use of descriptive statistics

		Level of Measurement	
	Nominal	Ordinal	Interval or Ratio
Measure of Central Tendency	mode	median	mean
Measure of Variability	range	semiquartile range	standard deviation/variance

(nominal level). Generally it is not advisable to select a statistic that is suitable to a lower level of data, but circumstances may warrant it, as in the case of using a median with a severely skewed distribution.

□
Bivariate descriptive statistics: contingency tables and correlation

The discussion has so far focused on a description of single variables. The mean, mode, standard deviation, and so forth are all used in describing data for one variable at a time. We have been examining what is referred to as *univariate* (one-variable) statistics. As indicated throughout this text, research usually is concerned with relationships between variables. What is needed then, is some method of describing such relationships. In this section we will look at *bivariate* (two-variable) descriptive statistics.

Contingency tables

A contingency table is essentially a two-dimensional frequency distribution in which the frequencies of two variables are cross-tabulated. Suppose we had data on subjects' sex and responses to a question on whether they were nonsmokers, light smokers, or heavy smokers. We might be interested in learning if there is a tendency for members of one sex to smoke more heavily than members of the opposite sex. Some fictitious data on these two variables are presented in Table 20-5. It is difficult to make sense of these data in their present form. In order to describe the data we need a method of organizing this mass of numbers. The best way to do so in a manner that highlights the research question is to construct a contingency table.

A contingency table for the data in Table 20-5 is presented in Table 20-6. Six "cells" are created by placing one variable (sex) along the vertical dimension and the other variable (smoking status) along the horizontal dimension. The system of bars and cross hatches can then be used to tabulate the number of subjects belonging in each cell. The first subject, who has a code of 1 for sex and 1 for smoking status, would be marked in the upper left-hand cell, and so on. After all subjects have been "assigned" to the appropriate cells, the frequencies can be tabulated and percentages computed. This simple procedure allows us to see at a glance that, in this particular sample, women were more likely to be nonsmokers and less likely to be heavy smokers than males. Contingency tables, or cross-tabulations as they are sometimes called, are easy to construct and have the ability to communicate a lot of information. The use of contingency tables usually is restricted to nominal data or to ordinal data that have few levels or ranks. In the present example, sex is a nominal measure and smoking status is an ordinal measure. We will encounter contingency tables again in the chapter on inferential statistics.

Table 20-5
Fictitious data on sex/smoking relationship

Subject Sex*	Smoking Status†	Subject Sex	Smoking Status	Subject Sex	Smoking Status
1	1	2	2	2	1
2	3	2	3	1	1
2	1	1	1	2	2
1	2	2	2	1	2
1	1	1	2	1	1
2	2	1	1	2	2
2	1	1	3	2	3
2	3	1	2	2	3
1	1	2	2	2	2
2	3	2	1	1	2
1	2	1	3	1	1
1	3	2	3	2	1
1	1	1	1	1	2
2	3	1	3	2	2
2	1	1	2		

* 1 = female; 2 = male
† 1 = nonsmoker; 2 = light smoker; 3 = heavy smoker

Correlation

The most common method of describing the relationship between two measures is through correlation procedures. The computation of a correlation coefficient is normally performed with either ordinal, interval, or ratio data. Correlation coefficients were briefly described in Chapter 17, and this section extends that discussion.

The correlation question asks: to what extent are two variables related to each other? For example, to what extent are height and weight related? To what degree are anxiety test scores and blood pressure measures related? These questions can be answered graphically or, more commonly, by the calculation of an index that describes the magnitude of a relationship.

The graphic representation of a correlation between two variables is called a *scatter plot* or scatter diagram. In order to construct a scatter plot, one first sets up a scale for the two variables constructed at right angles, making a rectangular coordinate graph. The range of values for one variable (X) is scaled off along

Table 20-6
Contingency table for sex/smoker relationship

	Nonsmoker (1)	Light Smoker (2)	Heavy Smoker (3)	Total
Female (1)	∣ ∣ ∣ ∣ ∣ ∣ ∣ ∣ 10 (45% of females)	∣ ∣ ∣ ∣ ∣ ∣ ∣ 8 (36% of females)	∣ ∣ ∣ ∣ 4 (18% of females)	22 (50% of sample)
Males (2)	∣ ∣ ∣ ∣ ∣ 6 (27% of males)	∣ ∣ ∣ ∣ ∣ ∣ ∣ 8 (36% of males)	∣ ∣ ∣ ∣ ∣ ∣ ∣ 8 (36% of males)	22 (50% of sample)
TOTAL	16 (36% of sample)	16 (36% of sample)	12 (27% of sample)	44 (100% of sample)

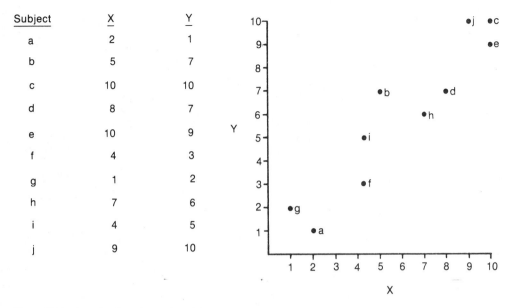

Subject	X	Y
a	2	1
b	5	7
c	10	10
d	8	7
e	10	9
f	4	3
g	1	2
h	7	6
i	4	5
j	9	10

Figure 20-8. Construction of a scatter plot.

the horizontal axis, while the same is done for the second variable (Y) along the vertical axis. Such a graph is presented in Figure 20-8. To locate the position for subject a, one goes over two units along the X-axis, and up one unit on the Y-axis. The same procedure is followed for all subjects, resulting in the scatter plot shown. The letters shown on the plot in this figure have been included to help identify each point. Normally only the "dots" appear on the diagram.

From a scatter plot it is possible to determine both the direction and approximate magnitude of a correlation. The direction of the slope of points indicates the direction of the correlation. It may be recalled from Chapter 17 that correlations can be either positive or negative in direction. A positive correlation is obtained when high values on one variable are associated with high values on the second variable. If the slope of points begins at the lower left corner and extends to the upper right corner, the relationship is positive. In the present example, we would say that X and Y

are positively related. Inspection of the values shows that, indeed, persons who have a high score on variable X also tend to have a high score on variable Y, while low-scorers on X tend to score low on Y.

A negative relationship is one in which high values on one variable are related to low values on the other. On a scatter plot, negative relationships are depicted by points that slope from the upper left corner to the lower right corner. A negative correlation is shown in graphs A and D of Figure 20-9.

Relationships are described as "perfect" when it is possible to know precisely a person's score on one variable by knowing his or her score on the other. For instance, if all persons who were 6′2″ tall weighed 180 pounds, and all people who were 6′1″ tall weighed 175 pounds, and so on, then we could say that weight and height were perfectly, positively related. In such a situation, one would only need to be informed of a person's height in order to know his or her weight, or vice versa. On a scatter plot, a perfect relationship is rep-

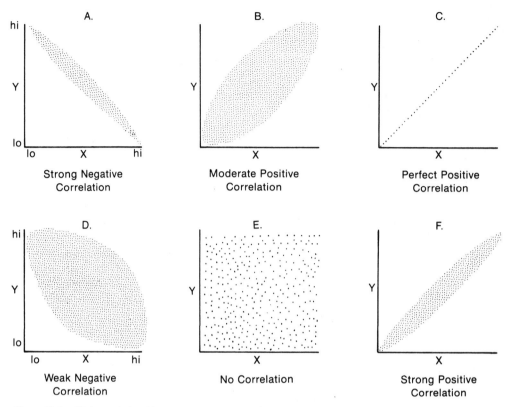

Figure 20-9. *Various relationships graphed on scatter plots.*

resented by a sloped straight line, as shown in Figure 20-9, graph C. When a relationship is not perfect, as is usually the case, one can interpret the degree of correlation from a scatter plot by seeing how closely the points cluster around a straight line. The more closely packed the points are about a diagonal slope, the higher the correlation. When the points are scattered all over the graph, the relationship is very low or nonexistent. Various degrees and directions of relationships are presented in the six graphs of Figure 20-9.

Usually it is more convenient and more succinct to express the direction and magnitude of a linear relationship by means of a numerical index that is called a correlation coefficient. A correlation coefficient, it may be re-

called, is an index whose values range from −1.0 for a perfect negative correlation, through zero for no relationship, to +1.0 for a perfect positive correlation. All correlations that fall between 0.0 and −1.0 are negative, while all correlations that fall between 0.0 and +1.0 are positive. The higher the absolute value of the coefficient (that is, the value disregarding the sign), the stronger the relationship. A correlation of −.80, for instance is stronger than a correlation of +.20.

The most commonly used linear correlation index is the *product moment correlation coefficient,* also referred to as *Pearson's r.* This coefficient is computed when the variables being correlated have been measured on either an interval or ratio scale. The calculation of the *r* statistic is rather laborious and seldom performed by hand.*

Perfect correlations ($+1.00$ and -1.00) are extremely rare in research with humans. It is difficult to offer guidelines on what should be interpreted as strong or weak relationships. This determination depends, to a great extent, on the nature of the variables. If we were to measure patients' body temperatures both orally and rectally, a correlation of .70 between the two measurements would be considered low. For most variables of a social or psychological nature, however, an *r* of .70 is quite high.

□
The computer and descriptive statistics

In the previous sections we introduced the basic concepts of statistics used to organize, summarize, and describe data. In this section we work through a fictitious example of a study and illustrate these concepts through the use of computer printouts. The intent of this section is both to make the concepts less abstract by illustrating them with some data and to familiarize the reader with printout from a standard computer program (SPSS*). Information regarding the use of such programs is described in greater detail in Chapter 23.

Suppose that a nurse researcher were interested in improving the childbirth outcomes

---

* For those who may wish to understand how a correlation coefficient is computed, we offer the following formula:

$$r_{xy} = \frac{\Sigma(X - \overline{X})(Y - \overline{Y})}{\sqrt{[\Sigma(X - \overline{X})^2][\Sigma(Y - \overline{Y})^2]}}$$

where r_{xy} = the correlation coefficient for variables X and Y

X = an individual score for variable X
$\overline{X}$ = the mean score for variable X
Y = an individual score for variable Y
$\overline{Y}$ = the mean score for variable Y
Σ = the sum of

---

among a group of young, low-income pregnant women. A program of intensive health care, nutritional counseling, and contraceptive counseling is developed, and an experiment is designed to test the effect of the program: half of a sample of pregnant girls, assigned randomly, will receive the special treatment, and the other half will be assigned to a group receiving routine care. The two outcomes that the researcher is primarily interested in are the birthweight of the infant and whether or not the young woman becomes pregnant again within 18 months of delivery. Some fictitious data for this example are presented in Table 20-7.

Figure 20-10 presents a frequency distribution printout for the birthweight variable. Under the term "VALUE," each birthweight in the sample is listed in ascending order. In the next column, "FREQUENCY," the number of occurrences of each birthweight is indicated. Thus, there was one 76-ounce baby, two 89-ounce babies, and so on. The next column, "PERCENT," indicates the percentage of birthweights in each class: 3.3 percent of the babies weighed 76 ounces at birth, 6.7 percent weighed 89 ounces, and so on. The next column, "VALID PERCENT," shows the percentage in each category after removing any missing data. In this example, birthweights were obtained for all 30 cases, but if one piece of data had been missing, the adjusted frequency for the 76-ounce baby would have been 3.4 percent (one divided by 29 rather than 30). The last column, "CUM PERCENT," adds the percent for a given birthweight value to the percent for all preceding values. Thus, we can tell by looking at the row for 99 ounces that, cumulatively, 33.3 percent of the babies weighed *under* 100 ounces in this example.

The bottom of this printout provides a number of the descriptive statistics discussed in this chapter. The MEAN is equal to 104.7, whereas the MEDIAN is 102.5, and the MODE is 99. This suggests that the distribution is

Table 20-7
Fictitious data on low-income pregnant young women

Group (1 = experimental; 2 = control)	Weight of Infant (in ounces)	Repeat Pregnancy (1 = yes; 0 = no)	Age of Mother
1	107	1	17
1	101	0	14
1	119	0	21
1	128	1	20
1	89	0	15
1	99	0	19
1	111	0	19
1	117	1	18
1	102	1	17
1	120	0	20
1	76	0	13
1	116	0	18
1	100	1	16
1	115	0	18
1	113	0	21
2	111	1	19
2	108	0	21
2	95	0	19
2	99	0	17
2	103	1	19
2	94	0	15
2	101	1	17
2	114	0	21
2	97	0	20
2	99	1	18
2	113	0	18
2	89	0	19
2	98	0	20
2	102	0	17
2	105	0	19

somewhat skewed in the positive direction. The RANGE is 52, which is equal to the MAXIMUM of 128 minus the MINIMUM of 76. The standard deviation (STD DEV) is 10.955, and the VARIANCE is 120.010 (10.955^2).

In addition to tabular information, such as that shown in Figure 20-10, many programs can produce graphic materials. Figure 20-11 presents a histogram for the variable of a mother's age. In this case, all of the values for age are shown on the vertical axis, and the frequency on the horizontal axis. The histo-gram shows at a glance that the modal age is 19 ($f = 7$) and that this variable is negatively skewed (i.e., there are fewer younger girls). Descriptive statistics shown at the bottom of the printout indicate that the mean age for this group was 18.167, with a standard deviation of 2.086.

If we were interested in comparing the repeat-pregnancy experience of the two groups of young women (experimental versus control), we would instruct the computer to cross-tabulate the two variables, as shown in the

WEIGHT   BIRTHWEIGHT OF BABY

VALUE LABEL	VALUE	FREQUENCY	PERCENT	VALID PERCENT	CUM PERCENT
	76	1	3.3	3.3	3.3
	89	2	6.7	6.7	10.0
	94	1	3.3	3.3	13.3
	95	1	3.3	3.3	16.7
	97	1	3.3	3.3	20.0
	98	1	3.3	3.3	23.3
	99	3	10.0	10.0	33.3
	100	1	3.3	3.3	36.7
	101	2	6.7	6.7	43.3
	102	2	6.7	6.7	50.0
	103	1	3.3	3.3	53.3
	105	1	3.3	3.3	56.7
	107	1	3.3	3.3	60.0
	108	1	3.3	3.3	63.3
	111	2	6.7	6.7	70.0
	113	2	6.7	6.7	76.7
	114	1	3.3	3.3	80.0
	115	1	3.3	3.3	83.3
	116	1	3.3	3.3	86.7
	117	1	3.3	3.3	90.0
	119	1	3.3	3.3	93.3
	120	1	3.3	3.3	96.7
	128	1	3.3	3.3	100.0
	TOTAL	30	100.0	100.0	

MEAN	104.700	STD ERR	2.000	MEDIAN	102.500
MODE	99.000	STD DEV	10.955	VARIANCE	120.010
KURTOSIS	.473	S E KURT	.833	SKEWNESS	-0.254
S E SKEW	.427	RANGE	52.000	MINIMUM	76.000
MAXIMUM	128.000	SUM	3141.000		

VALID CASES   30   MISSING CASES   0

Figure 20-10. SPSSˣ computer printout: frequency distribution.

contingency table in Figure 20-12. This cross-tabulation resulted in four cells: experimental subjects with no repeat pregnancy (upper left cell), control subjects with no repeat pregnancy (upper right), experimental subjects with a repeat pregnancy (lower left cell); and control subjects with a repeat pregnancy (lower right cell). Each cell contains four pieces of information, which we will explain for the first cell. The first number is the number of subjects in that cell. Ten experimental subjects did not have a repeat pregnancy within 18 months of their delivery. The next number is the *row* percentage: 47.6 percent of the girls who did not become pregnant again were in the experimental group (10 divided by 21). The next figure represents the *column* percent: 66.7 percent of the experimentals did not become pregnant (10 divided by 15). The last figure is the *overall* percent-

```
     COUNT       VALUE    ONE SYMBOL EQUALS APPROXIMATELY     .20 OCCURRENCES

        1        13.00    *****
        1        14.00    *****
        2        15.00    *********
        1        16.00    *****
        5        17.00    **************************
        5        18.00    *************************
        7        19.00    *************************************
        4        20.00    *******************
        4        21.00    *******************
                          I.........I.........I.........I.........I.........I
                          0         2         4         6         8        10
                                     HISTOGRAM FREQUENCY

MEAN           18.167     STD ERR         .381     MEDIAN          18.500
MODE           19.000     STD DEV        2.086     VARIANCE         4.351
KURTOSIS         .143     S E KURT        .833     SKEWNESS        -0.701
S E SKEW         .427     RANGE          8.000     MINIMUM         13.000
MAXIMUM        21.000     SUM          545.000


VALID CASES       30      MISSING CASES      0
```

Figure 20-11. SPSS[x] computer printout: histogram.

```
- - - - - - - - - - - - - - - - - - -   C R O S S T A B U L A T I O N   O F
    REPEAT                                              BY   GROUP
- - - - - - - - - - - - - - - - - - - - - - - - - - - - - - - - - - - - - - -

                        GROUP
              COUNT    |·
              ROW PCT  |EXPERIME CONTROL      ROW
              COL PCT  |NTAL                  TOTAL
              TOT PCT  |       1|        2|
REPEAT·                --------+--------+--------+
                 0     |    10  |    11  |       21
   NO REPEAT PREG      |  47.6  |  52.4  |     70.0
                       |  66.7  |  73.3  |
                       |  33.3  |  36.7  |
                       +--------+--------+
                 1     |     5  |     4  |        9
   REPEAT PREG         |  55.6  |  44.4  |     30.0
                       |  33.3  |  26.7  |
                       |  16.7  |  13.3  |
                       +--------+--------+
              COLUMN        15       15       30
              TOTAL       50.0     50.0    100.0
```

Figure 20-12. SPSS[x] computer printout: crosstabulation.

age of girls in that cell (10 divided by 30 equals 33.3 percent). This order need not be memorized. It is shown in the upper left corner of the table:

COUNT
ROW PCT
COL PCT
TOT PCT

Thus, this table indicates that a somewhat higher percentage of experimentals (33.3 percent) than controls (26.7 percent) experienced a repeat pregnancy. The row totals on the far right indicate that, overall, 30.0 percent of the sample (N = 9) had a subsequent pregnancy.

☐
Research example

Robb (1985) addressed the problem of verifying the amount and frequency of urinary incontinence in a sample of elderly men. A volunteer sample of 66 men aged 60 years or older — all community-dwelling veterans who had experienced urinary incontinence — constituted the sample. The amount of urinary loss was assessed using a 60-minute and a 3-day absorbent pad test. The pads, which were changed at intervals specified by the investigator, were weighed before and after use. To document frequency of incontinent episodes, subjects maintained a 7-day record of urinations (both continent and incontinent) and fluid intake.

A wide variety of descriptive statistics was reported to summarize some of the major findings of this study. For example, for the 60-minute test, it was found that the mean amount of urine loss per hour was 9.6 grams, with a range of 0.0 to 101.0 grams, and a standard deviation of 24.3. Thus, there was extensive intersubject variability, and the distribution of loss was very positively skewed. The 3-day amount test yielded similar results, although there was somewhat less variability ($\overline{X}$ = 10.1, SD =

18.3). The 60-minute test identified 57 percent of the men as being incontinent, compared to 59 percent of the men based on the 3-day test. However, only 59 percent of the men were classified the same way (abnormal or normal) by the two tests.

☐
Summary

Descriptive statistics enable the researcher to reduce, summarize, and describe data obtained from empirical observations and measurements. Raw data that have not been organized or analyzed are difficult, if not impossible, to interpret and communicate to others. A *frequency distribution* is one of the easiest methods of imposing some order on a mass of numbers. In a frequency distribution, numerical values are ordered from the lowest to the highest, with a count of the number of times each value was obtained. *Histograms* and *frequency polygons* are two common methods of displaying frequency information graphically.

A set of data may be completely described in terms of the shape of the distribution, central tendency, and variability. The most important attributes of the distribution's shape are its symmetry and modality. A distribution is *symmetrical* if its two halves are mirror images of each other. A *skewed distribution,* by contrast, is nonsymmetrical, with one "tail" longer than the other. The modality of a distribution refers to the number of peaks present: a *unimodal* distribution has one peak, while a *multimodal* distribution has more than one high point.

Measures of *central tendency* are indices, expressed as a single number, that represent the "average" or typical value of a set of scores. The *mode* is the numerical value that occurs most frequently in the distribution (or with greater frequency than other scores in its vicinity) The *median* is that point on a numerical scale above which and below which 50 percent of the cases fall. The mean is the arithmetic average of all the scores in the distribution. In general, the mean is the preferred measure of central tendency because of its stability and its usefulness in further statistical manipulations.

Variability refers to the spread or dispersion of the data. Measures of variability include the range, the semiquartile range, and the standard deviation. The *range* is the distance between the highest and lowest score values. The *semiquartile range* indicates one half of the range of scores within which the middle 50 percent of scores lie. The most commonly used measure of variability is the *standard deviation (SD)*. This index is calculated by first computing *deviation scores,* which represent the degree to which the scores of each person deviate from the mean. The standard deviation is designed to indicate how much, on the average, the scores deviate from the mean. A related index, the *variance,* is equal to the standard deviation squared.

Bivariate descriptive statistics describe the degree and magnitude of relationships between two variables. A *contingency table* is a two-dimensional frequency distribution in which the frequencies of two variables are cross-tabulated. When the scores have been measured on an ordinal, interval, or ratio scale, it is more common to describe the relationship between two variables with correlational procedures. A *correlation coefficient* can be calculated to express in numerical terms the direction and magnitude of a linear relationship. The values of the correlation coefficient range from −1.00 for a perfect negative correlation, through 0.0 for no relationship, to +1.00 for a perfect positive correlation. The most frequently used correlation coefficient is the *product-moment correlation coefficient,* also referred to as *Pearson's r.* The graphic representation of a relationship between two variables is called a *scatter plot* or scatter diagram.

☐
Study suggestions

1. Construct a frequency distribution for the following set of scores obtained from a scale to measure attitudes toward primary nursing:

   32 20 33 22 16 19 25 26 25 18
   22 30 24 26 27 23 28 26 21 24
   31 29 25 28 22 27 26 30 17 24

2. Construct a frequency polygon or histogram with the data from above. Describe the resulting distribution of scores in terms of symmetry and modality. How closely does the distribution approach a normal distribution?

3. What are the mean, median, and mode for the following set of data? Compute the range and standard deviation.

   13 12 9 15 7 10 16 8 6 11

4. Two hospitals are interested in comparing the tenure rates of their nursing staff. Hospital A finds that their present staff has been employed for a mean of 4.3 years, with a standard deviation of 1.5. Hospital B, on the other hand, finds that their nurses have worked there for a mean of 6.4 years, with a standard deviation of 4.2 years. Discuss what these results signify.

5. Suppose a researcher has conducted a study concerning lactose intolerance in children. The data revealed that 22 boys and 16 girls have lactose intolerance, out of a sample of 60 children of each sex. Construct a contingency table and calculate the percentages for each cell in the table. Discuss the meaning of these statistics.

6. A researcher has collected data on pulse rate and scores on a final exam for 10 students and would like to know if there is a relationship between the two measures. Compute Pearson's *r* for these data:

Pulse rate: 84 72 82 68 96 64 92 88 76 74
Test scores: 92 84 88 72 68 74 72 90 82 86

□

Suggested readings

Methodological references

Blalock, H.M., Jr. (1979). *Social statistics* (2nd ed.). New York: McGraw-Hill.

Games, P.A. & Klare, G.R. (1967). *Elementary statistics: Data analysis for the behavioral sciences.* New York: McGraw-Hill.

Glass, G.V. and Stanley, J.C. (1984). *Statistical methods in education and psychology* (2nd ed.). Englewood Cliffs, NJ: Prentice-Hall.

Knapp, R.G. (1984). *Basic statistics for nurses* (2nd ed.). New York: John Wiley & Sons.

Knapp, T.R. (1970). N vs N − 1. *American Educational Research Journal, 7,* 625–626.

McNemar, Q (1969). *Psychological statistics* (4th ed.). New York: John Wiley & Sons.

Runyon, R.P. & Haber, A. (1984). *Fundamentals of behavioral statistics* (5th ed.). Reading, MA: Addison-Wesley.

Sokal, R.R. & Rohlf, F.J. (1981). *Biometry: The principles and practice of statistics in biological research* (2nd ed.). San Francisco: W.H. Freeman.

Spence, J.T. *et al.* (1983). *Elementary statistics* (4th ed.). New York: Appleton-Century-Crofts.

Substantive references

Aberman, S. & Kirckhoff, K.T. (1985). Infant-feeding practices: Mothers decision making. *Journal of Obstetric, Gynecologic, & Neonatal Nursing, 14,* 394–398 (Percentages, cross-tabulations).

Aradine, C.R. (1983). Young children with long-term tracheostomies: Health and development. *Western Journal of Nursing Research, 5,* 115–124 (Means, standard deviations, ranges).

Archer, S.E. (1983). A study of nurse administrators' political participation. *Western Journal of Nursing Research, 5,* 65–75 (Percentages).

Engstrom, J.L. & Chen, E.H (1984). Prediction of birthweight by the use of extrauterine measurements during labor. *Research in Nursing and Health, 7,* 314–323 (Means, medians, standard deviations, ranges).

Ford, A.H. (1980). Use of automobile restraining devices for infants. *Nursing Research, 29,* 281–284 (Means, standard deviations, percentages).

Hurley, P.M. (1981). Communication patterns and conflict in marital dyads. *Nursing Research, 30,* 38–42 (Means, median, standard deviations).

Laschinger, S.J. (1984). The relationship of social support to health in elderly people. *Western Journal of Nursing Research, 6,* 341–350 (Means, standard deviations).

Norris, S., Campbell, L.A., & Brenkert, S. (1982). Nursing procedure and alterations in transcutaneous oxygen tension in premature infants. *Nursing Research, 31,* 330–336 (Means, SDs, ranges).

Robb, S.S. (1985). Urinary incontinence verification in elderly men. *Nursing Research, 34,* 278–282 (Percentages, cross-tabulations, means, SDs).

Updike, P.A., Accurso, F.J., & Jones, R.H. (1985). Physiologic circadian rhythmicity in preterm infants. *Nursing Research, 34,* 16–163 (Means, standard deviations).

Chapter 21
☐
Inferential statistics

Descriptive statistics such as means, standard deviations, and correlation coefficients are useful for summarizing univariate and bivariate sets of data. Usually, however, the researcher needs to do more than simply describe data obtained from a sample. Normally, subjects selected to participate in a research project are only a sample of individuals drawn from a population with certain characteristics. *Inferential statistical* methods provide a means for drawing conclusions about a population, given the data actually obtained for the sample. Inferential statistical reasoning would help us with such questions as "What do I know about the average Apgar score of premature babies (the population) after having learned that a sample of 50 premature babies had a mean Apgar score of 7.5?" or "What can I conclude about the differential need for health education among women over age 25 (the population) after having found in a sample of 500 women that 50 percent of college-educated women but only 20 percent of high school-educated women practiced breast self-examination? With the assistance of inferential statistics, researchers make judgments about or generalize to a large class of individuals based on information from a limited number of subjects.

Generally, the purpose of testing or measuring a sample is to gather data that allow us to make statements about the characteristics of a population. One estimates the parameters of a population from the statistics or attributes of the sample. These estimates are based upon laws of probability and, as we shall see, probabilistic estimates involve a certain degree of error. The difference between estimates based on inferential statistics and estimates arrived at through the ordinary thinking process is that the statistical method provides a framework for making judgments in a systematic, objective fashion. Different researchers working with identical data would be likely to come to the same conclusion after applying inferential statistical procedures.

☐
Sampling distributions

If a sample is to be used as a basis for making estimates of population characteristics, then it is clearly advisable to obtain as representative a sample as possible. As we saw in Chapter 12, random samples (that is, probability samples) are the most effective means of securing representative samples. Inferential statistical procedures are based upon the assumption of random sampling from populations.

Even when random sampling is used, however, it cannot be expected that the sample characteristics will be identical to those of the population. Suppose we have a population of 10,000 freshmen nursing students who have taken the Scholastic Aptitude Test (SAT). By applying descriptive statistics to the scores, we find that the mean for the entire population is 500 and the standard deviation is 100. Now, let us suppose that we do not know these parameters but that we must estimate them by using the scores from a random sample of 25 students. Should we expect to find a mean of exactly 500 and an *SD* of 100 for this sample? It would be extremely unlikely to obtain identical values. Let us say instead that we calculated a mean of 505. If a completely new sample were drawn and another mean computed, we might obtain a value such as 497. The tendency for the statistics to fluctuate from one sample to another is known as *sampling error*.

A researcher actually works with only *one* sample on which statistics are computed and inferences made. But to understand inferential statistics we must perform a small mental

exercise. With the population of 10,000 nursing students, consider drawing a sample of 25 individuals, calculating a mean and standard deviation, replacing the 25 students, and drawing a new sample. Each mean computed in this fashion will be considered a separate piece of data. If we draw 5000 such samples, we will have 5000 means or data points, which could then be used to construct a frequency polygon, as shown in Figure 21-1. This kind of frequency distribution has a special name: it is called a *sampling distribution* of the mean. A sampling distribution is a theoretical rather than actual distribution because one does not in practice draw consecutive samples from a population and plot their means. The concept of a theoretical distribution of sample means is basic to much of inferential statistics.

Characteristics of sampling distributions

When an infinite number of samples are drawn from an infinite population, the sampling distribution of means from those samples has certain known characteristics. Our example of a population of 10,000 students, and 5000 samples with 25 students each, deals with finite quantities, but the numbers are large enough to approximate these characteristics.

Statisticians have been able to demonstrate that sampling distributions of means follow a normal curve. Furthermore, the mean of a sampling distribution consisting of an infinite number of sample means is equal to the population mean. In the present example, the mean of the sampling distribution is 500, the same value as the mean of the population.

In the preceding chapter we discussed the standard deviation in terms of percentages of cases falling within a certain distance from the mean. When scores are normally distributed, 68 percent of the cases fall between $+1SD$ and $-1SD$ from the mean. Since a sampling distribution of means is normally distributed, we can make the same type of statement. The

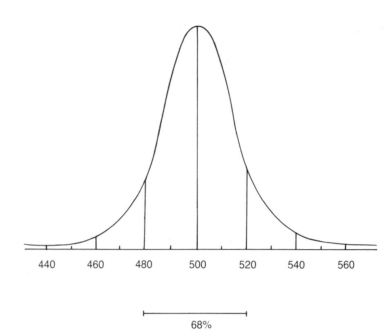

440   460   480   500   520   540   560

68%

95%

99.7%

Figure 21-1. Sampling distribution.

probability is 68 out of 100 that any randomly drawn sample mean lies within the range of values between $+1$SD and -1SD of the mean on the sampling distribution. The problem, then, is to determine the value of the standard deviation of the sampling distribution.

Standard error of the mean

The standard deviation of a theoretical distribution of sample means has a special name. It is called the *standard error of the mean.* The word "error" signifies that the various means comprising the distribution contain some error in their estimates of the population mean. The *standard* error indicates the magnitude of a standard, or average, error. The smaller the standard error—that is, the less

variable the sample means—the more accurate are those means as estimates of the population value.

Because one does not ever actually construct a sampling distribution, how can its standard deviation be computed? Fortunately, there is a formula for estimating the standard error of the mean from the data from a single sample. It has been shown that the value of the standard error (symbolized as $s_{\bar{x}}$) has a systematic relationship to the standard deviation of the population and to the size of the samples drawn from it. The population SD is estimated by the sample SD to yield the following equation.

$$s_{\bar{x}} = \frac{SD}{\sqrt{n}}$$

where SD = the standard deviation of the sample
n = sample size
$s_{\bar{x}}$ = standard error of the mean

If we use this formula to calculate the standard error of the mean in our present example we obtain:

$$s_{\bar{x}} = \frac{100}{\sqrt{25}} = 20.0$$

The standard deviation of the sampling distribution is 20, as shown in Figure 21-1. This statistic is an estimate of how much sampling fluctuation or sampling error there would be from one sample mean to another.

We can now use these calculations to estimate the probability of drawing a sample with a certain mean. With a sample size of 25, the chances are about 95 out of 100 that the mean would fall between the values of 460 and 540. Only 5 times out of 100 would the sample mean exceed 540 or be less than 460. In other words, only 5 times out of 100 would we be likely to draw a sample whose mean deviates from the population mean by more than 40 points.

From the formula for the standard error of the mean, it can be shown that, in order to increase the accuracy of our estimate of the population mean, we need only increase the sample size. Suppose that instead of using a sample of 25 nursing students to estimate the average SAT score, we used a sample of 100 students. With this many students, the standard error of the mean would be

$$s_{\bar{x}} = \frac{100}{\sqrt{100}} = 10.0$$

In such a situation, the probability of obtaining a sample mean greater than 520 or less than 480 would be about 5 in 100. The chances of drawing a sample with a mean very different from that of the population is reduced as the sample size increases because large numbers promote the likelihood that extreme cases will cancel each other out.

□
Estimation versus hypothesis testing

Statistical inference consists of two major types of techniques: estimation of parameters versus the testing of hypotheses. Of the two, hypothesis testing is more commonly encountered in research reports, but estimation plays an important role as well. Regardless of which approach is used, the overall goal remains the same: to use data from samples to draw conclusions about populations.

Estimation of parameters

Estimation procedures are used when the researcher has no preestablished hypothesis about the value of a population characteristic and desires to determine what that value might be. Suppose a new drug has been developed for persons sufferng from high blood pressure and a researcher administers the drug to a sample of patients. The researcher could use estimation procedures to estimate the average blood pressure of a population of persons with high blood pressure (or the average reduction in blood pressure) after administration of the drug. Estimation is the method used when no *a priori* prediction can be made about the attributes of a population, as would probably be the case for the effects of a new drug.

Estimation can take one of two forms: *point* or *interval estimation*. Point estimation involves the calculation of a single numerical value — a statistic — to estimate the unknown population parameter. To continue with the example used in the previous section, if we calculated the mean SAT score for a sample of 25 students and found that it was 510, then this number would represent the point estimation of the population mean.

The problem with point estimates is that they convey no information concerning the accuracy of the estimation. An interval estimate of a parameter is more useful because it indicates a range of values within which the parameter has a specified probability of lying. Interval estimates usually are referred to as *confidence intervals,* and the upper and lower limits of the range of values are called *confidence limits.*

The construction of a confidence interval around a sample mean establishes a range of values for a population parameter and also establishes a certain probability of being correct. In other words, we make the estimation with a certain degree of confidence. Although the degree of confidence one wishes to attain is somewhat arbitrary, researchers conventionally use either a 95 or a 99 percent confidence interval.

The calculation of the confidence limits involves the use of the standard error of the mean and the principles associated with the normal distribution. As shown in Figure 21-1, 95 percent of the scores in a normal distribution lie within about 2 standard deviations from the mean. The precise number of standard deviations is 1.96.

Returning to our example, let us say once again that the point estimation of the mean SAT score is 510, with a standard deviation of 100. The standard error of the mean for a sample of 25 would be 20. We can now build a 95 percent confidence interval by using the following formula:

$$\text{Conf. } (\overline{X} \pm 1.96 \ s_{\overline{x}}) = 95\%$$

That is, the confidence is 95 percent that the population mean lies between the values equal to 1.96 times the standard error, above and below the sample mean. In the example at hand we would obtain the following:

$$\text{Conf. } (510 \pm (1.96) \times (20.0)) = 95\%$$
$$\text{Conf. } (510 \pm (39.2)) \qquad\quad = 95\%$$
$$\text{Conf. } (470.8 \le \mu \le 549.2) \quad = 95\%$$

The final statement may be read as follows: the confidence is 95 percent that the population mean (symbolized by the Greek letter μ by convention) is greater than or equal to 470.8 but less than or equal to 549.2. Another way to interpret the confidence interval concept is in terms of a probabilistic statement. One could say that out of 100 samples with an *n* of 25, 95 out of 100 such confidence intervals would contain the parameter (the population mean).

The confidence interval reflects the degree of risk the researcher is willing to take of being wrong. With a 95 percent confidence interval, the researcher accepts the probability that she or he will be wrong 5 times out of 100. A 99 percent confidence interval sets the risk at only 1 percent by allowing a wider range of possible values. The formula is as follows:

$$\text{Conf. } (\overline{X} \pm 2.58 \ s_{\overline{x}}) = 99\%$$

The 2.58 reflects the fact that 99 percent of all cases in a normal distribution lie within ± 2.58 SD units from the mean. In the above example the 99 percent confidence interval would be:

$$\text{Conf. } (510 \pm (2.58) \times (20.0)) = 99\%$$
$$\text{Conf. } (510 \pm (51.6)) \qquad\qquad = 99\%$$
$$\text{Conf. } (458.4 \le \mu \le 561.6) \quad\ = 99\%$$

In 99 out of 100 samples with 25 subjects, the confidence interval so constructed would contain the population mean. One accepts a reduced risk of being wrong at the price of reduced specificity. Whereas in the case of the 95 percent interval the range between the confidence limits was only about 80 points, here the range of possible values is over 100 points. The risk of error that one is willing to accept depends upon the nature of the problem. In research that could affect the well-being of humans, it is not unusual to use stringent 99.9 percent confidence intervals, but for many research projects a 95 percent confidence interval is sufficient.

Hypothesis testing

Statistical hypothesis testing is essentially a process of decision-making. Suppose a nurse researcher hypothesized that structured information concerning a patient's condition would reduce the patient's level of anxiety to a greater degree than casual, unstructured information. Experimental and control samples of 25 subjects each are used and a self-report measure of anxiety obtained. The researcher finds that the mean anxiety level for the experimental group is 15.8 while that for the control group is 17.5. Should the researcher conclude that the hypothesis has been supported? True, the group differences are in the predicted direction, but the results might simply be due to sampling fluctuations. Statistical hypothesis testing helps researchers to make objective decisions concerning the results of their studies. Scientists need such a mechanism for helping them to decide which outcomes are likely to reflect only chance differences between groups and which are likely to reflect true population differences.

The null hypothesis
The procedures used in testing hypotheses are based upon rules of negative inference. This logic often seems somewhat awkward and peculiar to beginning researchers, so we will try to convey the concepts with a concrete illustration. In the above example, a nurse researcher used two methods of communicating information to patients and found that the structured experimental approach resulted in lower mean anxiety scores than the unstructured control approach. There are two explanations for this outcome: (1) the experimental treatment was successful in reducing patients' anxiety or (2) the differences were due to chance factors (such as differences in the pretreatment anxiety levels of the two groups). The first explanation is the researcher's scientific hypothesis, but the second explanation is known as the *null hypothesis*. The null hypoth-

esis is a statement that there is no actual relationship between variables and that any such observed relationship is only a function of chance, or sampling fluctuations. The need for a null hypothesis lies in the fact that statistical hypothesis testing is basically a process of rejection. It is not possible to demonstrate directly that the first explanation — the scientific hypothesis — is correct. But it is possible to show that the null hypothesis has a high probability of being incorrect, and such evidence lends support to the scientific hypothesis. The rejection of the null hypothesis, then, is what the researcher seeks to accomplish through statistical tests.

The null hypothesis is sometimes stated as a formal proposition, using the following symbols:

$$H_0 : \mu_A = \mu_B$$

The null hypothesis (H_0) predicts that the population mean for method A (μ_A) is the same as the population mean for method B (μ_B) with regard to, in this case, anxiety scores. The *alternative,* or research, *hypothesis* may also be stated in similar terms:

$$H_A : \mu_A \neq \mu_B$$

Although null hypotheses are accepted or rejected on the basis of sample data, the hypothesis is made about population values. The real interest in testing hypotheses, as in all statistical inference, is to use samples to draw conclusions about relationships within the population.

Type I and Type II errors
The researcher's decision about whether to accept or reject the null hypothesis is based upon a consideration of how probable it is that observed differences are due to chance alone. Since information concerning the entire population is not available, it is not possible to flatly assert that the null hypothesis is or is not true. The researcher must be content with the knowledge that the hypothesis is either proba-

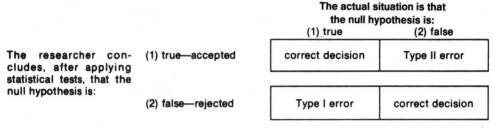

Figure 21-2. *Outcomes of statistical decision making.*

bly true or probably false. We make statistical inferences based on incomplete information, so that there is always a risk of making an error.

There are two types of errors that a researcher can commit: the rejection of a true null hypothesis or the acceptance of a false null hypothesis. The possible outcomes of a researcher's decision are summarized in Figure 21-2. When the investigator errs by concluding that the null hypothesis is false when it is in fact true, a Type I error is committed. For instance, if we concluded that the experimental treatment was more effective than the control treatment in alleviating patients' anxiety when in actuality observed sample differences were due only to sampling fluctuations, then we would have made a Type I error. In the reverse situation, we might conclude that observed differences in average group anxiety levels were due to chance, when in fact the experimental treatment had an effect on anxiety. This latter situation of accepting a false null hypothesis results in a Type II error.

Level of significance

The researcher does not know when an error in statistical decision-making has been committed. The truth or falseness of a null hypothesis could only be definitively ascertained by collecting information from the entire population, in which case there would be no need for statistical inference.

The degree of risk of a Type I error is controlled by the researcher. The selection of a *level of significance* determines the chance of making a Type I error. Level of significance is the phrase used to signify the probability of committing a Type I error. As in the case of confidence levels, the probability level can be established by the investigator.

The two most frequently used levels of significance are .05 and .01. If we say we are using a .05 significance level, this means that we are accepting the risk that out of 100 samples, a true null hypothesis would be rejected five times. With a .01 significance level, the risk of a Type I error is *lower:* in only 1 sample out of 100 would we erroneously reject the null hypothesis. The minimum acceptable level for significance level in scientific research generally is .05. A stricter level may be desirable for statistical tests when the decision has important consequences for humans.

Naturally, researchers would like to reduce the risk of committing both types of error. Unfortunately, lowering the risk of committing a Type I error increases the risk of a Type II error. The stricter the criterion we use for rejecting a null hypothesis the greater the probability that we will accept a false null hypothesis. There is a kind of trade-off that the researcher must consider in establishing criteria for statistical decision-making.

Tests of statistical significance

Within a hypothesis testing framework, the data collected in a study are used to compute a test statistic. For every test statistic there is a

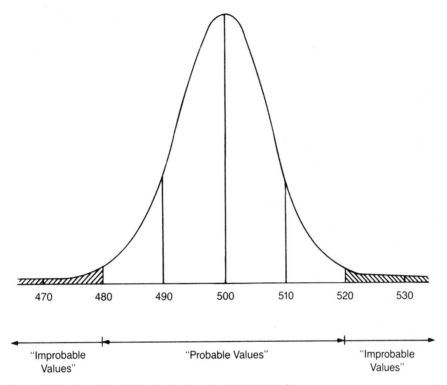

470   480   490   500   510   520   530

"Improbable   "Probable Values"   "Improbable
Values"   Values"

Figure 21-3. Sampling distribution for hypothesis test example.

related theoretical distribution. Hypothesis testing uses theoretical distributions to establish "probable" and "improbable" values for test statistics, which are in turn used as a basis for accepting or rejecting the null hypothesis.

A simple example will illustrate the process. Suppose a researcher wanted to test the hypothesis that the average SAT score for high school students who went on to a nursing program was higher than that for all high school students, whose mean score was 500. The null hypothesis is $H_0 : \mu_{NURS} = 500$, while the alternate hypothesis is $H_A : \mu_{NURS} \neq 500$. That is, our null hypothesis is that the population mean for students who went on to a nursing program is equal to 500; the alternative hypothesis is that the population mean is not equal to 500. To test this hypothesis, we draw a sample of 100 freshmen students in nursing programs. Let us

say that the mean score for this sample of students turns out to be 525, with an SD of 100. Using statistical procedures, we can assess the likelihood that a mean score this large represents a chance fluctuation from a true population mean of 500.

In hypothesis testing, one "assumes" that the null hypothesis is true and then gathers evidence to disprove it. Assuming a population mean of 500, a sampling distribution can be constructed with a mean of 500 and an SD equal to 10 ($s_{\bar{x}} = 100/\sqrt{100}$), as shown in Figure 21-3. Based upon our knowledge of normal distribution characteristics, we can determine "probable" and "improbable" values of sample means drawn from the nursing student population. If, as is assumed, the population mean is actually 500, then 95 percent of all sample means would fall between 480 and

520. The obtained sample mean of 525 is "improbable" given the null hypothesis, if we use as our criterion of "improbability" a significance level of .05. We would reject, therefore, the null hypothesis that the population mean for nursing students equals 500. We would not be justified in saying that we have "proved" the alternative hypothesis, because the possibility of having made a Type I error remains.

Researchers reporting the results of hypothesis tests often say that their findings were *statistically significant*. This terminology has a very precise meaning. The word "significant" should not be given the familiar interpretation of "important" or "meaningful." In statistics, significant means that given the hypothesis, the obtained results are unlikely to have been due to chance, at some specified level of probability. A nonsignificant outcome means that any difference between an obtained statistic and a hypothesized parameter could have been the result of a chance fluctuation.

The example used in this section was highly contrived; researchers rarely predict a specific value for a population mean. The use of theoretical distributions to determine "probable" and "improbable" values of a test statistic, however, is common to all tests of statistical significance.

One-tailed and two-tailed tests

In most hypothesis-testing situations, researchers apply what is known as *two-tailed tests*. This means that both ends, or "tails," of the sampling distribution are used to determine the range of "improbable values." In Figure 21-3, for example, the critical region that contains five percent of the area of the sampling distribution really involves 2.5 percent at one end of the distribution and 2.5 percent at the other. If the level of significance were .01, the critical regions would involve .5 percent of the distribution at both tails.

However, when the research has a strong basis for using a directional hypothesis (see Chapter 7), it might be justifiable to use what is referred to as a one-tailed test. For example, if a nurse researcher instituted an outreach program to improve the prenatal practices of low-income rural women, it might be hypothesized that women in the experimental program would not just be *different* from control women not exposed to the intervention (in terms of outcomes such as pregnancy complications, infant mortality, infant birthweight, and so on). One would expect the experimentals to have an advantage. It might make little sense to use the tail of the distribution that would signify *worse* outcomes among the experimental than the control mothers. In a one-tailed test, the critical region of improbable values is entirely in one tail of the distribution —the tail corresponding to the directionality of the hypothesis. Figure 21-4 illustrates that, in a one-tailed test, the region of "improbable values" lies entirely at one end of the distribution. When a one-tailed test is used, the critical area of .05 covers a bigger region of the specified tail, and for this reason, one-tailed tests are less conservative. This means that it is easier to reject the null hypothesis with a one-tailed test than with a two-tailed test.

The use of one-tailed tests has been the subject of considerable controversy. Most researchers follow the convention of using a two-tailed test, even if they have stated a directional hypothesis. In reading research reports, one can assume that a two-tailed test has been used, unless the investigator specifically mentions a one-tailed test. However, when there is a strong logical or theoretical reason for using a directional hypothesis and for assuming that findings opposite to the direction hypothesized are virtually impossible, a one-tailed test may be warranted.

In the remainder of this chapter, the examples that are worked out use two-tailed tests. It should also be noted that if a computer is used to perform statistical analyses, two-tailed hypothesis testing is almost always assumed.

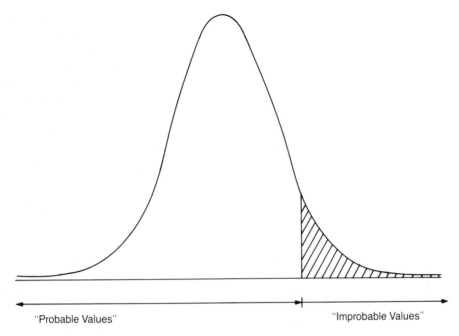

"Probable Values"   "Improbable Values"

Figure 21-4. Critical range for a one-tailed test.

Parametric and nonparametric tests

A distinction is often made between two classes of statistical tests. The bulk of the tests that we will consider in this chapter — and also the majority of tests used by researchers — are called *parametric tests*. Parametric tests are characterized by three attributes: (1) they involve the estimation of at least one parameter; (2) they require measurements on at least an interval scale; and (3) they involve several other assumptions about the variables under consideration, such as the assumption that the variables are normally distributed in the population.

Nonparametric tests may be contrasted with parametric tests in terms of several of these characteristics. This second class of statistical tests is not based upon the estimation of parameters. Nonparametric methods also involve less restrictive assumptions concerning the shape of the distribution of the critical variables than do parametric tests. For this reason,

nonparametric tests are sometimes called *distribution-free* statistics. Finally, nonparametric tests are usually applied when the data have been measured on a nominal or an ordinal scale.

Statisticians disagree about the utility and virtues of most nonparametric tests. Purists insist that if the strict requirements of parametric tests are not met, then parametric procedures are inappropriate. Many statistical research studies have shown, however, that the violation of the assumptions for parametric tests usually fails to affect statistical decision-making or the number of errors made. The more moderate position in this debate, and the one that we feel is reasonable, is that nonparametric tests are most useful when (1) the data under consideration cannot in any manner be construed as interval-level measures or (2) when the distribution of data is markedly non-normal. Parametric tests are usually more powerful and offer more flexibility than nonparametric tests and are, for these reasons, generally preferred.

Overview of hypothesis-testing procedures

In the pages that follow, various types of statistical procedures for testing research hypotheses are examined. The emphasis throughout is on explaining applications of statistical tests rather than on describing actual computations. One computational example is worked out to illustrate that numbers are not just "pulled out of a hat." However, calculators and computers have virtually eliminated the need for manual calculations, so that computational examples have been minimized. The serious researcher is urged to pursue other references for a fuller appreciation of statistical methods. In this basic text on research methods, our primary concern is to alert researchers to the potential use (or misuse) of statistical tests for different purposes.

Although each of the statistical tests described in the remaining sections of this chapter has a particular application and can be used only with particular kinds of data, the overall process of testing hypotheses is basically the same. The steps are essentially as follows:

1. *Determine the test statistic to be used.* Is a parametric test justified? What level of measurement was used for the measures? Is the distribution of data a reasonable approximation of a normal curve? The summarization in Table 21-6 may help in the selection of an appropriate test.
2. *Select the level of significance.* The .05 level will usually be acceptable. If a more stringent test is required, the significance level may be set at .01 or .001.
3. *Select a one-tailed or two-tailed test.* In most cases, a two-tailed test should be used to answer questions such as the following: Are the two groups different? Is there a relationship between the two variables? If the researcher has a firm basis for hypothesizing not only a difference or a relationship, but also the *nature* of that difference or relationship, then a one-tailed test may be appropriate.
4. *Compute a test statistic.* Using the values from the collected data, calculate a test statistic using the appropriate computational formulas. Or, alternatively, have the computer calculate the statistic using a program designed for this purpose.
5. *Calculate the degrees of freedom.* The term *degrees of freedom* is a concept used throughout hypothesis testing to refer to the number of observations free to vary about a parameter. The concept is too complex for full elaboration here, but fortunately the computation is extremely easy.
6. *Compare the test statistic to a tabled value.* Theoretical distributions have been developed for all test statistics. These theoretical distributions enable the researcher to discover whether obtained values are beyond the range of what is "probable" if the null hypothesis is true. That is, at some probability level specified by the researcher, the obtained value of the test statistic reflects a true relationship between variables (or a reliable estimate of a hypothesized population parameter) and not just a relationship or value that occurred in the sample by chance. The researcher examines a table appropriate for the test used, obtains the tabled value by entering the table at a point corresponding to the relevant degrees of freedom and level of significance, and compares the tabled value to the computed value of the statistic. If the tabled value is *smaller* than the absolute value of the test statistic, then the results are statistically significant. If the

tabled value is larger, then the results are nonsignificant.

When a computer program is used to test hypotheses, the researcher really only needs to follow the first step and then make the necessary commands to the computer. The computer will calculate the test statistic, the degrees of freedom, and the *actual* probability that the relationship being tested is due to chance. For example, the computer may print that the probability (p) of an experimental group doing better on a measure of postoperative recovery than the control group on the basis of chance alone is .025. This means that fewer than three times out of 100 (or only 25 times out of 1000) would a difference between the two groups as large as the one obtained reflect haphazard sampling differences rather than differences resulting from an experimental intervention. This computed probability level can then be compared with the investigator's desired level of significance. In the present example, if the significance level desired were .05, the results would be said to be significant, because .025 is more stringent than .05. If .01 were the significance level, the results would be nonsignificant (sometimes abbreviated NS). Any computed probability level greater than .05 (e.g., .20) indicates a nonsignificant relationship—that is, one that could have occurred on the basis of chance alone in more than five out of 100 samples.

In the sections that follow, a number of specific statistical tests and their applications are described. An example of a hypothesis test using computerized computations is provided at the end of the chapter.

□
Testing differences between two group means

A very common research situation is the comparison of two groups of subjects on the de-

pendent variable of interest. For instance, we might wish to compare the scores of an experimental and control group of patients on a measure of physical function. Or perhaps we would be interested in contrasting the average length of hospitalization for a sample of maternity patients in urban versus rural hospitals. This section will describe methods for testing the statistical significance of differences between two group means.

The basic parametric procedure for testing differences in group means is the *t-test*. A distinction must be drawn between the case in which the two groups are independent (such as an experimental and control group, or male versus female subjects) or dependent (as when a single group yields pretreatment and posttreatment scores). Procedures for handling independent samples are described below to illustrate the computation of a test statistic. In addition, several nonparametric procedures for comparing two groups will be reviewed.

t-Tests for independent samples

Suppose that a researcher wanted to test the effect of special instruction on pregnant women's attitudes toward breastfeeding. Twenty primiparas from a prenatal education program comprise the sample. Ten of these 20 women are randomly assigned to an experimental group, which will be exposed to special films and lectures on breastfeeding. The remaining ten women comprise the control group, which will not receive special instruction on breastfeeding. At the end of the experiment, both groups are administered a scale measuring attitudes toward breastfeeding. The hypotheses being tested are

$$H_0 : \mu_A = \mu_B \qquad H_A : \mu_A \neq \mu_B$$

In order to test these hypotheses, a statistic known as the *t*-statistic must be computed.

Table 21-1
Computation of the t-statistic for independent samples

Experimental Group A			Control Group B			
(1)	(2)	(3)	(4)	(5)	(6)	
X_A	x_A	$x_A{}^2$	X_B	x_B	$x_B{}^2$	
30	5	24	23	4	16	$t = \dfrac{25 - 19}{\sqrt{\dfrac{242 + 154}{(10 + 10 - 2)}\left(\dfrac{1}{10} + \dfrac{1}{10}\right)}} =$
27	2	4	17	−2	4	
25	0	0	22	3	9	
20	−5	25	18	−1	1	
24	−1	1	20	1	1	
32	7	49	26	7	49	$t = \dfrac{6}{\sqrt{(22.0)(.2)}} =$
17	−8	64	16	−3	9	
18	−7	49	13	−6	36	$t = \dfrac{6}{\sqrt{4.4}} =$
28	3	9	21	2	4	
29	4	16	14	−5	25	$t = \dfrac{6}{2.1} = 2.86$
$\Sigma X_A = 250$		$\Sigma x_A{}^2 = 242$	$\Sigma X_B = 190$		$\Sigma x_B{}^2 = 154$	
$\overline{X}_A = 25$			$\overline{X}_B = 19$			

With independent samples such as in the present example, the formula is

$$t = \frac{\overline{X}_A - \overline{X}_B}{\sqrt{\dfrac{\Sigma_{x_A}{}^2 + \Sigma_{x_B}{}^2}{n_A + n_B - 2}\left(\dfrac{1}{n_A} + \dfrac{1}{n_B}\right)}}$$

This formula looks rather complex and intimidating, but it boils down to simple components that can be calculated with elementary arithmetic. Let us work through one example with data shown in Table 21-1.

The first column of numbers presents the scores of the experimental group on a measure of attitudes toward breastfeeding. The mean score for group A is 25.0. In column 4, similar scores are shown for the control group, whose mean is 19.0. The question is: Is this six-point difference significant? What is the probability that a difference of this size is due to chance alone? The calcuation of the t-statistic will enable such questions to be answered. In columns 2 and 5, deviation scores are obtained for each subject: 25.0 is subtracted from each score in Group A and 19.0 is subtracted from each score in Group B. Then, each deviation score is squared (columns 3 and 6), and the

squared deviation scores are added. We now have all of the components for the formula presented above, as follows:

$\overline{X}_A = 25.0$	mean of Group A
$\overline{X}_B = 19.0$	mean of Group B
$\Sigma_{x_A}{}^2 = 242$	sum of Group A squared deviation scores
$\Sigma_{x_B}{}^2 = 154$	sum of Group B squared deviation scores
$n_A = 10$	number of subjects in Group A
$n_B = 10$	number of subjects in group B

When these numbers are used in the t-equation, the value of the t-statistic is computed to be 2.86, as shown in Table 21-1.

In order to ascertain whether this t-value is statistically significant, we need to consult a table that specifies the probability points associated with different t-values for the theoretical t-distributions. To make use of such a table, the researcher must have two pieces of information: the probability level sought — that is, the degree of risk of making a Type I error that one is willing to accept — and the number of degrees of freedom available. For independent samples, the formula for degrees of freedom is

$$df = n_A + n_B - 2$$

A table of *t*-values is presented in Table B-1 of Appendix B. The left-hand column lists various degrees of freedom, and the top row specifies different probability values. If we use as our decision-making criterion a two-tailed probability (*p*) level of .05, we find that with 18 degrees of freedom the tabled value of *t* is 2.10. This value establishes an upper limit to what is "probable," if the null hypothesis were true, while values in excess of 2.10 would be considered "improbable." Thus, our calculated *t* of 2.86* is improbable (i.e., statistically significant). We are now in a position to say that the subjects in the experimental group scored significantly higher than those in the control group on the attitude toward breast-feeding scale. The probability that the mean difference of six points was the result of chance factors is less than 5 in 100 ($p < .05$). The null hypothesis is rejected, therefore, and the alternative hypothesis retained.

Paired t-tests

In some studies the researcher may obtain two measures from the same subject or measures from paired sets of subjects. Whenever the criterion measures in the two comparison groups are not independent, then the procedures described above are inappropriate.

Suppose that we were interested in studying the effect of a special diet on the cholesterol level of adult males over the age of 60. A sample of 50 men is randomly selected to participate in the study. The cholesterol levels are measured before the start of the investigation and measured again after two months on the special diet. In this study the central concern is

---

* The tabled *t*-value should be compared with the absolute value of the calculated *t*.

the change in the cholesterol levels—the average difference in cholesterol values before and after the treatment. The hypotheses being submitted to a statistical test are

$$H_0 : \mu_X = \mu_Y \qquad H_A : \mu_X \neq \mu_Y$$

In these hypotheses, μ_X is the population mean for pretreatment cholesterol levels, while μ_Y is that for posttreatment cholesterol levels.

As in the previous example, a *t* statistic would be computed from the pretest and posttest measures (using, however, a different formula).* The obtained *t* would be compared with the *t* values in Table A of Appendix B. For this particular type of *t*-test, the degrees of freedom equal the number of paired observations minus one ($df = n - 1$).

Other two-group tests

In certain two-group situations the *t*-statistic might be inappropriate. If the researcher is working with nominal- or ordinal-level data, or if the distribution is markedly nonnormal, then a nonparametric test may be preferred. We will mention a few such tests here without actually working out examples.

The *median test* involves the comparison of two independent groups on the basis of deviations from the median rather than the mean. In the median test the scores for both samples are

---

* The *t*-statistic for paired measures is computed according to the following equation:

$$t = \frac{\overline{D}_{x-y}}{\sqrt{\dfrac{\Sigma d^2}{n(n-1)}}}$$

where D_{x-y} = the difference between two paired scores
   $\overline{D}_{x-y}$ = the mean difference between the paired scores
   d = the deviation scores for the difference measure
   Σd^2 = sum of the squared deviation scores
   n = number of pairs

combined and the overall median calculated. Then the number of cases above and below this median is counted separately for each sample, resulting in a 2 × 2 contingency table; (above/below median) × (sample A/sample B). From such a contingency table, a statistic can be computed to test the null hypothesis that the medians are the same for the two populations.

The *Mann-Whitney U test* is another nonparametric procedure for testing the difference between two independent samples. The test is based upon the assignment of ranks to the two groups of measures. The sum of the ranks for the two groups can be compared by calculating the *U* statistic. The Mann-Whitney *U* test tends to throw away less information than a median test and, therefore, is more powerful.

When data are paired rather than independent, either the *sign test* or the *Wilcoxon signed-rank test* can be used. The sign test is an extremely simple procedure, involving the assignment of a "+" or "−" to the differences between a pair of scores, depending on whether X is larger than Y or vice versa. The Wilcoxon test involves taking the difference between paired scores and ranking the absolute difference.

Compared with *t*-tests, all of these nonparametric tests are computationally quite easy. Since they are generally less powerful, however, the ease of computation should not be used as the basis for choosing which statistic is most appropriate.

☐
Analysis of variance

The procedure known as *analysis of variance* (ANOVA) is one of the most commonly used statistical tests reported in research journals at the present time. Like the *t*-test, ANOVA is a parametric procedure, utilized to test the significance of differences between means. However, analysis of variance is not restricted to two group situations: the means of three or more groups can be compared with ANOVA.

The statistic computed in an analysis of variance is the *F-ratio* statistic. Since the statistic is based on more than two groups, it should not be too surprising that the computation of an *F*-ratio is somewhat more complex than that for a *t*-statistic. A brief overview of the logic of analysis of variance might prove helpful.

Consider for the moment the raw scores shown in Table 21-1. The 20 scores—ten for each group—are not identical. The scores vary from one person to another. Some of that variability can be attributed to individual differences in feelings toward breastfeeding. Some of that variability could also be due to measurement error (unreliability), while some of it could be the result of the subjects' mood on that day and so forth. The research question is: can a significant portion of the variability be attributed to the independent variable, which in this case is exposure or nonexposure to special instruction on breastfeeding?

Analysis of variance decomposes the total variability of a set of data into two components: (1) the variability resulting from the independent variable and (2) all other variability, such as individual differences, measurement unreliability, and so on. Variation *between* treatment groups is contrasted with variation *within* groups, to yield an *F*-ratio. If the differences between groups receiving different treatments is large relative to random fluctuations within groups, then it is possible to establish the probability that the treatment is related to, or resulted in, the group differences.

One-way analysis of variance

Suppose that we were interested in comparing the effectiveness of different therapies to help individuals stop smoking. One group of smokers will undergo behavior modification therapy, which is based on reinforcement theory. A second group will be treated by means of hypnosis. A third group will serve as a control group and, therefore, will receive no special treatment. The dependent variable in this experiment will be cigarette consumption during the week following completion of the therapies. Thirty subjects who smoke regularly are randomly assigned to one of the three conditions. The analysis of variance will permit a test of the following hypotheses:

$$H_0 : \mu_A = \mu_B = \mu_C \qquad H_A : \mu_A \neq \mu_B \neq \mu_C$$

The null hypothesis asserts that the population means for posttreatment cigarette smoking will be the same for all three groups, while the alternative (research) hypothesis predicts inequality of means. Table 21-2 presents some hypothetical data for such a study.

For each of the three groups, the raw score for each subject is shown. Below the scores the means have been calculated. The mean number of posttreatment cigarettes consumed is 20, 25, and 28 for groups A, B, and C, respectively. These means are different but are they significantly different? Or are these differences attributable to random fluctuations?

The underlying concepts and terms for a one-way ANOVA will be briefly explained without working out the computations for this example. Again, the reader is urged to consult a statistics text for formulas and more detailed explanations. In calculating an *F*-statistic, the total variability within the data is broken down into two sources, as mentioned above. The portion of the variance resulting from group membership (that is, from exposure to different treatments) is arrived at by calculating a component known as the *sum of squares between groups*, or SS_B. This SS_B represents the sum of squared deviations of the individual group means from the overall mean for all the data. This SS_B term reflects the variability in individual scores attributable to group membership.

Table 21-2
Computation of a one-way ANOVA

Group A	Group B	Group C
X_A	X_B	X_C
28	22	29
0	31	40
17	26	23
20	30	35
35	34	28
19	37	20
24	0	17
0	19	38
41	24	24
16	27	26
$\Sigma X_A = 200$	$\Sigma X_B = 250$	$\Sigma X_C = 280$
$\overline{X}_A = 20$	$\overline{X}_B = 25$	$\overline{X}_C = 28$

The second component is the *sum of squares within groups*, or SS_W. This is an index of the sum of the squared deviations of each individual score from its own group mean. The SS_W term indicates variability attributable to individual differences, measurement error, and so on.

It may be recalled from the last chapter that the formula for calculating a variance is: $Var = \Sigma x^2 / n - 1$. The two sums of squares described above are analogous to the numerator of this equation. The sums of squares represent sums of squared deviations from means. Therefore, to compute the variance within and the variance between groups, we must divide by a quantity analogous to $(n - 1)$. This quantity is the degrees of freedom associated with each sum of squares. For between groups, $df = G - 1$, which is the number of groups minus one. For within groups, $df = (n_A - 1) + (n_B - 1) + \cdots (n_G - 1)$. That is, degrees of freedom within is found by adding together the number of subjects less 1 for each group.

In an analysis of variance context, the variance is conventionally referred to as the *mean square*. The formula for the mean square between groups and the mean square within groups is

$$MS_B = \frac{SS_B}{df_B} \qquad MS_W = \frac{SS_W}{df_W}$$

The *F*-ratio is the ratio of these mean squares, or

$$F = \frac{MS_B}{MS_W}$$

All of these computations for the data in Table 21-2 are presented in the summary table shown in Table 21-3.

The last step is to compare the obtained *F*-statistic with the value from a theoretical *F*-distribution. Table B-2 in Appendix B contains the upper limits of "probable" values for distributions with varying degrees of freedom. The first part of the table lists these values for a significance level of .05, while the second and third parts list those for .01 and .001 significance levels. Let us say that we have chosen the .05 probability level. To enter the table, we find the column headed by our between-groups *df* (2), and go down this column until we reach the row corresponding to the within-groups *df* (27). The tabled value of *F* with 2 and 27 degrees of freedom is 3.35. Because our obtained *F*-value of 3.90 exceeds 3.35, we reject the null hypothesis that the population means are equal. The differences in the number of cigarettes smoked after treatment are beyond chance expectations. In fewer than 5 samples out of 100 would differences of this magnitude be obtained by chance alone. The data support the hypothesis that the therapies affect cigarette-smoking behaviors.

The ANOVA procedure does not allow us to say that each group differed significantly from all other groups. We cannot tell from these results if Treatment A was significantly more effective than Treatment B. Some researchers incorrectly use *t*-tests to compare the different pairs of means (A vs. B, A vs. C, B. vs. C) when this type of information is required. There are methods known as *multiple comparison procedures* that should be used in such situations. The function of these procedures is to isolate the comparisons between group means that are responsible for the rejection of the ANOVA null hypothesis. Multiple comparison methods are described in most intermediate statistical textbooks.

The techniques described in this section are suitable only in the case in which the samples are independent. When three or more measures are obtained from the same set of subjects, a repeated measure analysis is called for. The treatment of repeated measures is beyond the scope of this book, but a full explanation and description of the necessary computations may be found in Winer (1971).

Multifactor ANOVA

The type of problem described above is known as a one-way analysis of variance because it deals with the effect of one independent variable (the different therapies) on a dependent variable. In Chapter 7 it was pointed out that hypotheses are sometimes complex and make predictions about the effect of two or more independent variables on a dependent variable. The analysis of data from such studies is often performed by means of a multifactor ANOVA.

Table 21-3
ANOVA summary table

Source of Variance	SS	df	MS	F	P
Between groups	326.7	2	163.4	3.90	<.05
Within groups	1130.0	27	41.9		
Total	1456.7	29			

Table 21-4
Fictitious data for a two-way (2 × 2) ANOVA

Factor B — Sex	Factor A — Treatment			
	Behavior Modification (1)		Hypnosis (2)	
Female (1)	24 28 22 19 27 25 18 21 0 36	Group 1 $\overline{X} = 22$	27 0 45 19 22 23 18 20 12 14	Group 2 $\overline{X} = 20$	Females $\overline{X}_{B1} = 21$
Male (2)	10 21 17 0 33 16 18 13 15 17	Group 3 $\overline{X} = 16$	36 31 28 32 25 22 19 30 35 42	Group 4 $\overline{X} = 30$	Males $\overline{X}_{B2} = 23$
	Treatment 1	$\overline{X}_{A1} = 19$	Treatment 2	$\overline{X}_{A2} = 25$	$\overline{X}_G = 22$

In this section we will describe some of the principles underlying a two-way analysis of variance. As above, the actual computations will not be worked out. Let us suppose that we were interested in determining whether the two therapies discussed above were equally effective in helping both men and women stop smoking. We could design an experiment using a randomized block design, with four groups: women and men would be randomly assigned, separately, to the two therapy conditions. After the experimental period, each subject would be required to report the average daily number of cigarettes smoked. Some fictitious data for this problem are shown in Table 21-4.

With two independent variables, there is more than one hypothesis to be tested. First,

we are testing whether, for both sexes, the behavior modification therapy is more effective than hypnosis as a means of reducing smoking or vice versa. Second, we are analyzing for sex differences in smoking behavior for individuals exposed to either therapeutic treatment. Third, we are examining the differential effect of the two treatments on males and females. This last hypothesis is the *interaction hypothesis.* Interaction is concerned with whether the effect of one independent variable is consistent for every level of a second independent variable. In other words, do the two therapies have the same effect on both sexes?

The data in Table 21-4 reveal the following: that, overall, subjects in Treatment 1 smoked less than those in Treatment 2 (19 vs. 25), that females smoked less than males (21 vs. 23);

and that males smoked less when exposed to Treatment 1 but females smoked less when exposed to Treatment 2. By performing a two-way analysis of variance on these data, it would be possible to ascertain the statistical significance of these differences.

Multifactor analysis of variance is an extremely important analytic technique. Human behaviors, conditions, and feelings are complex, and the ability to examine the combined effects of two or more independent variables permits this complexity to be incorporated into research designs. Multifactor ANOVA is not restricted to two-way schemes. Theoretically, any number of independent variables is possible, although in practice studies with more than four factors are rare because of the prohibitive number of subjects required.

Nonparametric "ANOVA"

Nonparametric tests do not, strictly speaking, analyze variance. There are, however, non-parametric procedures analogous to the parametric ANOVA for use with ordinal-level data or when a markedly nonnormal distribution renders parametric tests questionable. When the number of groups is greater than two and a one-way test for independent samples is desired, one may use a statistic developed by statisticians named Kruskal and Wallis. The *Kruskal-Wallis test* is a generalized version of the Mann-Whitney U test, based on the assignment of ranks to the scores from the various groups. When the researcher is working with paired groups, or when several measures are obtained from a single sample, then the *Friedman test* for "analysis of variance" by ranks may be applied. These tests are described in Hays (1973) and Siegel (1956).

□
The chi-square test

The chi-square statistic is used when we have categories of data and hypotheses concerning the proportions of cases that fall into the various categories. In the last chapter we discussed the construction of contingency tables to describe the frequencies of cases falling in different classes. The chi-square (χ^2) statistic is applied to contingency tables to test the significance of different proportions.

Consider the following example. A researcher is interested in studying the effect of planned nursing instruction on patients' compliance with a self-medication regimen. An experimental group of 100 patients is instructed by nurses who are implementing a new instructional approach. A second (control) group of 100 patients is cared for by nurses who continue their usual mode of instruction. The hypothesis being tested is that a higher proportion of subjects in the experimental group will report self-medication compliance than will subjects in the control group.

The chi-square statistic is computed by comparing two sets of frequencies: those observed in the collected data and those that would be expected if there were no relationship between two variables. The expected frequencies are calculated on the basis of the observed total frequencies for the rows and columns of a contingency table. Observed frequencies for the present example are shown in Table 21-5. As this table shows, 60% of the experimentals but only 30 percent of the controls reported self-medication compliance. The chi-square test will enable us to decide whether a difference in proportions of this magnitude is likely to reflect a real experimental effect or only chance fluctuations.

The chi-square statistic is computed* by summarizing differences between observed

---

* The formula for a χ^2 statistic is

$$\chi^2 = \Sigma \frac{(f_o - f_E)^2}{f_E}$$

where f_o = observed frequency for a cell

f_E = expected frequency for a cell

Σ = sum of the $(f_o - f_E)^2 / f_E$ ratios for all cells

(*Footnote continues on p. 413*)

Table 21-5
Observed frequencies for a chi-square example

	Compliance	Noncompliance	Total
Experimental	60	40	100
Control	30	70	100
Total	90	110	200

and expected frequencies for each cell. In this example there are four cells, and thus χ^2 will be the sum of four numbers. More specifically, $\chi^2 = 18.18$ in the present case. As usual, we need to compare this test statistic with the value from a theoretical chi-square distribution. A table of chi-square values for various degrees of freedom and significance levels is provided in Table B-3 in Appendix B. For the chi-squre statistic, the degrees of freedom are equal to $(R - 1)(C - 1)$, or the number of rows minus 1 times the number of columns minus 1. In the present case, $df = 1 \times 1$, or 1. With 1 degree of freedom, the value that must be exceeded in order to establish significance at the .05 level is 3.84. The obtained value of 18.18 is substantially larger than would be expected by chance. Thus, we can conclude that a significantly larger proportion of patients in the experimental group than in the control group complied with self-medication instructions.

□
Correlation coefficients

In the previous chapter the computation and interpretation of the Pearson product-moment correlation coefficient were explained. The Pearson r statistic is both descriptive and inferential. As a descriptive statistic, the correlation

---

$f_E = \dfrac{f_R f_C}{N}$ where f_R = observed frequency for the given row
f_C = observed frequency for the given column
N = total number of subjects

coefficient summarizes the magnitude and direction of a relationship between two variables. As an inferential statistic, r is used to test hypotheses concerning population correlations, which are ordinarily symbolized by the Greek letter rho, or ρ. The most commonly tested null hypothesis is that there is no relationship between two variables. Stated formally,

$$H_0 : \rho = 0 \qquad H_A : \rho \neq 0$$

For instance, suppose we were studying the relationship between patients' self-reported level of stress (higher stress scores imply more stress) and the pH level of their saliva. With a sample of 50 subjects, we find that $r = -.29$. This value implies that there was a slight tendency for people who received higher stress scores to have lower pH levels than those with low stress scores. But we need to question whether this finding can be generalized to the population. Does the coefficient of $-.29$ reflect a random fluctuation, caused only by the particular group of subjects sampled, or is the relationship significant? The table of significant values in Table B-4 of Appendix B allows us to make the determination. Degrees of freedom for correlation coefficients are equal to the number of subjects minus 2, or $(n - 2)$. With $df = 48$, the critical value for r (for a .05 two-tailed test) lies between .2732 and .2875, or approximately .2803. Since the absolute value of the calculated r is .29, the null hypothesis can be rejected. Therefore, we may conclude that there is significant relationship between a person's self-reported level of stress and the acidity of her or his saliva.

Table 21-6
Summary of statistical tests

Name of Procedure	Test Statistic	Degrees of Freedom	Parametric (P) or Non-Parametric (NP)	Purpose	Levels of Measurement Var. 1 (Independent)	Levels of Measurement Var. 2 (Dependent)
t-Test for independent samples	t	$n_{Group\ A} + n_{Group\ B} - 2$	P	To test the difference between the means of 2 independent groups	Nominal	Interval or Ratio
t-Test for dependent (paired) samples	t	$n - 1$	P	To test the difference between the means of 2 related groups or sets of scores	Nominal	Interval or Ratio
Median Test	χ^2	$(\text{Rows} - 1) \times (\text{Columns} - 1)$	NP	To test the difference between the medians of 2 independent groups	Nominal	Ordinal
Mann-Whitney U Test	U	$n - 1$	NP	To test the difference in the ranks of scores of 2 independent groups	Nominal	Ordinal
Wilcoxon Signed-Rank Test	Z	$n - 2$	NP	To test the difference in the ranks of scores of 2 related groups or sets of scores	Nominal	Ordinal

Test	Statistic	Degrees of Freedom	P/NP	Purpose		
ANOVA	F	Between: n of groups $- 1$ Within: n of subjects $- n$ of groups	P	To test the difference among the means of 3 or more independent groups, or of more than 1 independent variable	Nominal	Interval or Ratio
Kruskal-Wallis Test	H (χ^2)	n of groups $- 1$	NP	To test the difference in the ranks of scores of 3 or more independent groups	Nominal	Ordinal
Friedman Test	χ^2	n of groups $- 1$	NP	To test the difference in the ranks of scores for 3 or more related sets of scores	Nominal	Ordinal
Chi-Square Test	χ^2	(Rows $- 1$) $\times$ (Columns $- 1$)	NP	To test the difference in proportions in 2 or more groups	Nominal	Nominal
Pearson's Product Moment Correlation	r	$n - 2$	P	To test that a correlation is different from zero (i.e., that a relationship exists)	Interval or Ratio	Interval or Ratio
Spearman's Rho	ρ	$n - 2$	NP	To test that a correlation is different from zero (i.e., that a relationship exists)	Ordinal	Ordinal
Kendall's Tau	τ	$n - 2$	NP	To test that a correlation is different from zero (i.e., that a relationship exists)	Ordinal	Ordinal

The Pearson *r* is a parametric statistic. When the assumptions for a parametric test are violated, or when the data are inherently ordinal-level, then the appropriate coefficient of correlation is either *Spearman's rho* or *Kendall's tau*. (See, for example, Siegel, 1956).

☐
Overview of various statistical tests

As we have seen in the preceding section, the selection and use of a statistical test depends on several factors. In some cases nonparametric tests are more appropriate than parametric tests. For some research problems, a two-way ANOVA rather than a one-way ANOVA will be required. To aid researchers in selecting a test statistic or evaluating statistical procedures used by researchers in the literature, a chart summarizing the major features of several commonly used tests is presented in Table 21-6.

☐
The computer and inferential statistics

As in the previous chapter, we have stressed the logic and uses of various statistics rather than the computational formulas and mathematical derivations.* Because the computer is increasingly called upon to perform the computations for hypothesis testing, and because it is important to be able to make sense of the printed information produced by the computer, we conclude this chapter with examples of computer-produced information for two of the tests described in this chapter.

We return to the example described in Chapter 20. A researcher has designed an experiment to test the effect of a special prenatal program on a group of young, low-income

* It is important to note that this introduction to inferential statistics has necessarily been superficial. We urge novice researchers to undertake further exploration of statistical principles.

women. The raw data for this example are shown in Table 20-7. Given these data, let us test some hyotheses.

Hypothesis one: t-test

Let us suppose that our first research hypothesis is

The babies of the experimental subjects will have higher birthweights than the babies of the control subjects.

Birthweight, the dependent variable, is measured on a ratio scale. Therefore, the *t*-test for independent samples is used to test our hypothesis. The null and alternative hypotheses can be stated as follows:

$$H_0 : \mu \text{ experimental} = \mu \text{ control}$$
$$H_A : \mu \text{ experimental} \neq \mu \text{ control}$$

Figure 21-5 presents the computer printout for the *t*-test. The left side of the figure presents some basic descriptive statistics for the birthweight variable, separately for the two groups. Thus, the birthweight of the babies in Group 1 (the experimental group) was 107.5 ounces, compared with 101.9 ounces for the babies in Group 2 (the control group). These data, then, are consistent with our research hypothesis—the weight of the experimentals is higher than the weight of the controls. But do the differences reflect the impact of the experimental intervention or do they merely represent random fluctuations? To answer this, we examine the results of the *t*-test, shown on the right side of the figure. The computer program calculated that the value of *t* is 1.44. With 28 degrees of freedom, this value is not significant. The two-tailed probability (p value) for this *t* value is .16. This means that in 16 samples out of 100, one could expect to find a difference in weights at least this large, as a result of chance alone. Therefore, we cannot conclude that the special in-

```
GROUP 1 - GROUP    EQ      1.
GROUP 2 - GROUP    EQ      .2.
                                                        *  POOLED VARIANCE ESTIMATE
                                                        *
VARIABLE          NUMBER                STANDARD   STANDARD  *   T    DEGREES OF 2-TAIL
                 OF CASES      MEAN    DEVIATION     ERROR   *  VALUE   FREEDOM   PROB.
------------------------------------------------------------*---------------------------
WEIGHT    BIRTHWEIGHT OF BABY
      GROUP 1      15        107.5333   13.378      3.454    *
                                                            *  1.44      28       .160
      GROUP 2      15        101.8667    7.239      1.869    *
                                                            *
```

Figure 21-5. *SPSS^x computer printout: t test.*

tervention was effective in improving the birthweights of the experimental groups.*

Hypothesis two: Pearson correlation

The second research hypothesis might be stated as follows:

Older mothers will have babies of higher birthweight than younger mothers.

In this case, both birthweight and age are measured on the ratio scale. Referring to Table 21-6, we find that the appropriate test statistic is Pearson's product-moment correlation. The hypotheses subjected to the statistical test are

$$H_0 : \rho \text{ birthweight/age} = 0$$
$$H_A : \rho \text{ birthweight/age} \neq 0$$

The printout for the test of the hypothesis is presented in Figure 21-6. This printout shows

* The difference in weights is fairly sizable and in the right direction. The researcher might wish to pursue this study by increasing the sample size or by controlling some other variables, such as the mother's age, through analysis of covariance (see Chapter 22).

a two-dimension *correlation matrix,* in which each variable specified is indicated on both a row and a column. To read a correlation matrix, one finds the row for one of the variables and reads across until the row intersects with the column indicating the second variable.

The correlation matrix in Figure 21-6 shows, in row one, the correlation of weight with weight and of weight with age; and in row two, the correlation of age with weight and of age with age. The correlation of interest to us for testing the hypothesis is weight with age (or age with weight—the result is the same). At the intersection of these two variables, we find three numbers. The first is the actual correlation coefficient, and the second shows the number of cases. In our example, $r = .5938$ and $N = 30$. The correlation indicates a moderately strong positive relationship: the older the mother, the higher the baby's weight tends to be, as hypothesized. Again, the data are consistent with the research hypothesis, but does this reflect a true relationship or merely chance fluctuations in the data? The third number at the intersection of age and weight shows the probability that the correlation oc-

```
- - - - - - - - - - - P E A R S O N   C O R R E L A T I O N   C O E F F I C I E N T S

              WEIGHT      AGE
WEIGHT       1.0000      .5938
            (    30)   (    30)
            S= #####   S= .000

AGE           .5938     1.0000
            (    30)   (    30)
            S= .000    S=#####
```

Figure 21-6. *SPSS^x computer printout: Pearson's Correlation Coefficient.*

curred by chance: S (for significance level) = .000. The printout only shows p levels to the nearest thousandth. In this case, the actual p value might be .0004 or .000001, but we do not know the actual p value. We *do* know, however, that $p < .001$. In other words, a relationship this strong would be found by chance alone in fewer than 1 out of 1000 samples of 30 young mothers. Therefore, the research hypothesis is accepted.

□
Research example

Jalowiec and Powers (1981) studied life stress and coping behavior among patients with acute illness (emergency room patients) and among those with chronic illness (hypertensive patients). The study compared the number and types of stressful life events reported by persons in these two groups for a 1-year period prior to illness onset and the methods they used in coping with stress. The researchers also explored the relationships among coping styles, levels of stress, and health status.

The investigators used a variety of statistical procedures to develop appropriate instruments and examine the research questions. For example, stress was measured by administering a stressful life event (SLE) questionnaire, which measures 76 different types of stresses. The number of stressful life events was compared for the acute and chronic patient groups using a t-test for independent means. The results indicated that emergency room patients had significantly more SLEs than hypertensive patients ($t = 2.37$, $df = 48$, $p < .05$). Using a measure of coping behavior developed by the investigators, it was found that hypertensive subjects used somewhat more coping methods than emergency room subjects, but the difference was not statistically significant ($t = 1.17$, $df = 48$, $p > .05$). The investigators also examined the relation-

ship between stress and coping on the one hand and background characteristics of the subjects on the other. For example, among emergency room patients there was a strong positive correlation between educational level and coping scores. That is, the higher the educational level, the greater the number of coping methods the subjects used. The correlation was significantly different from zero ($r = .63$, $df = 23$, $p < .001$). Educational level was not, however, found to be significantly associated with SLE scores in either group. That is, people of all educational levels were equally likely to be exposed to numerous stressful life events.

□
Summary

Inferential statistics provide a means for a researcher to make inferences about the characteristics of a poulation based upon data obtained in a sample. The reason that we cannot make such inferences directly from the data is that sample statistics inevitably contain a certain degree of error as estimates of population parameters. Inferential statistics offer the researcher a framework for deciding whether or not the sampling error is too high to provide reliable population estimates.

The *sampling distribution* of the mean is a theoretical distribution of the means of many different samples drawn from the same population. When an infinite number of samples is drawn from a population, the sampling distribution of means follows a normal curve. Because of this characteristic, it is possible to indicate the probability that a specified sample value will be obtained. The *standard error of the mean* is the standard deviation of the theoretical sampling distribution of the mean. This index indicates the degree of average error in a sample mean as an estimate of the population mean. The smaller the standard error of the mean, the more accurate are the estimates of the population value. Sampling distributions are the basis for inferential statistics.

Statistical inference consists of two major types of approaches: estimating parameters and testing hypotheses. When a researcher wants to discover the value of an unknown population characteristic, he or she may estimate the value by means of either point or interval estimation. *Point estimation* provides a single numerical value. *Interval estimation* provides the upper and lower limits of a range of values between which the population value is expected to fall, at some specified probability level. The researcher is able to establish the degree of confidence that the population value will lie within this range. Interval estimates are often referred to as *confidence intervals.*

The testing of hypotheses by statistical procedures enables researchers to make objective decisions concerning the results of their studies. The *null hypothesis* is a statement that no relationship exists between the variables and that any observed relationships are due to chance or sampling fluctuations. The null hypothesis, rather than the research hypothesis, is used in hyothesis testing. Failure to reject the null hypothesis means that any observed differences may be attributable to chance fluctuations. Rejection of the null hypothesis lends support to the research hypothesis.

It is possible to fail to reject a null hypothesis when, in fact, it should be rejected. Such an error is referred to as a *Type II error.* If a null hypothesis is rejected when it should not be rejected, the error is termed a *Type I error.* Researchers are able to control the risk involved in committing a Type I error by establishing levels of significance. A *level of significance* indicates the probability of making a Type I error. The two most commonly used levels of significance are .05 and .01. A significance level of .01 means that in only 1 out of 100 samples will the null hypothesis be rejected when, if fact, it should be retained.

Researchers report the results of hypothesis testing as being either statistically significant or nonsignificant. The phrase *statistically significant* means that the obtained results are not likely to be due to chance fluctuations at the specified level of probability. Although most hypothesis testing involves *two-tailed tests* in which both ends of the sampling distribution are used to define the region of "improbable values," a *one-tailed* test may be appropriate if the researcher has a strong rationale for a directional hypothesis.

Statistical tests are classified as parametric and nonparametric. *Nonparametric tests* require less stringent assumptions than parametric tests and usually are used when the level of data is either nominal or ordinal or when normality of the distribution cannot be assumed. *Parametric tests* involve the estimation of at least one parameter, the use of data measured on an interval or ratio level, and assumptions concerning the variables under consideration. Parametric tests are usually more powerful than nonparametric tests and generally are preferred.

The most common parametric procedures are the *t*-test and *analysis of variance* (ANOVA), both of which can be used to test the significance of the difference between group means. The *t*-test can only be applied to two-group situations whereas the ANOVA procedure can handle three or more groups, as well as more than one independent variable. The nonparametric test that is used most frequently is the *chi-square test,* which is used in connection with hypotheses relating to differences in proportions.

□
Study suggestions

1. A researcher has administered a Job Satisfaction Scale to a sample of 50 primary nurses and 50 team nurses. The mean score

on this scale for each group was found to be 35.2 for the primary nurses and 33.6 for the team nurses. A *t* statistic is computed and is found to be 1.89. Interpret this result, using the table for *t*-values in Appendix B.

2. Compute the chi-square statistic for the following contingency table:

Group	Number of Complications Following Surgery		
	None	One	More Than One
Experimental	38	72	54
Control	29	50	11

How many degrees of freedom are there? At the .05 level of significance, what may be concluded?

3. Answer the following:
Given: (a) Three groups of nursing school students, with 50 in each group; (b) Probability level = .05; (c) Value of test statistic = 4.43; (d) Mean scores on test to measure motivation to attend graduate school: 25.8, 29.3, and 23.4 for Groups A, B, and C, respectively.
Specify: (a) What test statistic would be used; (b) How many degrees of freedom there are; (c) Whether the test statistic is statistically significant; and (d) What the test statistic means.

4. What inferential statistic would you choose for the following sets of variables? Explain your answers. (Refer to Table 21-6.)
a. Variable 1 is the weights of 100 patients; variable 2 is the patients' resting heart rate.
b. Variable 1 is the patient's marital status; Variable 2 is the patient's level of preoperative stress.
c. Variable 1 is whether an amputee has a leg removed above or below the knee; Variable 2 is whether or not the amputee has shown signs of aggressive behavior during rehabilitation.

☐ Suggested readings

Methodological references

Armstrong, G. (1981). Parametric statistics and ordinal data: A pervasive misconception. *Nursing Research, 30,* 60–62.

Brogan, D.R. (1981). Choosing an appropriate statistical test of significance for a nursing research hypothesis or question. *Western Journal of Nursing Research, 3,* 337–363.

Glass, G.V. & Stanley, J.C. (1984). *Statistical methods in education and psychology* (2nd ed.). Englewood Cliffs, NJ: Prentice-Hall.

Hays, W.L. (1973). *Statistics for the social sciences* (2nd ed.). New York: Holt, Rinehart and Winston.

Hoel, P.G. (1983). *Elementary statistics* (4th ed.). New York: John Wiley and Sons.

Holm, K. & Christman, N.J. (1985). Post hoc tests following analysis of variance. *Research in Nursing and Health, 8,* 207–210.

Knapp, R.G. (1984). *Basic statistics for nurses* (2nd ed.). New York: John Wiley and Sons.

Marks, R.G. (1982). *Analyzing research data: The basic of biomedical research methodology.* Belmont, CA: Life Long Learning.

Milton, J.S. & Tsokos, J.O. (1983). *Statistical methods in the biological and health sciences.* New York: McGraw-Hill.

Siegel, S. (1956). *Nonparametric statistics for the behavioral sciences.* New York: McGraw-Hill.

Triola, M. (1983). *Elementary statistics.* Menlo Park, CA: Addison-Wesley.

Welkowitz, J., Ewen, R.B., & Cohen, J. (1982). *Introductory statistics for the behavioral sciences* (3rd ed.). New York: Academic Press.

Winer, B.J. (1971). *Statistical principles in experimental design* (2nd ed.). New York: McGraw-Hill.

Young, R.K. & Veldman, D.J. (1981). *Introductory statistics for the behavioral sciences* (4th ed.). New York: Holt, Rinehart and Winston.

Substantive references

Beck, C.T. (1983). Parturients' temporal experiences during the phases of labor. *Western Journal of Nursing Research, 5,* 283–295 (*t*-tests).

Bullough, B., Bullough, V., & Smith, R.W. (1985). Masculinity and feminity in transvestite, transsexual and gay males. *Western Journal of Nursing Research, 7,* 317–332 (ANOVA, chi-square test).

Cohen, M.Z. & Loomis, M.E. (1985). Linguistic analysis of questionnaire responses: Methods of coping with work stress. *Western Journal of Nursing Research, 7,* 357–366 (Spearman's rho, Kruskal-Wallis test).

Damrosch, S.P. (1981). How nursing students' reactions to rape victims are affected by a perceived act of carelessness. *Nursing Research, 30,* 168–170 (Two-way ANOVA).

Douglas, E. & Larson, E.L. (1985). The effect of a positive end-expiratory pressure adaptor on oxygenation during endotracheal suctioning. *Heart & Lung, 14,* 396–400 (Paired *t*-test).

Ellison, E.S. (1983). Parental support and school-aged children. *Western Journal of Nursing Research, 5,* 145–153 (*t*-tests).

Ford, A.H. (1980). Use of automobile restraining devices for infants. *Nursing Research, 29,* 281–284 (Chi-square, ANOVA).

Jalowiec, A. & Powers, M.J. (1983). Stress and coping in hypertensive and emergency room patients. *Nursing Research, 30,* 10–15 (*t*-tests, Pearson's *r*, Spearman's rho).

Mercer, R.T. (1986). The relationship of developmental variables to maternal behavior. *Research in Nursing and Health, 9,* 25–33 (ANOVA, *t*-tests, multiple comparison procedures, Pearson's *r*).

Reed, P.G. (1986). Religiousness among terminally ill and healthy adults. *Research in Nursing and Health, 9,* 35–41 (One-tailed *t*-test, chi-square, Pearson's *r*).

Tulman, L.J. (1985). Mothers' and unrelated persons' initial handling of newborn infants. *Nursing Research, 34,* 205–209 (Mann-Whitney U-test; Friedman two-way ANOVA).

Ziemer, M.M. (1983). Effects of information on postsurgical coping. *Nursing Research, 32,* 282–287 (Chi-square tests, *t*-tests, Pearson correlation coefficients, ANOVA).

Chapter 22
□
Advanced statistical procedures

The phenomena of interest to nurse researchers are generally complex. Patients' preoperative anxieties, a nurses's effectiveness in caring for people, the self-concept of a person with severe thermal injuries, the fears of a woman giving birth for the first time, or the abrupt elevation of a patient's body temperature are phenomena that have multiple facets and multiple determinants. Scientists, in attempting to explain, predict, and control the phenomena that interest them, have come increasingly to the recognition that a two-variable study is often inadequate for such purposes. The classical approach to data analysis and research design, which consists of studying the effect of a single independent variable on a single dependent variable, increasingly is being replaced by more sophisticated *multivariate** procedures. Whether one structures a study to be multivariate or not, the fact remains that most nursing phenomena are essentially and unalterably multivariate in nature. The modern researcher who is unfamiliar with multivariate techniques is at a serious disadvantage both as a designer of research studies and as a consumer of research reports.

Unlike the statistical methods reviewed in the previous two chapters, multivariate statistics are computationally formidable. However, the widespread availability of computers has made complex manual calculations obsolete. Therefore, we make no attempt to provide formulas for the multivariate statistical procedures described here. The purpose of this chapter is to provide a general under-

* We use the term multivariate in this chapter to refer generally to analyses dealing with at least three variables. Some statisticians reserve the term for problems involving more than one dependent variable.

standing of how, when, and why multivariate statistics are used rather than to explain their mathematical basis. References are available at the end of this chapter for those desiring to enlarge this understanding.

☐
Multiple regression/correlation

Multiple regression analysis is a method used for understanding the effects of two or more independent variables on a dependent measure. The terms multiple correlation and multiple regression will be used almost interchangeably in reference to this technique, given the strong bond between correlation and regression. In order to comprehend the nature of this bond, we will first explain simple regression—that is, bivariate regression —before turning to multiple regression.

Simple linear regression

Regression analysis is basically performed with the intention of making predictions about phenomena. In the health care field, as in many other fields, the ability to make accurate predictions has important implications for the quality of services rendered. For example, whenever a scarce resource such as a medication is to be allocated, then it is important to be able to predict who will most be in need of that resource.

In simple regression, one variable (X) is used to predict a second variable (Y). For instance, we could use simple regression to predict weight from height, blood pressure from age, nursing school achievement from SAT scores, or stress from noise levels. An important feature of regression is that the higher the correlation between the two variables, the more accurate the prediction. If the correlation between diastolic and systolic blood pressure were perfect (i.e., if $r = 1.00$), then one would only need to measure one to be

able to know the value of the other. Since most variables of interest to researchers are not perfectly correlated, most predictions made through regression analysis are not perfect.

A simple regression equation is a formula for making predictions about the numerical values of one variable based upon scores of another variable. The basic linear regression equation is:

$$Y' = a + bX$$

where Y' is a predicted value of variable Y, *a* is the intercept constant, *b* is the regression coefficient, or slope of the line, and X is the score on variable X. Regression analysis solves for *a* and *b*, so that for values of X, predictions about Y can be made. Those readers with recollection of high school algebra may remember that the above equation is the algebraic equation for a straight line. Linear regression is essentially a method for determining a straight line to fit the data in such a way that deviations from the line are minimized.

An illustration may help to clarify some of these points. Two sets of scores for five subjects are shown in columns 1 and 2 of Table 22-1. Application of the formula for Pearson's *r* reveals that the scores are strongly related, $r = .90$. What we wish to do is develop a way of predicting Y scores for a *new* group of subjects from whom we will only have information on the variable X. In order to do this, we must use the five sets of scores to solve for *a* and *b* in the regression equation.

The equation for these two components are as follows:

$$b = \frac{\Sigma xy}{\Sigma x^2} \qquad a = \overline{Y} - b\overline{X}$$

where *b* = regression coefficient
  a = intercept constant
  $\overline{Y}$ = mean of variable Y
  $\overline{X}$ = mean of variable X
  x = deviation scores from $\overline{X}$
  y = deviation scores from $\overline{Y}$

Table 22-1
Computations for simple linear regression

(1) X	(2) Y	(3) x	(4) x²	(5) y	(6) y²	(7) xy	(8) Y'	(9) e	(10) e²
1	2	−4	16	−4	16	16	2.4	− .4	.16
3	6	−2	4	0	0	0	4.2	1.8	3.24
5	4	0	0	−2	4	0	6.0	−2.0	4.0
7	8	2	4	2	4	4	7.8	.2	.04
9	10	4	16	4	16	16	9.6	.4	.16
$\Sigma X = 25$	$\Sigma Y = 30$		40		40	36		0	7.6
$\overline{X} = 5$	$\overline{Y} = 6$								

$$r = .90$$

$$\Sigma e^2 = 7.6$$

$$b = \frac{\Sigma xy}{\Sigma x^2} = \frac{36}{40} = .90$$

$$a = \overline{Y} - b\overline{X} = 6 - (.9)(5.0) = 1.5$$

$$Y' = a + bX \qquad Y' = 1.5 + .9X$$

The calculations required for the various elements of these equations are worked out for the present example in columns 3 through 7 of Table 22-1. As shown at the bottom of the table, the solution to the regression equation is $Y' = 1.5 + .9X$. What does one do with this information? Suppose for the moment that the X scores in column 1 were the only data available for the five subjects and that we wanted to predict their scores for variable Y. For the first subject with an $X = 1$, we would predict that $Y' = 1.5 + (.9)(1)$, or 2.4. Column 8 shows similar computations for each X value. These figures show that Y' does not exactly equal the actual values obtained for Y. Most of the errors of prediction (e) are quite small, as shown in Column 9. The errors of prediction result from the fact that the correlation between X and Y is not perfect. Only when $r = 1.00$ or -1.00 does $Y' = Y$. The regression equation solves for a and b in such a way as to minimize such errors. Or, more precisely, the solution minimizes the sums of squares of the prediction errors, which is why standard regression analysis is said to use a *least-squares principle*. In column 10 of Table 22-1 the error terms — usually referred to as the *residuals* — have been squared and summed to yield a value of 7.6. Any values of a and b other than those obtained above would have yielded a larger sum of the squared residuals.

The solution to this regression analysis example is displayed graphically in Figure 22-1. The actual X and Y values from the table are plotted on the graph with circles. The line running through these points is the representation of the regression solution. The intercept (a) is the point at which the line crosses the Y axis, which in this case is 1.5. The slope (b) is the angle of the line, relative to the X and Y axes. With $b = .90$, the line slopes in such a fashion that for every 4 units on the X axis, we must go up 3.6 units ($.9 \times 4$) on the Y axis. The line, then, embodies the whole regression equation. To find a predicted value for Y, we could go to the point on the X axis for an obtained X score, find the point on the regression line vertically above the score, and read the predicted Y value horizontally from the Y axis. For example, with an X score of 5, we would predict a Y' of 6, as shown by the star designating that point on the figure.

The connection between correlation and regression can be made more evident by point-

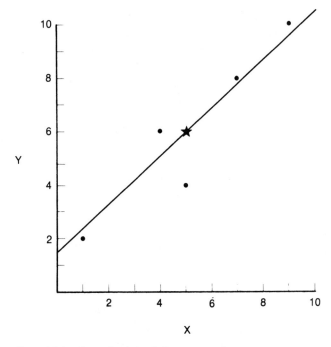

Figure 22-1. Example of simple linear regression.

ing out an important aspect of a correlation coefficient. The correlation coefficient, as described before, is an index of the degree to which variables are related with one another. Relationships, from a statistical point of view, are concerned with how variations in one score are associated with variations in another score. The *r* statistic enables us to specify how much variability can be "explained" or "accounted for" by two correlated variables. The square of *r* (*r²*) tells us the proportion of the variance in Y that can be accounted for by X. In the above example, *r* = .90, so *r²* = .81. This means that 81 percent of the variability in the Y scores can be understood in terms of the variability in the X scores. The remaining 19 percent constitutes variability resulting from some other source of influence.

Returning to the regression problem, it was found that the sum of the squared residuals (error terms) was 7.6. Column 6 of Table 22-1 also informs us that the sum of the squared deviations of the Y scores from the mean of Y (Σy^2) was 40.0. To demonstrate that the residuals constitute 19 percent of the unexplained variability in Y, we can compute the following ratio:

$$\frac{7.6}{40.0} = .19 = 1 - r^2$$

Although the computations are not shown, the sum of the squared deviations of the Y′ scores from the mean of Y′ ($\Sigma y'$) is equal to 32.4. As a proportion of the variability in the *actual* Y scores, this would equal

$$\frac{32.4}{40.0} = .81 = r^2$$

These calculations reinforce a point made earlier: the stronger the correlation the better the prediction. To put this another way, the stronger the correlation, the greater the percentage of variance accounted for.

Multiple linear regression

Since the correlation between two variables rarely is perfect, it is often desirable to try to improve one's ability to predict a Y score by including more than one X score as predictor variables. Suppose that we were interested in predicting graduate nursing students' grade point average. Since there are a limited number of students who can be accepted into graduate programs, there is naturally a concern for selecting those individuals who will have the greatest chance of success. Suppose from previous experience it has been found that those students who perform well on the verbal portion of the Graduate Record Examination (GRE) tend to obtain higher grades in graduate school than those with lower GRE scores. The correlation between the GRE-Verbal scores and graduate grade point average has been calculated as .50. With only 25 percent ($.50^2$) of the variance of graduate grade point average accounted for, there will be many errors of prediction made: many admitted students will not perform as well as anticipated, while many rejected applicants would have made successful students. It may be possible, by using additional information about students, to make more accurate predictions. Multiple linear regression can assist us by developing a regression equation that provides the best prediction possible, given the correlations among several variables. The basic multiple regression equation is:

$$Y' = a + b_1X_1 + b_2X_2 + \ldots b_kX_k$$

where Y′ is the predicted value for variable Y, a is the intercept constant, k is the number of predictor (independent) variables, b_1 to b_k are the regression coefficients for the k variables, and X_1 to X_k are the scores on the k variables.

When the number of predictor variables exceeds two, the computations required to solve this equation are prohibitively laborious and complex. Therefore, we will restrict our discussion to hypothetical rather than worked-out examples. Our major interest is to facilitate the use and interpretation of multiple regression statistics.

In the example in which we wished to predict graduate nursing students' grade point average, suppose we decided that information on undergraduate grade point average and scores on the quantitative portion of the GRE should be added to the prediction equation. The resulting equation might be:

$$Y' = .4 + .05 \, (GPA - U) + .003$$
$$(GRE - Q) + .002 \, (GRE - V)$$

For instance, suppose an applicant had a verbal GRE score of 600, a quantitative GRE score of 550, and an undergraduate grade point average of 3.2. The predicted graduate grade point average would be

$$Y' = .4 + (.05) \, (3.2) + .003 \, (550)$$
$$+ .002 \, (600) = 3.41$$

We can assess the degree to which the addition of two independent variables improved our ability to predict graduate school performance through the use of the multiple correlation coefficient. In bivariate correlation, the index expressing the magnitude of a relationship is the Pearson r. When two or more independent variables are used, the index of correlation is the multiple correlation coefficient, symbolized as R. Unlike r, R does not have negative values. R varies only from 0.0 to 1.0, showing the *strength* of the relationship between several independent and a dependent variable but not *direction*. It would make no sense to indicate direction, since X_1 could be positively related to Y, while X_2 could be negatively related to Y. The R statistic, when squared, indicates the proportion of variance

Table 22-2
Correlation matrix

	GRA-GRAD	GPA-U	GRE-Q	GRE-V
GPA-Graduate	1.00			
GPA-Undergraduate	.60	1.00		
GRE-Q	.55	.40	1.00	
GRE-V	.50	.50	.70	1.00

in Y accounted for by the combined simultaneous influence of the independent variables. Sometimes R^2 is referred to as the *coefficient of determination.*

The calculation of R^2 provides a direct means of evaluating the accuracy of the prediction equation. Let us say that with the three predictor variables used in the present example the value of $R = .71$. This means that 50 percent ($.71^2$) of the variability in graduate students' grades can be explained in terms of their verbal and quantitative GRE scores and their grades as undergraduates. The addition of two predictors doubled the variance accounted for by the single independent variable, from .25 to .50.

We should point out that the multiple correlation coefficient cannot be less than the highest bivariate correlation between the dependent variable and one of the independent variables. Table 22-2 presents the Pearson correlation coefficients for all of the variables in this example, taken as pairs. Such a table is called a *correlation matrix.* It can be seen that all of the values on the diagonal are 1.00, resulting from the fact that every variable is "perfectly correlated" with itself. The independent variable that is correlated most strongly with graduate performance is undergraduate grade point average, $r = .60$. The value of R could not have been less than .60.

A second important point is that R tends to be larger when the independent variables have relatively low correlations among themselves. In the present case the lowest correlation coefficient is between GRE-Q and undergraduate grades ($r = .40$) and the highest is between GRE-Q and GRE-V ($r = .70$). All correlations here are fairly substantial, a fact that helps to explain why R is not much higher than the r between the dependent variable and undergraduate grades alone. This somewhat puzzling phenomenon can be explained in terms of redundancy of information among predictors. When correlations among the independent variables are high, they tend to add little predictive power to each other because they are redundant. When the correlations are low, each variable has the ability to contribute something unique to the prediction of the dependent variable.

In Figure 22-2, a Venn diagram illustrates this concept. Each circle represents the total variability inherent in a variable. The circle on the left (Y) is the dependent variable whose scores we are trying to predict. The overlap between this circle and the other circles represents the amount of variability that the variables have in common. If the overlap were complete—if the entire graduate GPA circle were covered by the other circles—then R would equal 1.00. As it is, only 50 percent of the circle is covered, because $R^2 = .50$. The hatched area on this figure designates the independent contribution of undergraduate GPA toward explaining graduate performance. This contribution amounts to 36 percent of Y's variance ($.60^2$). The remaining two independent variables do not contribute as much as one would anticipate by considering their bivariate correlation with graduate GPA (r for GRE-V $= .50$; r for GRE-Q $= .55$). In fact, their

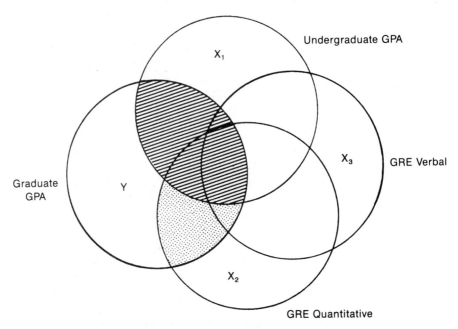

Figure 22-2. *Visual representation of multiple regression example.*

combined additional contribution is only 14 percent (.50 − .36 = .14), designated by the dotted area on the figure. The contribution is small because the two GRE scores have redundant information once the undergraduate grades are taken into consideration. The implication of this principle is that in selecting predictor variables, the researcher should choose independent variables that are strongly correlated with the dependent variable, but weakly correlated with each other.

A related point about multiple correlation is that, as more independent variables are added to the regression equation, the increment to R tends to decrease. It is rare to find many predictor variables that correlate well with a criterion measure while correlating only slightly with one another. Redundancy is difficult to avoid as more and more variables are added to the prediction equation. The inclusion of independent variables beyond the first four or five typically does little to improve the accuracy of prediction.

It should be noted that the dependent variable in multiple regression analysis, as in ANOVA, should as a rule be measured on an interval or ratio scale. The independent variables, on the other hand, can either be continuous interval-level or ratio-level variables or dichotomous variables. A text such as that of Pedhazur (1982) should be consulted for information on how to handle and interpret dichotomous "dummy" variables.

Tests of significance

In multiple correlation, as in simple correlation, researchers wishing to generalize their results must ask: is the calculated R the result of chance fluctuations or is it statistically significant? In order to test the null hypothesis that the population multiple correlation coefficient is equal to zero, we can compute a statistic that can be compared with tabled values for the F distribution.

We stated in Chapter 21 that the general form for calculating an F-ratio is as follows:

$$F = \frac{SS_{between}/df_{between}}{SS_{within}/df_{within}}$$

In the case of multiple regression, the form is similar:

$$F = \frac{SS_{due\ to\ regression}/df_{regression}}{SS_{of\ residuals}/df_{residuals}}$$

In both cases the basic principle is the same: the variance resulting from the independent variables is contrasted with variance attributable to error or chance. To calculate the *F*-statistic for regression, we can use the following alternative formula:

$$F = \frac{R^2/k}{(1 - R^2)/(N - k - 1)}$$

where *k* equals the number of predictor variables and *N* equals the total sample size. In the example used throughout this section, suppose that the r^2 of .50 had been calculated from a sample of 100 graduate students. The value of the *F*-statistic would be:

$$F = \frac{.50/3}{.50/96} = 32.05$$

The tabled value of *F* with 3 and 96 degrees of freedom for a significance level of .01 is approximately 4.0. Thus, the probability that the *R* of .71 was due to chance fluctuations is considerably less than .01.

Another question that researchers often seek to answer is: does adding X_k to the regression equation significantly add to the prediction of Y over that which is possible with X_{k-1}? In other words, how effective is, say, a third predictor in increasing our ability to predict Y after two predictors have already been used? An *F*-statistic can also be computed for answering this question.

Let us remember each independent variable in the example at hand, in order according to its correlation with Y: X_1 = GPA-undergraduate; X_2 = GRE-Q; and X_3 = GRE-V. We can then symbolize various correlation coeffi-

cients as follows: $R_{y \cdot 1}$ = the correlation of Y with undergraduate GPA; $R_{y \cdot 12}$ = the correlation of Y with GPA-U *and* GRE-Q and $R_{y \cdot 123}$ = the correlation of Y with all 3 predictors. The values of these *R*s are as follows.

$$\begin{array}{ll} R_{y \cdot 1} = .60 & R^2_{y \cdot 1} = .36 \\ R_{y \cdot 12} = .71 & R^2_{y \cdot 12} = .50 \\ R_{y \cdot 123} = .71 & R^2_{y \cdot 123} = .50 \end{array}$$

These figures show at a glance that the verbal scores of the Graduate Record Exam made no independent contribution to the correlation coefficient. The value of $R_{y \cdot 12}$ is identical to the value of $R_{y \cdot 123}$. Figure 22-2 illustrates this point: if the circle for GRE-V were completely removed, the area of the Y circle covered by X_1 and X_2 would remain the same.

We cannot tell at a glance, however, whether adding X_2 to X_1 *significantly* increases the prediction of Y. What we want to know, in effect, is whether or not X_2 would be likely to improve predictions in a new sample, or did the added predictive power in this particular sample result from chance? The general formula for the *F*-statistic for testing the significance of variables added to the regression equation is:

$$F = \frac{(R^2_{y \cdot 12 \ldots k_1} - R^2_{y \cdot 12 \ldots k_2})/(k_1 - k_2)}{(1 - R^2_{y \cdot 12 \ldots k_1})/(N - k_1 - 1)}$$

where $R^2_{y \cdot 12 \ldots k_1}$ is the squared multiple correlation coefficient for Y correlated with k_1 predictor variables (the larger number of predictors), $R^2_{y \cdot 12 \ldots k_2}$ is the squared *R* for Y correlated with k_2 predictor variables, and k_2 is the smaller of the two sets of predictors.

In the present example, the calculated *F-statistic* for testing whether the addition of GRE-Q scores results in significant improvement of prediction over GPA-U alone would be:

$$F = \frac{(.50 - .36)/1}{.50/97} = 27.16$$

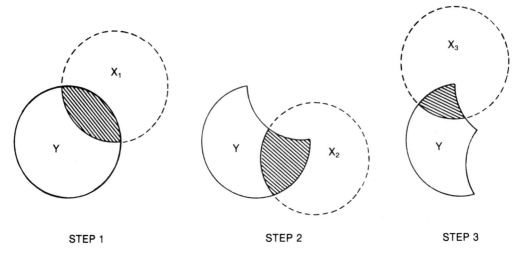

STEP 1   STEP 2   STEP 3

Figure 22-3.   Visual representation of stepwise multiple regression analysis.

Consulting Table B-2 in the Appendix, we find that with $df = 1$ and 97 and a significance level of .01, the critical value is approximately 6.90. Therefore, the addition of GRE-Q to the regression equation significantly improved the accuracy of predictions of graduate grade point averages.

Stepwise multiple regression

If the researcher had ten independent variables available for use in a regression equation, the process of testing all possible combinations to determine which set of variables was significant, while at the same time yielding the highest R^2, would be exceedingly time-consuming. Stepwise multiple regression is a method by which all potential predictors can be considered and through which the combination of variables providing the most predictive power can be chosen.

The computational aspects of stepwise multiple regression are too involved to discuss here, but some major features of this procedure can be pointed out. In stepwise multiple regression, predictors are stepped into the regression equation sequentially, in the order that produces the greatest increments to R^2.

The first step involves the selection of the single best predictor of the dependent variable, which is the independent variable with the highest bivariate correlation coefficient with Y. The second variable to enter the regression equation is the one that produces the largest increase to R^2 when used simultaneously with the variable selected in the first step. The procedure continues until no additional predictor can significantly increase the value of R^2.

The basic principles of stepwise multiple regression are illustrated in Figure 22-3. The first variable to enter the regression, X_1, is correlated .45 with Y ($r^2 = .20$). No other predictor variable is correlated more strongly with the dependent variable. The variable X_1 accounts for the portion of the variability of Y represented by the hatched area in the first step of the figure. This hatched area is, in effect, removed from further consideration as far as subsequent predictors are concerned. This portion of Y's variability is "explained" or "accounted for." Therefore, the variable chosen in Step 2 is not necessarily the X variable with the second largest correlation with Y. The selected variable will be the predictor that explains the largest portion of what *remains* of

Y's variability after X_1 has been taken into the account. Variable X_2, in turn, removes a second part of Y, so that the independent variable selected in Step 3 will be the variable that accounts for the most variability in Y after *both* X_1 and X_2 are controlled.

Relative contribution of predictors

Scientists are concerned not only about the prediction of phenomena but about their explanation as well. Predictions can be made in the absence of understanding. For instance, in our graduate school example, we could predict performance moderately well without really understanding how the variables were functioning or what underlying factors were responsible for students' success. For practical applications, it may be sufficient to make accurate predictions, but scientists typically desire to understand the world around them and to make contributions to knowledge.

In multiple regression problems, one aspect of understanding the phenomenon under investigation is the determination of the relative importance of the independent variables. Unfortunately, the problem of determining the relative contributions of various independent variables in predicting a dependent variable is one of the thorniest issues in regression analysis. When the independent variables are correlated, as they usually are, there is really no ideal way to untangle the effects of the variables in the equation.

It might appear that a solution could be found by comparing the contributions of the independent variables to R^2. In our graduate school example, undergraduate grades accounted for 36 percent of Y's variance, and GRE-Q explained an additional 14 percent of the variance. Should we conclude that undergraduate grades are about two and one-half times as important as GRE scores in explaining graduate school grades? This conclusion would be inaccurate because the order of entry of variables in a regression equation affects their apparent contribution. If these two predictor variables were entered in reverse order, with GRE-Q first, the R^2 would remain unchanged at .50; but GRE-Q's share would then be $.30(.55^2)$ and the undergraduate GPA's contribution would be $.20(.50 - .30)$. This circumstance is due to the fact that whatever variance the independent variables share in common is attributed to the first variable entered in the regression analysis.

Another approach to assessing the relative importance of the predictors is to compare the regression coefficients. Earlier the regression equation was given as:

$$Y' = a + b_1X_1 + b_2X_2 + \ldots b_kX_k$$

where b_1 to b_k are the regression coefficients. These *b* values are not directly comparable because they are in the units of raw scores, which differ from one X to another. X_1 might be in inches, X_2 in dollars, and so forth. The use of *standard scores* eliminates this problem by transforming all variables to scores with a mean of zero and a standard deviation of one. The formula that accomplishes this standardization* is:

$$z_X = \frac{X - \overline{X}}{SD_x}$$

In standard score form, the regression equation is:

$$z_{Y'} = \beta_1 z_{x1} + \beta_2 z_{x2} + \ldots \beta_k z_{xk}$$

where $z_{Y'}$, is the predicted value of the standard score for Y, β_1 to β_k are the standardized regression weights for the *k* independent variables, and z_{x1} to z_{xk} are the standard scores for the *k* predictors.

With all of the βs (sometimes known as *Beta weights*) in the same measurement units, is it possible that their relative size could shed

---

* For a complete discussion of standard scores, an elementary statistical text should be consulted.

light on how much weight or importance to attach to the predictor variables? Many researchers have interpreted Beta weights in this fashion, but there are problems in doing so. These regression coefficients will be the same no matter what the order of entry of the variables. The difficulty, however, is that regression weights are highly unstable. The values of Beta tend to fluctuate considerably from sample to sample. Moreover, when a new variable is added to or subtracted from the regression equation, the Beta weights change. Since there is nothing absolute about the values of the regression coefficients, it is difficult to attach much theoretical importance to them.

Another method of disentangling relationships is path analysis. This procedure is a very important tool in the testing of theoretical expectations about relationships. Path analysis is described later in this chapter.

□
Analysis of covariance

A significant portion of this chapter has been devoted to multiple regression analysis both because it is one of the most widely used multivariate techniques and because an understanding of it should facilitate comprehension of other related multivariate statistics. Analysis of covariance is a good example of a related procedure: it is a combination of analysis of variance and regression.

Analysis of covariance (ANCOVA) is used as a means of providing statistical control for one or more extraneous variables. This approach is especially appropriate in certain types of research situations. For example, when random assignment to treatment groups is not feasible, a quasi-experimental design is often adopted. The initial equivalency of the comparison groups in such studies is always questionable; therefore, the researcher must consider whether the obtained results were influenced by preexisting differences in the comparison groups. When experimental control such as the ability to randomize is lacking, ANCOVA offers the possibility of post hoc statistical control. Even in true experiments, analysis of covariance can play a role in permitting a more precise estimate of group differences. When randomization procedures are used, there are typically slight differences between groups. Analysis of covariance can adjust for initial differences so that the final analysis will reflect more precisely the effect of an experimental intervention.

In both of these situations, the researcher is concerned with the possibility that the comparison groups differ in some respect at the beginning of the study. That is, the groups might differ with regard to an attribute or attributes that could affect the dependent variables and, hence, the outcome of the study. In order to use analysis of covariance, a researcher must anticipate what those attributes are and must measure them at the outset of the study. For instance, suppose a researcher wanted to test the effectiveness of biofeedback therapy on patients' anxiety. An experimental group in one hospital is exposed to the treatment, while a comparison group of patients in another is not. If the researcher wanted to be sure of the initial equivalance of the two groups, the anxiety levels of all subjects could be measured both prior to and after the intervention. The initial anxiety score could be statistically controlled through ANCOVA. In such a situation, the posttest anxiety score is the dependent variable, experimental/comparison group status is the independent variable, and the pretest anxiety score is referred to as the *covariate*. Covariates can either be continuous variables (e.g., anxiety test scores) or dichotomous variables (male/female). However, the independent variables are categorical, that is, nominal-level variables.

The covariate or covariates should be selected with care. The variables chosen should be ones that the researcher strongly suspects

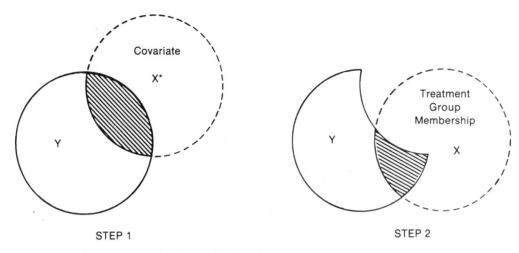

Figure 22-4. Visual representation of analysis of covariance.

are correlated with the dependent variable. A pretest measure is often selected as the controlled variable. A pretest is simply a measure of the same variable as the criterion variable, taken before a treatment is instituted. When pretests are not feasible, other related attributes can be controlled. For instance, if we were comparing the licensure exam scores for nursing students who had or had not attended schools using an integrated curriculum, there would be no possibility of a pretest, but other tests of academic aptitude or intelligence such as scores on the Scholastic Aptitude Test could be used to control for initial differences in ability.

Analysis of covariance tests the significance of differences between group means after first adjusting the scores on the dependent variable to eliminate the effects of the covariate. The adjustment of scores utilizes regression procedures. In essence, the first step in ANCOVA is the same as the first step in a stepwise multiple regression analysis. The variability in the dependent measure that can be explained by the covariate is removed from further consideration. Analysis of variance is performed on what remains of Y's variability to see whether, once

the covariate is controlled, significant differences between the groups remain. Figure 22-4 illustrates this two-step design.

A concrete example may help to further explore aspects of the analysis of covariance procedure. Suppose that we wanted to compute the effectiveness of three different types of diets on overweight individuals. Although the sample of 30 subjects is randomly assigned to one of the three treatment groups, an analysis of covariance, using pretreatment weights, permits a more sensitive analysis of weight change than a simple ANOVA. Some hypothetical data for such a study are displayed in Table 22-3.

Two aspects of the weight scores in this table are immediately discernible. First, despite random assignment to the treatment groups, the initial group means are different. Subjects assigned to Diet B differ from those assigned to Diet C by an average of ten pounds (175 versus 185 pounds). This difference is not significant* but rather reflects chance sampling fluctuations. Second, the posttreat-

---

* Calculations demonstrating nonsignificance are not shown. The calculated F = .45. With 2 and 27 *df,* p > .05.

Table 22-3
Analysis of covariance example

Diet A (X_A)		Diet B (X_B)		Diet C (X_C)	
X_A^*	Y_A	X_B^*	Y_B	X_C^*	Y_C
195	185	205	200	175	160
180	170	150	140	210	165
160	150	145	135	150	130
215	200	210	190	185	170
155	145	185	185	205	180
205	195	160	150	190	165
175	165	190	175	160	135
180	170	165	150	165	140
140	135	180	165	180	160
195	185	160	160	230	195
1800	1700	1750	1650	1850	1600
$\overline{X}_A = 180$	$\overline{Y}_A = 170$	$\overline{X}_B = 175$	$\overline{Y}_B = 165$	$\overline{X}_C = 185$	$\overline{Y}_C = 160$

X = independent variable (diet); X^* = covariate (pretreatment weight); Y = dependent measure (post-treatment weight)

ment means are similarly different by a maximum of only ten pounds. It can be noted, however, that the mean number of pounds *lost* ranged from ten pounds for Diets A and B to 25 pounds for Diet C.

An ordinary analysis of variance for group differences in posttreatment means results in a nonsignificant F value. The ANOVA summary table is presented in part A of Table 22-4. Based on the analysis of variance results, we would conclude that all three diets were equally effective in influencing weight loss.

The second part of Table 22-4 presents the summary table for the analysis of covariance. The first step of the analysis breaks the total variability of the posttreatments weights into two components: (1) that which can be accounted for by the covariate, which in this case is the pretreatment weights; and (2) residual variability. As the table shows, the covariate

Table 22-4
Comparison of ANOVA and ANCOVA results

	Source of Variation	Sum of Squares	df	Mean Square	F	p
A. Summary Table for ANOVA						
	Between groups	500.0	2	250.0	55	>.05
	Within groups	12300.0	27	455.6		
	Total	12800.0	29			
B. Summary Table for ANCOVA						
Step 1	Covariate	10563.1	1	10563.1	132.23	<.01
	Residual	2236.9	28	79.9		
	Total	12800.0	29			
Step 2	Between groups	1284.8	2	642.4	17.54	<.01
	Within groups	952.1	26	36.6		
	Total	2236.9	28			

accounted for a significant amount of the variance, which is not surprising in light of the strong relationship between the pretreatment and posttreatment weights ($r = .91$). In the second phase of the analysis, the residual variance is broken down to reflect the between-group and within-group contributions. With 2 and 26 degrees of freedom, the F of 17.54 is significant beyond the .01 level. The conclusion is that, after controlling for the initial weight of the subjects, there is a significant difference in weight loss resulting from exposure to different diets.

The fictitious example presented here was deliberately contrived so that a result of "no difference" could be altered by the addition of a covariate to yield a significant difference. Most actual results are less dramatic than this example might suggest. Nonetheless, it is true that if the researcher can select meaningful covariates, a more sensitive statistical test will always be made than if an ordinary ANOVA is performed. The increase in sensitivity results from the fact that the covariate reduces the error term (the within-group's variability), against which treatment effects are compared. In Part A of Table 22-4, it can be seen that the within-group's term is extremely large, thereby masking the contribution made by the experimental treatments.

Theoretically, it is possible to use any number of covariates. It is probably unwise to use more than five or six in practice, however. For one thing, the inclusion of more than five or six covariates is probably unnecessary because of the typically high degree of redundancy beyond the first few variables. Moreover, it may be to the researcher's disadvantage to add covariates that do not explain a statistically significant portion of the variability of a dependent variable. Each covariate "uses up" a degree of freedom, leaving the balance for the within-group's term. Fewer degrees of freedom means that a higher computed F is required for significance. For instance, with 2

and 26 df, an F of 5.53 is required for significance at the .01 level, but with 2 and 23 df (i.e., adding three covariates), an F of 5.66 is needed.

In sum, the analysis of covariance procedure is an extremely powerful and useful analytic technique for controlling extraneous or confounding influences on dependent measures. Strictly speaking, analysis of covariance should not be used with intact groups because one of the underlying assumptions of ANCOVA is randomization. However, this assumption is frequently violated because no other alternative analysis works as effectively. Random assignment should always be done when possible but, in many situations in which randomization is not feasible, analysis of covariance could make an important contribution to the internal validity of a study.

Multiple classification analysis

As shown in Panel B of Table 22-4, an ANCOVA table provides information relating to significance testing. The table indicates that at least one of the three groups had a posttreatment weight that is significantly different from the overall grand mean, after adjusting for pretreatment weights. Sometimes it is extremely useful to examine *adjusted means*—that is, mean values on the dependent variable by group, after adjusting for covariates. It is possible to compute such adjusted means from information provided from regression analyses, as described in Pedhazur (1982). When several covariates are used to statistically control extraneous variables, however, manual computations become laborious.

Multiple classification analysis (MCA) is a versatile variant of multiple regression that will result in information about a dependent variable after adjustment for covariates, on one or more independent variables. MCA is versatile because it allows for (a) dichotomous or

Table 22-5
Example of information from multiple classification analysis

Dependent variables	Postintervention diastolic blood pressure
Independent variables	Race (white/nonwhite)
	Age group (21–25; 26–30)
Covariates	Preintervention diastolic blood pressure
	Marital status (married/not married)
	Number of prior pregnancies
	Number of years of schooling

Grand Mean = 80

Variable/Category		Unadjusted	Adjusted for Independents and Covariates
Race:	White	−10	−2
	Nonwhite	+ 5	+3
Age:	21–25	− 5	−4
	26–30	+10	+8
Multiple R			.866
Multiple R^2			.750

continuous covariates, (b) correlated independent variables and/or covariates; and (c) nonlinear relationships between dependent and predictor variables (Andrews et al., 1973). In MCA, like ANCOVA, the independent variables are nominal-level. MCA can be performed on some standard statistical programs, such as SPSS[x] (see next chapter).

Let us take as an example a researcher who wanted to examine whether there were differences by age group and race among hypertensive pregnant women who had participated in an educational program that encouraged ongoing self-monitoring of blood pressure during the pregnancy. The researcher collected information on preintervention blood pressure readings, as well as information on a number of background variables, such as number of prior pregnancies, number of years of schooling, and marital status. All four variables could be used as the covariates in a multiple classification analysis.

Table 22-5 presents some hypothetical results. Overall, the mean posttreatment diastolic blood pressure (DBP) of the two groups was 80 (grand mean). By adding or subtracting deviations from the grand mean we can deter-

mine group differences. The first column shows unadjusted group deviations, that is, the raw posttreatment group means. Thus, without any covariate adjustments, white women had a mean DBP of 70 (80 − 10) and nonwhite women had a mean of 85 (80 + 5). However, some of the posttreatment differences between these two groups might reflect initial nonequivalences, rather than a differential benefit of the intervention. The second column indicates that, after adjusting for four covariates *and* age, the white and nonwhite women had more similar postintervention DBP readings: 78 for whites and 83 for blacks. ANCOVA would indicate whether this difference is significant. (In the SPSS[x] program, ANCOVA and MCA can be performed simultaneously). The R^2 at the bottom of the table indicates the proportion of variance in posttreatment DBP accounted for by all independent variables and covariates.

MCA provides a very useful method of displaying the results of complex analyses, especially to audiences that might be unfamiliar with sophisticated analytic techniques. Table 22-6 illustrates how the results from Table 22-5 could be presented in a report of research findings, after incorporating information on statistical testing from an ANCOVA. Tables such as this are generally easier to read and more meaningful than the numbers produced in an ANCOVA, such as shown in Table 22-4.

□
Factor analysis

Factor analysis is a somewhat controversial multivariate procedure because it involves a higher degree of subjectivity than one ordinarily finds in a statistical technique. It is, nevertheless, a highly powerful and widely applied procedure and, therefore, merits attention. Factor analysis is related to multiple regression analysis in that both analyses develop equations that are linear combinations of the variables. The two procedures have little apparent resemblance, however, because factor analysis does not deal with relationships between variables that the researcher classifies as dependent and independent variables.

The major purpose of factor analysis is to reduce a large set of variables into a smaller, more manageable set of measures. Factor analysis disentangles complex interrelationships among variables and identifies which variables "go together" as unified concepts. The underlying dimensions thus identified are called *factors*. As an example, consider a researcher who has prepared 100 Likert-type items aimed at measuring women's attitudes toward menopause. Suppose that the research goals was to compare the attitudes of women in different religious, racial, and ethnic groups. If the researcher does not combine some of the items to form a scale, it would be necessary to calculate 300 chi-square statistics. The formation of a scale is preferable, but it involves adding together the scores from several individual items. The problem is, which items are to be combined? Would it be meaningful to combine all 100 items? Probably not, because the 100 questions are not all asking

Table 22-6
Example of table displaying MCA results

Adjusted Group Means* for Posttreatment Diastolic Blood Pressure		
Group	Adjusted Mean	P
White women	78.0	NS
Nonwhite women	83.0	
Younger women (21–25)	76.0	p < .05
Older women (26–30)	88.0	

* The means presented in this table have been adjusted through multiple classification analysis for subjects' pretreatment diastolic blood pressure, parity, education, and marital status.

exactly the same thing. There are various aspects, or various "themes" to a woman's attitude toward menopause. One aspect may relate to the problem of aging, while another aspect is concerned with a loss of the ability to reproduce. Other questions may touch upon the general issue of sexuality, and yet others may concern the release from monthly pain or bother. There are, in short, multiple dimensions to the issue of attitudes toward menopause, and these dimensions should serve as the basis for scale construction. The identification of these dimensions can be made *a priori* by the researcher, but the difficulty is that different researchers may read different concepts into the items. Factor analysis offers an empirical method of elucidating the underlying dimensionality of a large number of measures.

A factor, mathematically, is a linear combination of the variables in a data matrix. A data matrix contains the scores of N persons on k different measures. For instance, a factor might be defined by the following equation:

$$F = b_1X_1 + b_2X_2 + b_3X_3 + \ldots b_kX_k$$

where F is a factor score, X_1 to X_k are original variables from the matrix and b_1 to b_k are weights. The development of such an equation for a factor permits the reduction of the X_k

Table 22-7
Summary of factor extraction results

Factor	Eigenvalue	Percentage of variance explained	Cumulative percentage of variance explained
1	12.32	29.2	29.2
2	8.57	23.3	52.5
3	6.91	15.6	68.1
4	2.02	8.4	76.5
5	1.09	6.2	82.7
6	.98	5.8	88.5
7	.80	4.5	93.0
8	.62	3.1	96.1
9	.47	2.2	98.3
10	.25	1.7	100.0

scores to one (or perhaps several) factor scores.

Factor extraction

Most factor analyses consist of two separate phases. The first step is to condense the variables in the data matrix into a smaller number of factors. Sometimes this first phase is referred to as the *factor extraction* phase. The factors usually are derived from the intercorrelations among the variables in the correlation matrix. The general goal is to seek clusters of highly interrelated variables within the matrix. There are various methods of performing the first step, each of which uses different criteria for assigning weights to the variables. Probably the most widely used method of factor extraction is called *principal components* (or principal factor or principal axes), but other methods that a researcher may come across are the image, alpha, centroid, maximum likelihood, and canonical techniques.

The result of the first step of the factor analysis is a *factor matrix* (sometimes labeled as the unrotated factor matrix), which contains coefficients or weights for each variable in the original data matrix on each extracted factor. Since unrotated factor matrices are difficult to interpret, we will postpone a detailed discussion of factor matrices until the second factor analysis phase is described. In the principal components method, weights for the first factor are defined such that the average squared weight is a maximum, thereby permitting a maximum amount of variance to be extracted by the first factor. The second factor, or linear combination, is formed in such a way that the highest possible amount of variance is again extracted from what remains after the first factor has been taken into account. The factors thus delineated represent independent sources of variation in the data matrix.

In extracting factors in this fashion, some criterion must be applied to delimit the number of factors or underlying dimensions. Factoring should continue until there is no further meaningful variance left. There are several criteria available from which the researcher can choose to specify when factoring should cease. It is partly the availability of so many different criteria or justifications for halting factor extraction that makes factor analysis a semisubjective process. Several of the most commonly used criteria can be described by illustrating information that is usually output from factor analysis programs. Table 22-7 presents hypothetical values for eigenvalues, percentages of variance accounted for, and cumulative percentages of variance accounted for, for ten factors. *Eigenvalues* are values equal to the sum of the squared weights for each factor. Many researchers establish as their cutoff point for factor extraction eigenvalues less than 1.00. In the example in the table, this would mean that the first five factors or dimensions would meet this criterion. Another cutoff rule that is adopted sometimes is a minimum of 5 percent of explained variance, in which case six factors would qualify for inclusion in our present example. Yet another criterion is based upon a principle of discontinuity. According to this procedure, a sharp drop in the percentage of explained variance indicates the appropriate termination point. In Table 22-7, one might argue that there is considerable discontinuity between the third and fourth factors. The general consensus seems to be that it is probably better to extract too many factors than too few.

Factor rotation

The factor matrix produced in the first phase of factor analysis usually is rather difficult to interpret. For this reason a second phase known as *factor rotation* is almost invariably performed on those factors that have met one or more of the criteria for inclusion. The concept of rotation is complex and can perhaps be best explained graphically. Figure 22-5 shows two coordinate systems, marked by axes A1 and A2, and B1 and B2. The primary axes (A1 and A2) represent factors I and II, respectively, as they are defined prior to rotation. The points 1 through 6 represent 6 variables in this two-dimensional space. The weights associated with each variable can be determined in reference to the appropriate axis. For instance, before rotation variable 1 is assigned a weight of .80 on Factor I and .85 on Factor II, while variable 6 has a weight of − .45 on Factor I and .90 on Factor II. The unrotated reference frames are designed to account for a maximum of variance but rarely provide a structure that has conceptual meaning. However, by rotating the

axes in such a way that clusters of variables are distinctly associated with a factor, interpretability is enhanced. In the figure, B1 and B2 represent the rotated factors. The rotation has been performed in such a way that variables 1, 2, and 3 would be assigned large weights on Factor I and small weights on Factor II, while the reverse would be true for variables 4, 5, and 6.

There are two general classes of rotation procedures from which a researcher must choose. Figure 22-5 illustrates *orthogonal rotation,* in which the factors are kept at right angles to one another. Orthogonal rotations maintain the independence of factors. That is, orthogonal factors are uncorrelated with one another. *Oblique rotations,* on the other hand, permit the rotated axes to depart from a 90 degree angle. In our figure, an oblique rotation would have put axis B1 between variables 2 and 3 and axis B2 between variables 5 and 6. This placement of the axes strengthens the clustering of variables around an associated factor. The result is that oblique rotation produces correlated factors. Some researchers insist that orthogonal rotation leads to greater theoretical clarity, while others claim that it is unrealistic. Those advocating oblique rotation point out that if the concepts *are* correlated, then the analysis should be permitted to reflect this fact. In practice, studies have revealed that similar conclusions are often reached by both rotational procedures.

The rotated factor matrix is what the researcher normally works with in interpreting the factor analysis. An example of such a matrix is displayed in Table 22-8 for discussion purposes. To make this discussion less abstract, let us say that the 10 variables listed in this table are the first 10 of the 100 items to measure attitudes toward menopause. The entries under each factor are the weights on that factor, which are actually called factor *loadings.* For orthogonally rotated factors, factor loadings can be readily interpreted. Like correlation coefficients, they range from − 1.00 to

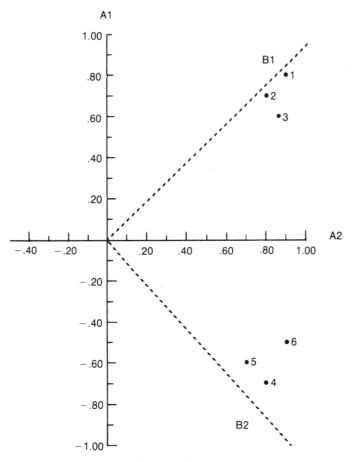

Figure 22-5. *Illustration of factor rotation.*

+ 1.00. In fact, they can be interpreted in much the same way as a correlation coefficient. Factor loadings express the correlations between individual variables and factors (underlying dimensions). In this example, variable 1 is fairly highly correlated with the first factor, .75. Therefore, it is possible to find which variables "belong" to a factor. For Factor I, variables 1, 3, 8, and 10 have fairly sizeable loadings. Normally, a cutoff value of about .40 or .30 is used for such determinations. The researcher is now in a position to interpret the underlying dimensionality of the data. By inspecting items 1, 3, 8, and 10, it is usually pos-

sible to find some common theme that makes the variables go together. Perhaps these four questions have to do with the link between menopause and infertility. And perhaps items 2, 5, and 6 (Factor II) are related to sexuality. The "naming" of factors is essentially a process of identifying theoretical constructs.

Factor scores

In some cases in which the main purpose of factor anlaysis is to delineate the conceptual makeup of a set of measures, the analysis may

Table 22-8
Rotated factor matrix

Variable	Factor I	Factor II	Factor III
1	.75	.15	.23
2	−.02	.61	.18
3	−.59	−.11	.03
4	.05	.08	.48
5	.21	.79	.02
6	−.07	−.52	−.29
7	.08	.19	.80
8	.68	.12	−.01
9	−.04	.08	−.61
10	−.43	−.13	.06

end at this point. Frequently, however, the researcher will want to use the information obtained to develop *factor scores* for use in subsequent analyses. For instance, the factor analysis of the 100 menopause items might demonstrate that there are five principal dimensions or concepts being tapped. By reducing 100 variables to five variables, the analysis of ethnic group differences via some procedure such as analysis of variance will be greatly simplified.

Several types of methods can be used to form factor scores. One procedure is to weight the variables according to their factor loading on each factor. For example, a factor score for the first factor in Table 22-8 could be computed for each subject by the following formula:

$$F_1 = .75X_1 - .02X_2 - .59X_3$$
$$+ .05X_4 + .21X_5 - .07X_6 + .08X_7$$
$$+ .68X_8 - .04X_9 - .43X_{10} \ldots b_{100}X_{100}$$

where all of the X values* are the subject's scores on the 100 items. Some factor analysis computer programs have the capability of directly computing this type of factor score.

A second method of obtaining factor scores is to select certain variables to represent the

* Standardized *(z)* scores are often used in lieu of raw scores in computing factor scores when the means and standard deviations of the variables differ substantially.

factor and to combine them with unit weighting. This composite estimate method would produce a factor score on the first factor of our example in the following fashion:

$$F_1 = X_1 - X_3 + X_8 - X_{10} \pm \ldots$$

The variables here are those with high loadings on Factor I (the "± . . ." indicates the inclusion of any of the other 90 variables with high loadings). This procedure is both computationally and conceptually simpler than the first approach, and both have been found to yield similar results.

To illustrate the composite estimate approach more concretely, let us consider the rotated factor matrix in Table 22-8 and assume that factor scores were to be computed on the basis of this 10-item analysis. Suppose that two respondents had the following scores on these ten items:

Subject 1: 7, 1, 1, 5, 1, 6, 7, 6, 3, 2
Subject 2: 2, 5, 6, 3, 7, 3, 2, 3, 4, 4

Factor I has fairly high loadings on items 1, 3, 8, and 10. Thus, the two subjects' factor scores on Factor 1 would be:

$$7 - 1 + 6 - 2 = 10$$
$$2 - 6 + 3 - 4 = -5$$

The minus signs reflect the negative loadings on items 3 and 10.* The same procedure would be performed for all three factors, yielding the following factor scores:

Subject 1: 10, −3, 9
Subject 2: −5, 9, 1

Factor scores would similarly be computed for

* Researchers forming scale scores with Likert items often reverse the directionality of the scoring on negatively loaded items before forming the factor score, in order to eliminate negative scores. Directionality of an item can be reversed by subtracting the raw score from the sum of 1 + the maximum item value. For example, in a 7-point scale, a score of 2 would be reversed to 6 ((1 + 7) − 2). When such reversals have been done, all raw scores can be *added* in forming factor scores.

all respondents, and these scores could then be used in the subsequent analyses.

☐ Related multivariate techniques

In addition to analysis of covariance, several other multivariate techniques are closely related to least-squares multiple regression analysis. In this section the methods known as discriminant function analysis, canonical correlation, and multivariate analysis of variance will be introduced. The introduction will be brief and computations will be entirely omitted, because these procedures are exceedingly complex. The intent of this brief review is to acquaint the reader with the types of research situations for which these methods are appropriate. Advanced statistical texts such as the ones listed in the references may be consulted for additional information.

Discriminant analysis

In multiple regression, the dependent variable being predicted is normally a measure on either the interval or ratio scale of measurement. The regression equation makes predictions about scores that take on a large range of values. *Discriminant analysis,* by contrast, makes predictions about membership in categories or groups. The groups are identified by the researcher, and the purpose of the analysis is to distinguish the groups from one another on the basis of the independent variables available for prediction purposes. For instance, we may wish to develop a means of predicting membership in or affiliation with such groups as complying versus noncomplying cancer patients; or graduating nursing students versus dropouts; or normal pregnancies versus those terminating in a miscarriage.

Discriminant analysis develops a regression equation—called a *discriminant function*—for a categorical dependent variable, with in-

dependent variables that are either categorical or continuous The researcher begins with data from subjects whose group membership is known. The intent is to develop an equation that can be used to predict membership for new subjects for whom measures of the independent variables only are available. The discriminant function indicates to which group each subject will probably belong.

Discriminant analysis with two classification groups is relatively simple and can be interpreted in much the same fashion as a multiple regression. When there are more than two groups or categories, the calculations and interpretations are more complicated. When the number of groups is three or larger, then the possible number of discriminant functions is either the number of groups minus one or the number of independent variables, whichever is smaller. The first discriminant function is the linear combination of predictors that maximizes the ratio of between-group's variance to within-group's variance. The second function derived is the linear combination that maximizes this ratio, after the effect of the first function is removed. Since the independent variables are assigned different weights on the various functions, it is possible to develop theoretical interpretations based on the knowledge of which predictors are important in discriminating among different groups.

Discriminant analysis shares several features in common with multiple regression analysis, aside from the fact that prediction equations based on a linear combination of independent variables are developed. For one thing, it is possible to use a stepwise approach in entering predictors into the equation. Also, the analysis produces an index designating the proportion of variance in the dependent variable accounted for by the predictor variables. The index is known as Wilks' lambda (λ). Actually, λ indicates the proportion of variance *un*accounted for by predictors, or $\lambda = 1 - R^2$.

In sum, discriminant analysis has potential

for being quite useful to researchers particularly those with practical problems of classification or diagnosis. An excellent and relatively simple guide to this procedure has been prepared by Tatsuoka (1970).

Canonical correlation

Canonical correlation is the most general multivariate technique, of which other procedures are special cases. Canonical correlation analyzes the relationship between two or more independent variables and two or more dependent variables. Conceptually, one can think of this technique as an extension of multiple regression to more than one dependent variable. Mathematically and interpretatively, the gap between multiple regression and canonical correlation is greater than this statement suggests.

Like other techniques described in this chapter, canonical correlation uses the least squares principle to partition and analyze variance. Basically, two linear composites are developed, one of which is associated with the dependent variables, the other of which is for the independent variables. The relationship between the two linear composites is expressed by the canonical correlation coefficient, R_c. As in the case of the coefficient of determination (R^2), R_c^2 indicates the proportion of variance accounted for in the analysis. When there is more than one source or dimension of covariation in the two sets of variables, more than one canonical correlation can be found.

Examples of research utilizing canonical correlation are relatively rare. Perhaps the method is not well known, and it requires a higher degree of mathematical sophistication than is needed for most statistical techniques. Still, when a study involves multiple dependent and independent variables, canonical correlation may be the most suitable way to analyze the data.

Multivariate analysis of variance

Multivariate analysis of variance, sometimes abbreviated MANOVA, is the extension of analysis of variance procedures to more than one dependent variable. This procedure is used primarily to test the significance of differences between the means of two or more dependent variables, considered simultaneously. Like ordinary analysis of variance, MANOVA was developed for use in experimental situations in which at least one independent variable has been manipulated. For instance, if we wanted to examine the effect of two methods of exercise (A_1 and A_2 and two lengths of exercise treatment (B_1 and B_2) on both diastolic and systolic blood pressure (Y_1 and Y_2) then a multivariate analysis of variance would be appropriate. Researchers often analyze such data by performing two separate univariate ANOVAs. Strictly speaking, this practice is not correct. Separate analyses of variance imply that the dependent variables have been obtained independently of one another. In fact, the dependent measures have been obtained from the same subjects and are, therefore, correlated. Multivariate analysis of variance takes the intercorrelations of the dependent variables into account in computing the test statistics.

The analogy might be made that multiple regression is to canonical correlation as analysis of variance is to multivariate analysis of variance. This analogy, while correct, obscures a point that the astute reader has perhaps already suspected, and that is the close affinity between multiple regression and analysis of variance. Pedhazur (1982) has observed that the two procedures are virtually identical. Both techniques are concerned with analyzing the variability in a dependent measure and contrasting the proportion of the variability attributable to one or more independent variables with that attributable to unexplained sources of variation, or "error." Multiple regression and ANOVA use a somewhat different approach and employ different symbols and terminology, but both analyses boil down to a final *F*-ratio. By tradition, experimental data are typically analyzed by ANOVA while ex post facto data are analyzed by regression procedures. Nevertheless, it should be realized that any data for which ANOVA is appropriate could also be analyzed by multiple regression, although the reverse is not true. In many cases multiple regression is preferable because it can be used with a broader range of data and because it provides more information, such as a prediction equation and an index of association, *R*.

□
Path analysis

Path analysis is a regression-based method for studying patterns of causation among a set of variables in ex post facto studies. Path analysis usually begins with a theory or causal model that dictates the type of data to be collected. It is not a method for discovering causes; rather it is a method applied to a prespecified model formulated on the basis of prior knowledge and theory.

Path analysis is a complex topic to which entire books have been devoted. Therefore, we will briefly describe some of the key concepts without discussing actual analytic procedures. Path analytic reports often use a *path diagram* to display their results and we will use such a diagram (Figure 22-6) to illustrate important concepts. This model postulates that patients' length of hospitalization (V4) is the result of their capacity for self-care (V3); this, in turn, is affected by nursing actions (V1) and the severity of their illness (V2).

In path analysis, a distinction is often made between exogenous and endogenous variables. An *exogenous variable* is a variable whose determinants lie outside the model. In Figure 22-6, nursing actions (V1) and illness

severity (V2) are exogenous; no attempt is made in the model to elucidate what causes different nursing actions or different degrees of illness. An *endogenous variable,* by contrast, is one whose variation is determined by other variables in the model. In our example, self-care capacity (V3) and length of hospitalization (V4) are endogenous.

In path analysis, causal linkages are illustrated by arrows, drawn from the presumed causes to the presumed effects. In our illustration, severity of illness is hypothesized to affect length of hospitalization both directly (path p42) and indirectly through the *mediating variable* self-care capacity (paths p32 and p43). Correlated exogenous variables are indicated by curved lines, as shown by the curved line between nursing actions and illness severity.

Ideally, the model would totally explain the outcome of interest, in this case, the length of hospitalization. In practice, this almost never happens, because causal theories are rarely comprehensive when dealing with human phenomena. There are usually other determinants, which are generally referred to as *residual variables*. In Figure 22-6, there are two boxes labeled "e," which denote a composite of all determinants of self-care capacity and hospitalization stay that are not in the model. The residuals summarize our "ignorance" of the causes of endogenous variables; if we can identify and measure additional causative forces, they should be in the model.

It should be noted that Figure 22-6 represents what is referred to as a *recursive model*. This means that the causal flow is unidirectional and without feedback loops. In other words, it is assumed that variable 2 is a cause of variable 3, and that variable 3 is *not* a cause of variable 2.

In Figure 22-6, causal paths are indicated by symbols denoting that a given variable (e.g., V3) is caused by another (e.g., V2), yielding a path labeled p32. In research reports, the path

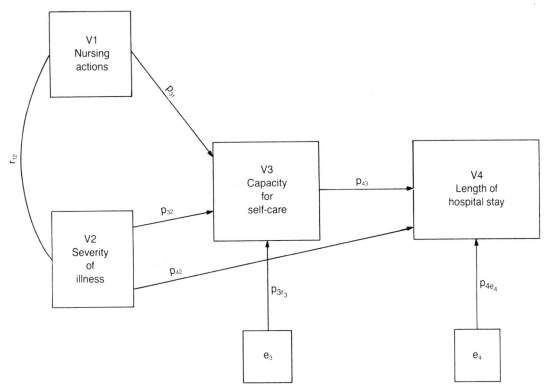

Figure 22-6. *A path diagram.*

symbols would be replaced by actual numbers developed by applying regression procedures. The numbers shown are called *path coefficients,* which are standardized partial regression slopes. For example, path p32 is equal to $\beta 32.1$ — the Beta weight between variables 2 and 3, holding variable 1 constant. Because path coefficients are in standard form, they indicate the proportion of a standard deviation difference in the caused variable that is directly attributable to a one SD difference in the specified causal variable. Thus, the path coefficients give us some indication of the relative importance of various determinants.

Path analysis involves estimation of the path coefficients through the use of *structual equations.* The structural equations for Figure 22-6 are as follows:

$$z_1 = e_1$$
$$z_2 = e_2$$
$$z_3 = p_{31} z_1 + p_{32} z_2 + e_3; \text{ and}$$
$$z_4 = p_{43} z_3 + p_{42} z_2 \quad e_4$$

These equations indicate that z_1 and z_2 (standard scores for variables 1 and 2) are determined by outside variables; that z_3 depends directly on z_1 and z_2 plus outside variables; and that z_4 depends directly on z_2, z_3, and outside variables. In our example, the structural equations could be solved to yield path coefficients by performing two multiple regressions: (1) by regressing variable 3 on variables 1 and 2; and (2) by regressing variable 4 on variables 2 and 3.

The model presented in Figure 22-6 may or may not be a reasonable construction of the hospitalization process. Path analysis involves a number of procedures for testing causal models and for determining effects. Pedhazur (1982) provides a good overview of path analytic techniques and the advanced student should refer to books such as that by Blalock (1972).

☐
Power analysis

Many published and unpublished nursing studies result in nonsignificant findings — that is, one or more of the researcher's main hypotheses are not supported. While standard statistical texts pay considerable attention to the problem of Type I errors, (wrongly rejecting a *true* null hypothesis), virtually no attention is paid to Type II errors (wrongly accepting a *false* null hypothesis). We suspect that in many nursing studies, Type II errors are being committed. *Power analysis* represents a method for reducing the risk of Type II errors.

As indicated in the previous chapter, the probability of committing a Type I error is established by the investigator as the level of significance, which is often referred to as α. The probability of a Type II error is β. The complement of β $(1 - \beta)$ is the *probability of obtaining a significant result,* and is referred to as the *power* of a statistical test.

In performing a power analysis, there are four components, at least three of which must be known to or estimated by the researcher; power analysis solves for the fourth component. The four major factors are as follows:

- *The significance criterion, α.* Other things being equal, the more stringent this criterion, the lower the power.
- *The sample size, n.* As sample size increases, power increases.
- *The population effect size, γ (gamma).* As discussed below, γ is a measure of how

"wrong" the null hypothesis is, that is, how strong the effect of the independent variable is on the dependent variable in the population. All else equal, as γ increases, so does power increase.
- *Power, or $1 - \beta$.* This is the probability of rejecting the null hypothesis.

Researchers typically use power analysis for two purposes: (1) to solve for the sample size needed in a study to increase the likelihood of demonstrating significant results; and (2) to determine the power of a statistical test. In this section, which is only a brief summary of power analysis, we will focus on the first of these purposes.

In order to solve for a needed sample size, the researcher must specify α, γ, and $1 - \beta$, as indicated above. Usually, the researcher establishes α, the risk of a Type I error, as (at most) .05; in some cases a lower (stricter) criterion such as .01 may be required. Just as .05 has been adopted as the standard for the α criterion, a conventional standard for $1 - \beta$ is .80. This means that the risk of committing a Type II error is .20. While this risk may seem rather high, a stricter criterion would require sample sizes much larger than most nurse researchers could manage. The majority of nursing studies being conducted probably have a power of well below .50, thus making it very difficult to avoid a Type II error.

With α and $1 - \beta$ selected, the only other piece of information needed to solve for n is γ, the population effect size.

The value of γ is arrived at differently depending on the nature of the data and the statistical test to be performed. We will provide formulas for two situations only: testing the difference between two group means (i.e., situations requiring a *t*-test); and testing the significance of a linear relationship (i.e., situations requiring a Pearson *r*). Cohen (1977) discusses power analysis in the context of many other situations.

Sample size estimates for test of difference between two independent means

Suppose you were interested in testing the hypothesis that cranberry juice reduces the urinary pH of diet-controlled patients. In your study, you plan to randomly assign some subjects to a control condition (no cranberry juice) and others to an experimental condition in which they would be given 200 ml of cranberry juice with each meal for five days. How large a sample is needed for this study, given an α of .05 and power equal to .80?

To answer this question, we must first estimate γ. In a two-group situation in which the difference of means is of interest, the formula for γ is:

$$\gamma = \frac{\mu^1 - \mu^2}{\sigma}$$

That is, γ is the difference between the population means, divided by the population standard deviation. But how can the researcher ever know this information? If you knew, for example, the mean urinary pH of all subjects who had or had not ingested cranberry juice, there would not be much point to the study. Nevertheless, the researcher must *estimate* the population means and standard deviation, based on whatever information is available. This could come from a pilot study or from findings from similar studies. In our present example, suppose you found an earlier ex post facto study that compared the urinary pH of subjects who had or had not ingested cranberry juice in the previous 24 hours. The previous and current studies are quite different. In the ex post facto study, the diets are uncontrolled; there may be selection biases in who drinks or does not drink cranberry juice; the length of ingestion is only one day; and so on. However, this study may be your only starting point. Suppose the results of the earlier study were as follows:

$$\overline{X}_1 \text{ (no cranberry juice)} = 5.70$$
$$\overline{X}_2 \text{ (cranberry juice)} \quad = 5.50$$
$$\sigma \text{ (pooled SD)} \qquad\quad = .50$$

Thus, the value of γ would be .40:

$$\gamma = \frac{5.70 - 5.50}{.50} = .40$$

Table 22-9 presents sample size requirements for various effect sizes and powers, and two values of α, in a two-group mean-difference situation. In the upper half of the table for $\alpha = .05$, we find that the *n* needed for an effect size of .40 and a power of .80 is 98 subjects per group. That is, assuming that the earlier study provided roughly accurate estimates of population values, the number of subjects required in the new study would be 196; 98 would be assigned to the control group (no cranberry juice) and 98 would be assigned to the experimental group. A sample size much smaller than 200 would have a good chance of leading to a Type II error.

Usually, a researcher will be able to find more than one piece of research from which the effect size can be estimated. In such a case, the estimate should be based on the study that yields the most stable and reliable results and/or whose design most closely approximates that of the new study. In some cases in which equally good (or equally bad) prior research is available, it may be necessary to combine information from multiple studies to develop an effect size estimate.

What can the researcher do if there is *no* prior research? Although this is rarely the case, the researcher can, as a last resort, estimate on the basis of readings or experience whether the expected effect is small, moderate, or large. By convention, the value of γ in a two-group test of mean differences is estimated at .20 for "small" effects, .50 for "medium" effects, and .80 for "large" effects. With an α value of .05 and power of .80, the *total* sample size (number of subjects in both groups) for

Table 22-9
Sample size* estimates for test of difference of two independent means

Power	Estimated Effect†									
	.10	.15	.20	.25	.30	.40	.50	.60	.70	.80
Part A: $\alpha = .05$										
.60	977	434	244	156	109	61	39	27	20	15
.70	1230	547	308	197	137	77	49	34	25	19
.80	1568	697	392	251	174	98	63	44	32	25
.90	2100	933	525	336	233	131	84	58	43	33
.95	2592	1152	648	415	288	162	104	72	53	41
.99	3680	1636	920	589	409	230	147	102	75	58
Part B: $\alpha = .01$										
.60	1602	712	400	256	178	100	64	44	33	25
.70	1922	854	481	308	214	120	77	53	39	30
.80	2339	1040	585	374	260	146	94	65	48	37
.90	2957	1324	745	477	331	186	119	83	61	47
.95	3562	1583	890	570	396	223	142	99	73	56
.99	4802	2137	1201	769	534	300	192	133	98	75

* Sample size requirements for *each* group; total sample size would be twice the number shown.
† Estimated effect (γ) is the estimated population group differences, divided by the estimated population SD, or:

$$\gamma = \frac{\mu_1 - \mu_2}{\sigma}$$

studies with expected small, medium, and large effects would be 784, 126, and 60, respectively. It is probably safe to say that the majority of nursing studies cannot expect effect sizes in excess of .50, and those in the range of .20 to .40 are probably most common. Cohen (1977) has noted that in new areas of research inquiry, effect sizes are likely to be small. A medium effect should be estimated only when the effect is so substantial that it can be detected by the naked eye (i.e., without formal research procedures).

Sample size estimates for bivariate correlation tests

Suppose you wanted to study the effect of social support on primaparas' acceptance of the motherhood role. You plan to administer two scales to women who have had a normal vagi-

nal delivery of full-term infants. One scale measures the amount of social support available to the mother in her family and community; the other scale measures the woman's positive and negative reactions to her new role. The hypothesis is that women who have more social support available to them will be more accepting of the role transition to motherhood. How many women should be included in the study, given an α of .05 and power of .80?

As in the case above, we need an estimate of γ. In this situation, we have two measures on an interval scale, and the relationship between them would be tested using a Pearson r. The estimated value of γ here is actually ρ, that is, the expected population correlation coefficient.

Suppose you found an earlier study that correlated a simple measure of social support

Table 22-10
Sample size estimates for bivariate correlation

Power	Estimated Effect*									
	.10	.15	.20	.25	.30	.40	.50	.60	.70	.80
Part A: $\alpha = .05$										
.60	489	218	123	79	55	32	21	15	11	9
.70	616	274	155	99	69	39	26	18	14	11
.80	785	349	197	126	88	50	32	23	17	13
.90	1050	468	263	169	118	67	43	30	22	17
.95	1297	577	325	208	145	82	53	37	27	21
.99	1841	819	461	296	205	116	75	52	39	30
Part B: $\alpha = .01$										
.60	802	357	201	129	90	51	33	23	17	14
.70	962	428	241	155	108	61	39	28	21	16
.80	1171	521	293	188	131	74	48	33	25	19
.90	1491	663	373	239	167	94	61	42	31	24
.95	1782	792	446	286	199	112	72	50	37	28
.99	2402	1068	601	385	267	151	97	67	50	39

* For bivariate correlations, the estimated effect (γ) is the estimated population correlation (ρ).

(the number of persons subjects felt they could "count on" in times of stress) with an observational measure of maternal warmth. Neither of these measures perfectly captures the variables in the new study, but they are conceptually close and, if no better information were available, they would provide a useful approximation. Suppose the completed study found $r = .18$, which we will use as our estimate of ρ, and hence of γ. Table 22-10 shows sample size requirements for various powers and effect sizes in situations in which Pearson's r is used. With an α of .05 and power of .80, the sample size needed in this study would lie between 197 (for an effect size of .20) and 349 (for an effect size of .15) Extrapolating for an effect size of .18, you would need a sample of about 250 subjects to achieve a power of .80 with an alpha of .05. With a sample this size, you would wrongly reject the null hypothesis only five times out of 100 and wrongly retain the null hypothesis 20 times out of a hundred. In order to increase the power to .95 (wrongly retaining the null hypothesis only five times out of 100), you would need a sample of about 400 women.

When no prior estimates of effect size are available, the conventional values of small, medium, and large effect sizes in a bivariate correlation situation are .10, .30, and .50, respectively. It is wise to be fairly conservative in estimating effect size in the absence of evidence supporting a moderate or strong effect.

□
Research example

Muhlenkamp and her colleagues (1985) investigated nursing clinic clients' health beliefs, health values, and background characteristics in relation to health promotion activities. The subjects in this study were 175 clients of a nursing clinic who were administered instruments that measured health locus of control, health values, health-related elements of their personal lifestyle, and demographic variables such as marital status, religion, sex, education, income, and age.

The lifestyle variables were measured with a 24-item Likert scale developed by the investigators—the Personal Lifestyle Questionnaire, or PLQ. The Likert statements were designed to reflect health-related preferences and activities in six areas: relaxation, substance use, health promotion, safety, nutrition, and exercise. Responses to the PLQ were factor analyzed to determine its dimensionality. The factor analysis confirmed that six separate dimensions were being measured, supporting the calculation of six subscale scores. However, a total PLQ score was computed by adding the scores on all six subscales. The total score reflected the degree to which subjects engaged in an overall health-promoting lifestyle.

The PLQ total score was used as a dependent variable in a multiple regression analysis designed to shed light on factors that could predict healthful lifestyles. Both demographic and attitudinal variables (such as the scores on the locus of control scale) were used as the predictor variables. Using stepwise multiple regression, five variables were found to be significantly related to the PLQ total score: sex, age, education, belief in chance as a determinant of health, and self-rated health status. Education was found to be the best predictor— the better educated the subject, the higher his or her lifestyle score. Overall, the five predictor variables accounted for only 16 percent of the variance in PLQ scores, suggesting that there were numerous unmeasured factors that led subjects to engage (or not engage) in a health-promoting lifestyle.

☐
Summary

The *multivariate* statistical procedures explored in this chapter are used to untangle complex relationships among three or more variables. One of the most versatile multivariate procedures is *multiple correlation/regression,* which is a statistical method for understanding the effects of two or more independent variables on a dependent variable. Regression analysis provides a mechanism for researchers to make predictions about phenomena. A simple regression equation is a formula for making predictions about the numerical values of one variable based on the values of a second variable. The researcher can often improve the precision of the predictions by including more than one predictor (independent) variable in the regression equation. The multiple correlation coefficients is symbolized by R. The multiple correlation coefficient, when squared (R^2), indicates the proportion of the variance of the dependent variable that is "explained" or "accounted for" by the combined influences of the independent variables. R^2 is sometimes referred to as the *coefficient of determination.* The versatility of multiple regression analysis is demonstrated by its various related analyses and special options. For example, in *stepwise multiple regression,* the researcher can select from a pool of potential predictor variables those variables that in combination have the greatest predictive power.

Analysis of covariance (ANCOVA) is a procedure that permits the researcher to control extraneous or confounding influences on dependent variables. ANCOVA combines the principles of multiple regression and analysis of variance. The effect of one or more variable (called the *covariate*) is statistically controlled or removed before testing for group differences via traditional ANOVA procedures. ANCOVA is often used in ex post facto or quasi-experimental designs to control for potential pretreatment differences but can also be used in experimental designs to provide more precise estimates of experimental effects.

Multiple classification analysis (MCA) is a variant of regression that produces information about a dependent variable after adjusting for covariates. The information is usually provided in the form of values for the grand mean of the dependent variable and adjusted deviations from it.

Factor analysis is used to reduce a large set of variables into a smaller set of underlying dimensions, called *factors.* Mathematically, each factor represents a linear combination of the variables contained in a data matrix. The first phase of factor analysis, called *factor extraction,* identifies clusters of variables with a high degree of communality, or redundancy, and condenses the larger set of variables into a smaller number of factors. The second phase of factor analysis involves *factor rotation,* which enhances the interpretability of the factors by aligning variables more distinctly with a particular factor. The *factor loadings* shown in a rotated factor matrix can then be examined to identify and "name" the underlying dimensionality of the original set of variables and to compute *factor scores.*

Discriminant analysis is essentially a multiple regression analysis in which the dependent variable is categorical (i.e., nominal level of measurement). This procedure is useful for making predictions about memberships in groups on the basis of two or more predictor variables. *Canonical correlation* is the most general of all the multivariate procedures: it analyzes the relationship between two or more independent *and* two or more dependent variables. *Multivariate analysis of variance* (MANOVA) is the extension of analysis of variance principles to cases in which there is more than one dependent variable. All of the procedures reviewed here are closely related methods that have as a common goal the identification, control, and prediction of variance.

Path analysis is a regression-based procedure for testing causal models. The researcher first prepares a *path diagram* that stipulates hypothesized causal linkages among variables. Using regression procedures applied to a series of *structural equations,* a series of *path coefficients* are developed. These path coefficients represent weights associated with a causal path in standard deviation units. The

simplest form of a causal model is one that is *recursive,* that is, one in which causation is presumed to be unidirectional.

Power analysis refers to techniques for estimating either the likelihood of committing a Type II error or sample size requirements. Power analysis involves four components: a desired significance level (α), power ($1 - \beta$), sample size (n), and an estimated *effect size* (γ). In order to calculate needed sample size, all three other components must be specified by the researcher. The most difficult part is estimating the effect size, but there is usually at least one existing study that can provide rough guidelines for the estimate. The application of power analysis would probably greatly reduce the number of nonsignificant findings reported in the nursing literature.

☐
Study suggestions

1. Suppose that you were investigating job satisfaction among nurses. You have collected information on 12 variables concerning nurse satisfaction. After submitting these variables to factor analysis, you obtain the following information:

Factor	Eigenvalue	Percent of Variance	Cumulative Percentage
1	9.03	28.0	28.0
2	6.39	20.4	48.4
3	4.82	17.1	65.5
4	1.09	6.3	71.8
5	.98	5.8	77.6
6	.93	5.6	83.2
7	.87	4.9	88.1
8	.60	3.5	91.6
9	.52	2.8	94.4
10	.48	2.6	97.0
11	.30	1.8	98.8
12	.26	1.2	100.0

According to these data, how many dimensions underlie job satisfaction? On what did you base this decision?

2. Refer to Figure 22-1. What would the value of Y' be for the following X values: 8, 1, 3, 6?
3. A researcher has examined the relationship between preventive health care attitudes on the one hand and the person's educational level, age, and sex on the other. The multiple correlation coefficient is .62. Explain the meaning of this statistic. How much of the variation in attitudinal scores has been explained by the three predictors?
4. Which multivariate statistical procedure would you recommend using in the following situations:
   a. A researcher wants to test the effectiveness of a nursing intervention for reducing stress levels among surgical patients, using an experimental group of patients from one hospital and a control group from another hospital.
   b. A researcher wants to predict which students are at risk of venereal disease by using background information such as sex, socioeconomic status, religion, grades in sex education course, and attitudes toward sex.
   c. A researcher wants to test the effects of three different diets on blood sugar levels and blood pH.
5. Estimate the required sample sizes for the following situations.
   a. Comparison of two group means: $\alpha = .01$; power = .90; $\gamma = .35$.
   b. Comparison of two group means: $\alpha = .01$; power = .70; $\gamma = .45$.
   c. Correlation of two variables: $\alpha = .01$; power = .85; $\gamma = .27$.

☐
Suggested readings

Methodological references

Anderson, S. *et al.,* (1980). *Statistical methods for comparative studies.* New York: John Wiley and Sons.

Andrews, F.M. *et al.,* (1973). *Multiple classification analysis.* Ann Arbor, MI: University of Michigan Institute for Social Research.

Bennett, S. & Bowers, D. (1978). *An introduction to multivariate techniques for the social and behavioral sciences.* New York: John Wiley and Sons.

Blalock, H.M., Jr. (1972). *Causal inferences in nonexperimental research.* New York: W.W. Norton.

Cohen, J. & Cohen, P. (1983). *Applied multiple regression: Correlation analysis for behavioral sciences* (2nd ed.). New York: Halsted Press.

Cohen, J. (1977). *Statistical power analysis for the behavioral sciences.* New York: Academic Press.

Draper, N. & Smith, H. (1981). *Applied regression analysis* (2nd ed.). New York: John Wiley and Sons.

Goodwin, L.D. (1984). The use of power estimation in nursing research. *Nursing Research, 33,* 118–120.

Goodwin, L.D. (1984). Increasing efficiency and precision of data analysis: Multivariate vs. univariate statistical techniques. *Nursing Research, 33,* 247–249.

Huitema, B.E. (1980). *The analysis of covariance and its alternatives.* New York: John Wiley and Sons.

Kerlinger, F.N. (1973). *Foundations of behavioral research* (2nd ed.) (Chapters 35, 36, and 37). New York: Holt, Rinehart and Winston.

Kim, J. & Mueller, C. (1978). *Factor analysis: Statistical methods and practical issues.* Beverly Hills: Sage Publications.

Maxwell, A.E. (1978). *Multivariate analysis in behavioral research: For medical and social science students* (2nd ed.). New York: Methuen.

Pedhazur, E.J. (1982). *Multiple regression in behavioral research* (2nd ed.). New York: Holt, Rinehart & Winston.

Rummel, R.J. (1970). *Applied factor analysis.* Evanston, IL: Northwestern University Press.

Tatsuoka, M. (1970). *Discriminant analysis: The study of group differences.* Champaign, IL: Institute for Personality and Ability Testing.

Tatsuoka, M. (1971). *Multivariate analysis: Techniques for educational and psychological research.* New York: John Wiley and Sons.

Verran, J. A. & Ferketich, S.L. (1984). Residual analysis for statistical assumptions of regression equation. *Western Journal of Nursing Research, 6,* 27–40.

Volicer, B. J. (1981). *Advanced statistical methods with nursing applications.* Bedford, MA: Merestat Press.

Weisberg, S. (1985). *Applied linear regression* (2nd ed.). New York: John Wiley and Sons.

Welkowitz, J., Ewen, R. B., & Cohen, J. (1982). *Introductory statistics for the behavioral sciences* (3rd ed.). New York: Academic Press (pp. 216–233).

Substantive references

Alexy, B. (1985). Goal setting and health risk reduction. *Nursing Research, 34,* 283–292 (ANCOVA).

Bowles, C. (1986). Measure of attitude toward menopause using the semantic differential model. *Nursing Research, 35,* 81–85 (Factor analysis, multiple regression).

Greenleaf, N. P. (1983). Labor force participation among registered nurses and women in comparable occupations. *Nursing Research, 32,* 306–322 (Discriminant function analysis; canonical correlation).

Heidt, P. (1981). Effect of therapeutic touch on anxiety level of hospitalized patients. *Nursing Research, 30,* 32–37 (ANCOVA).

Ide, B.A. (1983). Social network support among low-income elderly: A two-factor model? *Western Journal of Nursing Research, 5,* 235–244 (Factor analysis).

Miller, P., Sr. *et al.* (1985). Indicators of medical regimen adherence for myocardial infarction patients. *Nursing Research, 34,* 268–272 (Multiple regression).

Mulhlenkamp, A., Brown A., Sands, D. (1985). Determinants of health promotion activities in nursing clinic clients. *Nursing Research, 34,* 327–332 (Factor analysis; multiple regression).

Munro, B. H. (1983). Job satisfaction among recent graduates of schools of nursing. *Nursing Research, 32,* 350–355 (Factor analysis, multiple regression).

Murphy, S.A. (1984). Stress levels and health status of victims of a natural disaster. *Research in Nursing and Health, 7,* 205–215 (Discriminant function analysis).

Pardue, S.F. (1979). Blocked- and integrated-content baccalaureate nursing programs: A comparative study. *Nursing Research, 28,* 305–311 (MANOVA).

Ruiz, M.C.J. (1981). Open–closed mindedness, intolerance of ambiguity and nursing faculty attitudes toward culturally different patients. *Nursing Research, 30,* 177–181 (Factor analysis).

Ryden, M.B. (1984). Morale and perceived control in institutionalized elderly. *Nursing Research, 33,* 130–136 (Path analysis).

Sime, A.M. & Libera, M. B. (1985). Sensation information, self-instruction and responses to dental surgery. *Research in Nursing and Health, 8,* 41–47 (MANOVA).

Van Os, D. K. (1985). Life stress and cystic fibrosis. *Western Journal of Nursing Research, 1,* 301–315 (Multiple regression).

Young, K. J. (1984). Professional commitment of women in nursing. *Western Journal of Nursing Research, 6,* 11–26 (Path analysis).

Chapter 23
□
Computers and scientific research

High-speed electronic computers have evolved and expanded at a tremendous rate since their development in the 1940s. Few aspects of our society have remained untouched by the impact of computers: bills are sent out, weather is predicted, literature sources are retrieved, classroom schedules are determined, production machines are controlled, medical records are maintained, and diagnoses are made—all with the assistance of computers. With the advent of microcomputers, computers have, indeed, become ubiquitous.

The use of computers in scientific research, as one might suspect, is substantial and inevitably growing. Computers have, in fact, revolutionized research by making possible the kinds of operations that could not conceivably have been attempted with human labor alone. One of the most important applications of the computer in scientific investigations is the analysis of data. While many other important applications have been developed, the discussion here will be geared to the person seeking to analyze information obtained during the course of a research project.

The purpose of this chapter is to introduce the reader to some of the basic principles of computer operations. While computers are electronically complex machines, the basic logic of computers is not difficult to comprehend. One of the most striking features of modern computer technology is that computer users do not need to understand in detail how a computer works in order to benefit from its labor-saving computations. Computers have become accessible to broader and broader classes of users. It is hoped that an acquaintance with some of the basic characteristics of computers will be sufficient to demonstrate that computer analysis is within the reach of all readers of this book.

□
Powers and limitations of computers

Computers are machines of tremendous power. Without any doubt, they are indispensable to modern scientists because of the characteristics we describe below. Computers are not, however, on the verge of making human intelligence obsolete. Respect for the computer's potency must be balanced by a recognition of its limitations.

Computer capabilities

The most noteworthy characteristic of computers is unquestionably their remarkable speed. The fact that computers are fast probably is familiar to everyone, but it is difficult to grasp how incredibly speedy computers actually are. The most sophisticated computers can perform elementary arithmetic calculations such as addition and subtraction in billionths of a second. In other words, in a single second computers are capable of executing tens of millions of operations. A large computer can perform more arithmetic in one second than a human could perform working 40-hour weeks for several years. The speediness of computers, therefore, removes the drudgery and delays of doing computations manually.

Not only are computers fast but they also are accurate. Highly complex calculations can be performed without error. By contrast, human "calculators" are fallible. The person who spends an hour calculating a statistic such as a correlation coefficient would probably have to spend at least as much time checking for computational errors. A computer could perform the same calculation, error-free, in a fraction of a second.* An additional advantage of computers is that they are dependably accurate. They can work hour after hour without making a mistake.

The memory capacity of large computers is impressive. The memory of a computer can store immense files of symbols to which it can gain access in a fraction of a second. Some memory devices can store millions of digits. What is even more impressive, the information stored in memory is not permanent but can be erased and replaced with new information. In other words, the memory can be used over and over again to solve new problems.

Another noteworthy aspect of computers is their flexibility. Most computers have been built for a variety of purposes. A university computer, for instance, does the payroll, produces income tax forms, keeps track of scholarship monies, bills students, produces grade reports, analyzes data from faculty research, and so forth.

Finally, we should point out that while computers do break down, they behave for the most part as our faithful servants. They do exactly what they are told to do, day in and day out, no matter how boring or repetitive the task might be.

Computer limitations

One of the most conspicuous limitations of computers is their utter and complete stupidity. Computers are sometimes referred to as "giant brains," but computers have absolutely no innate intelligence. They do only those operations that they are told to do by human

---

* The accuracy of a computer is limited to numbers of a certain size, owing to limitations in the computer's memory. Usually numbers can be accurate to 16 significant digits (e.g., 0.000000000000001), which is sufficiently accurate for virtually all nursing research applications.

beings. The computer's inability to think can result in many frustrating experiences for its users. Unlike human beings, a computer is unable to make even the simplest of inferences. Consider the following equation: $1 + 1, = X$. The comma placed before the equal sign would probably not interfere with a 6-year-old's ability to come up with the answer "2." Yet most computers could not solve this equation. The computer would not be capable of inferring that the extraneous comma should be ignored. Actually, while this aspect of computers usually taxes the patience of computer users, it is often an advantage. In the above equation, perhaps the comma should actually have been a zero. In such a situation, it is preferable for the computer to alert the user to an error than to perform a faulty computation.

Computer time is quite costly, despite the downward trend of computer prices. Although costs vary markedly from one installation to another, it is not unusual for computer time to cost ten dollars per minute. Of course, the computer could perform an enormous quantity of operations in one minute. Thus, while computer costs may be high, they are really a bargain in comparison with the costs of human labor.

Another limitation of computers is the detail with which instructions must be described. When a human being is confronted with the task $2 + 2 = ?$, the solution is (at the conscious level at least) straightforward and simple. A computer normally requires several instructions to process such computations. Every logical and arithmetic operation must be "explained" to the computer in detail, a feature that makes most tasks seem more complex than they would to human beings. Fortunately, the average researcher does not have to worry about such matters for analyzing data. The detailed instructions are developed by experts who have taken pains to simplify the use of computers.

☐
Overview of computer components

A computer system is an elaborate complex consisting of numerous components that perform specialized functions. The components of a computer system can be classified as either hardware or software. *Hardware* is a term that refers to the physical equipment that stores, processes and controls information. *Software* refers to the instructions and procedures required to operate the computer. In this section, the major aspects of both hardware and software will be reviewed.

Computer hardware

A schematic diagram of computer hardware is presented in Figure 23-1. Essentially, the computer consists of five types of components. Information is fed into the computer through some type of *input device*. The information read in through an input device is composed of data, on the one hand, and instructions concerning how the data are to be processed, on the other. After the computer has performed its necessary calculations, the resulting information comes out through an *output device*. Input/output (sometimes abbreviated I/O) devices are in many cases the only parts of the machine with which a researcher comes in direct physical contact. Because it is more important for a researcher to become familiar with I/O devices than with other components of a computer, a separate section has been devoted to them.

The information that is read into the computer is stored in a device called *memory*. The computer memory is composed of a series of cells, which may be likened to a set of pigeon holes or post office boxes. Each cell of memory can store either an instruction or a numerical value. The cells are organized into a series and assigned a number so that any piece of

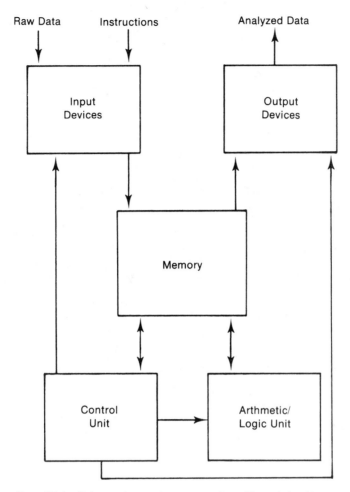

Figure 23-1. Scheme of computer components and interrelationships.

information stored in memory can be located by its "address." The memory unit of a computer is designed to store large amounts of information and to allow rapid access to any specific portion of that information.

From the memory, the instructions are sent to the *control unit.* This component coordinates the functions of the other components. The control unit interprets the instructions, determines the sequence of operations of the computer, and controls the movements of information from one component to another.

The control unit and arithmetic/logic unit are together referred to as the *central processing unit,* or CPU. It is in the central processing unit where all of the decisions and calculations are performed. The *arithmetic/logic unit* is the component in which arithmetic operations are accomplished.

Most universities, hospitals, and other large institutions own what is referred to as a *mainframe computer,* which is a large multiuser system that usually has I/O devices located at multiple sites. Figure 23-2 presents a picture

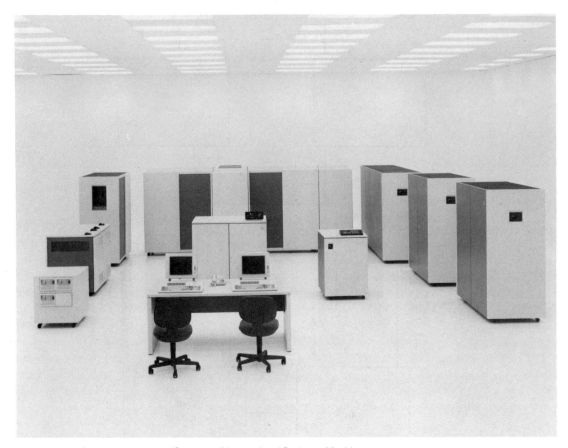

Figure 23-2. *Computer hardware. (Courtesy of International Business Machines Corporation.)*

of the main components of such a mainframe computer.

Microcomputers or *personal computers* are becoming increasingly popular both in institutions and in private homes and offices. Personal computers are slower, have less memory, and are generally restricted to just one user (or a handful of users) who can use the machine at any given time. Yet personal computers are inexpensive and generally easy to use and are becoming especially useful for certain applications, such as word processing. Figure 23-3 shows an example of a personal computer. Both mainframes and smaller computers consist of the same five basic components described above.

Computer software

The software components of a computer include the instructions for performing operations and the documentation for those instructions. A set of instructions is referred to as a *program.* The ability of a computer to solve problems is dependent upon computer programs, which specify clearly and precisely what operations the machine is to perform and how to perform them.

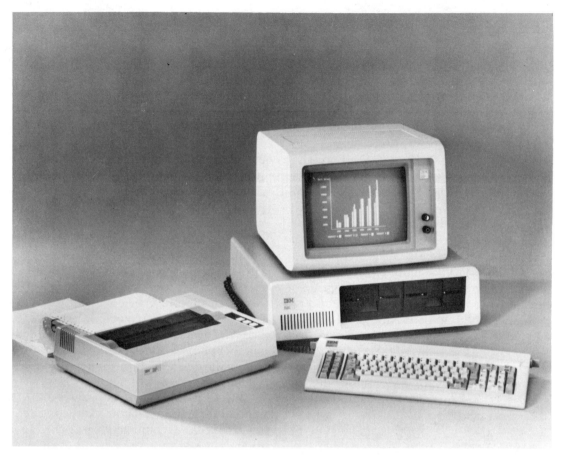

Figure 23-3. A personal computer. (Courtesy of International Business Machines Corporation.)

In order to give the computer a set of commands, people must be able to communicate with the machine. Computers, unfortunately, do not "speak" or understand natural languages such as English. Direct machine language that a computer *can* comprehend is extremely complex and accessible to only programming experts. Happily, various *programming languages* have been developed that are reasonably easy to learn and that are structured in a manner comfortable to human communicators. The instructions to the computer can be written in a programming lan-guage, and then another program called a *compiler* translates the instructions into an equivalent machine language program that the computer can comprehend and execute.

Various programming languages are available to computer users. Many of these languages have been developed for a specific type of application. The language most commonly used in scientific applications is FOR-TRAN, which is an acronym for FORmula TRANslation. The language known as PL/1 (Programming Language 1) is becoming increasingly popular in the scientific community. It includes many features of FORTRAN, but has additional new features and capabilities that make it attractive for use with scientific and social scientific problems. One of the simplest languages for beginning programmers to learn is BASIC (Beginners All-purpose Symbolic Instruction Code).

Most researchers can make ample use of computers without ever having to learn a computer language. This is because there are standard programs available for most types of statistical analysis. It would be inefficient to have every researcher write a program to compute an average or percentage, when a single program could be used by thousands of individuals.

Despite the fact that most readers will never need to master a programming language, a brief and simplified example of a BASIC program might help to demystify the process of computer functioning. Suppose that we had information concerning the weights of 100 subjects and that we wanted to know the average weight of the sample. We could obtain the average by means of a program with eight statements as follows:

```
10 LET N = 0
20 LET S = 0
30 INPUT X
40 LET S = S + X
50 LET N = N + 1
60 IF N < 100 THEN GO TO 30
70 LET A = S/N
80 PRINT A
```

In this program, the numbers 10,20 . . . 80 are merely labels to help identify different commands. The symbol S is used to represent the sum of the subjects' weights, N represents the number of subjects, X stands for an individual datum (the weight of a subject), and A is the average weight of the sample. The first two statements set the initial values of N and S to zero, as one would normally do when using a

pocket calculator. Statement 30 tells the computer to read in the weight (X) of the first subject. The sum is incremented by the value of X in line 40. If the first person weighed 120 pounds, S would at this point be equal to 120 pounds. In line 50 the value of N is increased by 1, in order to keep track of the number of subjects whose weights have been added to the sum. The first time through, N would be set equal to 1. In line 60 the computer is instructed to make a decision. If the number of cases processed is less than 100, then the computer is instructed to return to statement 30, where another case is read in. Once again, the weight would be added to the sum and the number counter would be increased. The cyclical process would continue until all 100 cases had been read into the computer. When N was equal to 100, the computer would proceed to execute statement 70, which calculates the average by dividing the sum by the number of cases. Finally, the computer would output the desired information by printing the average weight of the sample.

This short example demonstrates that there is nothing mysterious about instructing a computer to perform computational operations, although most computer tasks are considerably more complex than the task used here as an illustration. A great deal of skill and effort are normally required to develop efficient and sophisticated programs, but the logical processes underlying programming are much the same from one application to another.

The increasing availability of software packages to perform a variety of analytic jobs has made it possible for large numbers of nonprogrammers to profit from the advantages that computers offer. Knowledge of a programming language is definitely an asset to researchers. There are numerous operations that a packaged program does not perform, and researchers may also find that some specialized computation is required for their data. Nevertheless, for the typical researcher, igno-

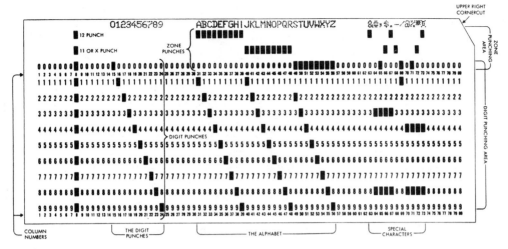

Figure 23-4. *An IBM punch card. Courtesy of International Business Machines Corporation.*

rance of a computer language is not an adequate reason to avoid computer analysis.

□

Input and output devices

Both data and programs must be transmitted to the computer through some input medium. Similarly, the computer communicates back to the user through an output medium. Usually, researchers interact with the computer through input and output devices without having to worry too much about what happens inside the computer itself. Since researchers do operate and work with I/O devices, it is appropriate to describe them more fully than other hardware components.

Input media and devices

Input devices convert alphabetical and numerical characters to a form amenable to storage in the computer's memory. A variety of input devices exist, and most computer installations have more than one type of device available for use. One input medium is the *punched card,* an illustration of which is presented in Figure 23-4. These cards contain eighty columns and twelve rows for storing information that is either data or program instructions. The information is coded on the card in machine-readable form through a process known as *keypunching.* A keypunch machine is similar to a typewriter, except that as the keypunch operator types onto the keyboard, holes are punched onto successive columns of the card. Each column represents a single character.

Perhaps the most widely used method of input today is through direct communication devices. These devices transmit information via electronic impulses and permit the user to communicate directly with the computer without the use of cards or other input devices. Direct communication devices take the form of a teletype, terminal, or console with a keyboard onto which the user types the relevant information.

There are several other kinds of input media used in the analysis of scientific data that serve both as methods of inputting information into the computer and as storage devices. In mainframe settings, the two most common devices for input and storage are magnetic tapes and magnetic disks. In the case of *magnetic tapes,* information is stored on reels similar to the reels for a tape recorder. Magnetic tape can break or become unreadable, but it is a much more durable input medium than cards. Information is often put onto tape by a transfer from punched cards or from input from a terminal. The input device through which tape information is passed on to the computer is called a *tape drive.*

Magnetic disks are flat spinning objects, analogous to a record, with magnetizable surfaces. Information is stored on disks on concentric tracks. Disks are a more dependable medium for storing information than either punched cards or magnetic tapes. Information typed into a terminal is typically stored on disks. Like magnetic tapes, disks have the advantage that they can be erased and reused.

Several types of storage/input media are available for use with personal computers. Many have a built-in hard disk, analogous to the disks used by mainframes. However, most personal computers use *floppy disks* as a means of putting information into the computer. Floppy disks are small (3 inches or 5 1/4 inches in diameter), flexible circular objects that resemble a 45-rpm record, protected by a paper cover. Floppies can be erased and reused many times.

Output media and devices

Output devices transfer the problem solutions in the computer's memory to a form that is understandable to humans. The most common output medium is a permanent readable record of the results of the analysis. The *line printer* is typically a principal output device for mainframe computers. Printers usually create an entire line of print at once and can print over 1000 lines per minute. The copy produced by printers is usually called the *printout* or *printed output.*

Various visual display devices are often used to output information in direct communication systems. *Cathode ray tube* (CRT) devices are becoming increasingly common in many settings, including hospitals. The information transmitted on a CRT is not permanent, but may be photographed. *Plotters* are another output device that can be used for producing graphs and diagrams. When a teletype or terminal is used to communicate with the computer, a typewriter-like printing mechanism is often used to produce output in permanent, hard-copy form.

In some cases, a researcher wants the results of one part of an analysis stored on a medium that the computer can then read for subsequent analyses. In such cases, information can be transferred to tapes, disks, or floppy disks for later use.

□

Modes of communicating with a computer

Researchers can communicate with a computer in one of several modes. For many mainframe applications, instructions to the computer are processed in the *batch processing* mode. Batch processing refers to a method in which a batch of programs is assembled for execution during the same machine run. A batch program constitutes an independent, integral package. All of the data and instructions regarding the analysis of the data are entered into the computer as a package. After the package is read into the computer by some input device, the program is processed without any further intervention. The researcher must normally wait some time before getting the output from a batch processing job. The delay between the input of the job and the availability of the output, which is referred to as the *turn-*

around time, may be several minutes or several hours.

Some computer systems and software packages offer users the capability of interacting directly with the computer, in what is called the *interactive mode.* When direct communication devices such as terminals, consoles, or teletypes are used, a researcher may be able to type in information and receive feedback essentially immediately, either on a CRT display or on a typed copy. Microcomputers operate in an interactive mode. On large computer systems, direct communication between the computer and numerous users concurrently is made possible by a concept known as *time-sharing.* Time-sharing is a method of operation by means of which several different programs are interleaved, giving the users the impression that the jobs are being processed simultaneously. Time-sharing usually operates on a "round robin" system. The computer spends a small amount of time (perhaps only one hundredth of a second) on each program, passing onto the next user. Since an entire cycle takes only seconds, it appears to all users as though they are getting instantaneous, personal service. The slowness of the keyboard and the rapidity of the central processing unit have combined to make time-sharing feasible. The major advantages of the interactive mode are convenience, ease of use, and immediate feedback. By choosing an interactive mode, the user can communicate with the computer in a conversational way: to enter a program or commands, to enter data, to receive and answer questions from the computer, and to select a course of action to be followed. Because interactive terminals are connected to the computer by telephone lines, the terminals need not be in the same building or even the same city as the computer.

Programs written in the batch mode can often be executed on an interactive terminal. The researcher can, from a terminal, instruct the computer to load the program and data from some input storage device (for example, from a disk file), and then direct the computer to execute the program without further interaction.

☐
Available programs

A great boon to researchers unfamiliar with a programming language, as well as to those with programming skills, is the widespread availability of ready-made programs to perform standard statistical analyses. The computer centers at universities are particularly likely to have a variety of software packages available to their users. Most computer centers have a professional staff that is accessible for consultation concerning the computer's library of programs.

Many computer facilities have a variety of simple, easy-to-use statistical programs in their general library. Often there are a large number of such "canned" programs that can be run from an interactive terminal. The use of these programs requires no expertise at all on the part of the researcher. For example, a researcher could obtain some basic descriptive statistics about a set of data by a simple instruction, such as RUN TALLY. The terminal would ask questions that would then guide the researcher in providing the necessary information to the computer.

These simple library programs are excellent heuristic devices when a user is first learning to work with a computer. When a researcher has a large number of cases, a large number of variables or desires a sophisticated statistical procedure, however, a more complex statistical software package may be required.

The most widely used statistical software packages for use on mainframe computers include the Biomedical Computer Programs or BMD (Dixon, 1975), the Statistical Package for the Social Sciences, or SPSS[x] (SPSS, Inc., 1983) and Statistical Analysis System, or SAS (SAS Institute, 1979). Each of these packages contains programs to handle a broad variety of statistical analyses. The reference section at the end of this chapter identifies the major statistical capabilities currently available for each of the above packages. Since these packages are updated, refined, and expanded frequently, readers are advised to check with personnel at their computer facility for any modifications to the listing provided in this chapter. There are also a growing number of statistical packages for personal computers. SPSS, for example, has a personal computer version called SPSS-PC that is very similar to the mainframe SPSS[x] package.

Researchers using packaged programs do not need to know a programming language but still must be able to communicate to the computer some basic information about what their variables are and how the data are to be analyzed. This is accomplished by means of certain commands that are unique to each software package. To illustrate the kinds of commands the researcher would need to know, an example of a set-up for an SPSS[x] task (in the batch processing mode) will be presented. SPSS[x] was chosen because it is widely available, because it is fairly easy to learn, and because a version is available for personal computers.

Let us suppose that we wanted to analyze the data that we used as an example in Chapters 20 and 21 concerning the intervention for low-income pregnant young women. The data for 30 subjects are shown in Table 20-7. The four variables are group (experimental versus control); weight of the infant; repeat pregnancy; and the mother's age. These data could be keypunched onto cards or entered into the computer directly via a terminal. In either case, the data would be entered onto separate cards or records for each subject. In the case of cards, for example, we would have a deck of 30

cards, each with information on these four variables. On each record, the information for the research variables would have to be entered according to some plan. Suppose, for example, the data were to be entered as follows: an identification number would be assigned and entered in columns 1 and 2; designation of group status would be entered in column 3; the infant's birthweight would be entered in columns 4 through 6; whether the mother had a repeat pregnancy would be entered in column 7; and the mother's age would be entered in columns 8 and 9. (Chapter 24 explains how such decisions are made.)

In order to use SPSS[x] to analyze the data, we must tell the computer how we have set up our data, just as we had to communicate this information to you in the preceding paragraph. Figure 23-5 presents the SPSS[x] instructions and the data that would be entered into the computer. The first line (DATA LIST) tells the computer that we are about to define the variables that are in the data file. The next line contains all of the variable definition and variable location information. The first entry on the line (/1) tells the computer that, in this case, all of the information for a given subject is contained on a single record. (If we had collected information on 50 variables per subject, we might well have needed two records per subject, in which case the second line would have begun with /2.) Next, each variable is specified by name, followed by the designation of the columns in which data for that variable will appear. In SPSS[x], variable names can be up to eight alpha-numeric characters. In this example, we have called our variables ID, GROUP, WEIGHT, REPEAT, and MOMSAGE. Then, to the right of each variable name, we have entered the appropriate column number. For example, the data for mothers' age (MOMSAGE) is in columns 8 and 9.

The next two records, taken together, instruct the computer what statistical analysis to

```
DATA LIST
  /1  ID 1-2  GROUP 3  WEIGHT 4-6  REPEAT 7  MOMSAGE 8-9
FREQUENCIES  VARIABLES=WEIGHT,REPEAT,MOMSAGE/
  STATISTICS=ALL
BEGIN DATA
011107117
021101014
031119021
041128120
051089015
061099019
071111019
081117118
091102117
101120020
111076013
121116018
131100116
141115018
151113021
162111119
172108021
182095019
192099017
202103119
212094015
222101117
232114021
242097020
252099118
262113018
272089019
282098020
292102017
302105019
END DATA
FINISH
```

Figure 23-5. Instructions for an SPSSˣ program.

perform. These instructions will produce, for the variables WEIGHT, REPEAT, and MOMS-AGE, a frequency count of every value obtained, together with many basic descriptive statistics, such as the mean, median, and standard deviation. The printout produced by this program for the WEIGHT variable was presented in Figure 20-10. If we wanted more complex statistics, such as those described in Chapters 21 and 22, we would need only to replace the FREQUENCIES/STATISTICS instructions with other instructions.

Finally, the command BEGIN DATA tells the computer to begin reading the data records, which follow immediately. There are 30 records here, because there were 30 subjects. The command following the data records (END DATA) tells the computer that all of the data have been read in, and the final command (FINISH) informs the computer that there are no further instructions for that particular run.

Hopefully, this simple example has made it clear that a researcher need not be a computer whiz or mathematical genius in order to make use of a computer. SPSS^x has many features that were not described here, but these features are not difficult to understand either. Similarly, other packaged programs have commands that must be learned by users but that are designed to be easy to learn by persons with no or minimal computer skills.

Computers are an invaluable aid to researchers. They can also be lots of fun. Although not all researchers would agree that their computer experiences have been enjoyable, the fact remains that serious researchers must develop some knowledge of computers if they wish to avoid obsolescence.

☐
Logging on to a computer

Each mainframe computer installation has developed its own idiosyncratic procedures by which users gain access to computer facilities. If you are a first-time user of a system, you will need to learn exactly what steps must be taken to make use of the equipment. You may obtain such information from your instructors or from one of the many computer assistants who are generally available to guide you.

Generally, regardless of what your input mechanisms are, you will need to provide the computer with some administrative information that allows the computer to determine whether you should have access to it. If you are using cards, the first card (often called the JOB CARD) needs to include information about your user ID (the account that should be billed for use of the computer) and a password. If you are using an interactive terminal, the computer will request a user ID and password, which allows you to *log on,* or gain access, to

the computer. If you do not have this information, you will not be permitted to use the facilities.

Mainframe computers often have several options for interacting with the system and creating files. Two common options in university settings are TSO (Time-Sharing Option) and CMS (Conversational Monitoring System). You will need to learn which monitoring system is available at your installation and how to gain access to it. You will also need to learn what statistical software packages are available.

Personal computers generally do not have as many security precautions, so an identification number may not be required. Most software for personal computers is designed to be easy to learn to use through printed manuals and direct instructions from the computer. Easy-to-use programs are called "user-friendly."

☐
Summary

The advantages of computers to researchers include their speed, accuracy, and flexibility. On the other hand, computers are costly and require considerable attention to detail on the part of users.

The components of a computer system are broadly categorized as either hardware or software. The term *hardware* refers to the physical equipment that stores, processes, and controls information. Large, multiuser computer systems are often referred to as *mainframe computers,* while smaller machines for individual users are called *microcomputers,* or simply *personal computers. Software* refers to the instructions and procedures required to operate the computer.

The five essential components of computer hardware are the *input device, memory, control unit, arithmetic/logic unit,* and *output device.* The control unit and the arithmetic/

logic unit are collectively called the *central processing unit*. The input device is the means by which the researcher feeds information into the computer. The memory is the device that stores the information that is fed into the computer. The control unit coordinates the functions of the other components. The arithmetic/logic unit performs the arithmetic or logic operations requested. Finally, the output device produces the resulting information.

A *program* is a set of instructions informing the computer what to do. *Programming languages* make it possible for humans to communicate with computers. FORTRAN, PL/1, and BASIC are examples of programming languages. Many packaged software programs exist for the researcher who is not greatly skilled in a programming language.

The most commonly used input and storage media for research applications include *punched cards, magnetic tapes, magnetic disks, floppy disks* and direct communication by means of a terminal or console. The most commonly used output media are the paper *printout* (which is a permanent, readable record of the results of the analysis) and displays from plotters and cathode ray tubes.

Researchers are able to communicate with computers in several ways. *Batch processing* refers to a process in which a batch of programs is assembled for execution during the same computer run. Generally, there is a delay between feeding the information into the computer and the output phase. The delay is referred to as *turn-around time. Interactive mode* permits direct communication between the researcher and the computer through the use of consoles, terminals, or teletypes. Almost immediate feedback of information is possible when the interactive mode is used. *Time-sharing* is a method in which several programs are processed "simultaneously" by the computer, which spends a small amount on each program in a "round robin" fashion.

□
Study suggestions

1. Can you solve the following equation:
   ,10 − 3 = X
   Do you think a computer could? Why or why not?
2. Look at statement 40 in the BASIC program illustrated in this chapter (40 LET S = S + X). In which hardware component would this instruction actually be processed?
3. If you have access to a computer, find out how many cells or words of memory are available in your computer.
4. Visit a computer center. Check what types of input and output devices the computer has. Does the computer have a time-sharing system? If possible, learn how to operate a terminal. Ask someone what software packages are available for doing statistical analyses.
5. Suppose you had data from 50 subjects on the following four variables: age, sex (coded 1 for females, 2 for males), number of cigarettes smoked per day, and number of days absent from work in the past year. Write out SPSS[x] instructions that would produce a frequency listing for these four variables. (N.B. first determine in which columns the data would be entered.)

□
Suggested readings

General references

Capron, H.L. & Williams, B.K. (1984). *Computers and data processing* (2nd ed.). Menlo Park, CA: Benjamin/Cummings.

Chang, B.L. (1985). Computer use and nursing research. *Western Journal of Nursing Research, 7,* 142–144.

Edmunds, L. (1982). Teaching nurses to use computers. *Nurse Educator, 7,* 32–38.

McElmurry, B.J. & Newcomb, B.J. (1981). Clarification of the database concept. *Nursing Research, 30,* 155.

Moore, R.W. (1978). *Introduction to the use of computer packages for statistical analyses.* Englewood Cliffs, NJ: Prentice-Hall.

Silver, G.A. (1979). *The social impact of computers.* New York: Harcourt, Brace, Jovanovich.

Stern, R. & Stern, N. (1979). *Principles of data processing* (2nd ed.). New York: John Wiley and Sons.

Sweeney, M.A. & Olivieri, P. (1981). *An introduction to nursing research: Research, measurement and computers in nursing.* Philadelphia: J.B. Lippincott (Chapters 14–17).

Sweeney, M.A. (1985). *The nurse's guide to computers.* New York: Macmillan Publishing Co.

References on software packages

Dixon, W. J. (Ed.) (1975). *Biomedical computer programs.* Berkeley, CA: University of California Press. (Major programs include summary statistics, correlations, analysis of variance, analysis of covariance, multiple regression analysis, cluster analysis, factor analysis, canonical correlation, and discriminant analysis.)

SAS Institute (1979). *SAS user's guide.* Cary, NC: SAS Institute. (This package includes all basic descriptive and inferential statistics, plus additional programs for cluster analysis, Guttman scalogram analysis, multiple regression, factor analysis, discriminant function analysis, canonical correlation, logit/probit analysis and spectral analysis.)

SPSS, Inc. (1983). *SPSS^x user's guide.* New York: McGraw-Hill. (Major programs include descriptive statistics, frequency distributions, contingency tables and related measures of association, bivariate correlation and scatter diagrams, partial correlation, multiple regression analysis, *t*-tests, analysis of variance, analysis of covariance, multivariate analysis of variance, discriminant analysis, factor analysis, canonical analysis, survival analysis, loglinear analysis, and various nonparametric procedures.)

Chapter 24
□
Preparing data for computer analysis

Nurse researchers are increasingly using computers to help with their data analyses. This trend reflects both the widespread availability of appropriate software packages and the increasing complexity of nurse researchers' analytic and research designs. However, even relatively simple projects can benefit by the assistance of computers. For example, if a researcher asked a small sample of 50 subjects only 20 questions, there would be 1000 pieces of information to analyze, and a computer would be useful in doing this. This chapter is devoted to methods for preparing data for computer analysis.

□
Coding

If a computer is to be used to analyze data, the information typically must be converted to a machine-readable form. Computers cannot process verbatim responses to open-ended questions. It is similarly difficult for a computer to read and analyze information with verbal labels such as male or female, agree or disagree. *Coding* is the process by which basic research information is transformed into symbols compatible with computer analysis. It is possible to code information using alphabetical symbols. For example, the code for females could be F and the code for males could be M. However, we strongly urge that a completely numerical coding scheme be developed because some packaged programs cannot handle alphabetical coding.

Inherently quantitative variables

While the majority of data collected in the course of a project will need to be coded, there are certain variables whose measures are directly amenable to computer analysis because they are inherently quantitative. Variables such as age, weight, body temperature, and diastolic blood pressure do not normally require coding. Sometimes the researcher may ask for information of this type in a way that does call for the development of a coding plan. If a researcher asks respondents to indicate whether they are younger than 30, between the ages of 31 and 49, or over 50, then the responses would have to be coded before being entered into a computer file.

When the responses to questions such as age, height, income level, and so forth are given in their full, natural form, then the researcher should *not* reduce the information to coded categories for data entry purposes. As a general rule, it is better to maintain responses in as much detail as possible. It is always possible to collapse information for analytic purposes by instructing the computer to group together responses within a certain range. However, if the data are coded and entered into a few gross categories, it will be impossible for the computer to reconstruct the original responses.

Therefore, information that is "naturally" quantitative may need no coding whatsoever, but the researcher should inspect the data before having them entered. It is quite important that all of the responses be of the same form and precision. For instance, in entering a person's height, the researcher would need to decide whether to use feet and inches or to convert the information entirely to inches. Whichever method is adopted, it must be used consistently for all subjects. There must also be consistency in the method of handling information reported with differential precision. If a researcher asked a group of mothers to indicate the age of their youngest child, some mothers might report the age to the nearest month, while others would specify the age in years only. Probably the most reasonable solution in such a situation is to round off and use the less precise figure, since there might be no way to retrieve the full information. These decisions must be made prior to data entry so that all of the information for any particular variable is truly comparable.

Precategorized data

Much of the data from questionnaires, interviews, observation schedules, and psychological scales can be coded easily because of precategorization. Closed-ended questions that provide for response alternatives can easily be assigned a numerical code, as in the following example:

> From what type of program did you receive your basic nursing preparation?
> 1. Diploma school
> 2. Associate degree program
> 3. Baccalaureate degree program

Thus, if a nurse received his or her nursing preparation from a diploma school, the response to this question would be coded "1."

In many cases the codes will be arbitrary, as in the case of a variable such as gender. Whether a female is coded 1 or 2 will have no bearing on the subsequent analysis as long as females are consistently assigned one code and males another. Variables with arbitrary codes, it may be recalled, are measured on a nominal scale. Other variables will appear to have a more obvious coding scheme, as in the following example:

> How often do you suffer from insomnia?
> 1. almost never
> 2. once or twice a year
> 3. three to eleven times a year
> 4. at least once a month

Sometimes respondents may have the option of checking off more than one answer in reply to a single question, as in the following illustration:

To which of the following journals do you subscribe?
( ) American Journal of Nursing
( ) Nursing Forum
( ) Nursing Outlook
( ) Nursing Research

With questions of this type, it is not possible to adopt a simple 1-2-3-4 code because subjects may check several, or none, of the responses. The most appropriate procedure for questions such as the one on journal subscriptions is to treat each journal on the list as a separate question. In other words, the researcher would code the responses as though the item were four separate items asking "Do you subscribe to the American Journal of Nursing? Do you subscribe to Nursing Forum? . . ." A checkmark beside a journal would be treated as though the reply were "yes." In effect, the question would be turned into four dichotomous variables, with a code (perhaps "1") signifying a "yes" response and another code (perhaps "2") signifying a "no."

Uncategorized data

Qualitative data from open-ended questions, unstructured observations, and projective tests usually are not readily amenable to direct computer analysis. When this type of information is to be analyzed by the computer, it is usually necessary to categorize and code it. Sometimes it is possible for the researcher to develop a coding scheme in advance of data collection. For instance, a question might ask, "What is your occupation?" If the researcher knew the sample characteristics, he or she could probably predict such major categories as "Professional," "Managerial," "Clerical," and so forth.

Usually, however, unstructured formats for data collection are adopted specifically because it is difficult to anticipate the kind of information that will be obtained. In using open-ended questions, for instance, the researcher is expressing unwillingness to impose what might be an inappropriate constraint on the responses. In such a situation it is necessary to code responses after all the data are collected if a computer is to be used to analyze the information. The researcher should begin by scanning all of the responses, or a sizable sample of them, to get a feel for the nature of the replies. The researcher can then proceed to develop a scheme to categorize responses. The categorization scheme should be designed to reflect both the researcher's theoretical and analytic goals as well as the substance of the information. The amount of detail in the categorization scheme can vary considerably, but again the researcher should keep in mind that too much detail is better than too little detail. In developing a coding scheme for unstructured information, the only "rule" is that the coding categories should be both mutually exclusive and collectively exhaustive. Chapter 19 provides additional information on handling qualitative material.

Whenever the actual coding is performed by more than one person, it is imperative that precise instructions be developed for the coders. Coders, like observers and interviewers, must be properly trained. Intercoder reliability checks are strongly recommended.

Coding missing data

A code should be designated for every question or variable for every subject, even if in some cases no response or information is available. Missing data can be of various types. A person responding to an interview question may be undecided, refuse to answer, or say "don't know." An observer coding behavior may get distracted during a 10-second sampling frame, may be undecided about an appropriate categorization, or may observe behavior not listed on the observation schedule. In some cases it may be important to distinguish between various types of missing data by specifying separate codes, while in another case a single code may suffice. This decision must be made with the conceptual aims of the research in mind. A person who replied "don't know" to a question seeking to understand the public's familiarity with health maintenance organizations should probably be distinguished from the person who refused to answer the question. However, it might be less important to make a distinction between a "don't know" and a failure to answer a question such as "Do you generally approve or disapprove of unionization for nurses?"

Insofar as possible, it is desirable to code missing data in the same manner for all variables. If a "no response" is coded as a 4 on variable 1, a 6 on variable 2, a 5 on variable 3, and so forth, there is a greater risk of error than if a uniform code is adopted. The choice of what number to use as the missing data code is fairly arbitrary, but the number must be one that has not been assigned to an actual piece of information. Many researchers follow the convention of coding missing data as 9, since this value is normally out of the range of codes for true information. Others use blanks to indicate missing information. Some software packages require a specific handling of missing information. For example, SAS uses periods (.) for missing values.

☐
Entering coded data

For most types of computer analysis, the coded data are transferred onto a disk file by means of a console or terminal. Coded data are transferred to a computer file in accordance with a predesignated plan. The next section discusses the considerations to be made in designing and implementing such a plan.

Preparing data for data entry

In many cases, data files are set up to store 80 columns of information, analagous to an 80-column keypunched card. In this section, we will illustrate data preparation activities based on an 80-column scheme, but it is sometimes possible to use alternative schemes, depending on the software being used.

The researcher should plan in advance of the actual data entry the layout of information within the 80 columns. It is usually preferable to adopt what is known as a *fixed format,* which places the values for any specific variable in the same column for every case. Some packaged programs also permit data to be entered in a *free format,* in which there is no necessary correspondence between the variables entered in any particular column from one case to the next. However, it is often safer to use a fixed format because it is more widely acceptable. Moreover, fixed format is usually preferable for beginning researchers because it permits an easier check for errors.

With fixed format the researcher must specify in which columns all items of information are to be entered. Many variables will require no more than one column. That is, if a variable has a code whose maximum value is one digit, the variable can be assigned to a single column. Examples include variables whose responses are male/female, agree/disagree, or yes/no/maybe. Other variables, such as age, weight, and blood pressure measures, must occupy more than one column. Anytime the maximum value of a variable exceeds 9, the researcher must be sure to reserve two (or more, if the number is larger than 99) columns. The space allocated to a particular variable is referred to as a *field.*

The researcher must be careful in dealing with a variable whose values may be of different widths. For example, if we were recording a person's weight, we would need only two digits for persons weighing under 100 pounds, but three digits for those weighing 100 pounds or more. Since the maximum value would be three digits long, then three columns on the card would be required for all subjects. To record the weight of a person of 95 pounds, we would have to occupy the full three columns, so it would be necessary to enter 095. This procedure is known as *right-justifying* the data. Whenever a number smaller than the corresponding field is entered in fixed format, the number should be entered as far to the right as possible in the designated field. In the above example if columns 11, 12, and 13 were reserved for the weight measurement, 95 should be entered in columns 12 and 13. If, instead, 95 were entered in columns 11 and 12, the value would be read typically as 950.

In designing the layout for the data, the researcher should allocate space for recording an identification number. Each individual case (that is, the information from a single questionnaire, test, observation, and so forth) should be assigned a unique identifying number, and this number should be entered along with the actual data. This procedure will permit the investigator to go back to the original source if there are any difficulties with the data file. The numbering is completely arbitrary and is used only as a label. Usually, a consecutive numbering scheme is used, running from number 1 to the number of actual cases. The identification number normally is entered in the first columns of the record. If there are fewer than 100 subjects, the first two columns would be used, starting with subjects 01, 02, and so on. As in the case of other variables, the field width is determined by the maximum value of the identification number.

The researcher will often find that a single 80-column format is insufficient for recording all of the information obtained from a single case. There is no restriction on the number of records that may be used for a given case or subject. In fact, it is quite common to require two or three records to enter all of the data for each subject. When multiple records are needed, the identification number for a particular case is often entered onto all records for that case. If the file somehow got rearranged, it would then be possible to group together those records belonging to a single case. As an additional precaution, the researcher should also enter a number identifying the order of the records within a case. That is, the first record of a case would be identified with a "1," the second card with a "2," and so forth. The record sequence number is often entered either immediately after the ID number, or in column 80.

A number of procedures are available to facilitate the actual data entry process. The first is to transfer codes from the original source (such as a questionnaire) onto a specially prepared coding sheet. These sheets, which are available commercially, are ruled off into a grid with 80 columns and 20 to 40 rows. The columns correspond to the columns in a data file, and each row represents a single record. The researcher can use these sheets to write numbers representing the desired entries in the appropriate columns. It is fairly easy to enter data that have been recorded on code sheets.

A second procedure is to use a margin on the original source to write the appropriate numerical codes for the data entry person to follow. This *edge-coding* scheme may lead to fewer errors than the use of code sheets since the coder does not have to worry about losing his or her place in going back and forth between the original source and the code sheets. However, edge coding can also create problems because the coder may fail to code a variable without realizing it. Data entry from edge-coded materials usually proceeds more slowly than from coding sheets since the person entering must stop to turn pages and must pay attention to whether or not the data are being entered in the correct columns.

Other procedures exist for transferring data to computer files. Sometimes it is possible to enter data directly from an original source without edge coding if the source has been designed properly. Optical scanning sheets can, in some cases, be used to avoid manual data entry altogether.

Data entry and verification

The data entry operation can begin after the layout scheme has been developed and the codes have been specified for each variable. Data entry is a tedious and exacting task that is usually subject to numerous errors. Therefore, it is necessary to verify or check the entries to correct the mistakes that are inevitably made. Several verification procedures exist. The first is to visually compare the numbers printed on a printout of the data file with the codes on either the original source or the coding sheets. A second possibility is to enter all of the data twice and to compare the two sets of records. The comparison can be done either visually or with the assistance of the computer. Finally, there are special verifying machines that are designed to perform comparisons. The use of machine verification is recommended as the best method for eliminating data entry inaccuracies.

Data cleaning

Even after the records are verified, the data usually will contain a few errors. These errors could be due to data entry mistakes but could also arise from coding or reporting problems. Data are not ready for analysis until they have been cleaned. Data cleaning involves two types of checks. The first is a check for *outliers* or wild codes. Using a computer printout of the frequency counts associated with every value for every variable, the researcher checks for undefined code values. The variable sex might have the following three defined code values: 1 for female, 2 for male, 9 for not reported. If it were discovered that a code of 5 were entered in the column for sex, then it would be clear that an error had been made. The computer could be instructed to list the identification (ID) number of the culpable record, and the error could be corrected by checking the appropriate code on the original source.

Editing of this type will of course, never reveal mistakes that look "respectable" or plausible. If the gender of a male is mispunched as a 1, the mistake may never be detected. Since errors can have a profound effect on the analysis and interpretation of data, it is naturally quite important to perform the coding, punching, verifying, and cleaning with great care.

The second data-cleaning procedure involves performing consistency checks, which focus on internal data consistencies. That is, the researcher looks for data entry or coding errors by testing whether data in one part of a record are compatible with data in another part. For example, one question in a questionnaire might ask respondents their current marital status and another might ask how many times they had been married. If the data were internally consistent, subjects who responded "Single, never married" to the first question, should have a zero entered in the field for the second. As another example, if the respondent's sex were entered with the code for male, and there was an entry of "2" for the variable "number of pregnancies," one of those two fields would contain an error. The researcher should identify a number of such opportunities for checking the consistency of entered data.

Once the data have been cleaned to the researcher's satisfaction, a backup copy of the data file should be made immediately as a protection against loss or damage. The duplicate copy can be stored on any input medium such as magnetic tape, disk, or diskette.

□

Documentation

The decisions that a researcher makes concerning coding, field width, placement of data in columns, and so on should be documented in full. Documentation is essential for the proper handling of any data set. The researcher's own memory should not be trusted to store all of the required information. Several weeks after coding, the researcher may no longer remember if males were coded 1 and females 2, or vice versa. Moreover, colleagues may wish to borrow the data set to perform a secondary analysis. Whether one anticipates a secondary analysis or not, documentation should be sufficiently thorough that a person unfamiliar with the original research project could use the data.

A major portion of the documentation involves the preparation of a codebook. A *codebook* is essentially a listing of each variable, the column(s) in which the variable has been entered, and the codes associated with the various aspects or attributes of the variable. The codebook is often prepared before coding so that it can be used as a guide by coders. In the next section we present an example of a codebook. Additional documentation is required if any type of transformation has been effected after the data have been entered. For instance, researchers often combine two or more variables to form a composite index or scale. Scale construction, item reversals, recodes, and other types of changes to the data should be recorded in full. Finally, the documentation should include a description of central features of the data, such as the time when they were collected, sample characteristics, and so forth. If the data are stored on a magnetic tape file, information concerning access to that file should also be prepared.

□
A hypothetical example

Perhaps the concepts and recommendations presented in this chapter can be best understood by reference to a detailed example. Figure 24-1 presents a questionnaire that was contrived solely for the purpose of illustrating many of the points made in the preceding sections. This hypothetical instrument should not be taken as an example of good questionnaire design. The intent was to include a variety of item types to demonstrate how different coding problems could be handled.

On the left-hand margin of the questionnaire are the numerical codes to be transferred to a computer file. The first code—001—represents the identification number assigned to the respondent who completed the questionnaire. The three-digit number implies that at least 100 respondents participated in the study. Following the identification number are the codes corresponding to the subject's responses. In question 2, part B, the missing values code of 9 signifies the subject's failure to respond. With regard to question 5, each individual symptom is treated for data analysis purposes as a separate question, with a check or "X" being coded as "1" and no check coded as "2." It might also be noted that the subject's height, reported in question 10, has been converted into inches.

The data entry person using edge-coded questionnaires such as this would simply follow the numbers in the left margin, entering them in consecutive columns. To illustrate an alternative to edge coding, the same data have been transferred to the coding sheet presented in Figure 24-2. As this figure shows, the code sheets specify precisely the column in which each numerical code is to be entered. The total number of columns required to store the information from this fictitious questionnaire is 31. If there were 150 respondents, then there would be 150 records, all with information in the first 31 columns.

The example presented here involves a simple and straightforward coding scheme. Since all the questions are closed-ended, there is little confusion or ambiguity concerning how to code the various responses. Even for uncomplicated data, it is a good practice to de-

(Text continues on p. 478)

001 This questionnaire is part of a study on health-related habits and attitudes. We hope you will help us by answering the following questions.

1. Overall, how would you describe your health in comparison with that of others your age?

2
( ) above average health
(x) average health
( ) below average health

2. Have you been hospitalized within the past two years?

2
( ) yes —
(X) no

If yes: how many times have you been hospitalized?
9
( ) once
( ) two times
( ) more than two times

3. Do you smoke cigarettes?

1
(X) yes —
( ) no

If yes, how many cigarettes do you usually smoke per day?
1
(X) 1 pack or less
( ) between one and two packs
( ) two packs or more

4. How often do you drink alcoholic beverages?

4
( ) never   (X) 2 or 3 times a month
( ) 10 times a year or less   ( ) about once a week
( ) about once a month   ( ) several times a week
                                                  ( ) nearly every day

5. Below is a list of some common somatic complaints. Please check off those symptoms which have bothered you within the past month or so.

1 (x) headache
2 ( ) indigestion
1 (x) constipation
2 ( ) diarrhea
2 ( ) insomnia
2 ( ) lower back pains
2 ( ) lack of appetite

6. Which of the following statements best describes your health care practices?

( ) I go for regular physical checkups as a preventive health care measure.
2 (X) I see a health care professional only when I have a specific complaint.
( ) I have to be extremely ill before I will see a health care professional.

7. Please indicate how important the following things are to you by placing an "X" under the appropriate column:

		Extremely important	Somewhat important	Not too important
1	Abundant leisure time	X		
3	A long life			X
2	Financial success and security		X	
1	Good family relationships	X		
2	Good health		X	
2	Lots of friends, popularity		X	

38 8. What is your present age? ___38___ years.
135 9. How much do you weigh? ___135___ pounds.
66 10. How tall are you? ___5___ feet, ___6___ inches.
1 11. What is your sex?
(X) female
( ) male

Figure 24-1. *Example of a questionnaire with edge coding.*

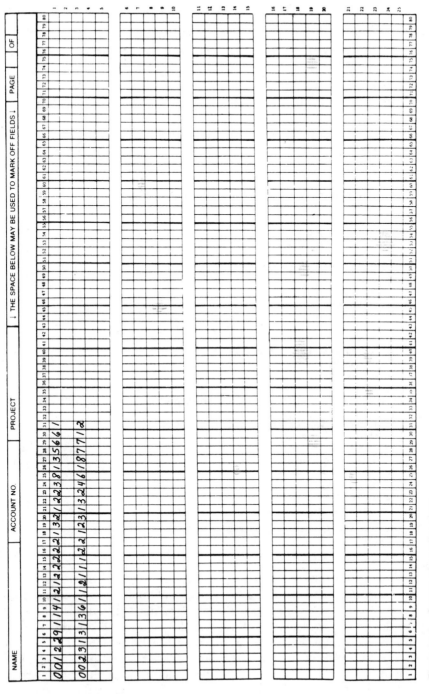

Figure 24-2. Sample of a coding sheet.

Card Column	Variable Description and Codes	Question Number
1-3	Respondent Identification Number (001 to 150)	
4	"Overall, how would you describe your health in comparison with that of others your age?" 1. above average health 2. average health 3. below average health 9. no response	1
5	"Have you been hospitalized within the past two years?" 1. yes 2. no 9. no response	2
6	"If yes: how many times have you been hospitalized?" 1. once 2. two times 3. more than two times 9. no response	2
7	"Do you smoke cigarettes?" 1. yes 2. no 9. no response	3
8	"If yes: how many cigarettes do you usually smoke per day?" 1. 1 pack or less 2. between one and two packs 3. two packs or more 9. no response	3
9	"How often do you drink alcoholic beverages?" 1. never 2. 10 times a year or less 3. about once a month 4. 2 to 3 times per month 5. about once a week 6. several times a week 7. nearly every day 9. no response	4

Figure 24-3. Example of a section of a codebook.

velop a codebook. The preparation of a codebook is not time-consuming and represents a permanent record of the researcher's major data preparation decisions. An example of a codebook setup is shown in Figure 24-3, which includes the information for the first four questions of this example only.

The example can also be used to illustrate

data cleaning. Figure 24-4 presents a computer listing of the frequency counts corresponding to all values entered for question 3, "Do you smoke cigarettes?" Of the 150 cases, 76 responses were entered, as "1," or "yes", and 68 responses were entered as "2" or "no." Three respondents apparently failed to answer (entered as "9"). The printout tells us that in two

```
 9-DEC-85    SPSS-X RELEASE 2.1 FOR VAX/VMS
15:31:09     BOSTON COLLEGE VAXCLUSTER              DEC VAX-11/780 VMS V4.1


SMOKE     DO YOU SMOKE CIGARETTES?
```

VALUE LABEL		VALUE	FREQUENCY	PERCENT	VALID PERCENT	CUM PERCENT
YES		1	76	50.7	51.7	51.7
NO		2	68	45.3	46.3	98.0
		3	2	1.3	1.4	99.3
		8	1	.7	.7	100.0
		9	3	2.0	MISSING	
		TOTAL	150	100.0	100.0	

MEAN	1.537	STD ERR	.062	MEDIAN	1.000	
MODE	1.000	STD DEV	.752	VARIANCE	.565	
KURTOSIS	36.298	S E KURT	.397	SKEWNESS	4.428	
S E SKEW	.200	RANGE	7.000	MINIMUM	1.000	
MAXIMUM	8.000	SUM	226.000			

```
VALID CASES    147    MISSING CASES    3
```

Figure 24-4. Hypothetical data for data cleaning example.

cases a "3" was incorrectly entered for question three, and in one case an "8" was entered. This computer listing has informed us that there are errors on three records in column seven. We could now go through the data file —either manually, with a printout, or by the computer—to find the three records in question. The records would indicate the ID number of the questionnaires to be rechecked, and the necessary corrections could then be made.

□
Summary

The focus of this chapter was on the preparation of data for computer analysis. Information collected in a research project must be converted to machine-readable form if a computer is to be used. *Coding* is the procedure of transforming research data into symbols compatible with computer analysis. Preferably, the coding scheme adopted is completely numerical. If the data are inherently quantitative (such as a person's weight), or if a precategorization scheme was used to collect the data, the coding task is straightforward. For uncategorized data, such as responses to open-ended questions, a coding system must be developed for analytic purposes. Special codes should be developed to signify missing data.

The researcher usually must plan in advance the layout of information on an 80-column record. In a *fixed-format* arrangement, which is commonly used for research data, each variable is entered onto the same column for every case. The width of the *field* (the space allocated to a particular variable) is determined by the maximum numerical value for that variable. The data should always be *right-justified,* or entered as far to the right as possible in the designated field. It is wise to identify each case with an identification number, which is typically entered onto the first few columns of the record.

The researcher may transfer the codes from the original source onto specially prepared *coding sheets,* which are ruled off into grids of 80 columns (one column per column on a data file) and about 20 rows (one row for each record). A second procedure is to use an *edge-coding* scheme, in which the numerical codes to be entered are written onto the margin of the original source.

Data entry is susceptible to a high error rate. Entered data therefore, should be checked or *verified* for errors. Even after the data are verified, they almost inevitably contain a few errors. Because of this fact, data should be *cleaned* before proceeding with the desired analyses. The cleaning process is primarily a check for *outliers* or numerical values that are not part of the coding scheme, and a check for internal consistency.

Finally, the researcher should document the decisions made concerning the coding, field placement, and so on. A fairly standard procedure is the preparation of a *codebook* that serves as a comprehensive, permanent record of the researcher's data processing decisions.

☐
Study suggestions

1. Prepare a codebook for the questionnaire presented on pages 64–65 of the 1984 volume (volume 33) of *Nursing Research* (Nursing Research Subscriber Profile).
2. Complete the questionnaire referenced in question 1. Code your responses and transfer them to a coding sheet.

3. If you have access to a terminal, enter the data from the hypothetical example presented in this chapter. Enter the data from both the edge-coded questionnaire and the coding sheet. Compare the amount of time spent on each. Verify your data entry by checking for discrepancies on the two records.
4. What field width would you need for the following variables: marital status, annual income, body temperature, number of children, white blood cell count, religious affiliation, days absent from work, Apgar score, time to first voiding, and pulse rate?

☐
Suggested readings

Babbie, E.R. (1973). *Survey research methods.* Belmont, CA: Wadsworth (Chapter 10).

Barhyte, D. & Bacon, L.D. (1985). Approaches to cleaning data sets. *Nursing Research. 34,* 62–65.

Harris, M.L. (1979). *Introduction to data processing* (2nd ed.) (Chapters 1, 2, & 3). New York: John Wiley and Sons.

Jacobsen, B.S. (1981). Know thy data. *Nursing Research, 30,* 254–255.

Marls, R.G. (1982). *Designing a research project: The basics of biomedical research methodology.* Belmont, CA: Life Long Learning.

Selltiz, C., Wrightsman, L.S., & Cook, S.W. (1976). *Research methods in social relations* (3rd ed.). New York: Holt, Rinehart and Winston (Chapters 13 & 14).

Sorin, M.D. (1982). *Data entry without keypunching: Improved preparation for social data analysis.* Lexington, MA: Lexington Books.

Tabachnick, B.G. & Fidell, L.S. (1983). *Using multivariate statistics.* New York: Harper & Row (Chapter 4).

Part VI

Communication in the research process

Chapter 25

☐

Interpreting and reporting research results

The final stages of a research project, like the beginning stages, are often more difficult than the intermediary steps of data collection and analysis. The interpretation and communication of the research results cannot be done mechanically by following methodological techniques that may at first seem cumbersome but that can be learned. To be sure, research skills are required for interpreting and reporting the findings of a study, but there is also a need for creativity, intellectual insights, logical reasoning, and theoretical grounding. These are not attributes that can be learned in a textbook. This chapter will offer some general guidelines for helping the researcher with the final steps in the scientific process, but it should be recognized that these guidelines tell only half the story of this challenging task.

☐

Interpretation of results

The results of statistical analyses are only numbers, with very little inherent meaning associated with them. It is the researcher's role to imbue these numbers with meaning. Interpretation of the statistical findings is essentially a search for the broader meaning and implications of those findings. The results of the analyses need to be interpreted with due consideration to the overall aims of the project, its theoretical underpinnings, the specific hypotheses being tested, the existing body of related research knowledge, and the limitations of the adopted research methods.

In this section we review issues relating to interpreting various kinds of research outcomes. In all cases, we urge that researchers carefully review relevant research and theory before trying to make sense of the results. If the research was conceived on the basis of a theory or conceptual model, it is important to relate the findings to that theoretical framework. That is, if a theoretical framework was truly the basis for the study, it should also provide a basis for trying to understand the data.

Interpreting hypothesized results

When the tests of statistical significance support the original research hypotheses, the task of interpreting the results is somewhat easier than when the hypotheses are challenged. In a sense, the interpretation has been partly accomplished beforehand in such a situation, because the researcher has already had to bring together prior research findings, a theoretical framework, and logical reasoning in the development of the hypotheses. This groundwork can then form the context within which more specific interpretations are made.

Naturally, researchers are gratified when the results of many hours of effort offer support for their predictions. There is a very decided preference on the part of individual researchers, advisers and journal reviewers for studies whose hypotheses have been supported. This preference is understandable, but it is important not to let personal predilections interfere with the critical appraisal that is appropriate in all interpretive situations. A few cautionary suggestions should be kept in mind.

First, it is preferable to be somewhat conservative in drawing conclusions from the data. The intrusion of personal viewpoints and subjective judgments is inevitable in making sense of research results, but they must be held in check as much as possible. It is sometimes tempting to go far beyond the data in developing explanations for what the results mean, but conscientious scientists avoid doing so. A simple example might help to explain what is meant by "going beyond the data." Suppose a nurse researcher hypothesized that a relationship existed between a pregnant woman's level of anxiety about the labor and delivery experience, and the number of children she has already borne. The data reveal that a negative relationship between anxiety levels and parity ($r = -.40$) does indeed exist. The researcher, therefore, concludes that increased experience with childbirth causes decreasing amounts of anxiety. Is this conclusion supported by the data? The conclusion appears to be logical but, in fact, there is nothing within the data that leads directly to this interpretation. An important, indeed critical, research precept is: *correlation does not prove causation*. The finding that two variables are related offers no evidence suggesting which of the two variables—if either—caused the other. In the present example perhaps causality runs in the opposite direction, i.e., that a woman's anxiety level influences how many children she bears. Or perhaps a third variable not examined in the study, such as the woman's social supports, "causes" or influences both anxiety and number of children.

Alternative explanations for the findings should always be considered. If these competing interpretations can be ruled out on the basis of the data or previous research findings, so much the better. However, every angle should be examined to see if one's pet explanation has been given adequate competition.

The fact that statistical significance was attained in testing the hypothesis does not necessarily mean that the results were important or of value to the nursing community and their clients. Statistical significance indicates that the results were unlikely to be a function of chance. This means that the observed group differences or observed relationships were probably real, but not necessarily important. With large samples, even modest relationships are statistically significant. For instance with a sample of 500, a correlation coefficient of .10 is significant at the .05 level, but a relationship of this magnitude might have little practical value. Researchers, therefore, must pay attention to the numerical values obtained in an analysis in addition to the significance level when assessing the implications of the findings.

The support of research hypotheses with empirical evidence never constitutes proof of their veracity. Hypothesis testing, as we have seen, is probabilistic. There always remains a possibility that the obtained relationships were due to chance. Therefore, one must be tentative about both the results and the interpretations given to those results. Care should also be taken in generalizing the results beyond the study sample, particularly if a nonrandom sampling plan has been used. In sum, even when the findings are in line with expectations, the researcher should exercise restraint in drawing conclusions.

Interpreting nonsignificant results

Failure to reject a null hypothesis is particularly problematic from an interpretative point of view. The statistical procedures currently prevalent are geared toward disconfirmation of the null hypothesis. The failure to reject a null hypothesis could occur for one or more reasons, and the researcher does not usually know which of these reasons pertains. First, the null hypothesis could actually be true. The nonsignificant result, in this case, would accurately reflect the absence of a relationship among the research variables. On the other hand, the null hypothesis could be false, in which case a Type II error would have been committed. The retention of a false null hypothesis can be attributed to several things, such as internal validity problems, the selection of a deviant sample, the use of a weak statistical procedure, or too small a sample. Unless the researcher has special justifications for attributing the nonsignificant findings to one of these factors, interpreting such results is a tricky business.

In any event, there is never justification for interpreting a retained null hypothesis as proof of a *lack* of relationship among variables. *The safest interpretation is that nonsignificant findings represent a lack of evidence for either truth or falsity of the hypothesis.* Thus, one can see that if the researcher's actual research hypothesis states that no differences or no relationships will be observed, traditional hypothesis testing procedures will not permit the required inferences.

When no significant results are found, there is sometimes a tendency to be overcritical of one's research strategy and methods and undercritical of the theory or logical reasoning on which the hypotheses were based. This is understandable: it is easier to say "My ideas were all right, I just didn't use the right approach to demonstrate this" than to admit that one has reasoned incorrectly. It is important to look for and identify flaws in the research methods, but it is equally important to search for theoretical shortcomings. The result of such endeavors should be recommendations for how the methods and/or theory could be improved.

Even though it is important to examine both theoretical and methodological issues in trying to understand nonsignificant findings, we suspect that the majority of nursing research studies in which the null hypothesis is not rejected are the consequence of insufficient power (usually reflecting too small a sample size). We encourage researchers to use power analyses (described in Chapter 22) prior to conducting research in order to minimize the risk of a Type II error.

Interpreting unhypothesized significant results

There probably is nothing more perplexing to a researcher than to obtain results opposite to those hypothesized. For instance, a nurse researcher might hypothesize that individualized patient teaching of breathing techniques is more effective than group instruction, but the results might reflect that the group method was better. Or a positive relationship might be predicted beween a nurse's age and level of job satisfaction but a negative relationship might be found.

It should go without saying that it is unethical to alter the hypothesis after the results are in. Although some researchers may view such situations as awkward or embarrassing, there is really little basis for such feelings. The purpose of research is not to corroborate the scientist's notions, but to arrive at truth and enhance understanding. There is no such thing as a study whose results "came out the wrong way," if the "wrong way" is the truth.

In the case of unhypothesized significant findings, it is less likely, though not impossible, that the methods are flawed than that the reasoning or theory is incorrect. As always, the interpretation that the researcher gives to the findings should involve comparisons with other research, a consideration of alternate theories, and a critical scrutiny of the data collection and analysis procedures. The final result of such an examination should be a tentative explanation for the unexpected findings, together with suggestions for how such explanations could be tested in other research projects.

Interpreting mixed results

The interpretive process is often confounded by mixed results. The investigator may find some hypotheses supported by the data, while others cannot be supported. Or a hypothesis may be accepted when one measure of the dependent variable is used but rejected when using a separate measure of the same variable. Of all the situations mentioned, mixed results are probably the most prevalent.

When only some results run counter to a theoretical position or conceptual scheme, the research methods are probably the first aspect of the study deserving of scrutiny. Differences in the validity and reliability of the various measures could account for such discrepancies, for example. On the other hand, mixed results could be indicative of how a theory needs to be qualified, or of how certain constructs within the theory need to be reconceptualized.

In sum, the interpretation of research findings is a demanding task, but offers the possibility of unique intellectual rewards. The researcher must in essence play the role of a scientific detective, trying to make pieces of the puzzle fit together so that a coherent picture emerges.

Other issues in interpretation

In addition to trying to make sense of the analyses, several other considerations emerge in interpreting study outcomes. The first concerns the generalizability of the results (i.e., the study's external validity). Researchers are rarely interested in discovering relationships among variables for a specific group of people at a specific point in time. The aim of research is typically to reveal enduring relationships, the understanding of which can be used to improve the human condition. If a nursing intervention under investigation is found to be successful, others will want to adopt the procedure. Therefore, an important interpretive question is whether the intervention will "work" or whether the relationships will "hold" in other settings with other people. Part of the interpretation process involves asking the question "To what groups, environments, and conditions can the results of the study be applied?"

A second issue concerns the use of the interpretation as a springboard for additional research. Interpretations are necessarily speculative: they represent one's best guess — albeit an educated guess — about what the data really mean. Therefore, the interpretation represents a good starting point for suggesting further lines of inquiry. Is a replication needed, and, if so, with what groups? Are methodological refinements needed to really test the hypothesis? If observed relationships are significant, what do we need to know next in order for the information to be maximally useful?

Finally, the interpretative task is not complete without considering the implications of the findings for nursing. Do the findings have implications for what is taught to nursing students, or for how nursing content should be taught? Are the results of potential use to clinical nurses? Typically, the results of an investigation can have several applications, and this should be kept in mind in trying to formulate an interpretation of the study's results. Of course, if the study is seriously flawed it may be that the results are not usable within the nursing profession. But they will probably be useful, nevertheless, in designing an improved new study for the same research question.

☐
The research report: content

No scientific project is ever complete until a research report has been written. The most brilliant piece of work is of little value to the scientific community unless that work is known. The task of writing the final report may appear to be anticlimatic: after all, the researcher has satisfied his or her curiosity. Nevertheless, the reporting of results adds to knowledge on some issue and is a scientist's responsibility. It is also to the researcher's advantage to have research findings known by others, because proper credit should be given to the work that has been completed.

Research reports are written for different audiences and for different purposes. A thesis or dissertation not only communicates the research strategy and results but also serves as documentation of the student's thoroughness and ability to perform scholarly empirical work. Theses and dissertations, therefore, are rather lengthy documents. Journal articles, on the other hand, are typically short because they must compete with other reports for limited journal space and because they will be read by busy professionals.

Despite these differences, the general form and content of research reports are quite similar. The major distinction lies in the amount of detail reported. In this section we review the type of material that is covered in the four major sections of a research report: the introduction, methods, results, and discussion sections. The important distinctions between the various kinds of reports are described later in the chapter.

The introduction

The purpose of the introductory section of a research report is to acquaint readers with the research problem on which the investigation has focused. A precise and unambiguous problem statement, phrased in question form, is of immense value in communicating to the reader the major objectives of the study. If formal hypotheses have been developed, they should also be identified in the introduction.

The researcher should explain enough of the background of the study to make clear the reasons that the problem was considered worth pursuing. The justification of a nursing research problem should ideally include both the practical and theoretical significance of the study. This ideal is not always feasible. Not all studies have a direct bearing on theoretical issues, nor should they all necessarily be expected to have such a bearing in a practicing profession such as nursing. With the present state of knowledge, no one should feel apologetic if a study can solve a practical problem but is not linked to a theory. Artificial attempts to contrive theoretical relevance do nothing to advance scientific knowledge and should be avoided. Of course, studies that are framed within a theoretical context are most likely to make enduring contributions to knowledge about nursing and the nursing process. The introductory section should make explicit such theoretical rationales when they exist.

The statement of the problem should also be accompanied by a summary of related research, so that the research may be seen in an appropriate context. The review of the literature helps to clarify the theoretical and practical foundations of the research problem. Chapter 5 described in greater detail the write-up of the literature review section.

Finally, the introductory section should incorporate definitions of the concepts under investigation. Sometimes complete operational definitions are reserved for the "Methods" section, but a reader should have a fairly good idea early in the report what the researcher had in mind with regard to such terms as "grief," "stress," "therapeutic touch," and so forth.

In sum, the purpose of the introduction is to set the stage for a description of what was done and what was discovered. The introductory section should answer the questions: "What did the researcher want to know?" "Why did he or she want to know it?" and "What is the likely significance of such a study?"

The methods section

The scientific reader needs to know what has been done to solve the problem. The methods section should have as its goal a description of what was done to collect and analyze the data in sufficient detail such that another researcher could replicate the study if desired. In theses and final reports to funding agencies, this goal should always be satisfied. In journal articles it is often necessary to condense the methods section. For example, it may be impossible to include a complete questionnaire, interview schedule or observation schedule. Nevertheless, the degree of detail should be sufficiently adequate to permit a reader to evaluate the manner in which the research problem was solved.

The methods section is often subdivided into several parts. The reader needs to know, first of all, who the subjects participating in the study were. The description of the subjects normally includes the specification and description of the population from which the sample was drawn. If the target and accessible populations are not identical, then both populations should be discussed. The method of sample selection, the reasons for the selection of this sampling design, and the sample size need to be clearly delineated so that the reader can estimate the generalizability of the findings. It is advisable to describe the basic characteristics of the subjects, such as their age, sex, and other relevant attributes, and to indicate, if known, the degree to which these characteristics are representative of the population. For instance, if it is known that a sample of nurses tends to underrepresent those who have not received a Bachelor's or higher degree, then this fact should be pointed out.

The design of the study is often given more detailed coverage in an experimental project than in a nonexperimental one. In an experiment, the researcher should indicate what variables were being manipulated, how subjects were assigned to groups, the nature of the experimental intervention, and the specific design adopted. In any type of study, it is essential to identify what steps were taken to control the research situation in general and extraneous variables in particular.

A critical component of the methods section is the description of the instruments used to measure the target variables. In rare cases, this description may be accomplished in three or four sentences, such as when a standard physiological measure has been utilized. More often, a detailed explanation of the instruments and a rationale for their use are required in order to communicate to the reader the manner in which the variables were operationalized. When it is not feasible to include the actual research instrument within the report, its form and content should be outlined in as much detail as possible. It is insufficient to merely say "A questionnaire containing questions on the research problem was administered to the subjects." How many questions did the instrument include? Were the items open-ended or closed-ended? What were the major sections of the instrument and how were these sections organized? Whenever the instrument is not incorporated in the report, it is courteous to indicate from whom a copy of the complete instrument could be obtained. If the measuring devices were constructed specifically for the research project, the report should describe how they were developed, the methods used for pretesting, revisions made as a result of pretesting, coding and scoring procedures, and guidelines for interpretation. Any information relating to the validity and reliability of the instruments should also be mentioned.

A procedure section provides information about what steps were followed in actually collecting the data. In an experiment, how much time elapsed between the intervention and the measurement of the dependent variable? In an interview study, where were the interviews conducted and how long, on the average, did each one last? In an observational study, what was the role of the observer vis à vis the subjects? When questionnaires are used, how were they delivered to respondents and were follow-up procedures used to increase the response rate? Any unforeseen events occurring during the collection of data that could affect the findings should be described and assessed. Those reading a report must be in a position to evaluate the quality of the data obtained, and a description of research procedures assists in this evaluation.

A delineation of the statistical analyses and, when applicable, the computer programs used to handle the data is sometimes incorporated into the methods section and sometimes put with the results of the analyses. From the reader's point of view, it is usually preferable to explain the analytic approach in the methods section so that he or she will be able to judge the appropriateness of the research methods taken as a whole. It is not necessary to give computational formulas or even references for commonly used statistical procedures. For unusual procedures, or unusual applications of a common procedure, a technical reference justifying your approach should be noted.

The results section

The results section summarizes the results of the analyses. If both descriptive and inferential statistics have been used, the descriptive statistics ordinarily come first. If both quantitative and qualitative analysis has been performed, the qualitative analyses are often placed later because of their ability to explain the meaning of statistical analyses. On the other hand, in some cases quantitative results may serve a useful summation or confirmatory function and may be more meaningful after a presentation of qualitative results. The researcher must be careful to report all results as accurately and completely as possible, whether or not the hypotheses were supported. If there are too many analyses for inclusion in the report, the criterion used to select analyses should be their relevance to the overall objectives of the study.

When the results of several analyses are to be presented, it is frequently useful to summarize the findings in a table. Good tables, with precise headings and titles, are an important way to economize on space and to avoid dull, repetitive statements. Important findings can then be highlighted in the text. Figures that present the results in graphic form are used less as an economy than as a means of dramatizing important findings and relationships. Tables and figures should be numbered for easy reference.

Although we will discuss style in a later section, it is difficult to avoid the mention of style here. The write-up of statistical results is often a difficult task for beginning researchers, because they are unsure both about what should be said and about the style in which to say it. A few suggestions may prove helpful. By now, it is hopefully clear that research evidence does not constitute proof of anything, but the point bears repeating here. The research report should never claim that the data "proved," "verified," "confirmed," or "demonstrated" that the hypotheses were correct or incorrect. Hypotheses are "supported" or "not supported," "accepted" or "rejected." It may seem a trivial point, but the presentation of results should be written in the past tense. For example, it is inappropriate to say "Nurses who receive special training perform triage functions significantly better than those without training." In this sentence, "receive" and "perform" should be changed to "received" and "performed." The present tense implies that the results are generalizable to all nurses, when in fact the statement pertains only to a particular sample whose behavior was observed in the past.

When the results of statistical tests are reported, three pieces of information are normally included: the value of the calculated statistic, the number of degrees of freedom, and the significance level. For instance, it might be stated: "A chi-square test revealed that patients who were exposed to the experimental intervention were significantly less likely to de-

velop decubitus ulcers than patients in a control group ($\chi^2 = 8.23$, $df = 1$, $p < .01$)." The researcher who is writing up a results section for the first time would profit from using as a model a research report published in a professional journal.

The discussion section

A bare report of the statistical findings is never sufficient to convey their full implications. The meaning that a researcher gives to the results plays a rightful and important role in the report. The discussion section is typically devoted to a consideration of interpretations, limitations, and recommendations.

The interpretation of the results, as discussed earlier, involves the "translation" of statistical findings into practical and conceptual meaning. The interpretative process is a global one, encompassing the investigator's knowledge of the results, the methods, the sample characteristics, related research findings, and theoretical issues. Included with the interpretations should be a statement of the population to which the results can reasonably be generalized. The researcher should justify the interpretations, explicitly stating why alternative explanations have been ruled out. If the findings conflict with those of earlier research investigations, tentative explanations should be offered.

Although the readers should be told enough about the methods of the study to identify its major weaknesses, report writers should point out the limitations themselves. The researcher is in the best position to detect and assess the impact of sampling deficiencies, design problems, instrument weaknesses, and so forth, and it is a professional responsibility to alert the reader to these difficulties. Moreover, if the writer shows that he or she is aware of the study's limitations, then the reader will know that these limitations were not ignored in the development of the interpretations.

The implications derived from a study are often speculative and, therefore, should be couched in tentative terms. For instance the kind of language appropriate for a discussion of the interpretations is illustrated by the following sentence: "The results suggest that it may be possible to improve nurse-physician interaction by modifying the medical student's stereotype of the nurse as the physician's handmaiden." The speculative nature of the researcher's interpretation should be demonstrated in another way. The interpretation is, in essence, a hypothesis and as such can presumably be tested in another research project. The discussion section, thus, should include recommendations for investigations that would help to test this hypothesis, as well as suggestions for other research to answer questions raised by the findings of the study.

Other aspects of the report

The materials covered in the four sections reviewed are found in some form in virtually all research reports, although the organization might differ slightly. In addition to these major divisions, some other aspects of the report deserve mention.

Every research report should have a title. The phrases "Research Report" or "Report of a Nursing Research Investigation" are not adequate. The title should indicate to prospective readers the nature of the study. Insofar as possible, the dependent and independent variables should be named in the title. It is also desirable to indicate the population studied. However, the title should be brief (no more than about fifteen words), so the writer must balance clarity with brevity. Some examples of titles include the following:

The Effect of Advance Information on Pain
Perception in Hospitalized Children
Attitudes Toward Preventive Health Care in
the Urban Working Class

Educational Preparation: Its Effects on Role
Conflict Among Nurses

If the title gets too unwieldy, its length can often be reduced by omitting unnecessary terms such as "A Study of . . . " or "An Investigation to Examine the Effects of . . . " and so forth. The title should communicate clearly and concisely the phenomena that were researched.

Journals and theses often require the preparation of an abstract to precede the main body of the report. *Abstracts* are brief descriptions of the problem, methods, and findings of the study, written so that a reader can assess whether the entire report should be read. Abstracts typically are as short as 100 or 200 words. Since the abstract may be the only part of the report that is read, the writer should describe only that which is essential in order for the reader to grasp what the study was all about. Sometimes a report concludes with a brief summary and the summary, in such cases, usually substitutes for the abstract.

□
Types of research reports

Although the general form and structure of a research report are fairly consistent across different types of reports, certain requirements vary. This section describes the content, structure, and features of three major kinds of research reports: theses and dissertations, journal articles, and papers for professional meetings. Reports for class projects are excluded not because they are unimportant but rather because they so closely resemble theses on a smaller scale. Final reports to agencies that have sponsored research are also not described. Most funding agencies issue guidelines for their reports and these guidelines can be secured from project officers. In most cases, reports to funding agencies require nearly as much detail and documentation as dissertations.

Theses and dissertations

Most doctoral degrees are granted upon the successful completion of an empirical research project. Empirical theses are sometimes required of master's degree candidates as well. Theses and dissertations typically document completely the steps performed in carrying out the research investigation. Faculty members overseeing the project must be able to judge whether the student has understood the research problem both substantively and methodologically. The majority of doctoral dissertations are between 150 and 250 pages long, double spaced.

Most universities have a preferred format for their dissertations, but the format shown below is fairly typical.

Preliminary Pages
    Title Page
    Acknowledgment Page
    Table of Contents
    List of Tables
    List of Figures
Main Body
    Chapter I. Introduction
    Chapter II. Review of the Literature
    Chapter III. Methods
    Chapter IV. Results
    Chapter V. Discussion and Summary
Supplementary Pages
    Bibliography
    Appendix

The preliminary pages for a dissertation are much the same as those for a scholarly book. The title page indicates the title of the study, the author's name, the degree requirement being fulfilled, the name of the university awarding the degree, the date of submission of the report, and the signatures of the dissertation committee members. The acknowledgment page gives the writer the opportunity to express appreciation to those who contributed to the completion of the project. The table of contents outlines the major sections and subsections of the report, indicating on which page the reader will find those sections of interest. The lists of tables and figures identifies by number, title, and page the tables and figures that appear in the text.

The main body of a dissertation incorporates those sections that were described earlier. The literature review often is so extensive for doctoral dissertations that a separate chapter may be devoted to it. When a short review is sufficient, the first two chapters may be combined. In some cases, a separate chapter may also be required to elaborate the study's conceptual framework.

The supplementary pages include a bibliography or list of references used to prepare the report, and one or more appendices. An appendix contains information and materials relevant to the study that are either too lengthy or too unimportant to be incorporated into the body of the report. Data collection instruments, listings of special computer programs, detailed scoring instructions, cover letters, permission letters, listings of the raw data, and unimportant statistical tables are examples of the kinds of materials included in the appendix. Some universities also require the inclusion of a brief *curriculum vitae,* or autobiography, of the author.

Journal articles

Progress in nursing research is dependent upon researchers' efforts to share their work with others. Dissertations and final reports to funders are rarely read by more than a handful of individuals. They are too lengthy and too inaccessible for widespread use. Publication in a professional journal ensures broadest possible circulation of scientific findings. From a personal point of view, it is exciting and professionally advantageous to have one or more publications.

A journal article generally follows the same form as that for the main body of a thesis, but articles are much shorter. The purpose of an article is not to demonstrate research competence but rather to communicate the contribution that the study makes to knowledge. Since readers are particularly interested in the findings of a research project, a relatively large proportion of the journal report normally is devoted to the results and discussion sections. For the sake of economy of journal space, the typical research article is only about 15 to 25 typed pages, double spaced.

Several nursing journals accept research articles for publication. *Nursing Research,* which is currently published six times annually, is one of the major communication outlets for research in the field of nursing. Other nursing journals that focus primarily on publishing empirical studies are *Advances in Nursing Science, Research in Nursing and Health,* and the *Western Journal of Nursing Research.* Nursing journals that are not devoted exclusively or even primarily to research but do accept research reports for publication include the *American Journal of Nursing, Heart and Lung, Nursing Forum, Nursing Outlook, Journal of Advanced Nursing, Journal of Obstetric, Gynecologic and Neonatal Nursing,* and *Journal of Gerontological Nursing.* Many journals not directly focusing on nursing also publish articles by nurse authors, such as *The American Journal of Public Health, Journal of School Health, Perceptual and Motor Skills, Family Planning Perspectives,* and numerous others. The prospective author should check through recent issues of journals under consideration for guidance concerning the journals' stylistic requirements and content coverage. Many publications make an explicit statement concerning the type of papers they are seeking. McCloskey and Swanson (1982) have prepared a valuable report on publishing

opportunities for nurses, which includes information on the circulation of the journal, number of copies of a paper required for submission, typical article word length, time for editorial decision and acceptance rate for 100 journals in nursing and related health fields.

Before submitting a paper to a journal, it is wise to let at least one person read and comment upon it. Usually an independent reader is able to spot weaknesses more readily than the authors. When the manuscript is finally prepared for journal submission, the required number of copies should be sent to the editor with a brief covering letter indicating the mailing address of at least one author.* Generally, the receipt of the manuscript is acknowledged immediately but the final decision concerning the paper's acceptance or rejection may require several months. Many journals have a policy of independent, blind reviews by two or more knowledgeable persons. By "blind," we mean that the reviewers do not know the identity of the authors of the article.

Accepted articles almost invariably are revised somewhat, either by the authors at the editor's request or by the editorial staff of the journal. If the paper is not accepted, authors are usually sent copies of the reviewers' comments or a summary of the reasons for its rejection. This information can be used to revise a manuscript before submitting it to another journal. A rejection by one journal should not discourage researchers from sending the manuscript to another journal. The competition for journal space is quite keen and a rejection does not necessarily mean that a study is unworthy of publication. Although it is considered unethical to submit an article to two journals simultaneously, manuscripts may need to

---

* By convention, the ordering of authors' names on a research report usually is alphabetical if authors have contributed equally, or in order of the importance of their contribution if otherwise. See Waltz *et al.* (1985) for a discussion of author credits.

be reviewed by several journals before final acceptance.

Papers read at professional conferences

Numerous professional organizations sponsor annual national meetings at which reports on research activities are read. The ANA is an example of an organization that holds meetings where nurses have an opportunity to share their knowledge with others interested in their research topic. Many local chapters of Sigma Theta Tau devote one or more of their yearly activities to research reports. Examples of regional organizations that sponsor research conferences are the Western Society for Research in Nursing, the Southern Council on Collegiate Education for Nursing, and the Eastern Conference on Nursing Research. Other nursing organizations such as the Society for Research in Nursing Education, the American Association of Critical Care Nurses, the American Association of Neurosurgical Nurses and the Congress of Nursing in Child Health have research conferences. Professional organizations such as the Association for the Care of Children's Health, the American Anthropological Association, the American Public Health Association, and the Orthopsychiatry Society have sessions that are of interest to nurses.

Reading a paper at a conference has at least two advantages over journal publication. First, there is generally less time elapsed between the completion of a research project and its communication to others when a presentation is made at a meeting. Second, there is an opportunity for dialogue between the researcher and the audience at a professional conference. The listeners can request clarification on certain points and can suggest interesting modifications to the research paradigm. Researchers also can take advantage of meeting and talking with others who are working on the same or similar problems in different parts of the country.

The mechanism for submitting a paper to a conference is somewhat simpler than in the case of journal submission. The association sponsoring the conference ordinarily publishes a "Call for Papers" in its newsletter or journal about 6 to 9 months prior to the meeting date. The notice indicates requirements and deadlines for submitting a paper. The journal *Nursing Research* publishes a "Call for Papers" section as one of its regular departments. Usually, an abstract of 500 to 1000 words is submitted rather than the full paper. If the paper is accepted for presentation, the researcher is committed to appear at the conference to read the report.

Papers of empirical work presented at professional meetings follow much the same format as a journal article. The report is typically quite condensed, inasmuch as the time allotted for presentation ranges from 10 to 20 minutes. Therefore, only the most important aspects of the study can be included in the paper. A handy rule of thumb is that a page of double-spaced text requires 2½ to 3 minutes to read aloud. Presentations are usually more effective, however, if they are informal summaries of research than if they are read verbatim from a written text.

☐
The style of a research report

A scientific report is not an essay but rather a factual account of how and why a problem was studied and what results were obtained. The report should generally not include overtly subjective statements, emotionally laden statements, or exaggerations. When opinions are stated, they should be clearly identified as such, with proper attribution if the opinion was expressed by another writer. In keeping with the goal of objective reporting, personal pronouns such as "I" and "my" and "we" are often avoided, because the passive voice and impersonal pronouns do a better job of conveying impartiality. However, some journals are beginning to break with this tradition and are encouraging a greater balance between active and passive voice and first person and third person narration. If a direct presentation can be made without sacrificing objectivity, a more readable and lively product usually will result.

It is not easy to write simply and clearly, but these are important goals of scientific writing. The use of pretentious words or technical jargon does little to enhance the communicative value of the report, although colloquialisms should be avoided. Similarly, complex sentence constructions are not necessarily the best way to convey ideas. The style should be concise and straightforward. If writers can add elegance to their reports without interfering with clarity and accuracy, so much the better, but the product is not expected to be a literary achievement. Needless to say, this does not imply that grammatical and spelling accuracy should be sacrificed. The research report should reflect scholarship, not pedantry.

With regard to references and specific technical aspects of the manuscript, various styles have been developed. The writer may be able to select a specific style but often such considerations are imposed by journal editors and university regulations. Specialized manuals such as those of Turabian (1973), the American Psychological Association (1983), and Linton (1972) are widely used. Two nursing research journals *(Nursing Research* and *Research in Nursing and Health)* use the reference style recommended by the American Psychological Association (APA), which is the reference style used in this book.

A common flaw in the reports of beginning researchers is inadequate organization. The overall structure is relatively inflexible and, therefore, should pose no difficulties, but the organization within sections and subsections needs careful attention. Sequences should be in an orderly progression with appropriate transition. Themes or ideas should not be introduced too abruptly nor abandoned suddenly. Continuity and logical thematic development are critical to good communication.

First drafts of research reports are almost never perfect. The assistance of a colleague or an adviser can be invaluable in improving the quality of a scientific paper. Objective criticism can often be achieved by simply putting the report aside for a few days and then rereading it with a fresh outlook. As a final check, one might try to subject one's work to an evaluation according to the guidelines presented in Chapter 26.

☐
Summary

The interpretation of research findings basically is a search for the broader meaning and implications of the results of an investigation. The results of the data analysis need to be scrutinized and reflected upon with consideration to the objectives of the project, the conceptual framework, the specific hypotheses that were tested, prior research findings, and the shortcomings of the methods used to answer the research questions. Whether one's hypotheses are supported or not, it is important to be objective, to avoid the temptation of reading too much into the results, to be critical of both conceptual and methodological weaknesses, and to consider alternative explanations for the obtained findings.

The research project is not complete until the results have been communicated in the form of a report. Despite some differences in the length, purposes, and audience of different types of research reports, the general form and content are similar. In general, the four major sections of a research report are the introduction, methods, results, and discussion.

The purpose of the introductory section is to acquaint the readers with the research problem. This section includes the problem statement, the research hypothesis, a justification of the importance or value of the research, a summary of relevant related literature, the identification of a theoretical framework, and definitions of the concepts being studied. The methods section acquaints the reader with what the researcher did to solve the research problem. This section normally includes a description of the subjects, how they were selected, the target and accessible populations, the study design, the instruments used to collect the data, the procedures used, and the techniques used to analyze the data. In the results section, the findings obtained from the analyses are summarized. Finally, the discussion section of a research report presents the researcher's interpretations of the results, together with a consideration of the study's limitations and recommendations for future research.

The major types of research reports are theses and dissertations, reports to funding agencies, journal articles, and papers presented at professional meetings. When space or time are at a premium—as in the case of journal articles and conference papers—detail should be kept to a minimum. In other types of reports, however, extensive documentation may be required.

Scientific communications should be written as simply and clearly as possible. Emotionally laden statements, overtly subjective statements, and exaggerations should be excluded from research reports. Various reference manuals exist to assist the researcher in selecting a consistent and acceptable style for noting references and handling other technical aspects of report writing. The style should be congruent with that of the university or journal to which the report is submitted.

☐
Study suggestions

1. Write an abstract for McCubbin's article "Nursing assessment of parental coping with cystic fibrosis," which appeared in the Fall 1984 issue of *Western Journal of Nursing Research* (Volume 6, No. 4, pp. 407–418). Compare your abstract with that written by a classmate.
2. Read the article by Roberts, Cerruti, and O'Reilly in the May-June 1976 issue of *Nursing Research* in which mixed results were obtained. How did they interpret the results? What are some other interpretations that could be made?
3. What are the similarities and differences of research reports that are written for journal publication and for presentation at a professional meeting?
4. Suppose that a researcher has found that women who experience severe cramps during menstruation are more likely than women who do not experience the discomforts of menstrual cramps to smoke cigarettes. Suggest two or three different ways that this finding might be interpreted.

☐
Suggested readings

American Psychological Association (1983). *Publication manual* (3rd ed.). *Washington: American Psychological Association.*

Campbell, W.G. (1969). *Form and style in thesis writing* (3rd ed.). Boston: Houghton Mifflin.

Carnegie, M.E. (1977). Avenues for reporting research (editorial). *Nursing Research, 26,* 83.

Fuller, E.O. (1983). Preparing an abstract of a nursing study. *Nursing Research, 32,* 316–317.

Huth, E.J. (1982). *How to write and publish papers in the medical sciences.* Philadelphia: Institute for Scientific Information.

Knafl, K. A. & Howard, M.T. (1984). Interpreting and reporting qualitative research. *Research in Nursing and Health., 7,* 17–24.

Kolin, P.C. & Kolin, J.L. (1980). *Professional writing for nurses in education, practice, and research*. St. Louis: C.V. Mosby.

Linton, M. (1972). *A simplified style manual for the preparation of journal articles in psychology, social sciences, education, and literature*. New York: Appleton-Century-Crofts.

Markmam, R.H. & Waddell, M.J. (1982). *Ten steps in writing the research paper* (rev. ed.). Woodbury, NY: Barron's Educational Series.

McCloskey, J.C. & Swanson, E. (1982). Publication opportunities for nurses: A comparison of 100 journals. *Image, 14,* 50–56.

Mirin, S.K. (1981). *The nurse's guide to writing for publication*. Wakefield, MA: Nursing Resources.

Sexton, D.L. (1984). Presentation of research findings: The Poster Session. *Nursing Research, 33,* 374–377.

Strunk, W., Jr. & White, E.B. (1972). *The elements of style* (2nd ed.). New York: Macmillan.

Turabian, K.L. (1973). *A manual for writers of term papers, theses, and dissertations* (4th ed.). Chicago: University of Chicago Press.

Van Till, W. (1985). *Writing for professional publication* (2nd ed.). Boston: Allyn & Bacon.

Waltz, C.F., Nelson, B., & Chambers, S.B. (1985). Assigning publication credits. *Nursing Outlook, 33,* 233–238.

Wilson, H.S. (1985). *Research in nursing*. Menlo Park, CA: Addison-Wesley (Chapter 17).

Chapter 26
□
Evaluating research reports

Research in a practicing profession such as nursing contributes not only scholarly knowledge but also concrete information concerning how that practice can be improved. Nursing research, then, has relevance for all nurses, not just the minority of nurses who actually engage in research projects. As professionals, nurses should possess skills with which to critically evaluate reports of research in their field. Hopefully, the preceding chapters have provided an adequate basis for the development of such skills. In this chapter more specific guidelines for the critical and intelligent review of research are presented.

Many consumers have the unfortunate impression that if a research report was accepted for publication, it must be a good study. On the contrary, most research has weaknesses and limitations. This does not mean that the results of most research should be ignored. It does mean that the value and usefulness of a study must be judged with due consideration to both its strengths and flaws. The most provocative findings are of little practical or theoretical significance if the results are spurious and unreplicable. Faulty research designs and procedures that leave many loopholes for interpreting the results cannot inspire confidence in the ultimate worth of the study.

The function of critical evaluations of a scientific work is not to dogmatically hunt for and expose mistakes. A good critique objectively identifies adequacies and inadequacies, virtues as well as faults. Sometimes the need for such balance is obscured by the terms "critique" and "critical appraisal," which connote unfavorable observations. The merits of a study are as important as its limitations in coming to conclusions about the worth of its findings. Therefore, the research critique should reflect a thoughtful, objective, and balanced consideration of the study's validity and significance.

For each component of a research report, there are various questions that can be asked concerning the adequacy of the study's plan and execution. Some of these questions are general and can be applied to almost all investigations, while others are specific to a certain type of research. In the presentation that follows, a number of general and method-specific questions are listed in order to facilitate an orderly research critique. This list is not exhaustive. Many additional questions will need to be raised in dealing with a particular piece of research.

☐
Evaluating the introduction

The introduction sets the stage for the readers of a report. The manner in which the introductory materials are presented is vital to the proper understanding and appreciation of what the researcher has done and how he or she has done it. If the introduction does not adequately identify what the problem is and why it is important, the reader will experience difficulties in determining whether the solution was appropriate. Various requirements or desiderata of a good introduction are identified below.

The problem

Is the problem clearly and concisely stated?

Is the problem too big or too complex to be solved in a single investigation?

Does the problem statement give precise information about the independent and dependent variables?

Is the research question one that can be answered with empirical evidence?

Are definitions of the terms needed for a clear understanding of the study included?

Is the significance of the problem to nursing discussed?

Is the problem likely to have relevance and importance beyond the local scene?

Review of related literature

Does the report tie the problem to previous related research?

Is there an overdependence on secondary sources when primary sources could have been obtained?

Have important relevant references been omitted?

Does the review include recent literature?

Is there an overemphasis on opinion articles or anecdotes and an underemphasis on empirical work?

Is the review paraphrased adequately or is it a string of quotations from the original sources?

Is the review merely a summary of past work or does it critically appraise and compare the contributions of key studies?

Is the review organized such that the development of ideas is clear?

Does the review conclude with a brief synopsis of the literature and its implications for the problem under investigation?

Conceptual framework

Does the report attempt to link the problem to a theoretical or conceptual framework?

Is the theoretical framework tied to the problem in a natural way, or does the link seem contrived?

Would an alternative conceptual framework be more appropriate?

Are the deductions from a theory or conceptual framework logical?

Hypotheses

Does the report identify the hypotheses to be tested?

Does each hypothesis express a predicted relationship between two or more variables?

Do the hypotheses flow logically from the theoretical rationale or review of the literature? If not, what justification is offered for the reseacher's predictions?

Are all of the hypotheses testable?

Are the hypotheses concisely and unambiguously stated?

Do the hypotheses indicate the general population of interest?

□

Evaluating the reseach methods

The heart of the research critique lies in the analysis of the procedures used to solve the research problems. For any given research question, a vast number of alternative strategies exist. Each aspect of a study's methods involves a decision. The methods of selecting subjects, measuring variables, controlling extraneous factors, minimizing internal validity threats, and so forth are all selected by the researcher. Faulty methods can arise through the researcher's failure to consider the range of available alternatives, from poor judgment, or from external constraints such as inadequate resources or insufficient time to complete the study. It may be important to deduce which of these reasons is applicable: it makes little sense to point out what the researcher "should have done" when the report indicates or suggests that alternate methods were unfeasible or ruled out for specific reasons. Of course, when the report fails to make explicit the rationale for the adopted procedures, there is considerably greater room for negative criticism. Thus, one of the first questions to be answered is, Does the report clearly indicate the rationale for methodological decisions?

Research design: general

Is the design of the study adequately described?

Is the general approach (i.e., experimental, quasi-experimental, or nonexperimental) the best approach for addressing the research questions?

Does the design adequately control for threats to the internal validity of the study?

Are threats to the external validity of the study given adequate consideration in the research design?

If a cross-sectional design is used, would a longitudinal design be more appropriate?

If a longitudinal design is used, are methods for minimizing attrition biases discussed?

Research design: specific approaches

Experimental studies

Were subjects assigned to groups by a completely random process?

Is the design adequately described and is it appropriate?

Is the rationale for the selection of the design specified?

Were pretreatment data collected? Should they have been?

Quasi-experimental and preexperimental studies

Was the most powerful design used, given that an experimental design was not?

Is the method for the selection of comparison groups (if any) described?

Were steps taken to ensure the equivalence of comparison groups and are those steps adequate?

Does the report indicate the degree to which comparison groups *are* equivalent?

If no comparison group is used, is a rationale provided for why this is the case?

If no comparison group is used, are methods used to facilitate the interpretability of the results? Are these methods appropriate and successful?

Nonexperimental studies

Is there a comparison group? Should there have been?

Is the method for the selection of comparison groups (if any) described?

Were steps taken (such as matching) to produce roughly equivalent comparison groups and are those steps adequate?

Does the report indicate the degree to which the comparison groups used (if any) *are* equivalent?

Are the attributes or experiences that differentiate comparison groups (if any) clearly defined?

Are important uncontrolled extraneous variables described?

Has the best possible design been used (e.g., prospective vs. retrospective)?

Research procedures

Are the procedures used to execute the design clearly described in sufficient detail to permit replication by another reseacher?

Are procedures for ensuring constancy of conditions described?

Are procedures for preventing contamination between treatment groups discussed?

Is the setting of the study (field versus laboratory) appropriate for the research question?

Were the rights of the subjects protected?

Subjects

Is the population identified and described?

Given the research problem and limitations on resources, is the target population appropriately designated?

Does the report indicate whether an entire population or a sample was studied?

Would a more limited population specification have controlled for important sources of extraneous variation not covered by the research design?

Are the sampling selection procedures clearly described?

Is the sample design one that is likely to produce a representative sample?

If the sampling design is relatively weak (such as in the case of nonprobability sampling), are potential sample biases identified?

Are the size and key characteristics of the sample described?

Is the sample size sufficiently large, given the heterogeneity of the population?

Was the sample size justified on the basis of a power analysis?

Does the report indicate the response rate (i.e., the percentage of contacted persons agreeing to participate in the study)?

Data collection methods: general

Are the data collection instruments clearly identified and described?

Given the research questions, were the data collection methods appropriate with regard to their degree of structure?

Are the data collection methods the most appropriate way possible to measure the critical variables (i.e., self-report, observation, etc.)?

If the instrument was developed specifically for the study, are the procedures for its development described?

If the instruments are new or adapted from earlier versions, have they been properly pretested?

Is evidence for the reliability of the instruments presented?

If yes, are the reliability coefficients of an acceptable magnitude? Is the type of reliability estimates obtained the most appropriate?

Is evidence for the validity of the instruments presented?

If yes, does the evidence indicate that the instruments are sufficiently valid for the use to which they are put?

Is the type of validity discussed (content, criterion-related, or construct) the most relevant for the instruments under consideration?

Are methods of coding unstructured materials described?

Data collection methods: specific major approaches

Interview schedules and questionnaires

Is the schedule or topic guide described or included in the report?

Do the questions adequately cover the complexities of the problem under investigation?

Are open-ended and closed-ended questions used effectively and with an appropriate admixture?

Are the questions simply and clearly phrased?

Do the questions tend to bias responses in a certain direction?

Are the directions for the interviews or respondents clear?

Are the qualifications and training of the interviews described?

Does the report indicate the place in which the interviews occurred?

Is the ordering of questions on the schedule meaningful and appropriate?

In closed-ended questions, do the responses adequately cover the alternatives?

Is the schedule or guide of an appropriate length?

Was confidentiality or anonymity of the respondents assured?

For questionnaires, are follow-up procedures described and, if so, were they suitable?

Scales

Is the rationale for selecting one scaling procedure as opposed to another explained (e.g., Likert vs. Guttman)?

Is the method for placing items on a scale judgmental or empirical (i.e., performed through factor analysis or item analysis)?

Are procedures for eliminating or minimizing response set biases described?

Are negative and positive items balanced?

Is the scale unidimensional?

Are directions to the respondents clear?

Is the scale sufficiently long?

If a preexisting scale was used, is its relevance to the objectives of the study clearly explained?

If a new scale was developed, is there adequate justification for failure to use an existing one?

Observational approach

Are the behaviors or conditions to be observed clearly defined?

Are the phenomena under observation the same phenomena described in the problem statement?

Is the unit of behavior adopted appropriate for the problem being studied?

Is the degree of concealment used consistent with the aims of the study and with ethical principles?

Is the category system (if any) adequately described and comprehensive?

Are observers required to make an inordinate amount of inferences?

Are observers required to code too many complex behaviors in too short a time frame?

Is the method of sampling behaviors discussed and is it appropriate?

Have the observers been sufficiently trained to use the observational methods?

Is interobserver reliability discussed and is it sufficiently high?

Are potential biases stemming from the observer or subject discussed?

Is the problem of subject reactivity and its implications discussed?

□
Evaluating the analysis and results

The results of a study are affected not only by the methods of collecting the data but also by the procedures used to analyze them. The data analysis should be consistent with the objectives of the study, the research design, the measurement level of the data, and with the assumptions underlying the use of a particular statistical test. Once these criteria are satisfied, it is desirable to use as powerful a procedure as possible. Beginning researchers may have some difficulty in handling this part of the critique if their statistical skills are weak, but many of the questions below are sufficiently general that an elementary knowledge of statistics should prove adequate for routine appraisals.

Data analysis: general

Were the data analyzed qualitatively, quantitatively, or both?

Was the type of analysis appropriate for the types of data that were collected?

If qualitative analysis was used, were appropriate steps taken to validate the findings?

Descriptive statistics

Are descriptive statistics presented?

Are the descriptive statistics appropriate for the data?

Were a sufficient number of descriptive statistics calculated to adequately summarize the major characteristics of the sample?

If only descriptive statistics are used, are they sufficient for the purposes of the research, or should inferential statistics be presented as well?

Are the statistics used appropriate for the level of measurement of the variables?

Inferential statistics

Are tests of statistical significance used to test hypotheses?

Are parametric tests used when the assumptions for parametric tests are patently violated?

Are nonparametric tests used when a more powerful parametric test would probably have been appropriate?

Is information unnecessarily thrown away by converting measures of a relatively high measurement level to lower-level measures (e.g., converting height in inches to the dichotomy tall/short)?

Are the tests of significance appropriate for testing the research hypotheses?

Does the report indicate the value of the computed statistic, the number of degrees of freedom, and the level of significance?

Findings

Are the results clearly presented?

Is the presentation of findings well organized?

Are tables and figures used effectively to highlight and streamline the results?

Are tables and figures well organized, properly labeled, and easy to understand?

Is there any evidence of bias in the reporting of the findings?

□
Evaluating the discussion

The discussion section of a research report provides the researcher with the opportunity to make sense of the various findings, to discuss the theoretical and practical implications of the findings, and to develop recommendations for new avenues of research. Inevitably, the discussion section is more subjective than other sections of the report. This subjectivity is not necessarily detrimental, because great insights spring from reseachers' personal experience, knowledge, and creative capacities—not from the data themselves. But subjectivity can often block insights if researchers read into the data only what they want to see.

Interpreting the findings

Are all of the important results discussed?

Is each result interpreted in terms of the original hypothesis to which it relates and to the conceptual framework?

Is each result interpreted in light of findings from similar research studies?

Are alternative explanations for the findings mentioned, and is the rationale for their rejection discussed?

Do the interpretations give due consideration to the limitations of the research methods?

Are the interpretations consistent with the results?

Are any unwarranted interpretations of causality made?

Is the language used in discussing the interpretations sufficiently tentative?

Are the interpretations organized in a meaningful fashion?

Is there evidence of bias in the interpretations?

Does the interpretation distinguish between practical and statistical significance?

Implications

Are implications of the study ignored, although a basis for them is apparent?

Are the implications of the study discussed in terms of the retention, modification, or rejection of a theory/conceptual framework?

Are the implications of the findings for nursing practice described?

Are the discussed implications appropriate?

Are generalizations made that are not warranted on the basis of the sample used?

Is due consideration given to the study's limitations in discussing its implications?

Recommendations

Are recommendations made concerning how the study's methods could be improved?

Are recommendations for specific nursing actions made on the basis of the implications?

Are recommendations for future research investigations made?

Are the recommendations thorough, consistent with the findings, and consistent with related research results?

□
Evaluating other aspects of the report

The issues raised in this section are of a relatively peripheral nature. Weaknesses detected in the main body of the report are naturally more critical to the success of the study than weaknesses found in supplementary materials. Similarly, methodological and conceptual flaws are more serious than stylistic shortcomings or grammatical errors. Still, a critique of the overall quality of the final product should bear in mind the questions noted below.

The title

Does the report have a title?

Is the title of a reasonable length?

Are important variables mentioned in the title?

Does the title suggest the population under investigation?

The summary or abstract

Does the report have a summary or abstract?

Is the abstract/summary too long or too short?

Does the abstract/summary restate the research problem?

Does the abstract/summary restate important findings?

Is the abstract/summary too vague or too detailed?

Bibliography and appendices

Is there a bibliographic entry for all cited references?

Is each bibliographic entry complete?

Are appendices used effectively to present lengthy or supplementay materials?

Stylistic considerations

Are the overall structure and format of the report good?

Is the overall report overly detailed or insufficiently detailed?

Is the writing style overly pompous or pretentious?

Is the writing style too personal and subjective?

Is sexist language avoided?

Are sentences inordinately complex?

Are transitions smooth and is the report characterized by continuity of thought and expression?

Are sentences grammatically correct?

Are words spelled correctly?

Stylistically, was the report pleasant to read?

□
Conclusion

In concluding this chapter, several points about the research critique should be made. It should be apparent to those who have glanced through the above questions that it will not always be possible to answer the questions satisfactorily on the basis of the research report. This is especially true for journal articles in which the need for economy often translates into a severe abridgement of methodological descriptions. Furthermore, there are many questions listed above that may have little or no relevance for a particular study. The inclusion of a question in the list does not necessarily imply that all reports should have all of the components mentioned. For instance, few reports (except perhaps theses) explicitly describe coding procedures. The questions are meant to suggest aspects of a study that often are deserving of consideration, and not meant to lay traps for identifying omitted and perhaps unnecessary details.

It must be admitted that the answers to many questions will call upon the reader's judgment as much as, or even more than, his or her knowledge. An evaluation of whether or not the most appropriate data collection procedure was used for the research problem necessarily involves a degree of subjectiveness. Issues concerning the appropriateness of various strategies and techniques are topics about which even experts disagree. One should strive to be as objective as possible and to indicate one's reasoning for the judgments made.

□
Summary

Evaluating research reports involves critically appraising both the merits and the limitations of the published report. A systematic assessment of the various sections of a research report is essential in judging the utility and value of a study. This chapter offers a series of questions for the introduction, methods, data analysis/results, and discussion sections of a research report.

☐
Study suggestions

1. Read the article by Rottkamp in *Nursing Research,* 1976, volume 25, pages 181–186. What limitations of the research methods does she offer? Do these limitations alter your acceptance of the findings?
2. Answer the general questions raised in this chapter concerning *Research Design* and the specific questions concerning quasi-experimental study design for the 1985 La-Montagne *et al.* study that appeared in *Nursing Research* (Volume 34, pp. 289–292). What is your evaluation of this study's research design?
3. Read an article from any issue of *Nursing Research* and systematically assess the article according to the questions contained in this chapter. What are the merits and limitations of the report?
4. Review the research critique presented in Polit and Hungler (1985), Chapter 19.

☐
Suggested readings

Aamodt, A.M. (1983). Problems in doing nursing research: Developing criteria for evaluating qualitative research. *Western Journal of Nursing Research, 5,* 398–402.

Downs, F.S. (1977). Elements of a research critique. In F.S. Downs & M.A. Newman (Eds.). *A source book of nursing research* (2nd ed.). Philadelphia: F.A. Davis, (pp.1–12).

Field, W.E. (1983). Clinical nursing research: A proposal of standards. *Nursing Leadership, 6,* 117–120.

Fleming, J.W. & Hayter, J. (1974). Reading research reports critically. *Nursing Outlook, 22,* 172–175.

Gehlbach, S.H. (1982). *Interpreting the medical literature.* Lexington, MA: The Collamore Press.

Horsley, J. & Crane, J. (1982). *Using research to improve nursing practice: A guide.* New York: Grune & Stratton.

Leininger, M.M. (1968). The research critique: Nature, function and art. *Nursing Research, 17,* 444–449.

Norbeck, J.S. (1979). The research critique. *Western Journal of Nursing Research, 1,* 296–306.

Parse, R., Coyne, A., & Smith, M. (1985). *Nursing research: Qualitative methods.* Bowie: Brady Communication Co. (Chapter 11).

Polit, D.F. & Hungler, B.P. (1985). *Essentials of nursing research: Methods and applications.* Philadelphia: J.B. Lippincott (pp. 39–48, 336–380)

Sherman, K.M. & Kirsch, A.K. (1978). Can nursing educators deal effectively with nursing students' difficulty in critiquing nursing research articles? How can critical thinking be fostered? *Nursing Research, 27,* 69–70.

Ward, M.J. & Felter, M.E. (1978). What guidelines should be followed in critically evaluating research reports? *Nursing Research, 27,* 120–126.

Chapter 27
□
Writing a research proposal

This concluding chapter brings us, in a sense, full circle: back to the beginning of a research project. A research proposal is a written document specifying what the investigator proposes to study and is, therefore, written before the project has commenced. Proposals serve to communicate the research problem, its significance, and planned procedures for solving the problem to some interested party.

Proposals are written for various reasons. A student enrolled in a research class is often expected to submit a brief plan to the professor before data collection actually begins. Most universities require a formal proposal and a proposal hearing for students about to engage in research for a thesis or dissertation. Funding agencies that sponsor research almost always award funds competitively and use proposals as a basis for their funding decisions. Proposals prepared for different reasons vary in the amount of detail expected but, like research reports, often have similar content. In the next section, we provide some general information regarding the content and preparation of research proposals. In a subsequent section, we offer more specific guidelines for the preparation of a proposal for the National Institutes of Health, the federal agency that sponsors a great number of nursing studies.

□
Overview of proposal preparation

Reviewers of research proposals, whether they are faculty, funding sponsors, or peer reviewers, want a clear idea of what the researcher plans to do, how and when various tasks are to be accomplished, and whether the reseacher is capable of successfully following a proposed plan of action. Proposals are generally evaluated on a number of criteria, including the importance of the research question, its theoretical relevance, the adequacy of the research methods, the availability of appropriate personnel and facilities, and, if money is being requested, the reasonableness of the budget. Below are some general guidelines for preparing research proposals.

Proposal content

A researcher preparing a proposal will almost always be given a set of instructions that indicate the format to be followed. Funding agencies often supply an application kit that includes forms to be completed and a specified format for organizing the contents of the proposal.

Although each institution and funding agency has its own method of structuring content, there is considerable similarity in the type of information that is expected. The major "ingredients" normally required in research proposals include the following:

Abstract
Proposals often begin with a brief synopsis of the proposed research. The abstract helps to establish a frame of reference for the reviewers as they begin to read the proposal. The abstract should be brief (about 200 words) and should concisely state the study objectives and methods to be used.

Statement of the problem
The problem that the intended research will address is ordinarily identified early in the proposal. The problem should be stated in such a way that its importance is apparent to the reviewer. On the other hand, the researcher should not promise more than can be produced. A broad and complex problem is unlikely to be solvable or manageable.

Significance of the problem
The proposal needs to clearly identify how the proposed research would make an important contribution to knowledge. The proposal should indicate the expected generalizability of the research, its contribution to theory, its potential for improving nursing practice and patient care, and possible applications or consequences of the knowledge to be gained.

Background of the problem
A section of the proposal is often devoted to an exposition of how the intended research builds upon what has already been done in an area. The background material should strengthen the author's arguments concerning the significance of the study, orient the reader to what is already known about the problem, and indicate how the proposed research will augment that knowledge, and serve as a demonstration of the researcher's command of current knowledge in a field.

Objectives
Specific, achievable objectives, presented in their approximate order of importance, provide the reader with clear criteria against which the proposed research methods can be assessed. Objectives stated as research hypotheses to be tested are often preferred. Whenever the theoretical background of the study, existing knowledge, or the researcher's experience permit an explicit prediction of outcomes, these predictions should be included in the proposal. Avoid the use of null hypotheses, which create an amateurish impression. In exploratory or descriptive research, the formulation of hypotheses might not be feasible. Objectives may, in such cases, be most conveniently phrased as questions.

Methods
The explanation of the research methods should be thorough enough that a reader

would have no question about how the research objectives will be addressed. A thorough methods section includes a description of the sampling plan, research design, instrumentation, specific procedures, and analytic strategies, together with a discussion of the rationale for the methods, potential methodological problems, and intended strategies for handling such problems.

The work plan

It is customary for the proposal to describe the plan according to which the various tasks and subtasks will be accomplished. In other words, the researcher must show the sequence of tasks to be performed, the anticipated length of time required for their completion, and the personnel required for their accomplishment. The work plan indicates to the reader how realistic and thorough the researcher has been in designing the study.

Personnel

In proposals addressed to funding agencies, the qualifications of key project personnel should be described. The research competencies of the project director and other team members are typically given major consideration in evaluating a proposal.

Facilities

The proposal should document the extent to which special facilities required by the project will be available. Access to physiological instrumentation, libraries, data processing equipment, computers, special documents or records, and so forth should be described in order to reassure sponsors or advisors that the project will be able to proceed as planned. The willingness of the institution with which the researcher is affiliated to allocate space, equipment, or services should also be indicated.

Budget

The budget translates the project activities into monetary terms. It is a statement of how much money will be required to accomplish the various tasks. A well-conceived work plan greatly facilitates the preparation of the budget. If there are inordinate difficulties in detailing financial needs, there may be reason to suspect that the work plan is not as tight and detailed as it should be.

General tips on proposal preparation

While it would be impossible to tell readers exactly what steps to follow in order to produce a successful proposal, there are some pieces of advice we can offer that might help to minimize some of the anxiety and frustration that often accompany proposal preparation. Many of the tips we provide below are especially relevant for researchers who are seeking to obtain funding for a research project.

1. Review a successful proposal

While there is no substitute for actually doing one's own proposal as a learning experience, beginning proposal writers can often profit considerably by actually seeing the "real thing." The information in this text is useful in providing some guidelines, but reviewing an actual successful proposal can do more to acquaint the novice with how all the pieces fit together than all the textbooks in the world.

Chances are some of your colleagues have written a proposal that has been accepted (either by a funding sponsor or by a dissertation committee), and many people are glad to share their successful efforts with others. Also, proposals funded by the federal government are generally in the public domain. That means that you can ask to see a copy of proposals that have obtained federal funding by writing to the sponsoring agency.

In recognition of the need of beginning researchers to become familiar with successful proposals, *The Western Journal of Nursing Research* has begun to publish proposals in their entirety (with the exception of administrative information such as budgets), together with the critique of the proposal prepared by a panel of expert reviewers. For example, the first such published proposal was a grant application to the Division of Nursing entitled "Couvade: Patterns, predictors, and nursing management" (Clinton, 1985). Another journal, called *Grants Magazine,* also publishes successful proposals.

2. Pay attention to reviewers' criteria

In most instances in which research funding is at stake, the funding agency will provide the researcher with information about the criteria that reviewers use in making funding decisions. In some cases, the criteria will simply be a listing of questions that the reviewers must address in making some global assessment of the proposal's quality. In other cases, however, the agency will be able to specify exactly how many points will be assigned to different aspects of the proposal on the basis of specified criteria. As an example, the National Institute of Child Health and Human Development funded some research projects relating to fertility regulation in 1985 using the following evaluation criteria:

A. *Conceptualization of the Problem.* Ability of the researcher to conceptualize the problem, including the operationalizing and quantifying of measures, and the development of a theoretical/conceptual framework.

(0 to 30 points)

B. *Project Staff Qualifications and Availability.* (1) Adequacy of the relevant training and experience of the proposed staff.

(0 to 15 points)

(2) Appropriateness of allocation of personnel and time to accomplish objectives of the project.

(0 to 10 points)

C. *Data Sources and Analysis.* Demonstration of capability for identifying and obtaining access to pertinent and relevant sources of data and adequacy of plans for data analysis.

(0 to 20 points)

D. *Review and Analysis of Literature.* Adequacy of the review and analysis of the literature in terms of scope and depth and extent to which research needs in theoretical, methodological, and analytical areas are delineated.

(0 to 15 points)

E. *Facilities and Equipment.* Adequacy of computer facilities and other equipment that would be needed in the performance of the research.

(0 to 10 points)

Different agencies establish different criteria for different types of research projects. The wise researcher will learn what those criteria are and pay careful attention to them in the development of the proposal. In the above example, there is a maximum of 100 points to be awarded for each competing proposal. The proposals with the highest scores would ordinarily be most likely to obtain funding. Therefore, the researcher should pay particular attention to those aspects of the proposal that contribute most to an overall high score. For example, it would make little sense to put 85 percent of your proposal development effort into the literature review section, when a maximum of 15 points can be given for this part of the proposal.

3. Be judicious in developing a research team

For projects that are funded, reviewers often give considerable weight to the qualifications of the people who will conduct the research. In the example of reviewers' criteria shown above, a full 25 of the 100 points were based on the expertise of the research personnel and their time allocations.

It is often wise for the person who is in the lead role (often referred to as the *Principal Investigator* or PI) to carefully scrutinize the qualifications of the research team. It is not enough to have a team of competent people. It is necessary to have the right mix of competence. A project team of three brilliant theorists without statistical skills in a project that proposes sophisticated multivariate techniques may have difficulty convincing reviewers that the project would be successful. Gaps and weaknesses can often be compensated for by the judicious use of consultants.

Another shortcoming of many project teams is that they often look as though there are too many "Chiefs" and too few "Indians." It is generally unwise to load up a project staff with five or more top-level professionals who are only able to contribute 5 to 10 percent of their time to the project. Such projects often run into management difficulties because no one person is ever really in control of the flow of work. While collaborative efforts are to be commended, you should be able to *justify* the inclusion of every staff person and to identify the unique contribution that each will make to the successful completion of the project.

4. Justify and document your decisions

Unsuccessful proposals often fail because they do not provide the reviewer with confidence that adequate thought and consideration have been given to a rationale for decisions. Almost every aspect of the proposal involves a decision—the problem selected, the population studied, the size of the sample, the data collection procedures to be used, the comparison group to be used, the extraneous variables to be controlled, the analytic procedures

to be used, the personnel who will work on the project, and so on. These decisions should be carefully made, weighing the costs and benefits associated with making an alternative decision. When you are satisfied that you have made the right decision, you should be ready to defend your decision by sharing the rationale with the reviewers. In general, insufficient detail is more detrimental to the proposal than an overabundance of detail.

Grant applications to NIH

The National Institutes of Health (NIH) funds a considerable number of nursing research studies through the National Center for Nursing Research and through other institutes and agencies within NIH. Most NIH-funded projects to nurse researchers are funded through Research Project Grants for investigations submitted by established nurse researchers or New Investigator Research Awards that support small studies by new investigators. In both cases, applications for funding are made by completing Public Health Service Grant Application Form PHS 398, which is available through the research offices of most universities and hospitals. Copies of the application kit can also be obtained by writing

Division of Research Grants
National Institutes of Health
Westwood Building
5333 Westbard Avenue
Bethesda, MD 20205

Both research project and new investigator applications follow the same schedule for the processing of grant applications. That schedule is shown in Table 27-1.

Proposals (grant applications) may be submitted on the proper forms at any time during the year. However, proposals received after

Table 27-1
Schedule for processing grant applications

Receipt Dates	Initial (Peer) Review Dates	National Advisory Council Review Dates	Earliest Possible Start Dates
February 1	May/June	September/October	December 1
June 1	October/November	January/February	April 1
October 1	February/March	May/June	July 1

one due date will be held for another cycle. That is, if a proposal is received by NIH on February 2, it will be considered with the proposals received by June 1, not February 1.

The review process

As the above schedule indicates, NIH uses a dual review system for making decisions about its grant applications. The first level involves a panel of peer reviewers (usually those who have already obtained funding from NIH), who evaluate the grant application for its scientific merit. This panel consists of about 10 to 15 scientists, often with interdisciplinary backgrounds. The second level of review is by a National Advisory Council, composed of both scientific and lay representatives. The National Advisory Council takes into consideration not only the scientific merit of an application but the relevance of the proposed study to the programs and priorities of the Division or Institute to which the application has been submitted.

The peer review panel, after discussing the strengths and weaknesses of a given application, normally makes one of three decisions: to approve an application; to disapprove an application; or to defer an application. Deferrals are relatively rare and usually involve an application that the review panel considers meritorious but missing some crucial information that would permit the panel to make a final determination. Most proposals are either approved or disapproved immediately. Review panels vary considerably in the proportion of applications that are approved. In part this reflects the quality of the proposals themselves, but it also reflects the "philosophy" of different panels. Because not all projects that are approved are actually funded, some panels decide to disapprove only a very small minority of applications, reserving their disapprovals for projects that are judged to potentially "set back science." In review groups in which 25 percent or more of the proposals are disapproved, the panel is simply providing the message that the application was not considered worthy of funding.

All applications that are *approved* are assigned a priority rating by each member of the review panel. The ratings range from 1.0 (the best possible score) to 5.0 (the least favorable score), in increments of 0.1. The individual ratings are then combined and standardized to range from 100 to 500—with 100 being the best possible score. Among all approved applications, only those with excellent priority scores actually obtain funding. Cutoff scores for funding vary from agency to agency and year to year. It is often necessary to obtain a rating of 200 or lower to become funded. Within NIH, fewer than 20 percent of all grant applications are actually funded.

Each applicant is sent a summary of the peer review panel's evaluation. These "pink sheets" (so called because they are printed on pink paper) summarize the reviewers' comments in six areas: (1) an overall description of the project; (2) a critique of the strengths and weaknesses of the methodological and conceptual aspects of the proposal; (3) an evaluation of the project team; (4) an evaluation of the facilities and resources; (5) an assessment of the reasonableness of the budget; and (6) a discussion of other considerations, with emphasis on the protection of the rights of human subjects and/or the welfare of animal subjects. The applicant is also advised of the panel's decision (approval, disapproval, or deferral), and the priority rating, if the application was approved. Unless the proposal is criticized in some very fundamental way (for example, the problem area was not judged to be significant), it is often worthwhile to resubmit an application, making revisions that reflect the concerns of the peer review panel. When a proposal is resubmitted, the next review panel is usually given a copy of the original application and the "pink sheet" so that they can evaluate the degree to which the original criticisms have been addressed.

Preparing a grant application for NIH

As indicated above, proposals to NIH must be submitted according to procedures described in the Public Health Service application kit. Each kit specifies exactly how the grant application should be prepared and what forms are to be used for supplying critical pieces of information. It is important to follow these instructions precisely. Below we describe the various components of an application and provide some tips that should be helpful in completing certain sections.

Section 1

The "frontmatter" of the grant application consists primarily of forms that help in the processing of the application or that provide administrative information about the conduct of the research. Proposal writers often fail to give this section the attention it merits, because all of the intellectual work is presented in Section 2. However, we urge researchers to pay as much attention to detail in this first section as in the second. Each component of Section 1 is briefly described to acquaint the reader with its contents.

- *Title Page*. Here the researcher provides the title of the application (not to exceed 56 spaces), the name of the Principal Investigator, the name of the PI's institutional affiliation, the amount of money requested, the length of the proposed project, and other administrative information.
- *Abstract of Research Plan*. Page 2 asks for a listing of the key professional personnel who would work on the study and a half-page abstract of the investigator's aims and methods. The abstract *must* fit into the space allocated.
- *Table of Contents*. Page 3 indicates on what pages various sections and subsections of the proposal are to be found.
- *Budget*. Pages 4 and 5 consist of budgetary forms. Page 4 asks for an itemization of all costs that would be incurred by the project during the first 12 months. Page 5 asks for a summary of the budget for the entire project period. For Research Project Grants, support can be requested for up to five years, but the majority of projects are completed in three years or fewer. Beginning at the bottom of Page 5, the researcher must provide a narrative justification of all budgeted items. New researchers often make the mistake of submitting a budget justification that is insufficiently detailed. Remember that the reviewers need to be able to tell whether the budget is reasonable, and part of your job is to convince them that you will use funding judiciously. Normally two or three single-spaced pages are needed to justify budgetary items. Figure 27-1 presents a hypothetical "Page 4" (detail of first-year expenditures), and Figure 27-2 presents a hy-

(Text continues on p. 516)

REMOVE AND USE FOR DRAFT COPY

PRINCIPAL INVESTIGATOR/PROGRAM DIRECTOR: White, C.M.

DETAILED BUDGET FOR FIRST 12 MONTH BUDGET PERIOD
DIRECT COSTS ONLY

FROM 12/1/87 THROUGH 11/30/89

DOLLAR AMOUNT REQUESTED *(Omit cents)*

PERSONNEL *(Applicant organization only)* NAME	POSITION TITLE	TIME/EFFORT %	TIME/EFFORT Hours per Week	SALARY	FRINGE BENEFITS	TOTALS
Cozette White	Principal Investigator	25		10,000	2,500	12,500
Alison Lupping	Co-Investigator	10		3,000	750	3,750
To Be Hired	Interviewer	100	(9 mos)	13,500	3,375	16,875
To Be Hired	Research Asst/Coder	25		3,750	938	4,688
To Be Hired	Secretary	40		5,200	1,300	6,500
			SUBTOTALS →	35,450	8,863	44,313

	TOTALS
CONSULTANT COSTS	
Paul Speckman 5 days @ $250 (Statistical Consultant)	1,250
Henry Mitchell 20 days @ $125 (Programming Consultant)	2,500
EQUIPMENT *(Itemize)*	
Computer Modem	500
SUPPLIES *(Itemize by category)*	
Office Supplies $75./Mo. X 12	900
Xerox $50./Mo. X 12	600
Postage $40./Mo. X 12	480
Printing Instruments	750
Telephone (Long Distance)	500
TRAVEL — DOMESTIC: 1 Conference and Interviewer Travel	1,750
TRAVEL — FOREIGN	
PATIENT CARE COSTS — INPATIENT	
PATIENT CARE COSTS — OUTPATIENT	
ALTERATIONS AND RENOVATIONS *(Itemize by category)*	
CONSORTIUM/CONTRACTUAL COSTS	
Subcontract to Woodlawn Hospital	9,375
OTHER EXPENSES *(Itemize by category)*	
Subject Stipends - 200 @ $15	3,000
Data Entry - 200 X $3	600
Work Processing - 100 Hrs. @ $5/Hr.	500
Computer Time (Preliminary Analyses)	500
TOTAL DIRECT COSTS *(Also enter on page 1, item 7)* →	$67,518

PHS 398 (Rev. 5/82) PAGE 4

Figure 27-1. Example of first-year budget.

BUDGET FOR ENTIRE PROPOSED PROJECT PERIOD
DIRECT COSTS ONLY

BUDGET CATEGORY TOTALS		1st BUDGET PERIOD *(from page 4)*	ADDITIONAL YEARS SUPPORT REQUESTED			
			2nd	3rd	4th	5th
PERSONNEL *(Salary and fringe benefits.)* *(Applicant organization only)*		44,313	60,309			
CONSULTANT COSTS		3,750	5,000			
EQUIPMENT		500	---			
SUPPLIES		3,230	2,480			
TRAVEL	DOMESTIC	1,750	1,500			
	FOREIGN					
PATIENT CARE COSTS	INPATIENT					
	OUTPATIENT					
ALTERATIONS AND RENOVATIONS						
CONSORTIUM/ CONTRACTUAL COSTS		9,375	4,250			
OTHER EXPENSES		4,600	5,800			
TOTAL DIRECT COSTS		67,518	79,339			

TOTAL FOR ENTIRE PROPOSED PROJECT PERIOD *(Also enter on page 1, item 8)* ⟶ $ 146,857

JUSTIFICATION (Use continuation pages if necessary): Describe the specific functions of the personnel and consultants. If a recurring annual increas in personnel costs is anticipated, give the percentage. For *all* years, justify any costs for which the need may not be obvious, such as equipment, foreig travel, alterations and renovations, and consortium/contractual costs. For any additional years of support requested, justify any significant increases i any category over the first 12 month budget period. In addition, for COMPETING CONTINUATION applications, justify any significant increases ov the current level of support.

Personnel

White, the Principal Investigator, will be responsible for overall project management, instrument development, data quality control, data analysis, and report preparation. She is budgeted for 25% effort in the first 18 months of the project. In the final 6 months, White will devote 50% of her time to the proposed project to perform the data analyses and prepare a final report.

Lupping, the Co-Investigator, will devote 10% of her time to the project throughout the 2-year period. She will participate in the instrumentation, training of the interviewer, development of a coding scheme, and analysis of the data.

The Interviewer will be hired in the fourth project month. She will work for 15 months at 100% effort and will be responsible for all data collection. A research assistant will be hired to assist with such tasks as library research, instrument pretests, and data coding. Her level of effort will be 25% throughout the project. A secretary will be hired at 40% effort to perform secretarial and clerical functions.

A 5% salary increase has been budgeted for all personnel in Year 2.

Consultants

Dr. Paul Speckman, a professor of statistics, will provide 5 days of consulting in Year 1 and 10 days of consulting in Year 2 relating to the analysis of research data.

Mr. Henry Mitchell, a doctoral student in computer sciences, will provide 20 days of consulting in both project years to assist with the establishment of data files and the processing of research data.

Equipment

A DC Hayes modem (300/1200 baud) will be purchased to permit communication between the project's mini-computer and the university mainframe. The modem will permit a more efficient analysis of the data.

Figure 27-2. Example of overall summary budget.

pothetical "Page 5" for a study that would require two years of support. The bottom of Figure 27-2 includes the beginning of a budget justification, showing the level of detail that is ordinarily considered appropriate. Note that the NIH budget forms should show direct project costs only. Indirect institutional costs (overhead) are not included in the budget.

- *Biographical Sketches.* Forms are provided to summarize salient aspects of the education and experience of key project personnel. The Principal Investigator and any other proposed staff who are considered important contributors to the project's success must have their biographical sketches included. A maximum of two pages is permitted for each person.
- *Other Support.* Key personnel must identify any sources of support they are now receiving or sources of support that they have pending in the form of other planned or submitted proposals. This page is designed to help reviewers determine whether important staff may be overcommitted and therefore potentially not able to devote a sufficient amount of time to the proposed project.
- *Resources and Environment.* On this form the author must designate the availability of needed facilities and equipment, such as office space, computers, laboratories, medical apparatus, and so on.

Section 2

Section 2 of the NIH grant application is reserved for the investigator's research plan. This section consists of eight subsections, not all of which are relevant to all applications.

- *Specific Aims.* The researcher must provide a very succinct summary of the research problem and the specific objectives to be undertaken during the course of the project. *This section must be limited to one page.* Researchers sometimes try to get around the page limitations by making some statement such as, "Due to the complexity of the research to be undertaken, it is necessary to expand this section to include information important to the reviewers." We strongly recommend that researchers adhere strictly to page limitations. Reviewers are busy professionals and often are responsible for reviewing between 50 and 100 applications in one panel meeting. There is no point in antagonizing a reviewer by disregarding instructions. Restrict your description of the aims of the study to one page and save elaborating details for a subsequent section or an appendix.
- *Significance.* It is in this section that the researcher must convince the review panel that the proposed study idea is sound and has important practical or theoretical relevance. It is also in this section that the researcher provides the context for the conduct of the study. In other words, this section ordinarily includes a brief review of critical work that leads to the need for and importance of the proposed new work. Beginning researchers often have an especially difficult time with this section because *it is restricted to a maximum of three pages.* In other words, the review of important literature must be compressed into three (single-spaced) pages that also include a description of the study's significance. This is often a challenging task, especially if you have a firm grasp on the broad range of literature relating to your topic. However, we again urge reseachers not to be tempted to exceed the three-page limitation. If you have completed a thorough review of the literaure and want to demonstrate your expertise, include a comprehensive literature review as an appendix.

• *Preliminary Studies.* This section, limited to eight pages, is reserved for a description of the project team's previous studies that are relevant to the new proposed investigation. Many novice researchers mistakenly believe that this section is designed for a literature review. If you make this mistake, it will only serve to indicate that you are a novice and unable to follow instructions. This section is an important one, because it provides an opportunity to convince the reviewers that you have the skills and background needed to do the research. Since the biographical sketch is limited to only two pages, the "Preliminary Studies" section provides a forum for the description of any relevant work you and other key staff have either completed or are in the process of doing. If the only relevant research you have completed is your dissertation, here is an opportunity to describe that research in full. If you have completed research that has led to a publication or presentation at a conference, you might want to reference that in this section, and include a copy of the paper as an appendix. Other items that might be described in this section include previous uses of an instrument or experimental procedure that will be used in the new study; relevant clinical or teaching experience; membership on task forces or in organizations that have provided you with a perspective on the research problem; or the results of a pilot study that involved the same research problem. The point is that this section is designed to allow you to demonstrate that the proposed work grew out of some ongoing commitment to, interest in, or experience with the topic.

• *Experimental Design and Methods.* It is in this section that you describe the methods you will use to conduct the study. This section should be succinct, but with sufficient detail to alert reviewers that you have a good rationale for all of your decisions. There are no page limitations, but superfluous information should be omitted. Because this section is really the heart of the grant application, we will try to provide a number of helpful tips.

The Methods section will consist of a number of subsections that vary from one application to another. Each subsection should be labeled clearly. It is often useful to begin with an outline. Here is an outline of the sections used in a successful grant application for a study of parenting behavior and family environments among low-income teenage mothers:

1. Conceptual Framework
2. Hypotheses
3. Overview of the Research Design
4. Sampling Considerations
5. Research Variables and Measuring Instruments
6. Data Collection Procedures
7. Data Analysis
8. Research Products
9. Project Schedule

If you have an elaborate conceptual framework, you might be unable to adequately describe it and how it relates to your proposed research in the Significance or Specific Aims sections. In such a case, it is often reasonable to begin the Methods section with an explication of the conceptual model and a description of the rationale underlying any hypotheses to be tested.

A number of things should be included in a section on sampling. The reviewer normally expects to find a thorough description of the population, the proposed sample, the sampling design, and the number of subjects to be included. This information has an important bearing on the generalizability of the results. The section should include both a description of the sampling plan and a justification for its use. If you cannot use random sampling, explain the constraints (e.g., the costs of implementing such a design), and discuss steps you would take to make the sample as representative as possible and to document any biases. Increasingly, review panels are beginning to expect power analyses that justify the adequacy of the specified sample size. It is also advisable to document your access to the specified subject pool. For instance, if the proposal indicates that patients and personnel from Park Memorial Hospital will participate in the study, a letter of cooperation from an administrator of the hospital should be included in an appendix. The reviewer needs to have confidence that the proposed study, if funded, would actually be done as planned.

If there is an experimental intervention, that intervention should be described in full. Protocols for the implementation of the intervention also need to be discussed. If there is to be a control group, clearly identify how the control group will be selected. If the control group is an intact group, you will need to discuss in detail your rationale for the selection of the specified group, any shortcomings in using this group, and why this group is preferable to some alternative. For example, if you were to study the psychological consequences of an abortion in an effort to determine the need for follow-up interventions, you might select one of the following as a control group: (a) same-aged, never-pregnant women; (b) same-aged women who had had a miscarriage; (c) same-aged women who were still pregnant and had not decided how to resolve the pregnancy; or (d) same-aged women who had delivered a baby. Each group might be expected to introduce different types of selection biases, so your rationale for selecting one

over the other would be a critical reflection of your conceptualization of the problem and your methodological sophistication.

The design section should also indicate how the research situation will be structured to control for extraneous variables. The proposal should specify what variables need to be controlled, which variables *will* be controlled (and how), why other variables will not be controlled, and what the probable impact of the uncontrolled variables on the study outcome will be. Krathwohl has observed, "Probably nobody knows better than the researcher the multiple sources of contamination which might affect the study. Convincingly indicate the nature and basis of the particular compromise which is being proposed and the reasons for accepting it" (1977, p. 31).

Normally, an entire subsection is devoted to instrumentation. The use of particular measuring instruments should be justified as appropriate for the purposes of the study. It is not sufficient to select a well-known measure without explicitly demonstrating its relevance and valued qualities. For established measures, the proposal should describe reported evidence of the measure's reliability and validity. If a new instrument is to be developed, the anticipated procedures for its development *and* evaluation should be described. If possible, sample items or the entire instrument should be included in an appendix.

A subsection should be addressed to the specific procedures that will be used to collect the research data. This subsection should include such information as where the data will be collected, how subjects will be recruited, how research personnel such as interviewers or observers will be trained, whether or not subjects will be paid a stipend for their time, what quality control procedures will be implemented to ensure the integrity of the data, and how the security of the data will be maintained. If the study is longitudinal, it is also important to describe in detail how the problem of attrition will be managed.

The grant application should include, in as much detail as possible, the plan for the analysis of data. This is typically one of the weakest sections of proposals. Some applications say little more than, "Trust me — I'll figure out what to do with the data once I have collected them." You may not be able to tell in advance every analytic strategy you will try, but you should be able to work through the general procedures you will use in testing the hypotheses. It is often useful to provide "dummy tables" — tables that are likely to be included in the final report, but without any data in them. Earlier in this section we presented an outline of a grant application relating to parenting among teenage mothers. The Data Analysis section of this grant application was five single-spaced pages in length and consisted of the following subsections:

7. Data Analysis
   a. Data Cleaning and Descriptive Analyses
   b. Exploratory Analyses
   c. Analysis of Bias
   d. Testing Individual Hypotheses
   e. Path Analysis

Although the grant application kit does not specifically request a project schedule or work plan, it is nevertheless wise to include one. It will help reviewers assess how realistic you have been in planning the project, and it should help you to develop an estimate of needed resources (i.e., your budget). Flowcharts and other diagrams are often useful for highlighting the sequencing and interrelationships of project activities. One of the simplest and most effective types of charts is called a *Gantt chart,* named after its inventor Henry Gantt. Figure 27-3 presents the Gantt chart used in the grant application for the 30-month study of teenage parents, to which reference has previously been made. Other more sophisticated charting techniques, such as the *Program Evaluation Review Technique* (PERT) and the *Critical Path Method,* are sometimes used for complex projects. These are briefly described by Krathwohl (1977).

- *Human Subjects.* If the research involves data collected from human subjects, this section must describe the procedures that would be used to protect their rights and to minimize the risks that they would take. The application kit specifies six questions that need to be addressed in this section (see Appendix A). The researcher would do well to obtain a copy of the guidelines for the protection of the rights of human subjects developed by the Department of Health and Human Services (usually available at all institutions receiving NIH funds or through the NIH Division of Research Grants). This section of the proposal often serves as the cornerstone of the document submitted to the Institutional Review Board (IRB) of your institution prior to funding (check with your office of research administration for IRB requirements).
- *Vertebrate Animals.* If your proposed research involves the use of vertebrate animals, this section must contain a justification of their use and a description of the procedures used to safeguard their welfare.
- *Consultants.* If you plan to include consultants to help with specific tasks on the proposed project, you must include a letter

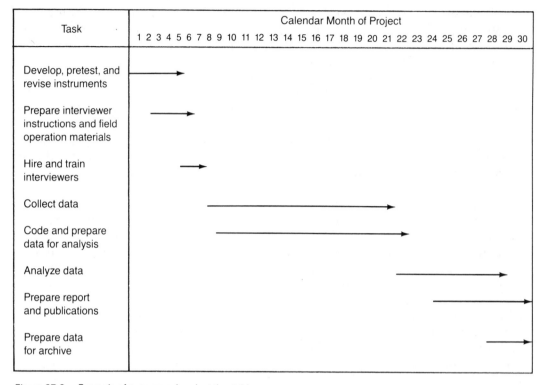

Task	Calendar Month of Project
	1 2 3 4 5 6 7 8 9 10 11 12 13 14 15 16 17 18 19 20 21 22 23 24 25 26 27 28 29 30
Develop, pretest, and revise instruments	
Prepare interviewer instructions and field operation materials	
Hire and train interviewers	
Collect data	
Code and prepare data for analysis	
Analyze data	
Prepare report and publications	
Prepare data for archive	

Figure 27-3. Example of a proposed project timetable.

from each consultant, confirming their willingness to serve on the project.
- *Literature Cited.* The final subsection of the Research Plan consists of a list of references used in the text of the grant application. Any reference style is acceptable.

Section 3.
The concluding section of the grant application is reserved for appended materials. This might include literature reviews, scoring instructions for instruments, coding instructions, a manual of interviewer instructions, actual instruments, proposed letters of consent, letters of cooperation from institutions that will provide access to subjects, relevant papers presented at conferences, or papers published in professional journals.

□
Funding for research proposals

Funding for research projects is becoming more and more difficult to obtain. The problem lies not only in research cutbacks and inflation but also in the extremely keen and growing competition among researchers. As increasing numbers of nurses become prepared to carry out significant research, so, too, will applications for research monies increase. Successful proposal writers need to have good research and proposal-writing skills, and they must also know how and from whom funding is available. The combined set of skills and knowledge is sometimes referred to as "grantsmanship."

Federal funding

The federal government is the largest contributor to the support of research activities. The two major types of federal disbursements are *grants* and *contracts*. Grants are awarded for proposals in which the research idea is developed by the investigator. The researcher who identifies an important research problem can seek federal monies through a grant program of one or more agencies of the government.

There are two basic mechanisms for the funding of federal grants. One mechanism is for agencies and institutes to issue broad objectives and priorities and to invite grant applications that address these objectives. For example, the overall purpose of the Division of Nursing grants program is "to enlarge the body of scientific knowledge that underlies nursing practice, nursing education, and nursing services administration, and to strengthen these areas through the utilization of such knowledge." Researchers apply for funding from this grants program through the process described in the preceding section.

There are several ways to find out about other grant programs. *The Catalogue of Federal Domestic Assistance* publishes information about all federal programs that provide any kind of aid. The programs of such agencies as National Institutes of Health (NIH), National Institute of Mental Health (NIMH), National Institute on Drug Abuse (NIDA), and so on are described in terms of objectives, types of assistance, award processes, and so on. *The Health Fields Directory* lists sources of federal funds that pertain specifically to health-related matters. Programs that seem particularly promising can then be contacted for further information.

The second grant-funding mechanism is a means for agencies to identify a topic area in which they are especially interested in receiving applications. An agency may announce, for instance, that it is soliciting grant applications for studies relating to infertility. Such an announcement is referred to as a *Request for Applications* or RFA. Unlike the more general grants programs, the RFA usually specifies a due date for the receipt of proposals. General guidelines and goals for the competition are also specified, but the researcher has considerable liberty to develop the specific research problem. Notices of such grant competitions are published in *The Federal Register*.

The second type of funding is in the form of contracts. An agency that identifies the need for a specific study issues a Request for Proposals (RFP), which details the work that the government wants done. Proposals in response to RFPs describe the methods the researcher would use in addressing the research problem, the project staff and facilities, and the cost of doing the study in the proposed way. Contracts are usually awarded to only one of the competitors. A summary of each federal RFP is printed in the *Commerce Business Daily,* which is published every government workday. Clearly, the contract method of securing research support severely constrains the kinds of work in which investigators can engage. For this reason, most nurse researchers probably will want to compete for grants rather than contracts. Nevertheless, many interesting RFPs have been issued by the National Institutes of Health. For example, one recent RFP called for proposals for a study of "Ethnic Differences in Life Style, Psychological Factors, and Medical Care During Pregnancy."

Private funds

Health-care research is supported by a number of philanthropic foundations and professional organizations. Many investigators prefer private funding to government support because there is less red tape. Private organizations typically are less rigid in their proposal regulations, their reporting requirements, clearance of instruments, and their monitoring of progress. Not surprisingly, private organizations are besieged with proposed research projects.

Information about philanthropic foundations that support research is available in *The Foundation Directory,* published by the Foundation Center. This volume, which is updated periodically, lists over 2500 foundations whose annual grants are at least half a million dollars. The directory lists the purposes and activities of the foundations and the addresses for contacting them.

Professional associations such as the American Nurses' Foundation, Sigma Theta Tau, the American Association of University Women, and the Social Science Research Council offer funds for conducting research. Health organizations such as the American Heart Association and the American Cancer Society also support research activities. Finally, funds for research are sometimes donated by private corporations, particularly those dealing with health-care products. Additional information concerning the requirements and interests of such groups should be obtained either from the organization directly or from personnel in research administration offices of universities, hospitals, or other agencies with which you are affiliated.

☐
Conclusion

Proposals represent the means for opening communication between researchers and parties interested in the conduct of research. Those "parties" may be funding agencies, faculty advisors, or institutional officers, depending upon the circumstances. An accepted proposal is a two-way contract: those accepting the proposal are effectively saying, "We are willing to offer our (emotional or financial) support, as long as the investigation proceeds as proposed," and those writing the proposal are saying "If you will offer support, I will conduct the project as proposed." Therefore, the proposal offers some assurance that neither party will be disappointed.

Beginning proposal writers sometimes forget that, in essence, they are selling a product: themselves and their ideas. It is not inappropriate, therefore, to do a little "marketing." If the researcher does not sound convinced that the proposed study is important and will be executed with skill, then the reviewers will not be convinced either. The proposal should be written in a positive, confident tone. Instead of saying "the study will *try to* . . . ," it is better to indicate more positively that the study *will* achieve some goals. Similarly, it is more optimistic to specify what the investigator *will* do, rather than what it *would* do, if approved. There is no need to brag or promise what cannot be accomplished. Rather, it is a question of putting the actual project accomplishments and significance in a positive light.

As another aspect of salesmanship, the proposal should be as physically attractive as possible. A neat and pleasing appearance invites the reviewer to read a proposal and suggests that care has been devoted to its preparation. Flashy and expensive binders, figures, and so forth are not necessary, but the physical presentation should not leave a bad impression on readers either.

Proposal writing, like research, is both a skill and an art. We hope we have been helpful in communicating some of what goes into the "skill" part and offer all readers our best wishes in cultivating the art of doing and writing about research.

☐
Study suggestions

1. Suppose that you were planning to study the problem of role conflict among nursing administrators.
   (a) Outline the methods you would recommend adopting.

(b) Develop a work plan.
(c) Prepare a hypothetical budget.
2. Suppose that you were interested in studying separation anxiety in hospitalized children. Using the references cited in this chapter, identify potential funding sources for your project.

☐
Suggested readings

Berthold, J.S. (1973). Nursing research grant proposals. What influenced their approval or disapproval in two national granting agencies. *Nursing Research, 22,* 292–299.

Bloch, D. *et al.* (1978). The Nursing Research Grants Program of the Division of Nursing. *Journal of Nursing Administration, 7,* 40–45.

Brodsky, J. (1976). *The proposal writer's swipe file II.* Washington: Taft Products.

Clinton, J. (1985). Couvade: Patterns, predictors and nursing management: A research proposal submitted to the Division of Nursing. *Western Journal of Nursing Research, 7,* 221–248.

Fuller, E.O. (1982). The pink sheet syndrome. *Nursing Research, 31,* 185–186.

Gortner, S. (1982). Research funding sources. *Western Journal of Nursing Research, 4,* 248–250.

Gortner, S. (1980). Researchmanship: The judges and their judgments. *Western Journal of Nursing Research, 2,* 434–437.

Jackson, N.E. (1982). Choosing and using a statistic consultant. *Nursing Research, 31,* 248–250.

Krathwohl, D.R. (1977). *How to prepare a research proposal* (2nd ed.). Syracuse: Syracuse University Bookstore.

Margolin, J.B. (1977). *About foundations: How to find the facts you need to get a grant.* New York: The Foundation Center.

Malasanos, L.J.Q. (1976). What is the pre-proposal? What are its component parts? Is it an effective instrument in assessing funding potential of research ideas? *Nursing Research, 25,* 223–224.

Oakley, D. (1981). A practical guide to political effectiveness: The case of federal funding for nursing research. *Nursing Research, 30,* 360–365.

Renz, L., Holt, S. & Read, P. (1984). *The Foundation Directory* (9th ed.). New York: The Foundation Center.

Stewart, R. & Stewart, A.L. (1984). *Proposal preparation.* New York: John Wiley and Sons.

White, V.P. (1975). *Grants: How to find out about them and what to do next.* New York: Plenum Press.

Wilson, H.S. (1985). *Research in nursing.* Menlo Park, CA: Addison-Wesley (Chapter 8).

Glossary

abstract   A brief description of a completed or proposed research investigation; in research journals, usually located at the beginning of an article.

accessible population   The population of subjects available for a particular study; often a nonrandom subset of the target population.

accidental sampling   Selection of the most readily available persons (or units) as subjects in a study; also known as *convenience sampling*.

active variables   Variables that the researcher creates or manipulates.

after-only design   An experimental design in which data are collected from subjects only after the experimental intervention is introduced.

analysis   Methods of organizing data in such a way that research questions can be answered.

analysis of covariance   A statistical procedure used to test the effect of one or more treatments on different groups while controlling for one or more extraneous variables (covariates); also referred to as ANCOVA.

analysis of variance   A statistical procedure for testing the effect of one or more treatments on different groups by comparing the variability between groups to the variability within groups; also referred to as ANOVA.

analytic induction   A method of analyzing qualitative data that involves an iterative approach to testing research hypotheses.

anonymity   Protection of the participant in a study such that even the researcher cannot link him or her with the information provided.

applied research   Research that concentrates

on finding a solution to an immediate practical problem.

assumptions Basic principles that are accepted as being true on the basis of logic or reason, without proof or verification.

attribute variables Preexisting characteristics of the entity under investigation, which the researcher simply observes and measures.

attrition The loss of participants during the course of a study; can introduce an unknown amount of bias by changing the composition of the sample initially drawn—particularly if more subjects are lost from one group than another; can thereby be a threat to the internal validity of a study.

basic research Research designed to extend the base of knowledge in a discipline for the sake of knowledge production or theory construction, rather than for solving an immediate problem.

before-after design An experimental design in which data are collected from research subjects both before and after the introduction of the experimental intervention.

bias Any influence that produces a distortion in the results of a study.

bivariate statistics Statistics derived from the analysis of two variables simultaneously for the purpose of assessing the empirical relationship between them.

canonical correlation A statistical procedure for examining the relationship between two or more independent variables *and* two or more dependent variables.

case study A research method that involves a thorough, in-depth analysis of an individual, group, institution or other social unit.

causal relationship A relationship between two variables such that the presence or absence of one variable (the "cause") determines the presence or absence, or value, of the other (the "effect").

cell The intersection of a row and column in a table with two or more dimensions. In an experimental design, a cell is the representation of an experimental condition in a schematic diagram.

central tendency A statistical index of the "typicalness" of a set of scores that comes from the center of the distribution of scores. The three most common indices of central tendency are the mode, the median, and the mean.

chi-square test A nonparametric test of statistical significance used to assess whether a relationship exists between two nominal-level variables. Symbolized as χ^2.

clinical research Research designed to generate knowledge to guide nursing practice.

closed-ended question A question that offers respondents a set of mutually exclusive and jointly exhaustive alternative replies, from which the one that most closely approximates the "right" answer must be chosen.

cluster sampling A form of multistage sampling in which large groupings ("clusters") are selected first (e.g., nursing schools), with successive subsampling of smaller units (e.g., nursing students).

codebook The documentation used in data processing that indicates the location and values of all the variables in a data file.

coding The process of transforming raw data into standardized form (usually numerical) for data processing and analysis.

coefficient alpha (Cronbach's alpha) A reliability index that estimates the internal consistency or homogeneity of a measure composed of several items or subparts.

cohort study A kind of trend study that focuses on a specific subpopulation (which is often an age-related subgroup) from which different samples are selected at different points in time (e.g., nursing students graduated in 1970–1974).

comparison group A group of subjects whose scores on a dependent variable are used as a basis for evaluating the scores of the target group or group of primary interest. The term comparison group is generally used instead of control group when the investigation does not use a true experimental design.

computer An electronic device that performs simple operations with extreme accuracy and speed.

computer program A set of instructions to a computer.

concept An abstraction based on observations of certain behaviors or characteristics (e.g., stress, death).

conceptual framework Interrelated concepts or abstractions that are assembled together in some rational scheme by virtue of their relevance to a common theme (see also *theory*).

concurrent validity The degree to which an instrument can distinguish individuals who differ on some other criterion measured or observed at the same time.

confidence interval The range of values within which a population parameter is estimated to lie.

confidence level The estimated probability that a population parameter lies within a given confidence level.

confidentiality Protection of participants in a study such that their individual identities will not be linked to the information they provided and publicly divulged.

consent form A written agreement signed by a subject and researcher concerning the terms and conditions of a subject's voluntary participation in a study.

construct An abstraction or concept that is deliberately invented (constructed) by re-

searchers for a scientific purpose (e.g., cognitive dissonance, locus of control).

construct validity The degree to which an instrument measures the construct under investigation.

content analysis A procedure for analyzing written, verbal, or visual materials in a systematic and objective fashion, typically with the goal of quantitatively measuring variables.

content validity The degree to which the items in an instrument adequately represent the universe of content.

contingency table A two-dimensional table that permits a crosstabulation of the frequencies of two nominal-level or ordinal-level variables.

control The process of holding constant possible influences on the dependent variable under investigation.

control group Subjects in an experiment who do not receive the experimental treatment and whose performance provides a baseline against which the effects of the treatment can be measured (see also *comparison group*).

convenience sampling Selection of the most readily available persons (or units) as subjects in a study; also known as *accidental sampling*.

convergent validity An approach to construct validation that involves assessing the degree to which two methods of measuring a construct are similar (i.e., converge).

correlation A tendency for variation in one variable to be related to variation in another variable.

correlation coefficient An index that summarizes the degree of relationship between two variables. Correlation coefficients typically range from +1.00 (for a perfect direct relationship) through 0.0 (for no relationship) to −1.00 (for a perfect inverse relationship).

correlational research Investigations that explore the interrelationships among variables of interest without any active intervention on the part of the researcher.

covariate A variable that is statistically controlled (held constant) in analysis of covariance. The covariate is typically an extraneous, confounding influence on the dependent variable or a pretest measure of the dependent variable.

criterion variable (criterion measure) The quality or attribute used to measure the effect of an independent variable; sometimes used instead of *dependent variable.*

criterion-related validity The degree to which scores on an instrument are correlated with some external criterion.

critical incident technique A method of obtaining data from study participants by in-depth exploration of specific incidents and behaviors related to the matter under investigation.

cross-sectional study A study based on observations of different age or developmental groups at a single point in time for the purpose of inferring trends over time.

crosstabulation A determination of the number of cases occurring when simultaneous consideration is given to the values of two or more variables (e.g., sex—male/female—crosstabulated with smoking status—smoker/nonsmoker). The results are typically presented in a table with rows and columns divided according to the values of the variables.

data The pieces of information obtained in the course of a study (singular is *datum*).

deductive reasoning The process of developing specific predictions from general principles (see also *inductive reasoning*).

degrees of freedom A concept used in tests of statistical significance, referring to the number of sample values that cannot be calculated from knowledge of other values and a calculated statistic (e.g., by knowing a sample mean, all but one value would be free to vary); degrees of freedom (df) is usually $N - 1$, but different formulas are relevant for different tests.

Delphi technique A method of obtaining judgments from a panel of experts. The experts are questioned individually, and a summary of the judgments is circulated to the entire panel. The experts are questioned again, with further iterations introduced as needed until there is some consensus.

dependent variable The outcome variable of interest; the variable that is hypothesized to depend on or be caused by another variable (called the *independent variable*); sometimes referred to as the *criterion variable.*

descriptive research Research studies that have as their main objective the accurate portrayal of the characteristics of persons, situations, or groups, and the frequency with which certain phenomena occur.

descriptive statistics Statistics used to describe and summarize the researcher's data set (e.g., mean, standard deviation).

dichotomous variable A variable having only two values or categories (e.g., sex).

directional hypothesis A hypothesis that makes a specific prediction about the direction (i.e., positive or negative) of the relationship between two variables.

discriminant function analysis A statistical procedure used to predict group membership or status on a categorical (nominal level) variable on the basis of two or more independent variables.

discriminant validity An approach to construct validation that involves assessing the degree to which a single method of measuring two constructs yields different results (i.e., discriminates the two).

double-blind experiment An experiment in which neither the subjects nor those who administer the treatment know who is in the experimental or control group.

effect size A statistical expression of the magnitude of the relationship between two variables, or the magnitude of the difference between two groups, with regard to some attribute of interest.

empiricism The process wherein evidence rooted in objective reality and gathered through the human senses is used as the basis for generating knowledge.

error of measurement The degree of deviation between true scores and obtained scores when measuring a characteristic.

ethics The quality of research procedures with respect to their adherence to professional, legal, and social obligations to the research subjects.

evaluation research Research that investigates how well a program, practice, or policy is working.

ex post facto research Research conducted *after* the variations in the independent variable have occurred in the natural course of events; a form of nonexperimental research in which causal explanations are inferred "after the fact."

experiment A research study in which the investigator controls (manipulates) the independent variable and randomly assigns subjects to different conditions.

experimental group The subjects who receive the experimental treatment or intervention.

exploratory research A preliminary study designed to develop or refine hypotheses, or to test and refine the data collection methods.

external validity The degree to which the results of a study can be generalized to settings or samples other than the ones studied.

extraneous variable Variables that confound the relationship between the independent and dependent variables and that need to be controlled either in the research design or through statistical procedures (e.g., in a study of the effect of a mother's age on the rate of premature deliveries, social class and ethnicity would be extraneous variables).

factor analysis A statistical procedure for reducing a large set of variables into a smaller set of variables with common characteristics or underlying dimensions.

factorial design An experimental design in which two or more independent variables are simultaneously manipulated; this design permits an analysis of the main effects of the independent variables separately, plus the interaction effects of these variables.

field study A study in which the data are collected "in the field" from individuals in their normal roles, with the aim of understanding the practices, behaviors and beliefs of individuals or groups as they normally function in real life.

focus group interview An interview in which the respondents are a group of ten to 20 individuals assembled to answer questions on a given topic.

focused interview A loosely structured interview in which the interviewer guides the respondent through a set of questions using a topic guide.

follow-up study A study undertaken to determine the subsequent development of individuals with a specified condition or who have received a specified treatment.

formative evaluation An ongoing assessment of a product or program as it is being developed, designed to optimize the ultimate quality of that product or program.

frequency distribution A systematic array of numerical values from the lowest to the highest, together with a count of the number of times each value was obtained.

Gantt chart A chart depicting the scheduling of activities (tasks) of a research study and highlighting the sequencing and interrelationships among activities.

generalizability The degree to which the research procedures justify the inference that the findings represent something beyond the specific observations on which they are based; in particular, the inference that the findings can be generalized from the sample to the entire population.

graphic rating scale A scale in which respondents are asked to rate something (e.g., a concept, issue, institution) along an ordered bipolar continuum (e.g., "excellent" to "very poor").

grounded theory An approach to collecting and analyzing qualitative data with the aim of developing theories and theoretical propositions "grounded" in real-world observations.

Guttman scale A method of measuring attitudes that makes use of a set of cumulative (monotone) items with which respondents are asked to agree or disagree.

Hawthorne effect The effect on the dependent variable caused by subjects' awareness that they are "special" participants under study.

heterogeneity The degree to which objects are dissimilar with respect to some attribute (i.e., characterized by high variability).

histogram A graphic presentation of frequency distribution data.

historical research Systematic studies designed to establish facts and relationships concerning past events.

history A threat to the internal validity of a study; refers to the occurrence of events external to the treatment but concurrent with it, which can affect the dependent variable of interest.

homogeneity (1) In terms of the reliability of an instrument, the degree to which the subparts are internally consistent (i.e., are measuring the same critical attribute). (2) More generally, the degree to which objects are similar (i.e., characterized by low variability).

hypothesis A statement of predicted relationships between the variables under investigation; hypotheses lead to empirical studies that seek to confirm or disconfirm those predictions.

independent variable The variable that is believed to cause or influence the dependent variable; in experimental research, the independent variable is the variable that is manipulated.

inductive reasoning The process of reasoning from specific observations to more general rules (see also *deductive reasoning*).

inferential statistics Statistics that permit us to infer whether relationships observed in a sample are likely to occur in a larger population of concern.

informed consent An ethical principle that requires researchers to obtain the voluntary participation of subjects, after informing them of possible risks and benefits.

Institutional Review Board (IRB) A group of individuals who convene to review proposed and ongoing studies with respect to ethical considerations.

instrument The device or technique that a researcher uses to collect data (e.g., questionnaires, tests, observation schedules, etc.).

instrumentation system The entire set of devices and apparatus used to collect in vivo physiological measurements; includes the subject, stimulus, sensing equipment, signal-conditioning equipment, display equipment, and recording equipment.

interaction effect The effect on a dependent variable of two or more independent variables acting in combination (interactively) rather than as unconnected factors.

internal consistency A form of reliability, referring to the degree to which the subparts of an instrument are all measuring the same attribute or dimension.

internal validity The degree to which it can be inferred that the experimental treatment (independent variable), rather than uncontrolled, extraneous factors, is responsible for observed effects.

interrater reliability The degree to which two raters, operating independently, assign the same ratings for an attribute being measured; such ratings normally occur in the context of observational research or in coding qualitative materials.

interval measure A level of measurement in which an attribute of a variable is rank ordered on a scale that has equal distances between points on that scale (e.g., Fahrenheit degrees).

intervention (1) In experimental research, the experimental treatment or manipulation. (2) More generally, the structure the investigator imposes on the research setting prior to making observations.

interview A method of data collection in which one person (an interviewer) asks questions of another person (a respondent); interviews are conducted either face-to-face or by telephone.

item A term used to refer to a single question on a test or questionnaire, or a single statement on an attitude or other scale (e.g., a final examination might consist of 100 items).

judgmental sampling A type of nonprobability sampling method in which the researcher selects subjects for the study on the basis of personal judgment about which ones will be most representative or productive; also referred to as *purposive sampling*.

key informant A person well-versed in the phenomenon of research interest and who is willing to share the information and insight with the researcher; key informants are often used in needs assessments.

known-groups technique A technique for estimating the construct validity of an instrument through an analysis of the degree to which the instrument separates groups that are predicted to differ on the basis of some theory or known characteristic.

Likert scale A type of composite measure of attitudes that involves summation of scores on a set of items (statements) to which respondents are asked to indicate their degree of agreement or disagreement.

literature review A critical summary of research on a topic of interest, generally prepared to put a research problem in context or to identify gaps and weaknesses in prior studies so as to justify a new investigation.

logical positivism The philosophy underlying the traditional scientific approach.

longitudinal study A study designed to collect data at more than one point in time, in contrast to a cross-sectional study.

mainframe A large, multi-user computer system.

manipulation An intervention or treatment introduced by the researcher in an experimental or quasi-experimental study; the researcher manipulates the independent variable to assess its impact on the dependent variable.

matching The pairing of subjects in one group with those in another group based on their similarity on one or more dimension, done in order to enhance the overall comparability of groups; when matching is performed in the context of an experiment, the procedure results in a randomized block design.

maturation A threat to the internal validity of a study that results when factors influence the outcome measure (dependent variable) as a result of time passing.

mean A descriptive statistic that is a measure of central tendency, computed by summing all scores and dividing by the number of subjects.

measurement The assignment of numbers to objects according to specified rules to characterize quantities of some attribute.

median A descriptive statistic that is a measure of central tendency, representing the exact middle score or value in a distribution of scores; the median is the value above and below which 50 percent of the scores lie.

methodological research Research designed to develop or refine procedures for obtaining, organizing, or analyzing data.

methods (research) The steps, procedures and strategies for gathering and analyzing the data in a research investigation.

meta-analysis A technique for quantitatively combining and thus integrating the results of multiple studies on a given topic.

methodological notes In unstructured observational studies, field notes regarding the methods used in collecting the data.

microcomputer A small computer used by individual users; also referred to as a personal computer.

mode A descriptive statistic that is a measure of central tendency; the score or value that occurs most frequently in a distribution of scores.

model A symbolic representation of concepts or variables, and interrelations among variables.

molar approach A way of making observations about behaviors that entails studying large units of behavior and treating them as a whole.

molecular approach A way of making observations about behavior that uses small and highly specific behaviors as the unit of observation.

mortality A threat to the internal validity of a study, referring to the differential loss of subjects (attrition) from different groups.

multiple classification analysis A variant of multiple regression that yields means on the dependent variable adjusted for the effects of covariates.

multiple correlation coefficient An index that summarizes the degree of relationship between two or more independent variables and a dependent variable; symbolized as R.

multiple regression A statistical procedure for understanding the simultaneous effects of two or more independent (or extraneous) variables on a dependent variable; the dependent variable must be measured on an interval or ratio scale.

multi-stage sampling A sampling strategy that proceeds through a set of stages from larger to smaller sampling units (e.g., from states, to nursing schools, to faculty members).

multitrait–multimethod matrix approach A method of establishing the construct validity of an instrument that involves the use of multiple measures for a set of subjects; the target instrument is valid to the extent that there is a strong relationship between it and other measures purporting to measure the same attribute *(convergence)* and a weak relationship between it and other measures purporting to measure a different attribute *(discriminability)*.

multivariate statistics Statistical procedures designed to analyze the relationships among three or more variables; commonly used multivariate statistics include multiple regression, discriminant function analysis, and factor analysis.

N Often used to designate the total number of subjects in a study (e.g., "the total N was 500").

n Often used to designate the number of subjects in a subgroup or in a cell of a study (e.g., "each of the four groups had an n of 125, for a total N of 500").

needs assessment A study in which a researcher collects data for estimating the needs of a group, community, or organization; usually used as a guide to resource allocation.

negative relationship A relationship between two variables in which there is a tendency for higher values on one variable to be associated with lower values on the other (e.g., as temperature increases, people's productivity may decrease); also referred to as an *inverse relationship.*

network sampling The sampling of subjects based on referrals from other subjects already in the sample.

nominal measure The lowest level of measurement that involves the assignment of characteristics into categories (e.g., males, category 1; females, category 2).

nondirectional hypothesis A research hypothesis that does not stipulate in advance the direction (i.e., positive or negative) of the relationship between variables.

nonequivalent control group A comparison group that was not developed on the basis of random assignment; when randomization is not used, there is no way of ensuring the initial equivalence among different groups.

nonexperimental research Studies in which the researcher collects data without introducing any new treatments or changes.

nonparametric statistics A general class of inferential statistics that does not involve rigorous assumptions about the distribution of the critical variables; most often used when the data are measured on the nominal or ordinal scales.

nonprobability sampling The selection of subjects or sampling units from a population using nonrandom procedures; examples include accidental, judgmental, and quota sampling.

normal distribution A theoretical distribution that is bell-shaped and symmetrical.

null hypothesis The hypothesis that states there is no relationship between the variables under study; used primarily in connection with tests of statistical significance as the hypothesis to be rejected.

objectivity A desired quality of research using the scientific approach; refers to the extent to which two independent researchers would arrive at similar judgments or conclusions (i.e., judgments not biased by personal values or beliefs).

observational notes In field studies, the observer's descriptions about observed events and conversations.

observational research Studies in which the data are collected by means of observing and recording behaviors or activities of interest.

obtained score The actual score or numerical value assigned to a subject on a measure.

one-tailed test A test of statistical significance in which only values at one extreme (tail) of a distribution are considered in determining significance; used when the researcher has predicted the direction of a relationship (see *directional hypothesis*).

open-ended question A question in an interview or questionnaire that does not restrict the respondents' answers to preestablished alternatives.

operational definition The definition of a concept or variable in terms of the operations or procedures by which it is to be measured.

ordinal measure A level of measurement that yields rank orders of a variable along some dimension.

outcome measure A term sometimes used to refer to the dependent variable (i.e., the variable that the researcher is attempting to predict, explain, or understand).

outliers Wild codes or numerical values that are not a part of the coding scheme.

panel study A type of longitudinal study in which the same subjects are used to provide data at two or more points in time.

parameter A characteristic of a population (e.g., the mean age of all U.S. citizens).

parametric statistics A class of inferential statistics that involves (a) assumptions about the distribution of the variables, (b) the estimation of a parameter, and (c) the use of interval measures.

participant observation A method of collecting data through the observation of a group or organization in which the researcher participates as a member.

path analysis A regression-based procedure for testing causal models.

personal notes In field studies, comments about the observer's own feelings during the research process.

phenomenology An approach to human inquiry that emphasizes the complexity of human experience and the need to study that experience holistically as it is actually lived.

pilot study A small scale version, or trial run, done in preparation for a major study.

population The entire set of individuals (or objects) having some common characteristic(s) (e.g., all RNs in the state of California); sometimes referred to as *universe*.

positive relationship A relationship between two variables in which there is a tendency for high values on one variable to be associated with high values on the other (e.g., as physical activity increases, pulse rate also increases).

posttest The collection of data after the introduction of an experimental intervention.

power The ability of a research design to detect existing relationships among variables.

power analysis A procedure for estimating either the likelihood of committing a Type II error or sample size requirements.

predictive validity The degree to which an instrument can predict some criterion observed at a future time.

preexperimental design A research design that does not include controls to compensate for the absence of either randomization or a control group.

pretest (1) The collection of data prior to the experimental intervention; sometimes referred to as *baseline data*. (2) The trial administration of a newly developed instrument to identify flaws or assess time requirements.

probability sampling The selection of subjects or sampling units from a population using random procedures; examples include simple random sampling, cluster sampling, and systematic sampling.

probing Eliciting more useful or detailed information from a respondent in an interview than was volunteered in the first reply.

problem statement The statement that identifies the key research variables, specifies the nature of the population, and suggests the possibility of empirical testing.

projective techniques Methods for measuring psychological attributes (values, attitudes, personality) by providing respondents with unstructured stimuli to which to respond.

proposal A document specifying what the researcher proposes to study; it communicates the research problem, its significance, planned procedures for solving the problem, and, when funding is sought, how much the research will cost.

prospective study A study that begins with an examination of presumed causes (e.g., cigarette smoking) and then goes forward in time to observe presumed effects (e.g., lung cancer).

purposive sampling A type of nonprobability sampling method in which the researcher selects subjects for the study on the basis of personal judgment about which ones will be most representative or productive; also referred to as *judgmental sampling*.

Q-sort A method of scaling in which the subject sorts statements into a number of piles (usually nine or 11) according to some bipolar dimension (e.g., most like me/least like me; most useful/least useful).

qualitative analysis The nonnumerical organization and interpretation of observations for the purpose of discovering important underlying dimensions and patterns of relationships.

quantitative analysis The manipulation of numerical data through statistical procedures for the purpose of describing phenomena or assessing the magnitude and reliability of relationships among them.

quasi-experiment A study in which subjects cannot be randomly assigned to treatment conditions, although the researcher does manipulate the independent variable and exercises certain controls to enhance the internal validity of the results.

quasi-statistics An "accounting" system used to assess the validity of conclusions derived from qualitative analysis.

questionnaire A method of gathering self-report information from respondents through self-administration of questions in a paper-and-pencil format.

quota sampling The nonrandom selection of subjects in which the researcher pre-specifies characteristics of the sample to increase its representativeness.

random number table A table of digits from 0 to 9 set up in such a way that each number is equally likely to follow any other; used in randomization or random sampling.

random sampling The selection of a sample such that each member of a population (or subpopulation) has an equal probability of being included.

randomization The assignment of subjects to treatment conditions in a random manner (i.e., in a manner determined by chance alone); also known as *random assignment*.

range A measure of variability, consisting of the difference between the highest and lowest values in a distribution of scores.

ratio measure A level of measurement in which there are equal distances between score units and which has a true meaningful zero point; the highest level of measurement (e.g., age).

reactivity A measurement distortion arising from the subject's awareness of being observed, or, more generally, from the effect of the measurement procedure itself.

regression A statistical procedure for predicting values of a dependent variable based on the values of one or more independent variables.

relationship A bond or a connection between two or more variables.

reliability The degree of consistency or dependability with which an instrument measures the attribute it is designed to measure.

repeated-measures design An experimental design in which one group of subjects is exposed to more than one condition or treatment.

replication The duplication of research procedures in a second investigation for the purpose of determining if earlier results can be repeated.

research Systematic inquiry that uses orderly scientific methods to answer questions or solve problems.

research design The overall plan for collecting and analyzing data, including specifications for enhancing the internal and external validity of the study.

response rate The rate of participation in a survey; calculated by dividing the number of persons participating by the number of persons sampled.

response set bias The measurement error introduced by the tendency of some individuals to respond to items in characteristic ways (e.g., always agreeing), independently of the item's content.

retrospective study A study that begins with the manifestation of the dependent variable in the present (e.g., lung cancer) and then links this effect to some presumed cause occurring in the past (e.g., cigarette smoking).

sample A subset of a population selected to participate in a research study.

sampling The process of selecting a portion of the population to represent the entire population.

sampling bias Distortions that arise from the selection of a sample that is not representative of the population from which it was drawn.

sampling distribution A theoretical distribution of a statistic using an infinite number of samples as a basis and the values of the statistic computed from these samples as the data points in the distribution.

sampling frame A list of all the elements in the population, from which the sample is drawn.

scale A composite measure of an attribute, consisting of several items that have a logical or empirical relationship to each other; involves the assignment of a score to place subjects on a continuum with respect to the attribute.

scatter plot A graphic representation of the relationship between two variables.

scientific approach A set of orderly, systematic, controlled procedures for acquiring dependable, empirical information.

secondary analysis A form of research in which the data collected by one researcher are reanalyzed by another investigator, usually to test new research hypotheses.

selection bias A threat to the internal validity of the study that results from pre-treatment differences between experimental and comparison groups.

self-report Any procedure for collecting data that involves a direct report of information by the person who is being studied (e.g., by interview or questionnaire).

semantic differential A technique used to measure attitudes that asks respondents to rate a concept of interest on a series of seven-point bipolar rating scales.

significance level The probability that an observed relationship could be caused by chance (i.e., because of sampling error); significance at the .05 level indicates the probability that a relationship of the observed magnitude would be found by chance only 5 times out of 100.

skewness A quality of a set of scores relating to their asymmetrical distribution around a central point.

snowball sampling The selection of subjects by means of nominations or referrals from earlier subjects.

software The instructions for performing operations made to a computer, and the documentation for those instructions.

Spearman–Brown prophecy formula An equation for making corrections to a reliability estimate that was calculated by the split-half method.

split-half technique A method for estimating the internal consistency (reliability) of an instrument by correlating scores on half of the measure with scores on the other half.

standard deviation The most frequently used statistic for measuring the degree of variability in a set of scores.

standard error The standard deviation of a sampling distribution.

standard scores Scores expressed in terms of standard deviations from the mean; raw scores are transformed to scores with a mean of zero and a standard deviation of one.

statistic An estimate of a parameter, calculated from sample data.

statistical significance A term indicating that the results obtained in an analysis of sample data are unlikely to have been caused by chance, at some specified level of probability.

strata Subdivisions of the population according to some characteristic (e.g., males and females); singular is *stratum.*

stratified random sampling The random selection of subjects from two or more strata of the population independently.

subject An individual who participates and provides data in a study; subjects are sometimes designated as *ss,* as "there were 50 ss in the experiment."

summative evaluation Research designed to assess the usefulness or worth of a program or practice after it is already in operation.

survey research A type of nonexperimental research that focusses on obtaining information regarding the status quo of some situation, often via direct questioning of a sample of respondents.

systematic sampling The selection of subjects such that every *k*th (e.g., every tenth) person (or element) in a sampling frame or list is chosen.

target population The entire population in which the researcher is interested and to which he or she would like to generalize the results of a study.

test statistic A statistic used to test for the statistical significance of relationships between variables; the sampling distributions of test statistics are known for circumstances in which the null hypothesis is true; examples include chi-square, F-ratio, *t,* and Pearson's *r.*

test–retest reliability Assessment of the stability of an instrument by correlating the scores obtained on repeated administrations.

theoretical notes In field studies, notes about the observer's interpretations of observed activities.

theory An abstract generalization that presents a systematic explanation about the relationships among phenomena.

Thurstone scale A type of attitude scale in which a panel of judges first rates the degree of favorability of a set of statements about some attitudinal object (e.g., abortion), and then subjects identify the statements with which they agree.

time sampling In observational research, the selection of time periods during which observations will take place.

time series design A quasi-experimental design that involves the collection of information over an extended period of time, with multiple data collection points both prior to and after the introduction of a treatment.

treatment A term used to refer to an experimental intervention or manipulation.

trend study A form of longitudinal study in which different samples from a population are studied over time with respect to some phenomenon (e.g., a series of Gallup polls of political preferences).

triangulation The use of multiple methods or perspectives to collect and interpret data about some phenomenon, in order to converge on an accurate representation of reality.

true score A hypothetical score that would be obtained if a measure were infallible; it is the portion of the observed score not due to random error or measurement bias.

t-test A parametric statistical test used for analyzing the difference between two means.

two-tailed test A test of statistical significance in which values at both extremes (tails) of a distribution are considered in determining significance; used when the researcher has not predicted the direction of a relationship (see *nondirectional hypothesis*).

Type I error A decision to reject the null hypothesis when it is true (i.e., the researcher concludes that a relationship exists when in fact it does not).

Type II error A decision to accept the null hypothesis when it is false (i.e., the researcher concludes that *no* relationship exists when in fact it does).

univariate statistics Statistical procedures for analyzing a single variable for purposes of description.

validity The degree to which an instrument measures what it is intended to measure.

variability The degree to which values on a set of scores are widely different or dispersed (e.g., one would expect higher variability of age within a hospital than within a nursing home).

variable A characteristic or attribute of a person or object that varies (i.e., takes on different values) within the population under study (e.g., body temperature, age, heart rate).

variance A measure of variability or dispersion, equal to the square of the standard deviation.

vignette A brief description of an event, person, or situation to which respondents are asked to react.

Appendix A
☐
Human subjects considerations

Appendix A-1
☐
Human Subjects Protocol*

(1) Describe the characteristics of the subject population, such as their anticipated number, age ranges, sex, ethnic background, and health status. Identify the criteria for inclusion or exclusion. Explain the rationale for the use of special classes of subjects, such as fetuses, pregnant women, children, institutionalized mentally disabled, prisoners, or others who are likely to be vulnerable.

1. Characteristics of the population. The sample for the proposed research will consist of approximately 300 women aged 18–22 who first became pregnant before the eighteenth birthday and who subsequently delivered a child. The women were interviewed initially in 1980–1981 as part of an evaluation of a special program for teenage mothers—Project Redirection. At the time of the initial interview, the women were residing in 6 communities: Phoenix, San Antonio, Fresno, Riverside (CA), Harlem and Bedford-Stuyvesant (NY).

---

* Grant applications under the Public Health Service (see Chapter 27) must include a section on the protection of human subjects, which must address six specific questions. This appendix contains the actual responses to those six questions for a funded study of parenting among low-income teenage mothers. Such a protocol often serves as the focal point of an evaluation by an Institutional Review Board.

The initial eligibility criteria for the Project Redirection study are indicated below:

- either pregnant or a parent;
- living in a household that met certain poverty guidelines;
- 17 years old or younger; and
- without a high school diploma or GED certificate.

The sample size for the proposed study is based on the teens in the six sites who completed three rounds of interviews thus far:

• Phoenix, AZ	81
• San Antonio, TX	86
• Harlem, NY	38
• Bedford-Stuyvesant, NY	54
• Riverside, CA	32
• Fresno, CA	38
TOTAL	329

This sample size is substantially larger than that used in most studies of teenage parenting and, as noted earlier, has the advantage of not depending on teens in a single site. The sample will also be heterogeneous with respect to ethnicity; of the 329 teens to be followed, the approximate ethnic distribution will be as follows: Blacks — 58%; Hispanics — 31%; and Whites — 11%.

(2) Identify the sources of research material obtained from individually identifiable living human subjects in the form of specimens, records, or data. Indicate whether the material or data will be obtained specifically for research purposes or whether use will be made of existing specimens, records, or data.

2. Sources of Data. Three rounds of interviews have already been completed with the research sample, and information from these earlier interviews will be used in the present study. Additionally, data will be gathered in a fourth round of in-home interviews, to be collected in 1986 – 1987 if the proposed research is funded. Data will be gathered by a combined interview/observation approach, using a specially constructed interview schedule and several standardized instruments.

(3) Describe plans for the recruitment of subjects and the consent procedures to be followed, including the circumstances under which consent will be sought and obtained, who will seek it, the nature of the information to be provided to prospective subjects and the method of documenting consent.

3. Recruitment and Consent. Subjects have already been recruited for this study — i.e., they were participants in three earlier rounds of interviewing as part of another research project. For the present study, letters will be mailed to respondents at their most recently known address and they will be asked to verify their current address and telephone number (if available). For respondents for whom there is no return postcard, tracking procedures to ascertain the respondents' present address will be undertaken.

For those respondents who are located through these procedures, an interviewer will contact them and explain the general nature and purpose of the research, the confidential nature of the interviews, the time commitments, and the stipend ($25) that would be paid to them in compensation for their time. The respondents will also be told that their children should be present at the time of the interview, so that appropriate observations can be made. Upon consent to be included in this wave of the research, an interview will be scheduled. At the time of the interview, the interviewers, who will receive extensive training for this project, will repeat the description of the research prior to commencing. The respondent will be told that her participation is voluntary; that no information she gives will be divulged to anyone other than research staff; that her participation will have no effect on any services that she might be receiving; that she can stop the interview at any time; and that she can decline to answer individual questions if she so chooses. This information will be included in a Consent Form, which each respondent will be requested to sign prior to the interview.

(4) Describe any potential risks — physical, psychological, social, legal, or other — and assess their likelihood and seriousness. Where appropriate, describe alternative treatments and procedures that might be advantageous to the subjects.

4. Risks. There is relatively minor risk, in interviewing these young women about their family life, that the interview will be stressful to them. Furthermore, our procedures are designed to minimize any discomfort on the respondents' parts. We will use female interviewers who will be trained not only with respect to the research instrument but also with regard to the stresses of parenthood in disadvantaged populations. In the event of any signs of distress during the interview, interviewers will be instructed to refrain from further questioning, proceeding only if the respondent desires. Our experience in dealing with this sample leads us to believe, however, that the women are more likely to find a conversation with an objective but sympathetic listener therapeutic rather than stressful.

(5) Describe the procedures for protecting against or minimizing any potential risks, including risks to confidentiality, and assess their likely effectiveness. Where appropriate, discuss provisions for insuring necessary medical or professional intervention in the event of adverse effects to the subjects. Also, where appropriate, describe the provisions for monitoring the data collected to insure the safety of subjects.

5. Confidentiality. Measures to protect the confidentiality of the respondents will be instituted throughout the course of this project. Data security procedures to protect the identity of individuals will be implemented during interviewer training, data collection, data analysis, and after completion of the project. Respondents will be fully informed as to these confidentiality procedures at the outset of the interview.

The issue of confidentiality and data security will be stressed during the training of data collectors. The need for confidentiality and the specific policies and procedures related to this issue will be explained to all interviewers. Thereafter, the interviewers will be required to sign a confidentiality statement prior to conducting interviews.

All identifying information will be removed from the interview schedule upon receipt from the field staff. Names, addresses, telephone numbers and any other identifying information will be recorded *only* on a cover sheet of the interview. The interview form itself, which will be kept in a locked file, will bear only a numeric identification code. The cover sheet will be removed from completed interviews and kept in a separate locked file. Access to this file will be restricted to key project personnel.

(6) *Discuss why the risks to subjects are reasonable in relation to the anticipated benefits to subjects and in relation to the importance of the knowledge that may reasonably be expected to result.*

6. Anticipated Benefits. In theory, no direct benefits to the respondents are anticipated. However, as mentioned above, we have found that respondents often enjoy the interview experience. Nevertheless, the primary benefit expected from the project is indirect. The study is expected to generate knowledge that will be useful in the formulation of social policy and in the design and delivery of appropriate services for young disadvantaged mothers and their children. Since we believe that the risks to subjects are negligible, we believe that the benefits provide justification for the conduct of this research.

Appendix A-2
☐
Sample Respondent's Consent Form

In signing this document, I am giving my consent to be interviewed by an employee of Humanalysis, Inc., a non-profit research organization. I understand that I will be part of a research study that will focus on the experiences and needs of mothers of young children in the United States. This study, supported by a grant from the U.S. Department of Health and Human Services, will provide some guidance to people who are trying to help mothers and their children.

I understand that I will be asked some questions about my experiences as a parent, my feelings about how to raise children, the characteristics of my oldest child, and my relations with my children. I also understand that the interviewer will ask to have my oldest child present during at least some portion of the interview. The interview will take about one and a half to two hours to complete.

This interview was granted freely. I have been informed that the interview is entirely voluntary, and that even after the interview begins I can refuse to answer any specific questions or decide to terminate the interview at any point. I have been told that my answers to questions will not be given to *anyone else* and no reports of this study will ever identify me in any way. I have also been informed that my participation/nonparticipation or my refusal to answer questions will have no effect on services that I or any member of this family may receive from health or social service providers.

This study will help develop a better understanding of the experiences of young mothers and the services that can be most helpful to them. I understand that the results of this research will be given to me if I ask for them and that Dr. Denise F. Polit (P.O. Box 1123, Jefferson City, MO 65102) is the person to contact if I have any questions about the study or about my rights as a study participant.

I acknowledge that I have received $25 for granting this interview.

_____   _____
Date   *Respondent's Signature*

                                      _____
                                      Interviewer

Appendix A-3
☐
Sample IRB Review/Approval Form

REVIEW OF SAFEGUARDS FOR HUMAN SUBJECTS

Proposal/Project Number: Internal ——————— Sponsor: ——————

Proposal/Project Title: —————————————————

—————————————————

Type of review:

—— Determination of Exemption   —— Full Board Proposal Review
—— Expedited Review   —— Ongoing research in certifi-
                                         cation of change

—— Other (Specify): —————————————————

After reviewing the above proposal/project:

Exemption —— The institutional official has determined that the research is exempt under 45 CFR 46.101 (b) or

Safeguards —— This Institutional Review Board (or member signing below in the case of expedited review) has determined by unanimous vote of the members present that:

—— Risks to subjects are minimized and are reasonable in relation to anticipated benefits. Selection of subjects is equitable, and the privacy of the subjects and confidentiality of the data are adequately protected. Approval is given.

—— Approval is given under the following conditions:

—— Approval is not given, for the following reasons:

Where applicable, attach summary of controverted issues and their resolution.

—————————————————

Date: ———————

Names of Members Present: *Signatures of Members Present:*

————————————   ————————————

————————————   ————————————

————————————   ————————————

————————————   ————————————

————————————   ————————————

Appendix B
□
Statistical tables

Table B-1
Distribution of t Probability

df	Level of Significance for One-Tailed Test					
	.10	.05	.025	.01	.005	.0005
	Level of Significance for Two-Tailed Test					
	.20	.10	.05	.02	.01	.001
1	3·078	6·314	12·706	31·821	63·657	636·619
2	1·886	2·920	4·303	6·965	9·925	31·598
3	1·638	2·353	3·182	4·541	5·841	12·941
4	1·533	2·132	2·776	3·747	4·604	8·610
5	1·476	2·015	2·571	3·365	4·032	6·859
6	1·440	1·943	2·447	3·143	3·707	5·959
7	1·415	1·895	2·365	2·998	3·449	5·405
8	1·397	1·860	2·306	2·896	3·355	5·041
9	1·383	1·833	2·262	2·821	3·250	4·781
10	1·372	1·812	2·228	2·764	3·169	4·587
11	1·363	1·796	2·201	2·718	3·106	4·437
12	1·356	1·782	2·179	2·681	3·055	4·318
13	1·350	1·771	2·160	2·650	3·012	4·221
14	1·345	1·761	2·145	2·624	2·977	4·140
15	1·341	1·753	2·131	2·602	2·947	4·073
16	1·337	1·746	2·120	2·583	2·921	4·015
17	1·333	1·740	2·110	2·567	2·898	3·965
18	1·330	1·734	2·101	2·552	2·878	3·922
19	1·328	1·729	2·093	2·539	2·861	3·883
20	1·325	1·725	2·086	2·528	2·845	3·850
21	1·323	1·721	2·080	2·518	2·831	3·819
22	1·321	1·717	2·074	2·508	2·819	3·792
23	1·319	1·714	2·069	2·500	2·807	3·767
24	1·318	1·711	2·064	2·492	2·797	3·745
25	1·316	1·708	2·060	2·485	2·787	3·725
26	1·315	1·706	2·056	2·479	2·779	3·707
27	1·314	1·703	2·052	2·473	2·771	3·690
28	1·313	1·701	2·048	2·467	2·763	3·674
29	1·311	1·699	2·045	2·462	2·756	3·659
30	1·310	1·697	2·042	2·457	2·750	3·646
40	1·303	1·684	2·021	2·423	2·704	3·551
60	1·296	1·671	2·000	2·390	2·660	3·460
120	1·289	1·658	1·980	2·358	2·617	3·373
∞	1·282	1·645	1·960	2·326	2·576	3·291

Table B-2
Significant values of F
$\alpha = .05$ (two-tailed) $\alpha = .025$ (one-tailed)

df_B / df_w	1	2	3	4	5	6	8	12	24	∞
1	161·4	199·5	215·7	224·6	230·2	234·0	238·9	243·9	249·0	254·3
2	18·51	19·00	19·16	19·25	19·30	19·33	19·37	19·41	19·45	19·50
3	10·13	9·55	9·28	9·12	9·01	8·94	8·84	8·74	8·64	8·53
4	7·71	6·94	6·59	6·39	6·26	6·16	6·04	5·91	5·77	5·63
5	6·61	5·79	5·41	5·19	5·05	4·95	4·82	4·68	4·53	4·36
6	5·99	5·14	4·76	4·53	4·39	4·28	4·15	4·00	3·84	3·67
7	5·59	4·74	4·35	4·12	3·97	3·87	3·73	3·57	3·41	3·23
8	5·32	4·46	4·07	3·84	3·69	3·58	3·44	3·28	3·12	2·93
9	5·12	4·26	3·86	3·63	3·48	3·37	3·23	3·07	2·90	2·71
10	4·96	4·10	3·71	3·48	3·33	3·22	3·07	2·91	2·74	2·54
11	4·84	3·98	3·59	3·36	3·20	3·09	2·95	2·79	2·61	2·40
12	4·75	3·88	3·49	3·26	3·11	3·00	2·85	2·69	2·50	2·30
13	4·67	3·80	3·41	3·18	3·02	2·92	2·77	2·60	2·42	2·21
14	4·60	3·74	3·34	3·11	2·96	2·85	2·70	2·53	2·35	2·13
15	4·54	3·68	3·29	3·06	2·90	2·79	2·64	2·48	2·29	2·07
16	4·49	3·63	3·24	3·01	2·85	2·74	2·59	2·42	2·24	2·01
17	4·45	3·59	3·20	2·96	2·81	2·70	2·55	2·38	2·19	1·96
18	4·41	3·55	3·16	2·93	2·77	2·66	2·51	2·34	2·15	1·92
19	4·38	3·52	3·13	2·90	2·74	2·63	2·48	2·31	2·11	1·88
20	4·35	3·49	3·10	2·87	2·71	2·60	2·45	2·28	2·08	1·84
21	4·32	3·47	3·07	2·84	2·68	2·57	2·42	2·25	2·05	1·81
22	4·30	3·44	3·05	2·82	2·66	2·55	2·40	2·23	2·03	1·78
23	4·28	3·42	3·03	2·80	2·64	2·53	2·38	2·20	2·00	1·76
24	4·26	3·40	3·01	2·78	2·62	2·51	2·36	2·18	1·98	1·73
25	4·24	3·38	2·99	2·76	2·60	2·49	2·34	2·16	1·96	1·71
26	4·22	3·37	2·98	2·74	2·59	2·47	2·32	2·15	1·95	1·69
27	4·21	3·35	2·96	2·73	2·57	2·46	2·30	2·13	1·93	1·67
28	4·20	3·34	2·95	2·71	2·56	2·44	2·29	2·12	1·91	1·65
29	4·18	3·33	2·93	2·70	2·54	2·43	2·28	2·10	1·90	1·64
30	4·17	3·32	2·92	2·69	2·53	2·42	2·27	2·09	1·89	1·62
40	4·08	3·23	2·84	2·61	2·45	2·34	2·18	2·00	1·79	1·51
60	4·00	3·15	2·76	2·52	2·37	2·25	2·10	1·92	1·70	1·39
120	3·92	3·07	2·68	2·45	2·29	2·17	2·02	1·83	1·61	1·25
∞	3·84	2·99	2·60	2·37	2·21	2·09	1·94	1·75	1·52	1·00

Table B-2 (continued)
Significant values of F
$\alpha = .01$ *(two-tailed)* $\alpha = .005$ *(one-tailed)*

$\dfrac{df_B}{df_w}$	1	2	3	4	5	6	8	12	24	∞
1	4052	4999	5403	5625	5764	5859	5981	6106	6234	6366
2	98·49	99·00	99·17	99·25	99·30	99·33	99·36	99·42	99·46	99·50
3	34·12	30·81	29·46	28·71	28·24	27·91	27·49	27·05	26·60	26·12
4	21·20	18·00	16·69	15·98	15·52	15·21	14·80	14·37	13·93	13·46
5	16·26	13·27	12·06	11·39	10·97	10·67	10·29	9·89	9·47	9·02
6	13·74	10·92	9·78	9·15	8·75	8·47	8·10	7·72	7·31	6·88
7	12·25	9·55	8·45	7·85	7·46	7·19	6·84	6·47	6·07	5·65
8	11·26	8·65	7·59	7·01	6·63	6·37	6·03	5·67	5·28	4·86
9	10·56	8·02	6·99	6·42	6·06	5·80	5·47	5·11	4·73	4·31
10	10·04	7·56	6·55	5·99	5·64	5·39	5·06	4·71	4·33	3·91
11	9·65	7·20	6·22	5·67	5·32	5·07	4·74	4·40	4·02	3·60
12	9·33	6·93	5·95	5·41	5·06	4·82	4·50	4·16	3·78	3·36
13	9·07	6·70	5·74	5·20	4·86	4·62	4·30	3·96	3·59	3·16
14	8·86	6·51	5·56	5·03	4·69	4·46	4·14	3·80	3·43	3·00
15	8·68	6·36	5·42	4·89	4·56	4·32	4·00	3·67	3·29	2·87
16	8·53	6·23	5·29	4·77	4·44	4·20	3·89	3·55	3·18	2·75
17	8·40	6·11	5·18	4·67	4·34	4·10	3·79	3·45	3·08	2·65
18	8·28	6·01	5·09	4·58	4·25	4·01	3·71	3·37	3·00	2·57
19	8·18	5·93	5·01	4·50	4·17	3·94	3·63	3·30	2·92	2·49
20	8·10	5·85	4·94	4·43	4·10	3·87	3·56	3·23	2·86	2·42
21	8·02	5·78	4·87	4·37	4·04	3·81	3·51	3·17	2·80	2·36
22	7·94	5·72	4·82	4·31	3·99	3·76	3·45	3·12	2·75	2·31
23	7·88	5·66	4·76	4·26	3·94	3·71	3·41	3·07	2·70	2·26
24	7·82	5·61	4·72	4·22	3·90	3·67	3·36	3·03	2·66	2·21
25	7·77	5·57	4·68	4·18	3·86	3·63	3·32	2·99	2·62	2·17
26	7·72	5·53	4·64	4·14	3·82	3·59	3·29	2·96	2·58	2·13
27	7·68	5·49	4·60	4·11	3·78	3·56	3·26	2·93	2·55	2·10
28	7·64	5·45	4·57	4·07	3·75	3·53	3·23	2·90	2·52	2·06
29	7·60	5·42	4·54	4·04	3·73	3·50	3·20	2·87	2·49	2·03
30	7·56	5·39	4·51	4·02	3·70	3·47	3·17	2·84	2·47	2·01
40	7·31	5·18	4·31	3·83	3·51	3·29	2·99	2·66	2·29	1·80
60	7·08	4·98	4·13	3·65	3·34	3·12	2·82	2·50	2·12	1·60
120	6·85	4·79	3·95	3·48	3·17	2·96	2·66	2·34	1·95	1·38
∞	6·64	4·60	3·78	3·32	3·02	2·80	2·51	2·18	1·79	1·00

Table B-2 (continued)
Significant values of F
α = .001 (two-tailed)   α = .0005 (one-tailed)

$\frac{df_B}{df_w}$	1	2	3	4	5	6	8	12	24	∞
1	405284	500000	540379	562500	576405	585937	598144	610667	623497	636619
2	998·5	999·0	999·2	999·2	999·3	999·3	999·4	999·4	999·5	999·5
3	167·5	148·5	141·1	137·1	134·6	132·8	130·6	128·3	125·9	123·5
4	74·14	61·25	56·18	53·44	51·71	50·53	49·00	47·41	45·77	44·05
5	47·04	36·61	33·20	31·09	29·75	28·84	27·64	26·42	25·14	23·78
6	35·51	27·00	23·70	21·90	20·81	20·03	19·03	17·99	16·89	15·75
7	29·22	21·69	18·77	17·19	16·21	15·52	14·63	13·71	12·73	11·69
8	25·42	18·49	15·83	14·39	13·49	12·86	12·04	11·19	10·30	9·34
9	22·86	16·39	13·90	12·56	11·71	11·13	10·37	9·57	8·72	7·81
10	21·04	14·91	12·55	11·28	10·48	9·92	9·20	8·45	7·64	6·76
11	19·69	13·81	11·56	10·35	9·58	9·05	8·35	7·63	6·85	6·00
12	18·64	12·97	10·80	9·63	8·89	8·38	7·71	7·00	6·25	5·42
13	17·81	12·31	10·21	9·07	8·35	7·86	7·21	6·52	5·78	4·97
14	17·14	11·78	9·73	8·62	7·92	7·43	6·80	6·13	5·41	4·60
15	16·59	11·34	9·34	8·25	7·57	7·09	6·47	5·81	5·10	4·31
16	16·12	10·97	9·00	7·94	7·27	6·81	6·19	5·55	4·85	4·06
17	15·72	10·66	8·73	7·68	7·02	6·56	5·96	5·32	4·63	3·85
18	15·38	10·39	8·49	7·46	6·81	6·35	5·76	5·13	4·45	3·67
19	15·08	10·16	8·28	7·26	6·61	6·18	5·59	4·97	4·29	3·52
20	14·82	9·95	8·10	7·10	6·46	6·02	5·44	4·82	4·15	3·38
21	14·59	9·77	7·94	6·95	6·32	5·88	5·31	4·70	4·03	3·26
22	14·38	9·61	7·80	6·81	6·19	5·76	5·19	4·58	3·92	3·15
23	14·19	9·47	7·67	6·69	6·08	5·65	5·09	4·48	3·82	3·05
24	14·03	9·34	7·55	6·59	5·98	5·55	4·99	4·39	3·74	2·97
25	13·88	9·22	7·45	6·49	5·88	5·46	4·91	4·31	3·66	2·89
26	13·74	9·12	7·36	6·41	5·80	5·38	4·83	4·24	3·59	2·82
27	13·61	9·02	7·27	6·33	5·73	5·31	4·76	4·17	3·52	2·75
28	13·50	8·93	7·19	6·25	5·66	5·24	4·69	4·11	3·46	2·70
29	13·39	8·85	7·12	6·19	5·59	5·18	4·64	4·05	3·41	2·64
30	13·29	8·77	7·05	6·12	5·53	5·12	4·58	4·00	3·36	2·59
40	12·61	8·25	6·60	5·70	5·13	4·73	4·21	3·64	3·01	2·23
60	11·97	7·76	6·17	5·31	4·76	4·37	3·87	3·31	2·69	1·90
120	11·38	7·31	5·79	4·95	4·42	4·04	3·55	3·02	2·40	1·56
∞	10·83	6·91	5·42	4·62	4·10	3·74	3·27	2·74	2·13	1·00

Table B-3
Distribution of χ^2 probability

df	Level of Significance				
	.10	.05	.02	.01	.001
1	2·71	3·84	5·41	6·63	10·83
2	4·61	5·99	7·82	9·21	13·82
3	6·25	7·82	9·84	11·34	16·27
4	7·78	9·49	11·67	13·28	18·46
5	9·24	11·07	13·39	15·09	20·52
6	10·64	12·59	15·03	16·81	22·46
7	12·02	14·07	16·62	18·48	24·32
8	13·36	15·51	18·17	20·09	26·12
9	14·68	16·92	19·68	21·67	27·88
10	15·99	18·31	21·16	23·21	29·59
11	17·28	19·68	22·62	24·72	31·26
12	18·55	21·03	24·05	26·22	32·91
13	19·81	22·36	25·47	27·69	34·53
14	21·06	23·68	26·87	29·14	36·12
15	22·31	25·00	28·26	30·58	37·70
16	23·54	26·30	29·63	32·00	39·25
17	24·77	27·59	31·00	33·41	40·79
18	25·99	28·87	32·35	34·81	42·31
19	27·20	30·14	33·69	36·19	43·82
20	28·41	31·41	35·02	37·57	45·32
21	29·62	32·67	36·34	38·93	46·80
22	30·81	33·92	37·66	40·29	48·27
23	32·01	35·17	38·97	41·64	49·73
24	33·20	36·42	40·27	42·98	51·18
25	34·38	37·65	41·57	44·31	52·62
26	35·56	38·89	42·86	45·64	54·05
27	36·74	40·11	44·14	46·96	55·48
28	37·92	41·34	45·42	48·28	56·89
29	39·09	42·56	46·69	49·59	58·30
30	40·26	43·77	47·96	50·89	59·70

Table B-4
Significant values of the correlation coefficient

df	Level of Significance for One-Tailed Test				
	.05	.025	.01	.005	.0005
	Level of Significance for Two-Tailed Test				
	.1	.05	.02	.01	.001
1	·98769	·99692	·999507	·999877	·9999988
2	·90000	·95000	·98000	·990000	·99900
3	·8054	·8783	·93433	·95873	·99116
4	·7293	·8114	·8822	·91720	·97406
5	·6694	·7545	·8329	·8745	·95074
6	·6215	·7067	·7887	·8343	·92493
7	·5822	·6664	·7498	·7977	·8982
8	·5494	·6319	·7155	·7646	·8721
9	·5214	·6021	·6851	·7348	·8471
10	·4973	·5760	·6581	·7079	·8233
11	·4762	·5529	·6339	·6835	·8010
12	·4575	·5324	·6120	·6614	·7800
13	·4409	·5139	·5923	·6411	·7603
14	·4259	·4973	·5742	·6226	·7420
15	·4124	·4821	·5577	·6055	·7246
16	·4000	·4683	·5425	·5897	·7084
17	·3887	·4555	·5285	·5751	·6932
18	·3783	·4438	·5155	·5614	·6787
19	·3687	·4329	·5034	·5487	·6652
20	·3598	·4227	·4921	·5368	·6524
25	·3233	·3809	·4451	·4869	·5974
30	·2960	·3494	·4093	·4487	·5541
35	·2746	·3246	·3810	·4182	·5189
40	·2573	·3044	·3578	·3932	·4896
45	·2428	·2875	·3384	·3721	·4648
50	·2306	·2732	·3218	·3541	·4433
60	·2108	·2500	·2948	·3248	·4078
70	·1954	·2319	·2737	·3017	·3799
80	·1829	·2172	·2565	·2830	·3568
90	·1726	·2050	·2422	·2673	·3375
100	·1638	·1946	·2301	·2540	·3211

Index